Lung Diseases: An Evidence-Based Approach

Lung Diseases: An Evidence-Based Approach

Editor: Nicholas Clarke

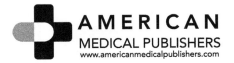

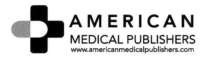

Cataloging-in-Publication Data

Lung diseases : an evidence-based approach / edited by Nicholas Clarke.
    p. cm.
Includes bibliographical references and index.
ISBN 979-8-88740-584-1
1. Lungs--Diseases. 2. Evidence-based medicine. 3. Lungs--Diseases--Diagnosis.
4. Lungs--Diseases--Treatment. I. Clarke, Nicholas.
RC756 .L86 2023
616.24--dc23

© American Medical Publishers, 2023

American Medical Publishers,
41 Flatbush Avenue,
1st Floor, New York,
NY 11217, USA

ISBN 979-8-88740-584-1 (Hardback)

This book contains information obtained from authentic and highly regarded sources. Copyright for all individual chapters remain with the respective authors as indicated. All chapters are published with permission under the Creative Commons Attribution License or equivalent. A wide variety of references are listed. Permission and sources are indicated; for detailed attributions, please refer to the permissions page and list of contributors. Reasonable efforts have been made to publish reliable data and information, but the authors, editors and publisher cannot assume any responsibility for the validity of all materials or the consequences of their use.

Trademark Notice: Registered trademark of products or corporate names are used only for explanation and identification without intent to infringe.

Contents

Preface.. VII

Chapter 1 **Perinatal Nutritional and Metabolic Pathways: Early Origins of Chronic Lung Diseases**.. 1
Celien Kuiper-Makris, Jaco Selle, Eva Nüsken, Jörg Dötsch
and Miguel A. Alejandre Alcazar

Chapter 2 **Opposing Effects of TGFβ and BMP in the Pulmonary Vasculature in Congenital Diaphragmatic Hernia**.. 22
Daphne S. Mous, Marjon J. Buscop-van Kempen, Rene M. H. Wijnen, Dick Tibboel,
Rory E. Morty and Robbert J. Rottier

Chapter 3 **An Experimental Model of Bronchopulmonary Dysplasia Features Long-Term Retinal and Pulmonary Defects but not Sustained Lung Inflammation**.................. 31
Lakshanie C. Wickramasinghe, Peter van Wijngaarden, Chad Johnson,
Evelyn Tsantikos and Margaret L. Hibbs

Chapter 4 **Updates on Functional Characterization of Bronchopulmonary Dysplasia – The Contribution of Lung Function Testing**.. 43
Anne Greenough and Anoop Pahuja

Chapter 5 **Intrauterine Growth Restriction Promotes Postnatal Airway Hyperresponsiveness Independent of Allergic Disease**.. 51
Jack O. Kalotas, Carolyn J. Wang, Peter B. Noble and Kimberley C. W. Wang

Chapter 6 **Stem Cells and their Mediators – Next Generation Therapy for Bronchopulmonary Dysplasia**.. 60
Marius A. Möbius and Bernard Thébaud

Chapter 7 **Sequential Exposure to Antenatal Microbial Triggers Attenuates Alveolar Growth and Pulmonary Vascular Development and Impacts Pulmonary Epithelial Stem/Progenitor Cells**.. 72
Helene Widowski, Niki L. Reynaert, Daan R. M. G. Ophelders, Matthias C. Hütten,
Peter G. J. Nikkels, Carmen A. H. Severens-Rijvers, Jack P. M. Cleutjens,
Matthew W. Kemp, John P. Newnham, Masatoshi Saito, Haruo Usuda,
Matthew S. Payne, Alan H. Jobe, Boris W. Kramer, Tammo Delhaas
and Tim G. A. M. Wolfs

Chapter 8 **The Future of Bronchopulmonary Dysplasia: Emerging Pathophysiological Concepts and Potential New Avenues of Treatment**...................................... 86
Jennifer J. P. Collins, Dick Tibboel, Ismé M. de Kleer, Irwin K. M. Reiss
and Robbert J. Rottier

Chapter 9 **Close Association Between Platelet Biogenesis and Alveolarization of the Developing Lung**.. 103
Xueyu Chen, Junyan Zhong, Dongshan Han, Fang Yao, Jie Zhao,
Gerry. T. M. Wagenaar, Chuanzhong Yang and Frans J. Walther

VI   Contents

Chapter 10   **The Extracellular Matrix in Bronchopulmonary Dysplasia: Target and Source**.................................111
Ivana Mižíková and Rory E. Morty

Chapter 11   **The Correlation Between Bronchopulmonary Dysplasia and Platelet
Metabolism in Preterm Infants**.................................131
Longli Yan, Zhuxiao Ren, Jianlan Wang, Xin Xia, Liling Yang, Jiayu Miao,
Fang Xu, Weiwei Gao and Jie Yang

Chapter 12   **A Breath of Fresh Air on the Mesenchyme: Impact of Impaired Mesenchymal
Development on the Pathogenesis of Bronchopulmonary Dysplasia**.................................138
Cho-Ming Chao, Elie El Agha, Caterina Tiozzo, Parviz Minoo and Saverio Bellusci

Chapter 13   **Early Life Microbial Exposure and Immunity Training Effects on Asthma
Development and Progression**.................................150
Andressa Daronco Cereta, Vinícius Rosa Oliveira, Ivan Peres Costa, Letícia Lopes
Guimarães, João Pedro Ribeiro Afonso, Adriano Luís Fonseca,
Alan Robson Trigueiro de Sousa, Guilherme Augusto Moreira Silva,
Diego A. C. P. G. Mello, Luis Vicente Franco de Oliveira and Renata Kelly da Palma

Chapter 14   **Understanding the Impact of Infection, Inflammation and their Persistence
in the Pathogenesis of Bronchopulmonary Dysplasia**.................................156
Jherna Balany and Vineet Bhandari

Chapter 15   **Etiologies of Hospitalized Acute Bronchiolitis in Children 2 Years of Age
and Younger: A 3 Years' Study during a *Pertussis* Epidemic**.................................166
Sainan Chen, Yuqing Wang, Anrong Li, Wujun Jiang, Qiuyan Xu, Min Wu,
Zhengrong Chen, Chuangli Hao, Xunjun Shao and Jun Xu

Chapter 16   **Affect of Early Life Oxygen Exposure on Proper Lung Development and Response
to Respiratory Viral Infections**.................................174
William Domm, Ravi S. Misra and Michael A. O'Reilly

Chapter 17   **Development and Functional Characterization of Fetal Lung Organoids**.................................187
Mandy Laube, Soeren Pietsch, Thomas Pannicke, Ulrich H. Thome
and Claire Fabian

Chapter 18   **Imaging Bronchopulmonary Dysplasia — A Multimodality Update**.................................206
Thomas Semple, Mohammed R. Akhtar and Catherine M. Owens

Chapter 19   **Mitochondrial Fission-Mediated Lung Development in Newborn Rats
with Hyperoxia-Induced Bronchopulmonary Dysplasia with Pulmonary
Hypertension**.................................213
Yuanyuan Dai, Binyuan Yu, Danyang Ai, Lin Yuan, Xinye Wang, Ran Huo,
Xiaoqin Fu, Shangqin Chen and Chao Chen

Chapter 20   **Aberrant Pulmonary Vascular Growth and Remodeling in Bronchopulmonary
Dysplasia**.................................223
Cristina M. Alvira

Permissions

List of Contributors

Index

Preface

The lungs are two air-filled and spongy organs that are situated on either side of the chest. The heart and lungs work together to make sure the body receives enough supply of oxygen. Lung diseases are a variety of conditions or diseases that impair the ability of the lungs to function normally. These diseases can have an impact on pulmonary function and the capacity to breathe. Lung diseases can be classified into three types, including lung circulation diseases, airway diseases and lung tissue diseases. The major causes of lung diseases include infections, air pollution and smoking. The other significant risk factor for these diseases is genetics. The most common types of lung diseases include asthma, bronchitis, pneumonia, chronic obstructive pulmonary disease (COPD), lung cancer, pulmonary fibrosis, etc. This book explores all the important aspects of lung diseases in the modern day. It will help new researchers by foregrounding their knowledge on these medical conditions. Such selected concepts that redefine the diagnosis and treatment of these diseases through an evidence-based approach have been presented in this book.

This book has been the outcome of endless efforts put in by authors and researchers on various issues and topics within the field. The book is a comprehensive collection of significant researches that are addressed in a variety of chapters. It will surely enhance the knowledge of the field among readers across the globe.

It gives us an immense pleasure to thank our researchers and authors for their efforts to submit their piece of writing before the deadlines. Finally in the end, I would like to thank my family and colleagues who have been a great source of inspiration and support.

Editor

Perinatal Nutritional and Metabolic Pathways: Early Origins of Chronic Lung Diseases

Celien Kuiper-Makris [1†], Jaco Selle [1†], Eva Nüsken [2], Jörg Dötsch [2] and Miguel A. Alejandre Alcazar [1,3,4,5*]

[1] Department of Pediatric and Adolescent Medicine, Translational Experimental Pediatrics—Experimental Pulmonology, Faculty of Medicine and University Hospital Cologne, University of Cologne, Cologne, Germany, [2] Department of Pediatric and Adolescent Medicine, Faculty of Medicine and University Hospital Cologne, University of Cologne, Cologne, Germany, [3] Center for Molecular Medicine Cologne (CMMC), Faculty of Medicine and University Hospital Cologne, University of Cologne, Cologne, Germany, [4] Excellence Cluster on Stress Responses in Aging-associated Diseases (CECAD), Faculty of Medicine and University Hospital Cologne, University of Cologne, Cologne, Germany, [5] Member of the German Centre for Lung Research (DZL), Institute for Lung Health, University of Giessen and Marburg Lung Centre (UGMLC), Gießen, Germany

*Correspondence:
Miguel A. Alejandre Alcazar
miguel.alejandre-alcazar@uk-koeln.de

[†] These authors share first authorship

Lung development is not completed at birth, but expands beyond infancy, rendering the lung highly susceptible to injury. Exposure to various influences during a critical window of organ growth can interfere with the finely-tuned process of development and induce pathological processes with aberrant alveolarization and long-term structural and functional sequelae. This concept of developmental origins of chronic disease has been coined as perinatal programming. Some adverse perinatal factors, including prematurity along with respiratory support, are well-recognized to induce bronchopulmonary dysplasia (BPD), a neonatal chronic lung disease that is characterized by arrest of alveolar and microvascular formation as well as lung matrix remodeling. While the pathogenesis of various experimental models focus on oxygen toxicity, mechanical ventilation and inflammation, the role of nutrition before and after birth remain poorly investigated. There is accumulating clinical and experimental evidence that intrauterine growth restriction (IUGR) as a consequence of limited nutritive supply due to placental insufficiency or maternal malnutrition is a major risk factor for BPD and impaired lung function later in life. In contrast, a surplus of nutrition with perinatal maternal obesity, accelerated postnatal weight gain and early childhood obesity is associated with wheezing and adverse clinical course of chronic lung diseases, such as asthma. While the link between perinatal nutrition and lung health has been described, the underlying mechanisms remain poorly understood. There are initial data showing that inflammatory and nutrient sensing processes are involved in programming of alveolarization, pulmonary angiogenesis, and composition of extracellular matrix. Here, we provide a comprehensive overview of the current knowledge regarding the impact of perinatal metabolism and nutrition on the lung and beyond the cardiopulmonary system as well as possible mechanisms determining the individual susceptibility to CLD early in life. We aim to emphasize the importance of unraveling the mechanisms of perinatal metabolic programming to develop novel preventive and therapeutic avenues.

Keywords: lung development and pulmonary diseases, perinatal nutrition, maternal obesity, intrauterine growth restriction, chronic lung disease, bronchopulmonary dysplasia (BPD)

INTRODUCTION

Chronic lung diseases (CLD) such as asthma, chronic obstructive pulmonary disease (COPD) and pulmonary arterial hypertension (PAH) have a major impact on global health, with COPD being the third leading cause of death worldwide (WHO Global Health Estimates, 2020). CLDs do not only have an enormous impact on the patient's quality of life, but also on health care costs (e.g., an average of $4147 per COPD patient per year) (1, 2). While the pathology of adult lung diseases and the influence of environmental factors such as smoking have been extensively studied, the mechanisms determining the individual susceptibility to CLD early in life remain elusive. This review will provide insights in the current knowledge on how perinatal nutritional and metabolic conditions adversely affect lung development and contribute to the origin of CLDs.

Maternal obesity and intrauterine growth restriction (IUGR) represent alterations of the antenatal, perinatal and postnatal nutritional and metabolic status with adverse consequences for the fetus and newborn. (1) First, both maternal obesity and IUGR increase the risk of pregnancy complications and prematurity of the offspring. Epidemiological studies have shown that not only the risk of pregnancy complications for overweight and obese mothers is higher; it is also associated with an early pregnancy loss, congenital malformations, premature birth and stillbirth (3). In addition, the offspring has an increased risk of being either macrosome or IUGR, both introducing their own risk of comorbidity. IUGR is diagnosed in 5–10% of all pregnancies, characterized as a rate of fetal growth less than the growth potential that is appropriate for the gestational age, and well-recognized as an additional risk factor for prematurity (4, 5). (2) Second, fetal and postnatal nutritional supply as well as maternal weight and metabolism can adversely affect the long-term health of the child. This is referred to as *perinatal or metabolic programming* (6, 7). This concept was initially coined by Barker as the *fetal origins* hypothesis, also known as *fetal programming*. Barker et al. proposed that the developing fetus adapts its growth rate and metabolism as a response to variations in the supply of nutrients (and oxygen), which may lead to permanent changes of organs' structure and physiology in the newborn (8). Over the past two decades, the developmental origins of health and disease have gained increasing scientific interest. There has been an enormous effort and an accumulation of studies devoted to elucidating the underlying mechanisms of perinatal (metabolic) programming of diseases as well as its prevention and therapy. (3) Lastly, maternal obesity and IUGR are associated with long-term alterations of lung function and lung structure. For example, clinical reports showed a positive linear trend between birth weight, adjusted for maternal factors, and lung function in adulthood (9). Furthermore, children that were exposed to maternal obesity during pregnancy or gestational diabetes mellitus (GDM) have an increased risk of developing asthma in childhood (10–12). These findings indicate the significant impact of body weight, nutrition, and metabolism during critical phases of pregnancy and the early postnatal period on the lung development and later pulmonary function of a child (13).

In addition to the adverse nutritive and metabolic influences, the time of exposure is of great importance with regard to the resulting lung pathology. There are different critical windows of lung development with diverse developmental biological processes. The lung develops in five stages, with the last (alveolarization) starting shortly before birth and continuing beyond infancy (14). The window and the nature of exposure to adverse influences render not only the prenatal, but also postnatal lung development highly susceptible to injury and CLDs (15). This basic principle of timing emphasizes the far-reaching complex consequences of antenatal, perinatal and postnatal nutrition. Here, we provide an overview of the impact and mechanisms of nutritive surplus with metabolic disorder (maternal obesity) as well as nutritive deprivation (e.g., IUGR) on the child's lung health (schematic representation in **Figure 1**).

THE IMPACT OF PERINATAL NUTRITIVE SURPLUS ON THE ORIGINS OF CHRONIC LUNG DISEASE

Obesity and overweight result from an imbalance of energy consumption and energy intake, causing fat accumulation in adipose tissue (16). The origin of obesity is multifactorial and comprises a complex interaction of genetic and life style factors (17, 18). It is widely accepted that each individual has a certain level of predisposition for obesity due to genetic and epigenetic adaptations along with modifying environmental factors that can in part contribute to familiar obesity (17). Two central endocrine pathways in obesity are those of insulin and leptin. Insulin is a critical regulator of adipocyte biology that promotes the uptake of glucose and fatty acids and stimulates lipogenesis while inhibiting lipolysis (19). In obesity, the glucose transport and adipocyte metabolism are decreased despite high circulating levels of insulin, also known as insulin resistance (20). Leptin is produced by adipose tissue and acts as a regulator of appetite and energy expenditure (21). Obesity is associated with high levels of circulating leptin combined with leptin resistance (22). Leptin and insulin directly interact with each other and in addition, leptin influences insulin sensitivity through the regulation of glucose metabolism (23). Interestingly, targeting the energy balance to favor weight loss might induce compensatory behavioral and metabolic actions that favor the maintenance of bodyweight (24). This is one of the explanations for the further increasing numbers of obesity, despite multiple broad scale attempts on lifestyle and dietary interventions. Instead, obesity has grown into a worldwide pandemic. Surveys conducted by the WHO in 2008 showed that around 1.5 billion adults worldwide suffer from overweight, which corresponds to a body mass index (BMI) of over 25. Of far greater concern are the ~200 million men and 300 million women with a BMI of more than 30, therefore considered to be obese (25). It is alarming that the prevalence of overweight and obesity is not only increasing dramatically among adults, but also children (26).

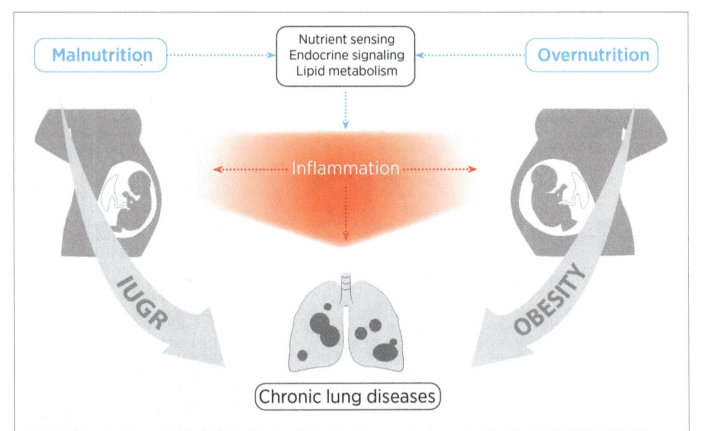

FIGURE 1 | Schematic representation of the structure of this review. We aim to provide a comprehensive overview of the influences of maternal obesity, early childhood obesity and intrauterine growth restriction (IUGR) on nutrient sensing as well as endocrine and inflammatory pathways, and how these adverse perinatal effects contribute to the early origins of chronic lung diseases.

Linking Maternal to Childhood Obesity: a Transgenerational Vicious Circle

Early childhood obesity has been proposed as a strong predictor of overweight in early adulthood (27). It has also been reported that maternal obesity and GDM can cause early-onset childhood obesity, which is associated with a higher prevalence of overweight or obesity in adulthood (28). In the USA, 17% of children are already considered obese (26, 29). Studies show that 1 to 2-year-old overweight children are more likely to be obese in their teenage and middle age years, and are prone to develop early-onset metabolic syndrome (30–33). Metabolic syndrome is characterized by obesity, type 2 diabetes, cardiovascular diseases, dyslipidemia and hypertension. As the prevalence of obesity amongst young adults continues to rise, the number of overweight/obese pregnant women is also steadily increasing. Interestingly, there is accumulating evidence of a transgenerational effect of obesity that adversely affects child health throughout life (34, 35). Specifically, maternal BMI shows a significant correlation with high offspring's birth weight and children's overweight (30, 36, 37). Thus, children of overweight mothers are at high risk of developing overweight later in life and tend to suffer from overweight-associated diseases (38). These findings are supported by experimental studies that show higher tendency for obesity and impaired insulin response in offspring of obese dams (39–41).

These transgenerational effects can be attributed, in part, to epigenetic changes in the offspring of obese mothers. The DNA is hypomethylated at the start of embryonic development, therefore, the developing embryo is particularly sensitive to epigenetic changes (e.g., DNA methylation, histone modification and microRNA expression) in response to the intrauterine environment (42). For example, maternal high-fat diet before, during and after pregnancy has been shown to alter miRNA expression and to induce a chronic dysregulation of insulin-like growth factor 2 (IGF-2) signaling in a mouse model (43). Such changes are not only detectable in adult mice (42), but also in human fetal umbilical cord blood (44). In addition, there are multiple reports of modified DNA methylation on sites of importance for metabolic processes after dysglycemia and/or high-fat diet during pregnancy (45–47).

In addition to metabolic consequences, the rising incidence of early childhood obesity is particularly concerning because of the association with respiratory symptoms and diseases in youth. One of the most common respiratory symptoms in childhood is wheezing, with ~30% of all children suffering from it (48). The risk of recurrent wheezing is especially high in children of obese mothers (49, 50). Obese children experience exertional dyspnea and often suffer from obstructive sleep apnea syndrome (OSAS) as well as obesity hypoventilation syndrome (OHS) (51, 52). In case of an emergency, obese children show dyspnea related to sedation and post-operative care (53). Furthermore, persistent asthma is strongly associated with high BMI throughout childhood (54–56), which manifests in a 92% higher prevalence of asthma in adult obese patients (57). In addition, the functional parameters of lung function such as respiratory muscle strength and endurance, airway resistance, lung volume and function or gas exchange are negatively influenced by obesity (58–60). Collectively, these studies indicate an adverse clinical course of respiratory diseases in children of obese mothers and after childhood obesity. In the following, we will discuss possible causes for the association between maternal obesity and child lung health.

Molecular Insights Into the Mechanical Effects of Obesity on Lung Function

Mechanical and physical influences on the lung play a significant role in the overall health of obese children and adults. Obese persons, including children, experience a lung restrictive syndrome, which goes along with increased overall body volume causing a narrowing of the upper airway and a reduced full inflation due to neck fat and an inadequate thoracic expansion, respectively (61). Accordingly, obese children suffer from obstructive sleep apnea hypoventilation syndrome (OSAHS) which is associated with hypoxemia, hypoventilation, sleep interruptions and chronic fatigue (62). Therefore, OSAHS has a drastic effect on oxygen supply and can induce hypoxia-associated changes in gene expression through the transcription factor hypoxia-inducible factor (HIF) (63). Under normoxia, prolyl hydroxylases (PHDs) hydroxylate proline residues on HIF-α subunits leading to subsequent proteasomal degradation through ubiquitination. In contrast, hypoxia reduces the O_2-dependent hydroxylation of HIF-α subunits by PHDs, resulting in nuclear HIF-α accumulation (64). In a murine model, the effects of hypoxia-mediated HIF activity have been reported to be involved in the pathogenesis of pulmonary arterial hypertension (PAH), in part by upregulating the vasoconstrictor endothelin-1 (65, 66). Deficiency of HIF-2α, however, partly protected from the increase in endothelin and PAH (65, 66). In addition, stabilization of HIF-α induces alveolar epithelial type 2 cell (ATII) apoptosis and subsequent fibrotic lung diseases (67). In contrast, the use of PHD inhibitors in vivo to stabilize HIF-α improved lung growth and function in a model of prematurity (68, 69).

It has been shown that HIF-1α in part sustains the Warburg effect (70, 71). The Warburg effect describes a condition in which the cells obtain their energy mainly through glycolysis with subsequent excretion of lactate. This alternative metabolic state for energy production is used by cancer cells, but also by healthy cells under hypoxia (anaerobic glycolysis). As described above, obesity-associated mechanical forces can lead to an activation of HIF, a mediator of hypoxia. HIF can cause a shift toward glycolysis rather than oxidative phosphorylation, in order to meet the energy demands under hypoxic conditions

(70). Interestingly, studies suggested a Warburg effect inversion, a condition in which cancer cells exposed to an adiposity environment increase energy production by aerobic respiration as well as gluconeogenesis (72). The authors suggest that the cells do not consume glucose in glycolysis, but produce glucose through gluconeogenesis. Moreover, it has been described that during hypoxia, mitochondria increase the production of reactive oxygen species (ROS) at complex III (73), leading to inhibition of PHD activity and subsequent stabilization of HIF-α (74, 75). The shift toward glycolysis by the Warburg effect and the increased production of ROS, both induced and maintained by hypoxia, resemble mitochondrial dysfunction (76, 77). Increasing evidence points toward a central role for mitochondrial dysfunction in the development of cancer as well as CLDs including asthma, COPD and PAH (71, 76, 77). Furthermore, recent studies have indicated that the hypoxia-induced increase of ROS in acute lung injury contributes to pulmonary fibrosis by triggering an epithelial-mesenchymal transition (EMT) (78, 79) via the stabilization of HIF-1α in several cell types, including alveolar epithelial cells (80).

These findings highlight the effect of obesity on oxygen sensing and energy metabolism as well as the subsequent consequences for the development of CLDs. HIF, as a central player in oxygen sensing, might serve as a potential therapeutic approach to target the rising incidences of obesity-related diseases. For example, preclinical data show that blocking HIF with digoxin in a mouse model prevented or slowed down the progression of PAH (81, 82). These promising findings demonstrate that not only preventing obesity itself, but also targeting specific metabolic processes might offer new preventive strategies for CLDs.

Cell Homeostasis and Inflammatory Response Under Obese Conditions

Obesity represents a state of low-grade chronic inflammation. The numbers of inflammatory cells such as $CD8^+$, $CD4^+$ and $CD68^+$ cells are significantly elevated in adipose tissue (83, 84). These immune cells along with adipocytes release a wide range of inflammatory factors including leptin, tumor necrosis factor-alpha (TNF-α) (85), interleukin 6 (IL-6), and IL-8 (86), C-reactive protein, monocyte chemoattractant protein-1 (MCP-1), and Plasminogen activator inhibitor-1 (PAI-1) (87–89). Exposure of the lung to these pro-inflammatory cytokines can occur in three different ways at different time points during lung development: (1) through transplacental transport from the obese mother to the fetus; (2) through breast milk of the obese mother during lactation; and (3) through the child's own adipose tissue as a result of (early) postnatal obesity. For example, maternal high-fat diet in a murine model during lactation [postnatal day 1 (P1) to P21] induced an early-onset obesity in the offspring with elevated inflammatory cytokines, such as IL-4, IL-6, IL-13, IL-17A, and TNF-α. The early inflammatory response was related to increased airway hyperreactivity, similar to asthma (90). The adverse effect of IL-6 on the lung was further supported by a study that showed that elevated IL-6 could in part account for the development of emphysema through IL-6 trans-signaling-mediated apoptosis of ATII. Blocking IL-6/gp130 signaling, however, prevented features of lung emphysema (91, 92). Furthermore, elevated IL-6 levels contribute to PAH (93). For example, IL-6 induces a downstream activation of Stat3, which in turn causes a phosphorylation of the transcription factor forkhead box O (FoxO) 1. Phosphorylation of FoxO1 leads to its cytoplasmatic sequestration, subsequent inactivation and ultimately to a hyperproliferation of bronchial smooth muscle cells (SMC) (93, 94). In addition to IL-6, TNF-α is also a notable adipocytokine that is elevated under obese conditions (95). TNF-α modulates the effects of G-protein coupled receptor (GPCR)-induced hyperreactivity in cultured murine airway SMCs and increases contractility (96). By this mechanism, TNF-α may be contributing to SMC responsiveness and the development of asthma. Consequently, the anti-inflammatory adiponectin reduces TNF-α-induced nuclear factor κ B (NFκB) signaling. Thus, the obesity-related decrease in adiponectin further contributes to a dysregulated TNF-α signaling (97). Due to its potential impact on the development of asthma, TNF-α is under intense investigation as a therapeutic target (98–100). Another important functional aspect of TNF-α is the ability to contribute to insulin resistance by inhibiting tyrosine phosphorylation of insulin receptor substrate-1 (IRS-1) (95). Similarly, PAI-1 is produced and secreted by adipocytes and elevated in obesity serum levels (89). In a mouse model of airway hyperresponsiveness, PAI-1 was involved in airway remodeling after LPS-induced lung injury (101). Chronically elevated levels of PAI-1 affect the extracellular matrix turnover and contribute to collagen deposition in the airways (102). Moreover, dysfunction of the adipose tissue after perinatal obesity can further contribute to the maintenance of *low-grade chronic inflammation*. For example, a recent study indicated that maternal obesity induces metabolic programming of adipocytes in the offspring with lifelong dysfunctional adipose tissue and obesity (103). Collectively, obesity represents a state of *low-grade chronic inflammation* exposing the developing lung to pro-inflammatory cytokines which could adversely affect lung growth as a first "hit" and increase susceptibility for CLDs in later life.

Nutrient Sensing and Leptin Signaling as a Mechanism of Perinatal Obesity

Under physiological conditions, leptin is integrated in the complex mechanisms of airway and bronchial maturation. A recent study highlighted the importance of physiological non-obese levels of leptin in lung maturation through the upregulation of the expression and the secretion of surfactant protein A (*Sftpa*) in ATII (104, 105). Similarly, leptin promoted maturation of lung structure and contributed to postnatal lung remodeling and enlargement of the alveolar surface area *via* the induction of the genes *Col1a1*, *Col3a1*, *Col6a3*, *Mmp2*, *Tieg1*, and *Stat1* (106). A lack of leptin signaling in *ob/ob* mice (induced by leptin deficiency) resulted in a significant reduction of alveolar surface, indicating a critical role of leptin in postnatal lung growth (106). These contradictory observations may be due to effects of high circulating concentrations of glucose and insulin during pregnancy in obese mothers, which might potentially

overrule the beneficial effect of leptin on lung development (107). In addition, long-term exposure to leptin before birth could affect the expression of pulmonary leptin receptors, disturbing leptin-signaling, leading to defective lung maturation and respiratory function at birth (108, 109).

Leptin has a central role in the immune response as well. Leptin was linked to asthma in adults as well as in children; the severity of asthma was correlated to serum leptin levels in a meta-analysis of 13 studies (110–113). High leptin levels increased the T-helper cell type 2 (Th2)-type immune response in airways *via* a leptin-mediated and XBP1 (X-box binding protein 1) s-dependent activation of mTOR (mechanistic target of rapamycin) as well as MAPK (mitogen-activated protein kinase) signaling (114). A shift toward the Th2-type immune response in airways is characteristic for the pathogenesis of asthma, thus providing a relevant link between obesity-induced high circulating leptin levels and the development of asthma (114, 115). Adiponectin acts as an anti-inflammatory agent, counteracting leptin (88, 89). Circulating adiponectin levels are known to be reduced in obesity, possibly further contributing to the pathogenesis of obesity-associated asthma (116).

There have been several attempts to alter the high leptin and low adiponectin levels in order to restore the metabolic balance. For example, pharmacological elevation of adiponectin levels in obese mice protected from hyperglycemia, glucose intolerance, and insulin resistance (117) as well as increasing insulin sensitivity (118). However, to date, the effect of adiponectin supplementation on pulmonary development and function remains elusive. In diabetes, thiazolidinedione (TZD) is possibly the most extensively characterized regulator of adiponectin expression. TZDs, such as pioglitazone and rosiglitazone increase adiponectin expression through the activation of peroxisome proliferator-activated receptor gamma (PPARγ) (119, 120). Since it is already a well-established therapeutic intervention for diabetes, targeting adiponectin might be a new promising therapeutic approach for the prevention of long-term consequences of obesity such as pulmonary remodeling and reduced lung function.

Lipid Metabolism and Perinatal Obesity

Obesity is characterized by a dysregulation of the energy and lipid metabolism. Lipoproteins are responsible for the transport of fatty acids, cholesterol and phospholipids. Therefore, the lipoproteins in obese patients show a change in circulating protein levels (121). For example, apolipoprotein E (ApoE), which is part of the low-density lipoprotein (LDL), is elevated in the obese and contributes to fat mass accumulation (122). LDL/ApoE is internalized into cells by its receptor, the low-density lipoprotein receptors (LDLRs), and is the main source of cholesterol and phospholipids efflux out of cells. In the lung, ApoE is produced by lung macrophages and acts on ciliated airway epithelial cells, where it can modulate airway hyperreactivity, mucin gene expression, and goblet cell hyperplasia (121). Thereby, it is involved in reducing the susceptibility to airway hyperresponsiveness (121, 123). In line with this, genetic modified mice with an ApoE deletion show reduced alveologenesis and abnormal pulmonary function with increased airway resistance as well as high dynamic and static compliance (124). PPARγ is a nuclear receptor and considered one of the master regulators of adipogenesis, showing a high expression pattern in adipose tissue and in the lung (125–127). PPARγ is essential for normal lung development *via* the induction of alveolar epithelial-mesenchymal paracrine signaling (128, 129). Murine studies with genetically deactivated PPARγ demonstrated a spontaneous development of PAH. Here, PPARγ has an anti-proliferative effect on smooth muscle cell proliferation, which might give the opportunity to use PPARγ agonists in treating PAH (130, 131). Moreover, unsaturated fatty acids and several eicosanoids are regulators of PPARγ and induce expression of genes encoding lipoprotein lipase, CD36, phosphoenolpyruvate carboxykinase, aquaporin 7 and adiponectin (132). This is of particular interest since the western style diet has high concentrations of poly-unsaturated fatty acids (133). In this context of western style diet and a higher rate of obese individuals in industrial western countries, elevated fatty acid levels in obesity may be important regulators and modulators of normal and aberrant lung development.

Glucose Metabolism and Hyperinsulemia

Obesity is intimately linked to insulin resistance, accompanied by elevated circulating insulin concentrations. The transduction of insulin signaling is in part mediated through the downstream phosphatidylinositol 3-kinase (PI3K)/protein kinase B (AKT) and mTOR pathways (134–137). The mTOR cascade is integral in orchestrating the complex mechanism of lung development, balancing nutrient and energy supply in the early stages of embryogenesis and fine-tuning tissue growth during organogenesis. An elaborated and comprehensive article by Land et al. provides a broad overview of the role of mTOR in lung development (138). High levels of insulin from diabetic mothers have the potential to inhibit the *Sftpa* gene expression in lung epithelial cells and thereby delay the fetuses' lung development. This insulin-induced inhibition acts *via* the rapamycin-sensitive PI3K signaling pathway and not *via* mitogen-activated protein kinase (MAPK) (139). This notion is further supported by the fact that inhibition of PI3K can contribute to insulin resistance and diabetes (140). Moreover, Ikeda and colleagues demonstrated that insulin reduces vascular endothelial growth factor (VEGF) expression and the transcriptional activity of HIF-2 on the VEGF promoter in an AKT-mTOR-dependent manner in cultured lung epithelial cells. They further demonstrated that activation of the AKT-mTOR pathway in mice reduced alveolar capillarization, stressing the importance of this pathway in lung epithelium and in the development of infant respiratory distress syndrome (RDS) (141). Interestingly, moderate physical activity of obese mothers can rescue maternal and the offsprings' insulin sensitivity, overall improving the metabolic, as well as potential pulmonary outcome in the obese mother as well as her offspring (142).

Insulin does not only affect the alveolar epithelial cells, but also increases the expression of genes related to the contractile phenotype of airway SMC through a Rho kinase- and PI3K-dependent mechanism (143). Apart from these direct effects on pulmonary cells, insulin is involved in the modulation of the immune response and thereby in the pathogenesis of asthma.

For example, in mast cells, insulin induces PI3K-dependent signaling, which could contribute to allergic bronchoconstriction (144). On the other hand, Viardot and colleagues demonstrated that insulin influences T cell differentiation promoting a shift toward a Th2-type response. They state, that this effect may contribute to insulin's anti-inflammatory role in chronic inflammation associated with obesity and type 2 diabetes (145). Insulin further exhibits anti-inflammatory properties in acute Th1-type inflammation, where insulin diminishes acute lung injury and reduces levels of inflammatory cytokines (146). Taken together, insulin plays an important role in physiological lung development, supporting alveolarization. In obese patients, however, elevated insulin levels interfere with lung development and maturation, while facilitating a pro-asthmatic immune environment, which could affect the outcome of CLDs in later life.

Collectively, these studies show that perinatal obesity resulting from maternal and early childhood obesity may determine individual susceptibility for CLDs later in life. In addition to mechanical factors due to increased body mass, adipose tissue dysfunction and its consequences play a particularly important role. *Low-grade chronic inflammation* with increased levels of adipocytokines, impaired insulin signaling, and altered lipid metabolism can be important in metabolic programming of CLDs. In the future, further elucidation of the fat-lung axis is imperative for a better understanding of metabolic mechanisms in the development of CLDs and to develop new preventive and therapeutic approaches.

THE IMPACT OF PERINATAL NUTRITIVE DEFICIENCY ON THE ORIGINS OF CHRONIC LUNG DISEASE

Nutrient Deprivation and Lung Development: the Role of Intrauterine Growth Restriction

Intrauterine growth restriction (IUGR) was first described as "dysmaturity" and indicates an abnormally low birth weight for the gestational age. Classically, IUGR was defined as a birthweight below 2,500 g (147). More recently, it has been characterized as "not reaching the biologically based potential," often due to reduced perfusion or malnutrition *in utero* (148–150). IUGR and "small for gestational age" (SGA, birthweight of-2 SD/mean) are often used interchangeably; however, SGA neither excludes nor proves IUGR but serves as an easily quantifiable proxy for IUGR. Pathological intrauterine circumstances induce IUGR, resulting in an infant with low birth weight, often followed by a period of rapid postnatal weight gain, also called "catch-up growth." Catch-up growth is associated with altered nutrient supply, and overlaps with the final stages of pulmonary alveolarization and vascular maturation (151, 152). Moreover, infants with catch-up growth after IUGR have a higher risk to become overweight or obese and to develop metabolic disorders later in life (4, 153). These clinical findings have been supported by experimental models of IUGR (154–157).

The etiology of IUGR can be divided in (1) *fetal origins*, such as genetic abnormalities (e.g., chromosomal abnormalities), (2) *maternal factors* (e.g., vascular diseases, persistent hypoxia or undernutrition, and toxins), and (3) *placental etiologies* (e.g., placental insufficiency, inflammation) (158). It is thought that 40% of birth weight is ascribable to genetic factors and that the remaining 60% is due to fetal environmental exposures (159). Several historical events have caused a surge of IUGR cases in a defined birth cohort, which has provided deeper insight into the clinical sequelae of IUGR. The latest temporary surge of IUGR caused by maternal malnutrition in Europe was caused by the Second World War. Investigations of the Dutch Famine Birth Cohort (Amsterdam, 1944-1946) have shown that low birth weight infants often have a lower FEV1 and FVC, but not FEV1/FVC ratios, indicative of restrictive lung alterations (160, 161). Other cohorts, however, including an Indian study demonstrate an association of small head circumference (indicative of early gestational growth restriction) with reduced FEV1/FVC ratios (162, 163). These data show the diverse impact of intrauterine nutrient deprivation on lung health that could be in part accounted to the window of injury or the type of nutrient restriction (e.g., protein, vitamins). Overall, these observational and experimental studies highlight that being born IUGR represents a pathologic condition with far-reaching consequences for the child's health and disease, especially regarding metabolism and the lung.

The Interplay Between IUGR and Obesity

Maternal obesity and GDM are often associated with macrosomic offspring (164). However, in uncontrolled or badly controlled GDM, diabetic vasculopathy and nephropathy may lead to placental insufficiency-induced IUGR (165, 166). In addition, experimental data have shown that overnutrition of pregnant sheep causes IUGR in the fetus, likely due to major restriction in placental growth and relative hypoglycemia and fetal hypoinsulinemia during late pregnancy (167). This might be partly related to fetal hypoxia, in turn inducing fetal catecholamine expression and reducing circulating insulin concentrations (168). On the contrary, IUGR induces metabolic changes to the growing fetus that cause a risk for developing obesity, diabetes and metabolic syndrome later in life (4, 153). These changes are passed onto the next generation; female IUGR rat offspring exhibit symptoms of gestational diabetes, and their offspring has increased fasting glucose and insulin levels despite having a normal birth weight when compared to controls (169). These transgenerational changes might be attributed to epigenetic changes, not only affecting the IUGR offspring, but also the second generation by direct exposition of the offspring germ-line to the IUGR environment (170, 171). More specifically, the increased risk for childhood and adult obesity in IUGR offspring could be in part due to *programming* of the adipocytes toward lipogenesis and proliferation (172, 173). Moreover, the combination of IUGR (induced by surgical bilateral artery ligation) with maternal obesity increased hepatic cholesterol accumulation and LDLR expression when compared to non-IUGR controls (156). These data further support the notion that maternal obesity along with IUGR provides an additional risk for metabolic complications.

The Adverse Effects of IUGR on Pulmonary Structure and Function

IUGR causes structural changes to the lung. Multiple animal studies have shown that IUGR impairs alveolar formation and lung growth, leading to reduced lung function (155, 174–179). In addition, a recent study from our group has demonstrated that IUGR also negatively influences angiogenesis and extracellular matrix formation (157). The intimate link between angiogenesis and alveologenesis has been shown in various animal studies, where alveolar formation was reduced after blocking angiogenesis (180–182). Conversely, the positive influence of angiogenesis on alveolar growth and regeneration is of great therapeutic importance (181, 183). Structural alveolar and vascular changes during lung development could account for the functional alterations that were reported after IUGR in epidemiological studies: several cohort studies have shown that school-children born IUGR have a significantly lower FEV1 and airway resistance as well as a higher susceptibility to airway infections, independent of catch-up growth (184–189). Moreover, in long-term follow-up studies it was shown that a low birthweight decreases lung function in adulthood, with a reduction of lung capacity and elasticity, resembling a COPD phenotype (9, 190). In summary, there is compelling epidemiological and experimental evidence that IUGR determines lung structure and function and could thereby predispose for CLDs.

Endocrine Effects of IUGR and Catch-Up Growth Resemble those of Obesity

Children born SGA have an increased risk of reduced embryonic β-cell growth, glucose intolerance, insulin resistance, type II diabetes and obesity in childhood as well as later in life (191–197). The effect of IUGR on the regulation of insulin levels has been extensively studied, as insulin is not only important for euglycemia in the fetus but also serves as a major fetal (pulmonary-) growth factor (159). The stable glucose flow over the placenta during healthy pregnancy causes fetal insulin secretion that regulates normal adipose tissue development and deposition (198). As stated before, IUGR fetus can exhibit hypoglycemia and hypoinsulinemia due to inhibition of endocrine signaling by catecholamines (168). In addition, the pancreatic function can be decreased after IUGR, resulting in lower levels of intrauterine insulin secretion as well (199). In contrast, reports on postnatal insulin levels in IUGR newborns are contradictive, they might be slightly lower or equal to healthy controls (200, 201). Thus, IUGR causes a deregulation of intrauterine insulin levels, an important mediator in adipose tissue development and fat deposition.

The phase of catch-up growth after IUGR appears to be a strong determinant of future (lung) health. A key fetal adaptation to nutrient deprivation is the intrauterine upregulation of the insulin receptor under hypoinsulinemic circumstances in fetal skeletal muscle (202). After birth and under nutrient surplus, this upregulated receptor is activated by an abundance of glucose and insulin, inducing accelerated body growth (202, 203). The closely related insulin-like growth factor 1 (IGF-1) is induced by growth hormone (GH)/somatropin and is an essential regulator of body growth. The inhibition of the GH/IGF-1 axis has been shown to dysregulate alveologenesis, mainly through disruption of the physiological deposition of the extracellular matrix (204). Work by our group has shown that inhibition of the GH/IGF-1 axis by IUGR was associated with an arrest of lung development; in contrast, catch-up growth caused a significant increase of GH/IGF-1 expression (174). Interestingly, recent work demonstrated that postnatal treatment with recombinant human IGF-1 improves lung growth and structure in a model for bronchopulmonary dysplasia (BPD) (205). In conclusion, there is a postnatal reactive upregulation of both the insulin receptor and the insulin-signaling (including IGF-1) pathway after IUGR, resulting in an initially increased insulin sensitivity during postnatal catch-up growth (4). However, school-aged and adolescent children with accelerated weight gain and catch-up growth after IUGR show increased levels of insulin and reduced insulin sensitivity, indicating the long-lasting effects of prenatal metabolic programming (206, 207).

In addition to the dysregulation of prenatal and postnatal insulin signaling, leptin has been identified to be dysregulated after IUGR as well. Animal studies have shown that IUGR rat pups rapidly develop leptin resistance during their catch-up growth, thereby stimulating weight gain through hyperphagia (208–210). An important molecular link between nutrient status, insulin/leptin signaling and metabolic outcome is the mTOR pathway, controlling cell growth in response to its environment (e.g., stress, oxygen, nutrient status) through protein synthesis as well as lipid, nucleotide, and glucose metabolism (211, 212). A study from our group has shown that nutrient sensing *via* the mTOR signaling pathway is dysregulated in lungs from a rat model of nutrient deprivation-induced IUGR (157). Recent reports demonstrated that the mTOR signaling pathway is also altered in the placenta of humans and in experimental IUGR studies, enforcing adaptive mechanisms from both the maternal nutrient supply and the fetus's energy demands (213, 214). These studies suggest that both the placenta and the fetus react to nutrient availability by regulating this key nutrient sensor. The mTOR pathway is postnatally essential for pancreatic β-cell and islet maturation (215). Furthermore, mTOR is a potent mediator of endocrine responses, translating signals from leptin and insulin to a negative feedback for insulin (216). Interestingly, studies demonstrate that mTOR is involved in lung development as well, by regulating cell growth for proper organ development (211, 212) and by interfering with essential developmental signaling pathways, such as pulmonary angiogenesis (VEGF) and extracellular matrix deposition (bone morphogenetic protein, BMP) (217, 218). Collectively, these data highlight the eminent impact of intrauterine nutrient deprivation on endocrine function. Of note are the converging similarities between IUGR and obesity with regard to the endocrine system and the long-term metabolic and pulmonary sequelae.

IUGR Causes Transgenerational Metabolic Programing

Epidemiological studies as well as animal studies have shown transgenerational effects of IUGR on metabolic function (219–221). In part, these effects can be attributed to epigenetic programming (222, 223). For example, Fu et al. as well as Tosh et al. described histone modification along the IGF-1 gene and subsequently altered mRNA expression of IGF-1 in a rat model for IUGR induced by placental insufficiency or maternal malnutrition, respectively (224, 225). In addition, Tosh et al. showed that the restriction of early postnatal nutrient intake partly prevents these epigenetic changes (224). Park et al. observed consistent epigenetic adaptations related to differential binding of dinucleotide methyl transferase 1 and 3a together with changes in histone acetylation and methylation in the promoter region of the *Pdx1* homeobox gene in a rat model of IUGR (226). Recent studies by Gonzalez-Rodriguez et al., demonstrated the genetic imprinting of H19/IGF2 in second-generation IUGR offspring. This genetic imprinting was associated with altered H19 and IGF2 expression, which is in turn related to an increased risk for obesity and associated metabolic diseases (220, 227). Interestingly, this effect is reversible with postnatal essential nutrient supplementation (220, 228). These studies highlight the influence of perinatal nutrition in the development but also the primary prevention of metabolic diseases, including their secondary pulmonary complications as described in the previous chapter. In summary, these data indicate the great potential of perinatal nutrition and metabolism as a preventive and therapeutic target for metabolic health and CLDs.

Chronic Inflammation in IUGR-Associated CLD

One of the vital connections between the metabolic consequences of intrauterine nutrient deprivation and altered lung development is chronic inflammation. Chronic inflammation has been associated with (1) IUGR (229–232), (2) obesity, type 2 diabetes and metabolic syndrome (233–235) as well as (3) CLDs (236–239). IUGR, followed by catch-up growth, shows similar endocrine dysregulation and activation of inflammatory mechanisms as obesity. For example, both obesity and IUGR exhibit similar levels of leptin and insulin resistance in response to their prenatal nutritional status and postnatal accelerated weight gain (191–197). A possible shift of the Th2 immune response might be another link between CLDs and metabolic changes, e.g., elevated leptin (240) and insulin (206, 207) levels after IUGR. Interestingly, a study in IUGR mice has shown that the Th2 shift and consequent recruitment of macrophages cause inflammation in the pancreatic β-cell islets, causing type 2 diabetes (230). To date, there is no conclusive evidence whether IUGR-associated chronic inflammation is causative for or a consequence of metabolic distress, but the reports support an intimate link between both conditions.

A clinical study on the cord blood of 20 SGA neonates showed that IUGR causes a low-grade inflammatory response: infants born IUGR had significantly increased levels of inflammatory markers IL-6, TNF-α, CRP and thrombopoetin

(232). Moreover, animal studies have demonstrated IUGR-associated systemic inflammation in various organs: adult (uteroplacental) IUGR rats exhibited increased pancreatic β-cell inflammation, increasing the risk of diabetes (230, 241); a sheep model for hypothermia-induced IUGR showed a decrease of NF-κB as key regulator of immune-responses (231); and finally, a recent study in IUGR lambs demonstrated increased inflammatory markers and expression of inflammatory as well as pro-apoptotic genes in liver tissue (229). Along with these reports, prior work from our group has shown that IUGR causes dysregulation of key developmental signaling pathways such as NPY(neuropeptide Y)/PKC(protein kinase C), IL-6/AMPKα and TGFβ (transforming growth factor β) signaling as well as the associated inflammatory response (178, 179, 242).

A highly relevant comorbidity for IUGR infants is prematurity. About 30–50% of all extremely premature infants display symptoms of IUGR (243, 244). The causes of prematurity are multifactorial, but there is a strong correlation with maternal obesity. A meta-analysis of 84 clinical studies has shown a significantly increased risk of (induced) preterm labor in overweight and obese pregnancies (245). In addition, the risk of neonatal respiratory complications after premature birth is higher in obese *vs.* non-obese pregnancies (246, 247).

Premature birth and perinatal inflammatory responses have been intimately linked to pathological processes (248). The lungs of preterm infants are often in the late-saccular to early-alveolar phase at birth and require respiratory support (249). Mechanical ventilation, continuous positive airway pressure (CPAP) or oxygen supplementation are necessary treatments, but cause inflammation, acute lung injury and lead to a neonatal CLD, also known as BPD (250–254). Lungs of infants with BPD are characterized by vascular and alveolar hypoplasia (255). As stated previously, IUGR alone adversely affects lung microvascular and alveolar formation. Interestingly, the combination of IUGR with the immature lung in premature infants increases the risk for the clinical manifestation of BPD (i.e., prolonged need of oxygen supplementation >36 weeks of gestation) (251, 256). These reports indicate that IUGR might be an initial "hit" to the organism, raising susceptibility to CLDs such as BPD.

In conclusion, similar to perinatal obesity and GDM, IUGR leads to acute as well as long-term functional and structural changes in the lung. A distinction must be made between an intrauterine and a postnatal phase in the process of perinatal programming caused by IUGR. While the intrauterine phase is characterized by nutritional deprivation, the postnatal phase is usually characterized by a catch-up growth. With regard to the pathomechanisms, metabolic signaling pathways, inflammation, and nutrient-sensing processes play an essential role, ultimately controlling alveolar and vascular formation and lung growth. However, the different phases of injury in IUGR also provide windows of opportunity for preventive strategies, therapeutic interventions and reprogramming in the future (**Figure 2**).

THE MICROBIOME AS A LINK BETWEEN NUTRITION AND LUNG HEALTH: OPPORTUNITY FOR INTERVENTION

As stated before, obesity represents a state of *low-grade chronic systemic inflammation*, as illustrated by the increased amount of circulating inflammatory cells (83, 84) as well as elevated expression levels of inflammatory factors (85–88). External influences on the lung health such as airway pollution and cigarette smoking have been extensively studied in the last decade. Recently however, another field of interest has gained momentum: the gut-lung microbiome. This represents an extremely important link between nutrition, chronic inflammation and pulmonary health. In the following, we will detail the role of the microbiome in the early origins of CLDs.

The infant's microbiome is predominantly established during and shortly after birth, where it is exposed to the maternal and environmental microbiome (257). The introduction of solid foods into the children's diet is the next essential step in the microbiome development. Western diet (rich in meat and fat) has been linked to decreased bacterial gut richness, whereas a diet-based on fruits and vegetables is associated with increased bacterial richness (258, 259). The human microbiome is closely related to the nutritional status and chronic inflammatory processes of the individual (260, 261). Studies have shown that it is possible to predict if an individual is lean or obese based on a classification of the gut microbiome with an accuracy of over 90% (262). In humans for example, the abundance of bacteria of the taxa *Christensenella* is negatively correlated with BMI; in contrast, in *in vivo* experiments feeding mice *Christensenella* bacteria induces weight loss (263). Another human study revealed that the gut microbiome can influence leptin concentrations, indicating that the microbiome might regulate appetite (264). Interestingly, it has been shown that the same dietary ingredients have different effects on the blood glucose levels in humans, which is thought to be mediated by the microbiome as well (265). In addition, new studies have shown that the fecal transplantation of lean to obese patients improves insulin sensitivity (266).

The microbiome alters the immune system and future immune response. For example, it has been shown that the yeast *Candida Albicans* in particular has a prominent effect on the TNF-α response of the host; and the palmitoleic acid metabolism of bacteria has been associated with lower systemic responses (267). An overall decrease of bacterial richness is linked to a variety of diseases including obesity, coronary vascular disease, metabolic syndrome insulin resistance, dyslipidemia, and inflammatory disorders (268, 269). When the development of the infants' microbiome is perturbed by the use of antibiotics it can lead to the development of obesity or asthma in later life (270). These examples highlight the mutual relationship between the immune system and the microbiome, creating a finely tuned balance (271). As a result, an imbalance between both creates a lifelong signature of the infants' microbiome (272).

The gut microbiome has been extensively studied, but the lung microbiome has only recently gained interest with the

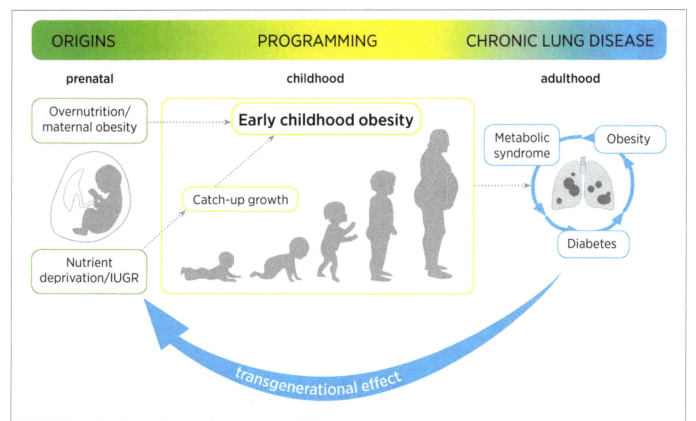

FIGURE 2 | Maternal obesity as well as intrauterine growth restriction (IUGR) increase the risk of (catch-up growth mediated) early childhood obesity. Maternal and early childhood obesity are associated with long-term adverse metabolic effects, including type 2 diabetes mellitus and metabolic syndrome. These pathological metabolic processes are not only intimately linked to an increased risk for pulmonary diseases, but can cause a transgenerational effect from mother to child, to second-generation offspring.

first reports of altered microbiome in asthma (273). The lung microbiome has a strong influence on the susceptibility to a wide array of chronic lung diseases, including COPD, asthma, Idiopathic Pulmonary Fibrosis (IPF) as well as altering the prognosis of cystic fibrosis (CF) (274). In healthy individuals, the lung microbiome is well-regulated by the environment (high clearance, low immigration and low nutrient availability). However, processes that favor alterations of the microbiome and inflammation include the increased production of mucus, creating a moist and warm bacterial niche, increased vascular permeability which increases the nutrient availability and selective growth promotion as well as selective clearance due to the altered immune response to airway colonization (275, 276). These factors promote the bacterial colonization of the airways as well as the selective overgrowth of certain well-adapted species, thereby creating a shift of the microbiome from healthy to diseased and inducing the "dysbiosis-inflammation cycle" as introduced by Dickson et al. (275–278). Thus, a perpetual cycle of microbial changes, possibly due to initial nutritional changes before and early after birth, along with inflammation has a significant impact on the development and prognosis of CLDs.

To date, the gut-lung axis remains elusive, especially with regard to clinical interventions. Nonetheless, several initial successes have been reported in the recent years. For example, stimulation of the gut microbiome with a high-fiber diet in COPD patients has been shown to increase the production of anti-inflammatory short chain fatty acids (SCFAs). These anti-inflammatory factors might reduce chronic inflammation of the lungs, prevent or decrease lung remodeling and therefore improve the lung health of COPD patients (279). Meanwhile, the Canadian Healthy Infant Longitudinal Development (CHILD) Study revealed that bacterial genera *Lachnospira*, *Veillonella*, *Faecalibacterium*, and *Rothia* are significantly reduced in infants at risk for asthma. Inoculation with these four bacteria reduced airway inflammation in a mouse model, possibly lowering the risk for asthma (280). These studies highlight the promising benefits of dietary changes or adjustment of the gut microbiome for the improvement of lung health.

The virome, including the genes of pathogenic viruses, resident viruses and bacteriophages, is of interest for CLDs as well (281, 282). Viral infection is the predominant reason for acute respiratory infections and the exacerbation of CLDs such as asthma, COPD and CF (283, 284). Next generation

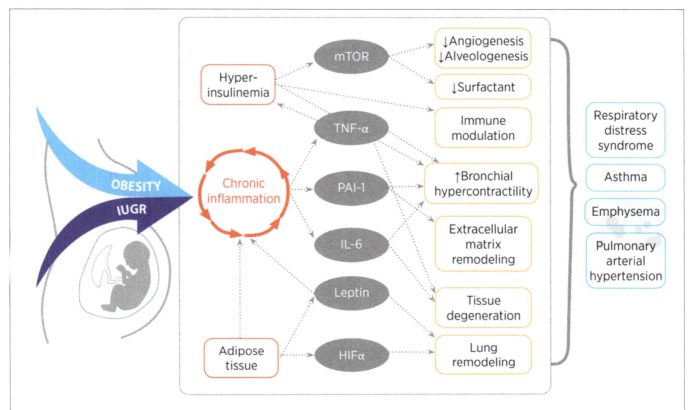

FIGURE 3 | Overview of the converging inflammatory signaling and nutrient sensing pathways of obesity and intrauterine growth restriction (IUGR). Obesity or IUGR lead to chronic inflammation and hyperinsulinemia, which induces mTOR, TNF-α, PAI-1, IL-6, Leptin, and HIF-α signaling. In the lung, these signaling molecules cause for example tissue remodeling, reduce alveolarization and induce smooth muscle cell hyperreactivity. These features are characteristics for a higher susceptibility to develop a chronic lung disease in later life. [mTOR (mechanistic target of rapamycin), TNF-α (tumor necrosis factor alpha), PAI-1 (plasminogen activator inhibitor-1), IL-6 (interleukin-6), HIF-α (hypoxia inducible hypoxia-inducible factor alpha)].

sequencing has made it possible to assess the viral DNA or RNA load in respiratory samples (285, 286). Obesity influences the virome of the host; it has been reported that increased viral RNA abundance is closely correlated to an increase of fat mass and hyperglycemia in mice (287). In line with this finding, obese patients show a higher susceptibility to dengue fever (288). Moreover, the adenovirus Ad-36 interferes with adipocyte differentiation, leptin production and glucose metabolism (289). Special interest is drawn to the fact that viral presence in the gut influences the host's immune response (290) by interfering with the host's microbiome and immune-modulatory actions (e.g., through the TNF-α pathway) (267, 291). This crosstalk between the bacterial microbiome and virome and their immune-modulating properties have also been reported in the lung (277, 292).

In conclusion, nutritional changes can directly and indirectly influence the intestinal and pulmonary microbiome (including the virome), modulating the immune response and increasing inflammation, and ultimately the risk of severe CLD. Targeting the microbiome might offer new preventive and therapeutic avenues for CLDs early in life.

SYSTEMIC CONSEQUENCES OF FETAL PROGRAMMING

Maternal obesity, maternal malnutrition or fetal nutrient deficiency through placental insufficiency naturally not only affect the lung, but all other organs as well. The organ-specific susceptibility to metabolic influences varies, and the "window of exposure" plays a crucial role. In other words, the timeframe during which organ development and/or -function is especially vulnerable differs from organ to organ. While a lot of research has been performed with traditional technologies, the ever-growing possibilities of bioinformatics will improve the longitudinal integration of transcriptomic, proteomic and lipidomic data with clinical parameters. These analyses will help to increase the understanding of the complex interaction of internal and external variables during development, resulting in a healthy individual or one with programmed disease. While the strength of animal models lies in the possibility to elucidate molecular mechanisms, it will be a challenge for clinicians to identify individuals at risk. Harmonization and standardization of cohorts like in the LifeCycle-Project (293) improves the epidemiological basis to translate hypotheses on the early origins of disease from animal models in to the human context and to confirm their clinical

TABLE 1 | Overview of the signaling molecules and pathways involved in the perinatal nutritional and metabolic origins of chronic lung diseases.

Disease	Regulator	Obesity	IUGR	Effector	Outcome and reference	
Pulmonary arterial hypertension (PAH)	HIF-α ↓	✓		Endothelin-1 ↑	Vascular remodeling (65, 66)	
	IL-6 ↑	✓	✓	Stat3 ↑ FoxO1 ↓	SMC proliferation (92, 93, 178)	
	PPARγ ↓	✓			Reduced SMC proliferation (130, 131)	Protective
	mTOR ↓		✓	VEGF ↓ BMP ↓	Reduced angiogenesis Altered ECM disposition (157, 218)	
COPD and emphysema	IL-6 ↑	✓	✓		ATII apoptosis (91, 232)	
	Leptin			Sftpa ↑	ATII maturation (104, 105)	Protective
	↑	✓	✓	Col1a1, Col3a1, Col6a3, Mmp2, Tieg1, Stat1 ↑	Enlarged alveoli (106, 157)	
Respiratory distress syndrome (RDS)	Insulin ↑	✓	✓	VEGF ↓ HIF-2 ↓ mTOR ↑	Reduced angiogenesis (141)	
		✓	✓	PI3K ↑ Sftpa ↓	Increased alveolar surface tension (139)	
			✓	GH/IGF-1 ↓ ↑	Reduced alveologenesis Lung- and bodygrowth (174, 204)	Protective
	PPARγ				Promotes Lung maturation (128, 129)	Protective
	Leptin ↓	✓	✓	Leptin resistance ↑ mTOR ↓	Reduced alveolar surface (173, 210, 213, 214)	
Asthma	TNF-α ↑	✓	✓	G-proteins ↑	Hyperreactivity in SMC (96, 232)	
	Adiponectin ↓	✓		NF-κB ↑	Enhanced TNF-α activity (97)	
	PAI-1 ↑	✓			Collagen, fibrin deposition (89)	
	Insulin ↑	✓	✓	Th2 shift	Enhanced immune response (145)	
		✓	✓	PI3K-signaling ↑	Contractile SMC phenotype (143)	
	Leptin ↑	✓	✓	mTOR ↑ MAPK ↑	Hyperreactivity (114)	

relevance. In this context, research on biomarkers is of high relevance to improve the diagnostic options in early detection of aberrant organ development. Candidates have been studied in clinical situations of known organ damage, e.g., BDP (294, 295) and neonatal kidney injury (296–298) and will have to be tested in the context of metabolic programming. Importantly, the goal is not to label an individual organ function as pathological beyond classical criteria but to identify individuals who are at risk to develop disease later in life in order to provide targeted prevention strategies.

Looking at molecular mechanisms, it is important to note that early metabolic origins of disease are based on a complex encounter of small-scale dysregulations rather than one single dysregulated pathway. Interestingly, apparently distinct causes of nutritional programming can cause similar molecular alterations. As discussed in detail for the lung, both IUGR (299) and maternal obesity-associated (300) models seem to induce inflammation in other organs as well. Briefly summarized, it is demonstrated that neuroinflammation is an important mechanism contributing to neurocognitive impairment after IUGR and maternal obesity (301, 302) and the window of vulnerability extends well-beyond

birth (303, 304). Circulating inflammatory proteins were even tested as biomarkers for later cognitive impairment in preterm infants (305). Experimental studies have also linked perinatal inflammation to adverse kidney development (306, 307) and cardiac dysfunction (308). Taken together, these studies highlight the need to consider inter-organ communication as an important contributor to health and disease.

CONCLUSION

The mission of this article was to provide a comprehensive review of the impact of perinatal nutrition and metabolism on lung development and early origins of CLD. The current literature provides compelling evidence that maternal obesity, early childhood obesity and IUGR are intimately linked to increased risk for lung disease. These perinatal nutritional alterations of the fetus and infant converge in similar metabolic, endocrine, nutrient sensing and inflammatory signaling pathways. Key regulators are insulin and leptin, and their respective downstream signaling cascades. Both hormones are essential for physiological growth and development during pregnancy; in contrast, interruption of the concerted interaction and balance of hormones, cytokines and growth factors during a critical window of development can disrupt developmental processes and adversely affect child (lung) health throughout life. For example, maternal obesity and early childhood obesity cause hyperinsulinemia and hyperleptinemia combined with insulin- and leptin-insensitivity. On the other hand, IUGR is characterized by a transient prenatal downregulation of insulin- and leptin signaling, followed by a postnatal upregulation during catch-up growth resulting in the same pathology as obesity. These two endocrine factors subsequently cause a cascade of pro-inflammatory programing with the release of (adipo-) cytokines and can contribute to metabolic and pulmonary disease (**Figure 3**, **Table 1**). These pulmonary sequelae span from aberrant alveolarization and angiogenesis to remodeling of the extracellular matrix and ultimately reducing lung function. While the present review primarily focused on the lung, other organs are affected as well, highlighting the importance of inter-organ communication. Beyond the metabolo-inflammatory stress response after perinatal nutritional alterations, smoking, air pollution as well as a consecutive dysbiosis of the intestinal and pulmonary microbiome contribute to the susceptibility and early origins of CLDs such as COPD, PAH and Asthma.

Both obesity-related comorbidities and CLDs are a relevant socioeconomic and individual burden. The alarmingly increasing rates of overweight and obese adults, pregnant women, and children emphasize the need to investigate and decipher the crosstalk between nutrition metabolism and the early origins of CLDs. Elucidation of the metabolo-pulmonary axis with subsequent identification of novel targets will provide new avenues to prevent metabolic programming and the early origins of CLDs.

AUTHOR CONTRIBUTIONS

CK-M, JS, EN, and MA conceived, designed, and drafted the manuscript. CK-M, JS, EN, JD, and MA edited and revised the manuscript and approved the final version of the manuscript. All authors contributed to the article and approved the submitted version.

ACKNOWLEDGMENTS

We greatly thank Mrs. Petra Kleinwächter (MedizinFoto Köln, University Hospital Cologne, University of Cologne) for her extraordinary support in graphical design and preparing the illustrations.

REFERENCES

1. May SM, Li JT. Burden of chronic obstructive pulmonary disease: healthcare costs and beyond. *Allergy Asthma Proc.* (2015) 36:4–10. doi: 10.2500/aap.2015.36.3812
2. Maleki-Yazdi MR, Kelly SM, Lam SY, Marin M, Barbeau M, Walker V. The burden of illness in patients with moderate to severe chronic obstructive pulmonary disease in Canada. *Can Respir J.* (2012) 19:319–24. doi: 10.1155/2012/328460
3. Poston L, Caleyachetty R, Cnattingius S, Corvalan C, Uauy R, Herring S, et al. Preconceptional and maternal obesity: epidemiology and health consequences. *Lancet Diabetes Endocrinol.* (2016) 4:1025–36. doi: 10.1016/S2213-8587(16)30217-0
4. Longo S, Bollani L, Decembrino L, Di Comite A, Angelini M, Stronati M. Short-term and long-term sequelae in intrauterine growth retardation (IUGR). *J Matern Fetal Neonatal Med.* (2013) 26:222–5. doi: 10.3109/14767058.2012.715006
5. Nardozza LM, Caetano AC, Zamarian AC, Mazzola JB, Silva CP, Marcal VM, et al. Fetal growth restriction: current knowledge. *Arch Gynecol Obstet.* (2017) 295:1061–77. doi: 10.1007/s00404-017-4341-9
6. Lucas A. Programming by early nutrition in man. *Ciba Found Symp.* (1991) 156:38–50.
7. Plagemann A. Perinatal programming and functional teratogenesis: impact on body weight regulation and obesity. *Physiol Behav.* (2005) 86:661–8. doi: 10.1016/j.physbeh.2005.08.065
8. Barker DJ. Intrauterine programming of adult disease. *Mol Med Today.* (1995) 1:418–23. doi: 10.1016/S1357-4310(95)90793-9
9. Edwards CA, Osman LM, Godden DJ, Campbell DM, Douglas JG. Relationship between birth weight and adult lung function: controlling for maternal factors. *Thorax.* (2003) 58:1061–5. doi: 10.1136/thorax.58.12.1061
10. Harpsoe MC, Basit S, Bager P, Wohlfahrt J, Benn CS, Nohr EA, et al. Maternal obesity, gestational weight gain, and risk of asthma and atopic disease in offspring: a study within the Danish national birth cohort. *J Allergy Clin Immunol.* (2013) 131:1033–40. doi: 10.1016/j.jaci.2012.09.008
11. Haataja P, Korhonen P, Ojala R, Hirvonen M, Paassilta M, Gissler M, et al. Asthma and atopic dermatitis in children born moderately and late preterm. *Eur J Pediatr.* (2016) 175:799–808. doi: 10.1007/s00431-016-2708-8
12. Aspberg S, Dahlquist G, Kahan T, Kallen B. Confirmed association between neonatal phototherapy or neonatal icterus and risk of childhood asthma. *Pediatr Allergy Immunol.* (2010) 21:e733–9. doi: 10.1111/j.1399-3038.2010.01038.x
13. Dyer JS, Rosenfeld CR. Metabolic imprinting by prenatal, perinatal, and postnatal overnutrition: a review. *Semin Reprod Med.* (2011) 29:266–76. doi: 10.1055/s-0031-1275521
14. Schittny JC. Development of the lung. *Cell Tissue Res.* (2017) 367:427–44. doi: 10.1007/s00441-016-2545-0
15. Burri PH. Structural aspects of postnatal lung development - alveolar formation and growth. *Biol Neonate.* (2006) 89:313–22. doi: 10.1159/000092868
16. Chooi YC, Ding C, Magkos F. The epidemiology of obesity. *Metabolism.* (2019) 92:6–10. doi: 10.1016/j.metabol.2018.09.005
17. Albuquerque D, Stice E, Rodriguez-Lopez R, Manco L, Nobrega C. Current review of genetics of human obesity: from molecular mechanisms to an evolutionary perspective. *Mol Genet Genomics.* (2015) 290:1191–221. doi: 10.1007/s00438-015-1015-9
18. Hopkins M, Blundell JE. Energy balance, body composition, sedentariness and appetite regulation: pathways to obesity. *Clin Sci.* (2016) 130:1615–28. doi: 10.1042/CS20160006
19. Kahn BB, Flier JS. Obesity and insulin resistance. *J Clin Invest.* (2000) 106:473–81. doi: 10.1172/JCI10842

20. Reaven GM. Pathophysiology of insulin resistance in human disease. *Physiol Rev.* (1995) 75:473–86. doi: 10.1152/physrev.1995.75.3.473

21. Schwartz MW, Woods SC, Porte D Jr, Seeley RJ, Baskin DG. Central nervous system control of food intake. *Nature.* (2000) 404:661–71. doi: 10.1038/35007534

22. El-Haschimi K, Pierroz DD, Hileman SM, Bjorbaek C, Flier JS. Two defects contribute to hypothalamic leptin resistance in mice with diet-induced obesity. *J Clin Invest.* (2000) 105:1827–32. doi: 10.1172/JCI9842

23. Kamohara S, Burcelin R, Halaas JL, Friedman JM, Charron MJ. Acute stimulation of glucose metabolism in mice by leptin treatment. *Nature.* (1997) 389:374–7. doi: 10.1038/38717

24. King NA, Caudwell P, Hopkins M, Byrne NM, Colley R, Hills AP, et al. Metabolic and behavioral compensatory responses to exercise interventions: barriers to weight loss. *Obesity.* (2007) 15:1373–83. doi: 10.1038/oby.2007.164

25. Ng M, Fleming T, Robinson M, Thomson B, Graetz N, Margono C, et al. Global, regional, and national prevalence of overweight and obesity in children and adults during 1980-2013: a systematic analysis for the Global burden of disease study 2013. *Lancet.* (2014) 384:766–81. doi: 10.1016/S0140-6736(14)60460-8

26. Ogden CL, Carroll MD, Fryar CD, Flegal KM. Prevalence of obesity among adults and youth: United States, 2011-2014. *NCHS Data Brief.* (2015) 219:1–8.

27. Venn AJ, Thomson RJ, Schmidt MD, Cleland VJ, Curry BA, Gennat HC, et al. Overweight and obesity from childhood to adulthood: a follow-up of participants in the 1985 Australian schools health and fitness survey. *Med J Aust.* (2007) 186:458–60. doi: 10.5694/j.1326-5377.2007.tb01436.x

28. Santangeli L, Sattar N, Huda SS. Impact of maternal obesity on perinatal and childhood outcomes. *Best Pract Res Clin Obstet Gynaecol.* (2015) 29:438–48. doi: 10.1016/j.bpobgyn.2014.10.009

29. Flegal KM, Carroll MD, Kit BK, Ogden CL. Prevalence of obesity and trends in the distribution of body mass index among US adults, 1999-2010. *JAMA.* (2012) 307:491–7. doi: 10.1001/jama.2012.39

30. Knight B, Shields BM, Hill A, Powell RJ, Wright D, Hattersley AT. The impact of maternal glycemia and obesity on early postnatal growth in a nondiabetic Caucasian population. *Diabetes Care.* (2007) 30:777–83. doi: 10.2337/dc06-1849

31. Cheng CW, Rifai A, Ka SM, Shui HA, Lin YF, Lee WH, et al. Calcium-binding proteins annexin A2 and S100A6 are sensors of tubular injury and recovery in acute renal failure. *Kidney Int.* (2005) 68:2694–703. doi: 10.1111/j.1523-1755.2005.00740.x

32. Parsons TJ, Power C, Manor O. Fetal and early life growth and body mass index from birth to early adulthood in 1958 British cohort: longitudinal study. *BMJ.* (2001) 323:1331–5. doi: 10.1136/bmj.323.7325.1331

33. Reilly MP, Rader DJ. The metabolic syndrome: more than the sum of its parts? *Circulation.* (2003) 108:1546–51. doi: 10.1161/01.CIR.0000088846.10655.E0

34. Han JC, Lawlor DA, Kimm SY. Childhood obesity. *Lancet.* (2010) 375:1737–48. doi: 10.1016/S0140-6736(10)60171-7

35. Godfrey KM, Reynolds RM, Prescott SL, Nyirenda M, Jaddoe VW, Eriksson JG, et al. Influence of maternal obesity on the long-term health of offspring. *Lancet Diabetes Endocrinol.* (2017) 5:53–64. doi: 10.1016/S2213-8587(16)30107-3

36. Ehrenberg HM, Mercer BM, Catalano PM. The influence of obesity and diabetes on the prevalence of macrosomia. *Am J Obstet Gynecol.* (2004) 191:964–8. doi: 10.1016/j.ajog.2004.05.052

37. Patel MS, Srinivasan M, Laychock SG. Metabolic programming: role of nutrition in the immediate postnatal life. *J Inherit Metab Dis.* (2009) 32:218–28. doi: 10.1007/s10545-008-1033-4

38. Eising JB, Uiterwaal CS, van der Ent CK. Maternal body mass index, neonatal lung function and respiratory symptoms in childhood. *Eur Respir J.* (2015) 46:1342–9. doi: 10.1183/13993003.00784-2014

39. Aalinkeel R, Srinivasan M, Song F, Patel MS. Programming into adulthood of islet adaptations induced by early nutritional intervention in the rat. *Am J Physiol Endocrinol Metab.* (2001) 281:E640–8. doi: 10.1152/ajpendo.2001.281.3.E640

40. Vadlamudi S, Hiremagalur BK, Tao L, Kalhan SC, Kalaria RN, Kaung HL, et al. Long-term effects on pancreatic function of feeding a HC formula to rats during the preweaning period. *Am J Physiol.* (1993) 265:E565–71. doi: 10.1152/ajpendo.1993.265.4.E565

41. Srinivasan M, Dodds C, Ghanim H, Gao T, Ross PJ, Browne RW, et al. Maternal obesity and fetal programming: effects of a high-carbohydrate nutritional modification in the immediate postnatal life of female rats. *Am J Physiol Endocrinol Metab.* (2008) 295:E895–903. doi: 10.1152/ajpendo.90460.2008

42. Bird A. DNA methylation patterns and epigenetic memory. *Genes Dev.* (2002) 16:6–21. doi: 10.1101/gad.947102

43. Zhang J, Zhang F, Didelot X, Bruce KD, Cagampang FR, Vatish M, et al. Maternal high fat diet during pregnancy and lactation alters hepatic expression of insulin like growth factor-2 and key microRNAs in the adult offspring. *BMC Genomics.* (2009) 10:478. doi: 10.1186/1471-2164-10-478

44. Jing J, Wang Y, Quan Y, Wang Z, Liu Y, Ding Z. Maternal obesity alters C19MC microRNAs expression profile in fetal umbilical cord blood. *Nutr Metab.* (2020) 17:52. doi: 10.1186/s12986-020-00475-7

45. Antoun E, Kitaba NT, Titcombe P, Dalrymple KV, Garratt ES, Barton SJ, et al. Maternal dysglycaemia, changes in the infant's epigenome modified with a diet and physical activity intervention in pregnancy: Secondary analysis of a randomised control trial. *PLoS Med.* (2020) 17:e1003229. doi: 10.1371/journal.pmed.1003229

46. Finer S, Mathews C, Lowe R, Smart M, Hillman S, Foo L, et al. Maternal gestational diabetes is associated with genome-wide DNA methylation variation in placenta and cord blood of exposed offspring. *Hum Mol Genet.* (2015) 24:3021–9. doi: 10.1093/hmg/ddv013

47. Moody L, Wang H, Jung PM, Chen H, Pan YX. Maternal and post-weaning high-fat diets produce distinct DNA methylation patterns in hepatic metabolic pathways within specific genomic contexts. *Int J Mol Sci.* (2019) 20:3229. doi: 10.3390/ijms20133229

48. Martinez FD, Wright AL, Taussig LM, Holberg CJ, Halonen M, Morgan WJ. Asthma and wheezing in the first six years of life. The group health medical associates. *N Engl J Med.* (1995) 332:133–8. doi: 10.1056/NEJM199501193320301

49. Zugna D, Galassi C, Annesi-Maesano I, Baiz N, Barros H, Basterrechea M, et al. Maternal complications in pregnancy and wheezing in early childhood: a pooled analysis of 14 birth cohorts. *Int J Epidemiol.* (2015) 44:199–208. doi: 10.1093/ije/dyu260

50. Kumar R, Story RE, Pongracic JA, Hong X, Arguelles L, Wang G, et al. Maternal pre-pregnancy obesity and recurrent wheezing in early childhood. *Pediatr Allergy Immunol Pulmonol.* (2010) 23:183–90. doi: 10.1089/ped.2010.0032

51. Arens R, Muzumdar H. Childhood obesity and obstructive sleep apnea syndrome. *J Appl Physiol.* (2010) 108:436–44. doi: 10.1152/japplphysiol.00689.2009

52. Rosen CL. Clinical features of obstructive sleep apnea hypoventilation syndrome in otherwise healthy children. *Pediatr Pulmonol.* (1999) 27:403–9. doi: 10.1002/(SICI)1099-0496(199906)27:6<403::AID-PPUL7>3.0.CO;2-811

53. Adams JP, Murphy PG. Obesity in anaesthesia and intensive care. *Br J Anaesth.* (2000) 85:91–108. doi: 10.1093/bja/85.1.91

54. Ekstrom S, Magnusson J, Kull I, Andersson N, Bottai M, Besharat Pour M, et al. Body mass index development and asthma throughout childhood. *Am J Epidemiol.* (2017) 186:255–63. doi: 10.1093/aje/kwx081

55. Black MH, Smith N, Porter AH, Jacobsen SJ, Koebnick C. Higher prevalence of obesity among children with asthma. *Obesity.* (2012) 20:1041–7. doi: 10.1038/oby.2012.5

56. Porter M, Wegienka G, Havstad S, Nageotte CG, Johnson CC, Ownby DR, et al. Relationship between childhood body mass index and young adult asthma. *Ann Allergy Asthma Immunol.* (2012) 109:408–11. e401. doi: 10.1016/j.anai.2012.09.009

57. Beuther DA, Sutherland ER. Overweight, obesity, and incident asthma: a meta-analysis of prospective epidemiologic studies. *Am J Respir Crit Care Med.* (2007) 175:661–6. doi: 10.1164/rccm.200611-1717OC

58. Koenig SM. Pulmonary complications of obesity. *Am J Med Sci.* (2001) 321:249–79. doi: 10.1097/00000441-200104000-00006

59. Lazarus R, Colditz G, Berkey CS, Speizer FE. Effects of body fat on ventilatory function in children and adolescents: cross-sectional findings from a random

population sample of school children. *Pediatr Pulmonol.* (1997) 24:187–94. doi: 10.1002/(SICI)1099-0496(199709)24:3<187::AID-PPUL4>3.0.CO;2-K

60. Li AM, Chan D, Wong E, Yin J, Nelson EA, Fok TF. The effects of obesity on pulmonary function. *Arch Dis Child.* (2003) 88:361–3. doi: 10.1136/adc.88.4.361

61. Watson RA, Pride NB, Thomas EL, Fitzpatrick J, Durighel G, McCarthy J, et al. Reduction of total lung capacity in obese men: comparison of total intrathoracic and gas volumes. *J Appl Physiol.* (2010) 108:1605–12. doi: 10.1152/japplphysiol.01267.2009

62. Gislason T, Benediktsdottir B. Snoring, apneic episodes, and nocturnal hypoxemia among children 6 months to 6 years old. An epidemiologic study of lower limit of prevalence. *Chest.* (1995) 107:963–6. doi: 10.1378/chest.107.4.963

63. Semenza GL, Wang GL. A nuclear factor induced by hypoxia via de novo protein synthesis binds to the human erythropoietin gene enhancer at a site required for transcriptional activation. *Mol Cell Biol.* (1992) 12:5447–54. doi: 10.1128/MCB.12.12.5447

64. Ivan M, Kondo K, Yang H, Kim W, Valiando J, Ohh M, et al. HIFalpha targeted for VHL-mediated destruction by proline hydroxylation: implications for O2 sensing. *Science.* (2001) 292:464–8. doi: 10.1126/science.1059817

65. Brusselmans K, Compernolle V, Tjwa M, Wiesener MS, Maxwell PH, Collen D, et al. Heterozygous deficiency of hypoxia-inducible factor-2alpha protects mice against pulmonary hypertension and right ventricular dysfunction during prolonged hypoxia. *J Clin Invest.* (2003) 111:1519–27. doi: 10.1172/JCI15496

66. Yu AY, Shimoda LA, Iyer NV, Huso DL, Sun X, McWilliams R, et al. Impaired physiological responses to chronic hypoxia in mice partially deficient for hypoxia-inducible factor 1alpha. *J Clin Invest.* (1999) 103:691–6. doi: 10.1172/JCI5912

67. Krick S, Eul BG, Hanze J, Savai R, Grimminger F, Seeger W, et al. Role of hypoxia-inducible factor-1alpha in hypoxia-induced apoptosis of primary alveolar epithelial type II cells. *Am J Respir Cell Mol Biol.* (2005) 32:395–403. doi: 10.1165/rcmb.2004-0314OC

68. Asikainen TM, Waleh NS, Schneider BK, Clyman RI, White CW. Enhancement of angiogenic effectors through hypoxia-inducible factor in preterm primate lung in vivo. *Am J Physiol Lung Cell Mol Physiol.* (2006) 291:L588–95. doi: 10.1152/ajplung.00098.2006

69. Asikainen TM, Chang LY, Coalson JJ, Schneider BK, Waleh NS, Ikegami M, et al. Improved lung growth and function through hypoxia-inducible factor in primate chronic lung disease of prematurity. *FASEB J.* (2006) 20:1698–700. doi: 10.1096/fj.06-5887fje

70. Levine AJ, Puzio-Kuter AM. The control of the metabolic switch in cancers by oncogenes and tumor suppressor genes. *Science.* (2010) 330:1340–4. doi: 10.1126/science.1193494

71. Burns JS, Manda G. Metabolic pathways of the warburg effect in health and disease: perspectives of choice, chain or chance. *Int J Mol Sci.* (2017) 18:2755. doi: 10.3390/ijms18122755

72. Luis C, Duarte F, Faria I, Jarak I, Oliveira PF, Alves MG, et al. Warburg effect inversion: adiposity shifts central primary metabolism in MCF-7 breast cancer cells. *Life Sci.* (2019) 223:38–46. doi: 10.1016/j.lfs.2019.03.016

73. Chandel NS, McClintock DS, Feliciano CE, Wood TM, Melendez JA, Rodriguez AM, et al. Reactive oxygen species generated at mitochondrial complex III stabilize hypoxia-inducible factor-1alpha during hypoxia: a mechanism of O2 sensing. *J Biol Chem.* (2000) 275:25130–8. doi: 10.1074/jbc.M001914200

74. Semenza GL. Targeting HIF-1 for cancer therapy. *Nat Rev Cancer.* (2003) 3:721–32. doi: 10.1038/nrc1187

75. Ivan M, Haberberger T, Gervasi DC, Michelson KS, Gunzler V, Kondo K, et al. Biochemical purification and pharmacological inhibition of a mammalian prolyl hydroxylase acting on hypoxia-inducible factor. *Proc Natl Acad Sci USA.* (2002) 99:13459–64. doi: 10.1073/pnas.192342099

76. Prakash YS, Pabelick CM, Sieck GC. Mitochondrial dysfunction in airway disease. *Chest.* (2017) 152:618–26. doi: 10.1016/j.chest.2017.03.020

77. Rowlands DJ. Mitochondria dysfunction: A novel therapeutic target in pathological lung remodeling or bystander? *Pharmacol Ther.* (2016) 166:96–105. doi: 10.1016/j.pharmthera.2016.06.019

78. Kim KK, Kugler MC, Wolters PJ, Robillard L, Galvez MG, Brumwell AN, et al. Alveolar epithelial cell mesenchymal transition develops in vivo during pulmonary fibrosis and is regulated by the extracellular matrix. *Proc Natl Acad Sci USA.* (2006) 103:13180–5. doi: 10.1073/pnas.0605669103

79. Zhou G, Dada LA, Wu M, Kelly A, Trejo H, Zhou Q, et al. Hypoxia-induced alveolar epithelial-mesenchymal transition requires mitochondrial ROS and hypoxia-inducible factor 1. *Am J Physiol Lung Cell Mol Physiol.* (2009) 297:L1120–30. doi: 10.1152/ajplung.00007.2009

80. Schroedl C, McClintock DS, Budinger GR, Chandel NS. Hypoxic but not anoxic stabilization of HIF-1alpha requires mitochondrial reactive oxygen species. *Am J Physiol Lung Cell Mol Physiol.* (2002) 283:L922–31. doi: 10.1152/ajplung.00014.2002

81. Zhang H, Qian DZ, Tan YS, Lee K, Gao P, Ren YR, et al. Digoxin and other cardiac glycosides inhibit HIF-1alpha synthesis and block tumor growth. *Proc Natl Acad Sci USA.* (2008) 105:19579–86. doi: 10.1073/pnas.0809763105

82. Abud EM, Maylor J, Undem C, Punjabi A, Zaiman AL, Myers AC, et al. Digoxin inhibits development of hypoxic pulmonary hypertension in mice. *Proc Natl Acad Sci USA.* (2012) 109:1239–44. doi: 10.1073/pnas.1120385109

83. Weisberg SP, McCann D, Desai M, Rosenbaum M, Leibel RL, Ferrante AW. Obesity is associated with macrophage accumulation in adipose tissue. *J Clin Invest.* (2003) 112:1796–808. doi: 10.1172/JCI200319246

84. Travers RL, Motta AC, Betts JA, Bouloumie A, Thompson D. The impact of adiposity on adipose tissue-resident lymphocyte activation in humans. *Int J Obes.* (2015) 39:762–9. doi: 10.1038/ijo.2014.195

85. Bullo M, Garcia-Lorda P, Salas-Salvado J. Plasma soluble tumor necrosis factor alpha receptors and leptin levels in normal-weight and obese women: effect of adiposity and diabetes. *Eur J Endocrinol.* (2002) 146:325–31. doi: 10.1530/eje.0.1460325

86. Bastard JP, Jardel C, Bruckert E, Blondy P, Capeau J, Laville M, et al. Elevated levels of interleukin 6 are reduced in serum and subcutaneous adipose tissue of obese women after weight loss. *J Clin Endocrinol Metab.* (2000) 85:3338–42. doi: 10.1210/jcem.85.9.6839

87. Roth CL, Kratz M, Ralston MM, Reinehr T. Changes in adipose-derived inflammatory cytokines and chemokines after successful lifestyle intervention in obese children. *Metabolism.* (2011) 60:445–52. doi: 10.1016/j.metabol.2010.03.023

88. Rajala MW, Scherer PE. Minireview: the adipocyte–at the crossroads of energy homeostasis, inflammation, and atherosclerosis. *Endocrinology.* (2003) 144:3765–73. doi: 10.1210/en.2003-0580

89. Nawrocki AR, Scherer PE. The delicate balance between fat and muscle: adipokines in metabolic disease and musculoskeletal inflammation. *Curr Opin Pharmacol.* (2004) 4:281–9. doi: 10.1016/j.coph.2004.03.003

90. Dinger K, Kasper P, Hucklenbruch-Rother E, Vohlen C, Jobst E, Janoschek R, et al. Early-onset obesity dysregulates pulmonary adipocytokine/insulin signaling and induces asthma-like disease in mice. *Sci Rep.* (2016) 6:24168. doi: 10.1038/srep24168

91. Ruwanpura SM, McLeod L, Dousha LF, Seow HJ, Alhayyani S, Tate MD, et al. Therapeutic targeting of the IL-6 trans-signaling/mechanistic target of rapamycin complex 1 axis in pulmonary emphysema. *Am J Respir Crit Care Med.* (2016) 194:1494–505. doi: 10.1164/rccm.201512-2368OC

92. Jones SA, Scheller J, Rose-John S. Therapeutic strategies for the clinical blockade of IL-6/gp130 signaling. *J Clin Invest.* (2011) 121:3375–83. doi: 10.1172/JCI57158

93. Savai R, Al-Tamari HM, Sedding D, Kojonazarov B, Muecke C, Teske R, et al. Pro-proliferative and inflammatory signaling converge on FoxO1 transcription factor in pulmonary hypertension. *Nat Med.* (2014) 20:1289–300. doi: 10.1038/nm.3695

94. Tamura Y, Phan C, Tu L, Le Hiress M, Thuillet R, Jutant EM, et al. Ectopic upregulation of membrane-bound IL6R drives vascular remodeling in pulmonary arterial hypertension. *J Clin Invest.* (2018) 128:1956–70. doi: 10.1172/JCI96462

95. Hotamisligil GS. Inflammatory pathways and insulin action. *Int J Obes Relat Metab Disord.* (2003) 27(Suppl. 3):S53–5. doi: 10.1038/sj.ijo.0802502

96. Chen H, Tliba O, Van Besien CR, Panettieri RA, Jr Amrani Y. TNF-[alpha] modulates murine tracheal rings responsiveness to G-protein-coupled receptor agonists and KCl. *J Appl Physiol.* (2003) 95:864–72. doi: 10.1152/japplphysiol.00140.2003

97. Ouchi N, Kihara S, Funahashi T, Matsuzawa Y, Walsh K. Obesity, adiponectin and vascular inflammatory disease. *Curr Opin Lipidol.* (2003) 14:561–6. doi: 10.1097/00041433-200312000-00003

98. Kim J, Remick DG. Tumor necrosis factor inhibitors for the treatment of asthma. *Curr Allergy Asthma Rep.* (2007) 7:151–6. doi: 10.1007/s11882-007-0013-3

99. Desai D, Brightling C. TNF-alpha antagonism in severe asthma? *Recent Pat Inflamm Allergy Drug Discov.* (2010) 4:193–200. doi: 10.2174/187221310793564218

100. Antoniu SA, Mihaltan F, Ulmeanu R. Anti-TNF-alpha therapies in chronic obstructive pulmonary diseases. *Expert Opin Investig Drugs.* (2008) 17:1203–11. doi: 10.1517/13543784.17.8.1203

101. Savov JD, Brass DM, Berman KG, McElvania E, Schwartz DA. Fibrinolysis in LPS-induced chronic airway disease. *Am J Physiol Lung Cell Mol Physiol.* (2003) 285:L940–8. doi: 10.1152/ajplung.00102.2003

102. Oh CK, Ariue B, Alban RF, Shaw B, Cho SH. PAI-1 promotes extracellular matrix deposition in the airways of a murine asthma model. *Biochem Biophys Res Commun.* (2002) 294:1155–60. doi: 10.1016/S0006-291X(02)00577-6

103. Litzenburger T, Huber EK, Dinger K, Wilke R, Vohlen C, Selle J, et al. Maternal high-fat diet induces long-term obesity with sex-dependent metabolic programming of adipocyte differentiation, hypertrophy and dysfunction in the offspring. *Clin Sci.* (2020) 134:921–39. doi: 10.1042/CS20191229

104. Chen H, Zhang JP, Huang H, Wang ZH, Cheng R, Cai WB. Leptin promotes fetal lung maturity and upregulates SP-A expression in pulmonary alveoli type-II epithelial cells involving TTF-1 activation. *PLoS ONE.* (2013) 8:e69297. doi: 10.1371/journal.pone.0069297

105. Kirwin SM, Bhandari V, Dimatteo D, Barone C, Johnson L, Paul S, et al. Leptin enhances lung maturity in the fetal rat. *Pediatr Res.* (2006) 60:200–4. doi: 10.1203/01.pdr.0000227478.29271.52

106. Huang K, Rabold R, Abston E, Schofield B, Misra V, Galdzicka E, et al. Effects of leptin deficiency on postnatal lung development in mice. *J Appl Physiol.* (2008) 105:249–59. doi: 10.1152/japplphysiol.00052.2007

107. Lock M, McGillick EV, Orgeig S, McMillen IC, Morrison JL. Regulation of fetal lung development in response to maternal overnutrition. *Clin Exp Pharmacol Physiol.* (2013) 40:803–16. doi: 10.1111/1440-1681.12166

108. Myers MG, Cowley MA, Munzberg H. Mechanisms of leptin action and leptin resistance. *Annu Rev Physiol.* (2008) 70:537–56. doi: 10.1146/annurev.physiol.70.113006.100707

109. Halaas JL, Boozer C, Blair-West J, Fidahusein N, Denton DA, Friedman JM. Physiological response to long-term peripheral and central leptin infusion in lean and obese mice. *Proc Natl Acad Sci USA.* (1997) 94:8878–83. doi: 10.1073/pnas.94.16.8878

110. Zhang L, Yin Y, Zhang H, Zhong W, Zhang J. Association of asthma diagnosis with leptin and adiponectin: a systematic review and meta-analysis. *J Investig Med.* (2017) 65:57–64. doi: 10.1136/jim-2016-000127

111. Guler N, Kirerleri E, Ones U, Tamay Z, Salmayenli N, Darendeliler F. Leptin: does it have any role in childhood asthma? *J Allergy Clin Immunol.* (2004) 114:254–9. doi: 10.1016/j.jaci.2004.03.053

112. Gurkan F, Atamer Y, Ece A, Kocyigit Y, Tuzun H, Mete N. Serum leptin levels in asthmatic children treated with an inhaled corticosteroid. *Ann Allergy Asthma Immunol.* (2004) 93:277–80. doi: 10.1016/S1081-1206(10)61501-3

113. Tanju A, Cekmez F, Aydinoz S, Karademir F, Suleymanoglu S, Gocmen I. Association between clinical severity of childhood asthma and serum leptin levels. *Indian J Pediatr.* (2011) 78:291–5. doi: 10.1007/s12098-010-0281-0

114. Zheng H, Wu D, Wu X, Zhang X, Zhou Q, Luo Y, et al. Leptin promotes allergic airway inflammation through targeting the unfolded protein response pathway. *Sci Rep.* (2018) 8:8905. doi: 10.1038/s41598-018-27278-4

115. Maffei M, Halaas J, Ravussin E, Pratley RE, Lee GH, Zhang Y, et al. Leptin levels in human and rodent: measurement of plasma leptin and ob RNA in obese and weight-reduced subjects. *Nat Med.* (1995) 1:1155–61. doi: 10.1038/nm1195-1155

116. Shore SA, Fredberg JJ. Obesity, smooth muscle, and airway hyperresponsiveness. *J Allergy Clin Immunol.* (2005) 115:925–7. doi: 10.1016/j.jaci.2005.01.064

117. Xu A, Wang H, Hoo RL, Sweeney G, Vanhoutte PM, Wang Y, et al. Selective elevation of adiponectin production by the natural compounds derived from a medicinal herb alleviates insulin resistance and glucose intolerance in obese mice. *Endocrinology.* (2009) 150:625–33. doi: 10.1210/en.2008-0999

118. Combs TP, Pajvani UB, Berg AH, Lin Y, Jelicks LA, Laplante M, et al. A transgenic mouse with a deletion in the collagenous domain of adiponectin displays elevated circulating adiponectin and improved insulin sensitivity. *Endocrinology.* (2004) 145:367–83. doi: 10.1210/en.2003-1068

119. Riera-Guardia N, Rothenbacher D. The effect of thiazolidinediones on adiponectin serum level: a meta-analysis. *Diabetes Obes Metab.* (2008) 10:367–75. doi: 10.1111/j.1463-1326.2007.00755.x

120. Amin RH, Mathews ST, Camp HS, Ding L, Leff T. Selective activation of PPARgamma in skeletal muscle induces endogenous production of adiponectin and protects mice from diet-induced insulin resistance. *Am J Physiol Endocrinol Metab.* (2010) 298:E28–37. doi: 10.1152/ajpendo.00446.2009

121. Yao X, Remaley AT, Levine SJ. New kids on the block: the emerging role of apolipoproteins in the pathogenesis and treatment of asthma. *Chest.* (2011) 140:1048–54. doi: 10.1378/chest.11-0158

122. Gao J, Katagiri H, Ishigaki Y, Yamada T, Ogihara T, Imai J, et al. Involvement of apolipoprotein E in excess fat accumulation and insulin resistance. *Diabetes.* (2007) 56:24–33. doi: 10.2337/db06-0144

123. Yao X, Gordon EM, Figueroa DM, Barochia AV, Levine SJ. Emerging roles of Apolipoprotein E and Apolipoprotein A-I in the pathogenesis and treatment of lung disease. *Am J Respir Cell Mol Biol.* (2016) 55:159–69. doi: 10.1165/rcmb.2016-0060TR

124. Massaro D, Massaro GD. Apoetm1Unc mice have impaired alveologenesis, low lung function, and rapid loss of lung function. *Am J Physiol Lung Cell Mol Physiol.* (2008) 294:L991–7. doi: 10.1152/ajplung.00013.2008

125. Chen H, Jackson S, Doro M, McGowan S. Perinatal expression of genes that may participate in lipid metabolism by lipid-laden lung fibroblasts. *J Lipid Res.* (1998) 39:2483–92. doi: 10.1016/S0022-2275(20)33329-0

126. Tontonoz P, Hu E, Spiegelman BM. Regulation of adipocyte gene expression and differentiation by peroxisome proliferator activated receptor gamma. *Curr Opin Genet Dev.* (1995) 5:571–6. doi: 10.1016/0959-437X(95)80025-5

127. Lazar MA. PPAR gamma, 10 years later. *Biochimie.* (2005) 87:9–13. doi: 10.1016/j.biochi.2004.10.021

128. Simon DM, Arikan MC, Srisuma S, Bhattacharya S, Tsai LW, Ingenito EP, et al. Epithelial cell PPAR[gamma] contributes to normal lung maturation. *FASEB J.* (2006) 20:1507–9. doi: 10.1096/fj.05-5410fje

129. Torday JS, Torres E, Rehan VK. The role of fibroblast transdifferentiation in lung epithelial cell proliferation, differentiation, and repair *in vitro. Pediatr Pathol Mol Med.* (2003) 22:189–207. doi: 10.1080/pdp.22.3.189.207

130. Hansmann G, de Jesus Perez VA, Alastalo TP, Alvira CM, Guignabert C, Bekker JM, et al. An antiproliferative BMP-2/PPARgamma/apoE axis in human and murine SMCs and its role in pulmonary hypertension. *J Clin Invest.* (2008) 118:1846–57. doi: 10.1172/JCI32503

131. Rabinovitch M. PPARgamma and the pathobiology of pulmonary arterial hypertension. *Adv Exp Med Biol.* (2010) 661:447–58. doi: 10.1007/978-1-60761-500-2_29

132. Koutnikova H, Cock TA, Watanabe M, Houten SM, Champy MF, Dierich A, et al. Compensation by the muscle limits the metabolic consequences of lipodystrophy in PPAR gamma hypomorphic mice. *Proc Natl Acad Sci USA.* (2003) 100:14457–62. doi: 10.1073/pnas.2336090100

133. Ailhaud G, Massiera F, Weill P, Legrand P, Alessandri JM, Guesnet P. Temporal changes in dietary fats: role of n-6 polyunsaturated fatty acids in excessive adipose tissue development and relationship to obesity. *Prog Lipid Res.* (2006) 45:203–36. doi: 10.1016/j.plipres.2006.01.003

134. Kanai F, Ito K, Todaka M, Hayashi H, Kamohara S, Ishii K, et al. Insulin-stimulated GLUT4 translocation is relevant to the phosphorylation of IRS-1 and the activity of PI3-kinase. *Biochem Biophys Res Commun.* (1993) 195:762–8. doi: 10.1006/bbrc.1993.2111

135. Czech MP, Corvera S. Signaling mechanisms that regulate glucose transport. *J Biol Chem.* (1999) 274:1865–8. doi: 10.1074/jbc.274.4.1865

136. Courtneidge SA, Heber A. An 81 kd protein complexed with middle T antigen and pp60c-src: a possible phosphatidylinositol kinase. *Cell.* (1987) 50:1031–7. doi: 10.1016/0092-8674(87)90169-3

137. Dibble CC, Manning BD. Signal integration by mTORC1 coordinates nutrient input with biosynthetic output. *Nat Cell Biol.* (2013) 15:555–64. doi: 10.1038/ncb2763

138. Land SC, Scott CL, Walker D. mTOR signalling, embryogenesis and the control of lung development. *Semin Cell Dev Biol.* (2014) 36:68–78. doi: 10.1016/j.semcdb.2014.09.023

139. Miakotina OL, Goss KL, Snyder JM. Insulin utilizes the PI 3-kinase pathway to inhibit SP-A gene expression in lung epithelial cells. *Respir Res.* (2002) 3:27. doi: 10.1186/rr191

140. Maffei A, Lembo G, Carnevale D. PI3Kinases in diabetes mellitus and its related complications. *Int J Mol Sci.* (2018) 19:4098. doi: 10.3390/ijms19124098

141. Ikeda H, Shiojima I, Oka T, Yoshida M, Maemura K, Walsh K, et al. Increased Akt-mTOR signaling in lung epithelium is associated with respiratory distress syndrome in mice. *Mol Cell Biol.* (2011) 31:1054–65. doi: 10.1128/MCB.00732-10

142. Fernandez-Twinn DS, Gascoin G, Musial B, Carr S, Duque-Guimaraes D, Blackmore HL, et al. Exercise rescues obese mothers' insulin sensitivity, placental hypoxia and male offspring insulin sensitivity. *Sci Rep.* (2017) 7:44650. doi: 10.1038/srep44650

143. Schaafsma D, McNeill KD, Stelmack GL, Gosens R, Baarsma HA, Dekkers BG, et al. Insulin increases the expression of contractile phenotypic markers in airway smooth muscle. *Am J Physiol Cell Physiol.* (2007) 293:C429–39. doi: 10.1152/ajpcell.00502.2006

144. Lessmann E, Grochowy G, Weingarten L, Giesemann T, Aktories K, Leitges M, et al. Insulin and insulin-like growth factor-1 promote mast cell survival via activation of the phosphatidylinositol-3-kinase pathway. *Exp Hematol.* (2006) 34:1532–41. doi: 10.1016/j.exphem.2006.05.022

145. Viardot A, Grey ST, Mackay F, Chisholm D. Potential antiinflammatory role of insulin via the preferential polarization of effector T cells toward a T helper 2 phenotype. *Endocrinology.* (2007) 148:346–53. doi: 10.1210/en.2006-0686

146. Shapiro H, Kagan I, Shalita-Chesner M, Singer J, Singer P. Inhaled aerosolized insulin: a "topical" anti-inflammatory treatment for acute lung injury and respiratory distress syndrome? *Inflammation.* (2010) 33:315–9. doi: 10.1007/s10753-010-9187-2

147. Wigglesworth JS. Foetal growth retardation. *Br Med Bull.* (1966) 22:13–5. doi: 10.1093/oxfordjournals.bmb.a070429

148. Kesavan K, Devaskar SU. Intrauterine growth restriction: postnatal monitoring and outcomes. *Pediatr Clin North Am.* (2019) 66:403–23. doi: 10.1016/j.pcl.2018.12.009

149. Gordijn SJ, Beune IM, Ganzevoort W. Building consensus and standards in fetal growth restriction studies. *Best Pract Res Clin Obstet Gynaecol.* (2018) 49:117–26. doi: 10.1016/j.bpobgyn.2018.02.002

150. Beune IM, Bloomfield FH, Ganzevoort W, Embleton ND, Rozance PJ, van Wassenaer-Leemhuis AG, et al. Consensus based definition of growth restriction in the newborn. *J Pediatr.* (2018) 196:71–6. e71. doi: 10.1016/j.jpeds.2017.12.059

151. Ong KK, Ahmed ML, Emmett PM, Preece MA, Dunger DB. Association between postnatal catch-up growth and obesity in childhood: prospective cohort study. *BMJ.* (2000) 320:967–71. doi: 10.1136/bmj.320.7240.967

152. Healy MJ, Lockhart RD, Mackenzie JD, Tanner JM, Whitehouse RH. Aberdeen growth study. I. The prediction of adult body measurements from measurements taken each year from birth to 5 years. *Arch Dis Child.* (1956) 31:372–81. doi: 10.1136/adc.31.159.372

153. Ravelli GP, Stein ZA, Susser MW. Obesity in young men after famine exposure *in utero* and early infancy. *N Engl J Med.* (1976) 295:349–53. doi: 10.1056/NEJM197608122950701

154. Rozance PJ, Seedorf GJ, Brown A, Roe G, O'Meara MC, Gien J, et al. Intrauterine growth restriction decreases pulmonary alveolar and vessel growth and causes pulmonary artery endothelial cell dysfunction in vitro in fetal sheep. *Am J Physiol Lung Cell Mol Physiol.* (2011) 301:L860–71. doi: 10.1152/ajplung.00197.2011

155. Joss-Moore L, Carroll T, Yang Y, Fitzhugh M, Metcalfe D, Oman J, et al. Intrauterine growth restriction transiently delays alveolar formation and disrupts retinoic acid receptor expression in the lung of female rat pups. *Pediatr Res.* (2013) 73:612–20. doi: 10.1038/pr.2013.38

156. Zinkhan EK, Zalla JM, Carpenter JR, Yu B, Yu X, Chan G, et al. Intrauterine growth restriction combined with a maternal high-fat diet increases hepatic cholesterol and low-density lipoprotein receptor activity in rats. *Physiol Rep.* (2016) 4:e12862. doi: 10.14814/phy2.12862

157. Kuiper-Makris C, Zanetti D, Vohlen C, Fahle L, Muller M, Odenthal M, et al. Mendelian randomization and experimental IUGR reveal the adverse effect of low birth weight on lung structure and function. *Sci Rep.* (2020) 10:22395. doi: 10.1038/s41598-020-79245-7

158. Brodsky D, Christou H. Current concepts in intrauterine growth restriction. *J Intensive Care Med.* (2004) 19:307–19. doi: 10.1177/0885066604269663

159. Devaskar SU, Chu A. Intrauterine growth restriction: hungry for an answer. *Physiology.* (2016) 31:131–46. doi: 10.1152/physiol.00033.2015

160. Lumey LH, Stein AD. Offspring birth weights after maternal intrauterine undernutrition: a comparison within sibships. *Am J Epidemiol.* (1997) 146:810–9. doi: 10.1093/oxfordjournals.aje.a009198

161. Lopuhaa CE, Roseboom TJ, Osmond C, Barker DJ, Ravelli AC, Bleker OP, et al. Atopy, lung function, and obstructive airways disease after prenatal exposure to famine. *Thorax.* (2000) 55:555–61. doi: 10.1136/thorax.55.7.555

162. Stein CE, Kumaran K, Fall CH, Shaheen SO, Osmond C, Barker DJ. Relation of fetal growth to adult lung function in south India. *Thorax.* (1997) 52:895–9. doi: 10.1136/thx.52.10.895

163. Lawlor DA, Ebrahim S, Davey Smith G. Association of birth weight with adult lung function: findings from the British Women's Heart and Health Study and a meta-analysis. *Thorax.* (2005) 60:851–8. doi: 10.1136/thx.2005.042408

164. Baeten JM, Bukusi EA, Lambe M. Pregnancy complications and outcomes among overweight and obese nulliparous women. *Am J Public Health.* (2001) 91:436–40. doi: 10.2105/AJPH.91.3.436

165. Hayes EK, Lechowicz A, Petrik JJ, Storozhuk Y, Paez-Parent S, Dai Q, et al. Adverse fetal and neonatal outcomes associated with a life-long high fat diet: role of altered development of the placental vasculature. *PLoS ONE.* (2012) 7:e33370. doi: 10.1371/journal.pone.0033370

166. Gutaj P, Wender-Ozegowska E, Iciek R, Zawiejska A, Pietryga M, Brazert J. Maternal serum placental growth factor and fetal SGA in pregnancy complicated by type 1 diabetes mellitus. *J Perinat Med.* (2014) 42:629–33. doi: 10.1515/jpm-2013-0227

167. Wallace JM, Bourke DA, Aitken RP, Palmer RM, Da Silva P, Cruickshank MA. Relationship between nutritionally-mediated placental growth restriction and fetal growth, body composition and endocrine status during late gestation in adolescent sheep. *Placenta.* (2000) 21:100–8. doi: 10.1053/plac.1999.0440

168. Limesand SW, Rozance PJ. Fetal adaptations in insulin secretion result from high catecholamines during placental insufficiency. *J Physiol.* (2017) 595:5103–13. doi: 10.1113/JP273324

169. Thamotharan M, Garg M, Oak S, Rogers LM, Pan G, Sangiorgi F, et al. Transgenerational inheritance of the insulin-resistant phenotype in embryo-transferred intrauterine growth-restricted adult female rat offspring. *Am J Physiol Endocrinol Metab.* (2007) 292:E1270–9. doi: 10.1152/ajpendo.00462.2006

170. Skinner MK. What is an epigenetic transgenerational phenotype? F3 or F2. *Reprod Toxicol.* (2008) 25:2–6. doi: 10.1016/j.reprotox.2007.09.001

171. Horsthemke B. A critical view on transgenerational epigenetic inheritance in humans. *Nat Commun.* (2018) 9:2973. doi: 10.1038/s41467-018-05445-5

172. Meng R, Lv J, Yu C, Guo Y, Bian Z, Yang L, et al. Prenatal famine exposure, adulthood obesity patterns and risk of type 2 diabetes. *Int J Epidemiol.* (2018) 47:399–408. doi: 10.1093/ije/dyx228

173. Desai M, Ross MG. Fetal programming of adipose tissue: effects of intrauterine growth restriction and maternal obesity/high-fat diet. *Semin Reprod Med.* (2011) 29:237–45. doi: 10.1055/s-0031-1275517

174. Nawabi J, Vohlen C, Dinger K, Thangaratnarajah C, Klaudt C, Lopez Garcia E, et al. Novel functional role of GH/IGF-I in neonatal lung myofibroblasts and in rat lung growth after intrauterine growth restriction. *Am J Physiol Lung Cell Mol Physiol.* (2018) 315:L623–37. doi: 10.1152/ajplung.00413.2017

175. Khazaee R, McCaig LA, Yamashita C, Hardy DB, Veldhuizen RAW. Maternal protein restriction during perinatal life affects lung mechanics and the surfactant system during early postnatal life in female rats. *PLoS ONE.* (2019) 14:e0215611. doi: 10.1371/journal.pone.0215611

176. Joss-Moore LA, Wang Y, Baack ML, Yao J, Norris AW, Yu X, et al. IUGR decreases PPARgamma and SETD8 Expression in neonatal rat lung and these

effects are ameliorated by maternal DHA supplementation. *Early Hum Dev.* (2010) 86:785–91. doi: 10.1016/j.earlhumdev.2010.08.026

177. Dravet-Gounot P, Morin C, Jacques S, Dumont F, Ely-Marius F, Vaiman D, et al. Lung microRNA deregulation associated with impaired alveolarization in rats after intrauterine growth restriction. *PLoS ONE.* (2017) 12:e0190445. doi: 10.1371/journal.pone.0190445

178. Alejandre Alcazar MA, Ostreicher I, Appel S, Rother E, Vohlen C, Plank C, et al. Developmental regulation of inflammatory cytokine-mediated Stat3 signaling: the missing link between intrauterine growth restriction and pulmonary dysfunction? *J Mol Med.* (2012) 90:945–57. doi: 10.1007/s00109-012-0860-9

179. Alejandre Alcazar MA, Morty RE, Lendzian L, Vohlen C, Oestreicher I, Plank C, et al. Inhibition of TGF-beta signaling and decreased apoptosis in IUGR-associated lung disease in rats. *PLoS ONE.* (2011) 6:e26371. doi: 10.1371/journal.pone.0026371

180. Thebaud B, Abman SH. Bronchopulmonary dysplasia: where have all the vessels gone? Roles of angiogenic growth factors in chronic lung disease. *Am J Respir Crit Care Med.* (2007) 175:978–85. doi: 10.1164/rccm.200611-1660PP

181. Tang JR, Markham NE, Lin YJ, McMurtry IF, Maxey A, Kinsella JP, et al. Inhaled nitric oxide attenuates pulmonary hypertension and improves lung growth in infant rats after neonatal treatment with a VEGF receptor inhibitor. *Am J Physiol Lung Cell Mol Physiol.* (2004) 287:L344–51. doi: 10.1152/ajplung.00291.2003

182. Jakkula M, Le Cras TD, Gebb S, Hirth KP, Tuder RM, Voelkel NF, et al. Inhibition of angiogenesis decreases alveolarization in the developing rat lung. *Am J Physiol Lung Cell Mol Physiol.* (2000) 279:L600–7. doi: 10.1152/ajplung.2000.279.3.L600

183. Yun EJ, Lorizio W, Seedorf G, Abman SH, Vu TH. VEGF and endothelium-derived retinoic acid regulate lung vascular and alveolar development. *Am J Physiol Lung Cell Mol Physiol.* (2016) 310:L287–98. doi: 10.1152/ajplung.00229.2015

184. Svanes C, Omenaas E, Heuch JM, Irgens LM, Gulsvik A. Birth characteristics and asthma symptoms in young adults: results from a population-based cohort study in Norway. *Eur Respir J.* (1998) 12:1366–70. doi: 10.1183/09031936.98.12061366

185. Rona RJ, Gulliford MC, Chinn S. Effects of prematurity and intrauterine growth on respiratory health and lung function in childhood. *BMJ.* (1993) 306:817–20. doi: 10.1136/bmj.306.6881.817

186. Greenough A, Yuksel B, Cheeseman P. Effect of in utero growth retardation on lung function at follow-up of prematurely born infants. *Eur Respir J.* (2004) 24:731–3. doi: 10.1183/09031936.04.00060304

187. Ronkainen E, Dunder T, Kaukola T, Marttila R, Hallman M. Intrauterine growth restriction predicts lower lung function at school age in children born very preterm. *Arch Dis Child Fetal Neonatal Ed.* (2016) 101:F412–7. doi: 10.1136/archdischild-2015-308922

188. Kotecha SJ, Watkins WJ, Heron J, Henderson J, Dunstan FD, Kotecha S. Spirometric lung function in school-age children: effect of intrauterine growth retardation and catch-up growth. *Am J Respir Crit Care Med.* (2010) 181:969–74. doi: 10.1164/rccm.200906-0897OC

189. He B, Kwok MK, Au Yeung SL, Lin SL, Leung JYY, Hui LL, et al. Birth weight and prematurity with lung function at ~17.5 years: "Children of 1997" birth cohort. *Sci Rep.* (2020) 10:341. doi: 10.1038/s41598-019-56086-7

190. Cai Y, Shaheen SO, Hardy R, Kuh D, Hansell AL. Birth weight, early childhood growth and lung function in middle to early old age: 1946 British birth cohort. *Thorax.* (2016) 71:916–22. doi: 10.1136/thoraxjnl-2014-206457

191. Simmons RA, Templeton LJ, Gertz SJ. Intrauterine growth retardation leads to the development of type 2 diabetes in the rat. *Diabetes.* (2001) 50:2279–86. doi: 10.2337/diabetes.50.10.2279

192. Ravelli AC, van Der Meulen JH, Osmond C, Barker DJ, Bleker OP. Obesity at the age of 50 y in men and women exposed to famine prenatally. *Am J Clin Nutr.* (1999) 70:811–6. doi: 10.1093/ajcn/70.5.811

193. Newsome CA, Shiell AW, Fall CH, Phillips DI, Shier R, Law CM. Is birth weight related to later glucose and insulin metabolism?–A systematic review. *Diabet Med.* (2003) 20:339–48. doi: 10.1046/j.1464-5491.2003.00871.x

194. Mohan R, Baumann D, Alejandro EU. Fetal undernutrition, placental insufficiency, and pancreatic beta-cell development programming in

utero. *Am J Physiol Regul Integr Comp Physiol.* (2018) 315:R867–78. doi: 10.1152/ajpregu.00072.2018

195. Laitinen J, Pietilainen K, Wadsworth M, Sovio U, Jarvelin MR. Predictors of abdominal obesity among 31-y-old men and women born in Northern Finland in 1966. *Eur J Clin Nutr.* (2004) 58:180–90. doi: 10.1038/sj.ejcn.1601765

196. Crume TL, Scherzinger A, Stamm E, McDuffie R, Bischoff KJ, Hamman RF, et al. The long-term impact of intrauterine growth restriction in a diverse US. cohort of children: the EPOCH study. *Obesity.* (2014) 22:608–15. doi: 10.1002/oby.20565

197. Barker DJ, Hales CN, Fall CH, Osmond C, Phipps K, Clark PM. Type 2 (non-insulin-dependent) diabetes mellitus, hypertension and hyperlipidaemia (syndrome X): relation to reduced fetal growth. *Diabetologia.* (1993) 36:62–7. doi: 10.1007/BF00399095

198. Illsley NP, Baumann MU. Human placental glucose transport in fetoplacental growth and metabolism. *Biochim Biophys Acta Mol Basis Dis.* (2020) 1866:165359. doi: 10.1016/j.bbadis.2018.12.010

199. Boehmer BH, Limesand SW, Rozance PJ. The impact of IUGR on pancreatic islet development and beta-cell function. *J Endocrinol.* (2017) 235:R63–76. doi: 10.1530/JOE-17-0076

200. Yada KK, Gupta R, Gupta A, Gupta M. Insulin levels in low birth weight neonates. *Indian J Med Res.* (2003) 118:197–203.

201. Wolf HJ, Ebenbichler CF, Huter O, Bodner J, Lechleitner M, Foger B, et al. Fetal leptin and insulin levels only correlate inlarge-for-gestational age infants. *Eur J Endocrinol.* (2000) 142:623–9. doi: 10.1530/eje.0.1420623

202. Muhlhausler BS, Duffield JA, Ozanne SE, Pilgrim C, Turner N, Morrison JL, et al. The transition from fetal growth restriction to accelerated postnatal growth: a potential role for insulin signalling in skeletal muscle. *J Physiol.* (2009) 587:4199–211. doi: 10.1113/jphysiol.2009.173161

203. Dunlop K, Cedrone M, Staples JF, Regnault TR. Altered fetal skeletal muscle nutrient metabolism following an adverse *in utero* environment and the modulation of later life insulin sensitivity. *Nutrients.* (2015) 7:1202–16. doi: 10.3390/nu7021202

204. Beyea JA, Sawicki G, Olson DM, List E, Kopchick JJ, Harvey S. Growth hormone (GH) receptor knockout mice reveal actions of GH in lung development. *Proteomics.* (2006) 6:341–8. doi: 10.1002/pmic.200500168

205. Seedorf G, Kim C, Wallace B, Mandell EW, Nowlin T, Shepherd D, et al. rhIGF-1/BP3 preserves lung growth and prevents pulmonary hypertension in experimental bronchopulmonary dysplasia. *Am J Respir Crit Care Med.* (2020) 201:1120–34. doi: 10.1164/rccm.201910-1975OC

206. Invitti C, Gilardini L, Mazzilli G, Sartorio A, Viberti GC, Ong KK, et al. Insulin sensitivity and secretion in normal children related to size at birth, postnatal growth, and plasma insulin-like growth factor-I levels. *Diabetologia.* (2004) 47:1064–70. doi: 10.1007/s00125-004-1565-6

207. Ibanez L, Potau N, Marcos MV, de Zegher F. Exaggerated adrenarche and hyperinsulinism in adolescent girls born small for gestational age. *J Clin Endocrinol Metab.* (1999) 84:4739–41. doi: 10.1210/jc.84.12.4739

208. Gurugubelli Krishna R, Vishnu Bhat B. Molecular mechanisms of intrauterine growth restriction. *J Matern Fetal Neonatal Med.* (2018) 31:2634–40. doi: 10.1080/14767058.2017.1347922

209. Desai M, Gayle D, Han G, Ross MG. Programmed hyperphagia due to reduced anorexigenic mechanisms in intrauterine growth-restricted offspring. *Reprod Sci.* (2007) 14:329–37. doi: 10.1177/1933719107303983

210. Coupe B, Grit I, Hulin P, Randuineau G, Parnet P. Postnatal growth after intrauterine growth restriction alters central leptin signal and energy homeostasis. *PLoS ONE.* (2012) 7:e30616. doi: 10.1371/journal.pone.0030616

211. Saxton RA, Sabatini DM. mTOR signaling in growth, metabolism, and disease. *Cell.* (2017) 169:361–71. doi: 10.1016/j.cell.2017.03.035

212. Kim J, Guan KL. mTOR as a central hub of nutrient signalling and cell growth. *Nat Cell Biol.* (2019) 21:63–71. doi: 10.1038/s41556-018-0205-1

213. Ganguly A, Collis L, Devaskar SU. Placental glucose and amino acid transport in calorie-restricted wild-type and Glut3 null heterozygous mice. *Endocrinology.* (2012) 153:3995–4007. doi: 10.1210/en.2011-1973

214. Brett KE, Ferraro ZM, Yockell-Lelievre J, Gruslin A, Adamo KB. Maternal-fetal nutrient transport in pregnancy pathologies: the role of the placenta. *Int J Mol Sci.* (2014) 15:16153–85. doi: 10.3390/ijms150916153

215. Sinagoga KL, Stone WJ, Schiesser JV, Schweitzer JI, Sampson L, Zheng Y, et al. Distinct roles for the mTOR pathway in postnatal morphogenesis,

maturation and function of pancreatic islets. *Development.* (2017) 144:2402–14. doi: 10.1242/dev.146316

216. Hu F, Xu Y, Liu F. Hypothalamic roles of mTOR complex I: integration of nutrient and hormone signals to regulate energy homeostasis. *Am J Physiol Endocrinol Metab.* (2016) 310:E994–1002. doi: 10.1152/ajpendo.00121.2016

217. Zhong H, Chiles K, Feldser D, Laughner E, Hanrahan C, Georgescu MM, et al. Modulation of hypoxia-inducible factor 1alpha expression by the epidermal growth factor/phosphatidylinositol 3-kinase/PTEN/AKT/FRAP pathway in human prostate cancer cells: implications for tumor angiogenesis and therapeutics. *Cancer Res.* (2000) 60:1541–5. doi: 10.1002/cyto.990020515

218. Wahdan-Alaswad RS, Song K, Krebs TL, Shola DT, Gomez JA, Matsuyama S, et al. Insulin-like growth factor I suppresses bone morphogenetic protein signaling in prostate cancer cells by activating mTOR signaling. *Cancer Res.* (2010) 70:9106–17. doi: 10.1158/0008-5472.CAN-10-1119

219. Pinheiro AR, Salvucci ID, Aguila MB, Mandarim-de-Lacerda CA. Protein restriction during gestation and/or lactation causes adverse transgenerational effects on biometry and glucose metabolism in F1 and F2 progenies of rats. *Clin Sci.* (2008) 114:381–92. doi: 10.1042/CS20070302

220. Gonzalez-Rodriguez P, Cantu J, O'Neil D, Seferovic MD, Goodspeed DM, Suter MA, et al. Alterations in expression of imprinted genes from the H19/IGF2 loci in a multigenerational model of intrauterine growth restriction (IUGR). *Am J Obstet Gynecol.* (2016) 214:625. doi: 10.1016/j.ajog.2016.01.194

221. Berends LM, Ozanne SE. Early determinants of type-2 diabetes. *Best Pract Res Clin Endocrinol Metab.* (2012) 26:569–80. doi: 10.1016/j.beem.2012.03.002

222. Aiken CE, Ozanne SE. Transgenerational developmental programming. *Hum Reprod Update.* (2014) 20:63–75. doi: 10.1093/humupd/dmt043

223. Joss-Moore LA, Lane RH, Albertine KH. Epigenetic contributions to the developmental origins of adult lung disease. *Biochem Cell Biol.* (2015) 93:119–27. doi: 10.1139/bcb-2014-0093

224. Tosh DN, Fu Q, Callaway CW, McKnight RA, McMillen IC, Ross MG, et al. Epigenetics of programmed obesity: alteration in IUGR rat hepatic IGF1 mRNA expression and histone structure in rapid vs. delayed postnatal catch-up growth. *Am J Physiol Gastrointest Liver Physiol.* (2010) 299:G1023–9. doi: 10.1152/ajpgi.00052.2010

225. Fu Q, Yu X, Callaway CW, Lane RH, McKnight RA. Epigenetics: intrauterine growth retardation (IUGR) modifies the histone code along the rat hepatic IGF-1 gene. *FASEB J.* (2009) 23:2438–49. doi: 10.1096/fj.08-124768

226. Park JH, Stoffers DA, Nicholls RD, Simmons RA. Development of type 2 diabetes following intrauterine growth retardation in rats is associated with progressive epigenetic silencing of Pdx1. *J Clin Invest.* (2008) 118:2316–24. doi: 10.1172/JCI33655

227. Deodati A, Inzaghi E, Liguori A, Puglianiello A, Germani D, Brufani C, et al. IGF2 methylation is associated with lipid profile in obese children. *Horm Res Paediatr.* (2013) 79:361–7. doi: 10.1159/000351707

228. Goodspeed D, Seferovic MD, Holland W, McKnight RA, Summers SA, Branch DW, et al. Essential nutrient supplementation prevents heritable metabolic disease in multigenerational intrauterine growth-restricted rats. *FASEB J.* (2015) 29:807–19. doi: 10.1096/fj.14-259614

229. Zhang H, Fan Y, Elsabagh M, Guo S, Wang M, Jiang H. Dietary supplementation of L-Arginine and N-carbamylglutamate attenuated the hepatic inflammatory response and apoptosis in suckling lambs with intrauterine growth retardation. *Mediators Inflamm.* (2020) 2020:2453537. doi: 10.1155/2020/2453537

230. Jaeckle Santos LJ, Li C, Doulias PT, Ischiropoulos H, Worthen GS, Simmons RA. Neutralizing Th2 inflammation in neonatal islets prevents beta-cell failure in adult IUGR rats. *Diabetes.* (2014) 63:1672–84. doi: 10.2337/db13-1226

231. Dodson RB, Powers KN, Gien J, Rozance PJ, Seedorf G, Astling D, et al. Intrauterine growth restriction decreases NF-kappaB signaling in fetal pulmonary artery endothelial cells of fetal sheep. *Am J Physiol Lung Cell Mol Physiol.* (2018) 315:L348–59. doi: 10.1152/ajplung.00052.2018

232. Amarilyo G, Oren A, Mimouni FB, Ochshorn Y, Deutsch V, Mandel D. Increased cord serum inflammatory markers in small-for-gestational-age neonates. *J Perinatol.* (2011) 31:30–2. doi: 10.1038/jp.2010.53

233. Fresno M, Alvarez R, Cuesta N. Toll-like receptors, inflammation, metabolism and obesity. *Arch Physiol Biochem.* (2011) 117:151–64. doi: 10.3109/13813455.2011.562514

234. Bhargava P, Lee CH. Role and function of macrophages in the metabolic syndrome. *Biochem J.* (2012) 442:253–262. doi: 10.1042/BJ20111708

235. Bastard JP, Maachi M, Lagathu C, Kim MJ, Caron M, Vidal H, et al. Recent advances in the relationship between obesity, inflammation, and insulin resistance. *Eur Cytokine Netw.* (2006) 17:4–12.

236. Vieira Braga FA, Kar G, Berg M, Carpaij OA, Polanski K, Simon LM, et al. A cellular census of human lungs identifies novel cell states in health and in asthma. *Nat Med.* (2019) 25:1153–63. doi: 10.1038/s41591-019-0468-5

237. Speer CP. Chorioamnionitis, postnatal factors and proinflammatory response in the pathogenetic sequence of bronchopulmonary dysplasia. *Neonatology.* (2009) 95:353–61. doi: 10.1159/000209301

238. Ramakrishna L, de Vries VC, Curotto de Lafaille MA. Cross-roads in the lung: immune cells and tissue interactions as determinants of allergic asthma. *Immunol Res.* (2012) 53:213–28. doi: 10.1007/s12026-012-8296-4

239. Bhat TA, Panzica L, Kalathil SG, Thanavala Y. Immune dysfunction in patients with chronic obstructive pulmonary disease. *Ann Am Thorac Soc.* (2015) 12(Suppl. 2):S169–75. doi: 10.1513/AnnalsATS.201503-126AW

240. Kyriakakou M, Malamitsi-Puchner A, Militsi H, Boutsikou T, Margeli A, Hassiakos D, et al. Leptin and adiponectin concentrations in intrauterine growth restricted and appropriate for gestational age fetuses, neonates, and their mothers. *Eur J Endocrinol.* (2008) 158:343–8. doi: 10.1530/EJE-07-0692

241. Rashid CS, Lien YC, Bansal A, Jaeckle-Santos LJ, Li C, Won KJ, et al. Transcriptomic analysis reveals novel mechanisms mediating islet dysfunction in the intrauterine growth-restricted rat. *Endocrinology.* (2018) 159:1035–49. doi: 10.1210/en.2017-00888

242. Thangaratnarajah C, Dinger K, Vohlen C, Klaudt C, Nawabi J, Lopez Garcia E, et al. Novel role of NPY in neuroimmune interaction and lung growth after intrauterine growth restriction. *Am J Physiol Lung Cell Mol Physiol.* (2017) 313:L491–506. doi: 10.1152/ajplung.00432.2016

243. Rosenberg A. The IUGR newborn. *Semin Perinatol.* (2008) 32:219–24. doi: 10.1053/j.semperi.2007.11.003

244. Regev RH, Reichman B. Prematurity and intrauterine growth retardation–double jeopardy? *Clin Perinatol.* (2004) 31:453–73. doi: 10.1016/j.clp.2004.04.017

245. McDonald SD, Han Z, Mulla S, Beyene J, Knowledge Synthesis G. Overweight and obesity in mothers and risk of preterm birth and low birth weight infants: systematic review and meta-analyses. *BMJ.* (2010) 341:c3428. doi: 10.1136/bmj.c3428

246. Lynch TA, Malshe A, Colihan S, Meyers J, Li D, Holloman C, et al. Impact of maternal obesity on perinatal outcomes in preterm prelabor rupture of membranes >/=34 weeks. *Am J Perinatol.* (2020) 37:467–74. doi: 10.1055/s-0039-1698833

247. Vincent S, Czuzoj-Shulman N, Spence AR, Abenhaim HA. Effect of pre-pregnancy body mass index on respiratory-related neonatal outcomes in women undergoing elective cesarean prior to 39 weeks. *J Perinat Med.* (2018) 46:905–12. doi: 10.1515/jpm-2017-0384

248. Goldenberg RL, Culhane JF. Prepregnancy health status and the risk of preterm delivery. *Arch Pediatr Adolesc Med.* (2005) 159:89–90. doi: 10.1001/archpedi.159.1.89

249. Smith LJ, McKay KO, van Asperen PP, Selvadurai H, Fitzgerald DA. Normal development of the lung and premature birth. *Paediatr Respir Rev.* (2010) 11:135–42. doi: 10.1016/j.prrv.2009.12.006

250. Kumar VH, Lakshminrusimha S, Kishkurno S, Paturi BS, Gugino SF, Nielsen L, et al. Neonatal hyperoxia increases airway reactivity and inflammation in adult mice. *Pediatr Pulmonol.* (2016) 51:1131–41. doi: 10.1002/ppul.23430

251. Jobe AH. The new bronchopulmonary dysplasia. *Curr Opin Pediatr.* (2011) 23:167–72. doi: 10.1097/MOP.0b013e3283423e6b

252. Dumpa V, Bhandari V. Surfactant, steroids and non-invasive ventilation in the prevention of BPD. *Semin Perinatol.* (2018) 42:444–52. doi: 10.1053/j.semperi.2018.09.006

253. Collins JJP, Tibboel D, de Kleer IM, Reiss IKM, Rottier RJ. The future of bronchopulmonary dysplasia: emerging pathophysiological concepts and potential new avenues of treatment. *Front Med (Lausanne).* (2017) 4:61. doi: 10.3389/fmed.2017.00061

254. Bustani P, Kotecha S. Role of cytokines in hyperoxia mediated inflammation in the developing lung. *Front Biosci.* (2003) 8:s694–704. doi: 10.2741/1113

255. Hwang JS, Rehan VK. Recent advances in bronchopulmonary dysplasia: pathophysiology, prevention, and treatment. *Lung.* (2018) 196:129–38. doi: 10.1007/s00408-018-0084-z

256. Garite TJ, Clark R, Thorp JA. Intrauterine growth restriction increases morbidity and mortality among premature neonates. *Am J Obstet Gynecol.* (2004) 191:481–7. doi: 10.1016/j.ajog.2004.01.036

257. Koenig JE, Spor A, Scalfone N, Fricker AD, Stombaugh J, Knight R, et al. Succession of microbial consortia in the developing infant gut microbiome. *Proc Natl Acad Sci USA.* (2011) 108(Suppl. 1):4578–85. doi: 10.1073/pnas.1000081107

258. Hehemann JH, Correc G, Barbeyron T, Helbert W, Czjzek M, Michel G. Transfer of carbohydrate-active enzymes from marine bacteria to Japanese gut microbiota. *Nature.* (2010) 464:908–912. doi: 10.1038/nature08937

259. Craig WJ. Health effects of vegan diets. *Am J Clin Nutr.* (2009) 89:1627S–33S. doi: 10.3945/ajcn.2009.26736N

260. Wu GD, Chen J, Hoffmann C, Bittinger K, Chen YY, Keilbaugh SA, et al. Linking long-term dietary patterns with gut microbial enterotypes. *Science.* (2011) 334:105–8. doi: 10.1126/science.1208344

261. Levy M, Kolodziejczyk AA, Thaiss CA, Elinav E. Dysbiosis and the immune system. *Nat Rev Immunol.* (2017) 17:219–32. doi: 10.1038/nri.2017.7

262. Knights D, Parfrey LW, Zaneveld J, Lozupone C, Knight R. Human-associated microbial signatures: examining their predictive value. *Cell Host Microbe.* (2011) 10:292–6. doi: 10.1016/j.chom.2011.09.003

263. Goodrich JK, Waters JL, Poole AC, Sutter JL, Koren O, Blekhman R, et al. Human genetics shape the gut microbiome. *Cell.* (2014) 159:789–99. doi: 10.1016/j.cell.2014.09.053

264. Zhang C, Yin A, Li H, Wang R, Wu G, Shen J, et al. Dietary modulation of gut microbiota contributes to alleviation of both genetic and simple obesity in children. *EBioMedicine.* (2015) 2:968–84. doi: 10.1016/j.ebiom.2015.07.007

265. Zeevi D, Korem T, Zmora N, Israeli D, Rothschild D, Weinberger A, et al. Personalized nutrition by prediction of glycemic responses. *Cell.* (2015) 163:1079–94. doi: 10.1016/j.cell.2015.11.001

266. Vrieze A, Van Nood E, Holleman F, Salojarvi J, Kootte RS, Bartelsman JF, et al. Transfer of intestinal microbiota from lean donors increases insulin sensitivity in individuals with metabolic syndrome. *Gastroenterology.* (2012) 143:913–6.e917. doi: 10.1053/j.gastro.2012.06.031

267. Schirmer M, Smeekens SP, Vlamakis H, Jaeger M, Oosting M, Franzosa EA, et al. Linking the human gut microbiome to inflammatory cytokine production capacity. *Cell.* (2016) 167:1897. doi: 10.1016/j.cell.2016.10.020

268. Le Chatelier E, Nielsen T, Qin J, Prifti E, Hildebrand F, Falony G, et al. Richness of human gut microbiome correlates with metabolic markers. *Nature.* (2013) 500:541–6. doi: 10.1038/nature12506

269. Cotillard A, Kennedy SP, Kong LC, Prifti E, Pons N, Le Chatelier E, et al. Dietary intervention impact on gut microbial gene richness. *Nature.* (2013) 500:585–8. doi: 10.1038/nature12480

270. Trasande L, Blustein J, Liu M, Corwin E, Cox LM, Blaser MJ. Infant antibiotic exposures and early-life body mass. *Int J Obes.* (2013) 37:16–23. doi: 10.1038/ijo.2012.132

271. Karczewski J, Poniedzialek B, Adamski Z, Rzymski P. The effects of the microbiota on the host immune system. *Autoimmunity.* (2014) 47:494–504. doi: 10.3109/08916934.2014.938322

272. Maynard CL, Elson CO, Hatton RD, Weaver CT. Reciprocal interactions of the intestinal microbiota and immune system. *Nature.* (2012) 489:231–41. doi: 10.1038/nature11551

273. Hilty M, Burke C, Pedro H, Cardenas P, Bush A, Bossley C, et al. Disordered microbial communities in asthmatic airways. *PLoS ONE.* (2010) 5:e8578. doi: 10.1371/journal.pone.0008578

274. O'Dwyer DN, Dickson RP, Moore BB. The lung microbiome, immunity, and the pathogenesis of chronic lung disease. *J Immunol.* (2016) 196:4839–47. doi: 10.4049/jimmunol.1600279

275. Siwicka-Gieroba D, Czarko-Wicha K. Lung microbiome - a modern knowledge. *Cent Eur J Immunol.* (2020) 45:342–5. doi: 10.5114/ceji.2020.101266

276. Dickson RP, Martinez FJ, Huffnagle GB. The role of the microbiome in exacerbations of chronic lung diseases. *Lancet.* (2014) 384:691–702. doi: 10.1016/S0140-6736(14)61136-3

277. Sencio V, Machado MG, Trottein F. The lung-gut axis during viral respiratory infections: the impact of gut dysbiosis on secondary disease outcomes. *Mucosal Immunol.* (2021) 14:296–304. doi: 10.1038/s41385-020-00361-8

278. Dickson RP, Erb-Downward JR, Huffnagle GB. The role of the bacterial microbiome in lung disease. *Expert Rev Respir Med.* (2013) 7:245–57. doi: 10.1586/ers.13.24

279. Vaughan A, Frazer ZA, Hansbro PM, Yang IA. COPD and the gut-lung axis: the therapeutic potential of fibre. *J Thorac Dis.* (2019) 11:S2173–80. doi: 10.21037/jtd.2019.10.40

280. Arrieta MC, Stiemsma LT, Dimitriu PA, Thorson L, Russell S, Yurist-Doutsch S, et al. Early infancy microbial and metabolic alterations affect risk of childhood asthma. *Sci Transl Med.* (2015) 7:307ra152. doi: 10.1126/scitranslmed.aab2271

281. Virgin HW, Wherry EJ, Ahmed R. Redefining chronic viral infection. *Cell.* (2009) 138:30–50. doi: 10.1016/j.cell.2009.06.036

282. Duerkop BA, Hooper LV. Resident viruses and their interactions with the immune system. *Nat Immunol.* (2013) 14:654–9. doi: 10.1038/ni.2614

283. Hewitt R, Farne H, Ritchie A, Luke E, Johnston SL, Mallia P. The role of viral infections in exacerbations of chronic obstructive pulmonary disease and asthma. *Ther Adv Respir Dis.* (2016) 10:158–74. doi: 10.1177/1753465815618113

284. Billard L, Le Berre R, Pilorge L, Payan C, Hery-Arnaud G, Vallet S. Viruses in cystic fibrosis patients' airways. *Crit Rev Microbiol.* (2017) 43:690–708. doi: 10.1080/1040841X.2017.1297763

285. van Boheemen S, van Rijn AL, Pappas N, Carbo EC, Vorderman RHP, Sidorov I, et al. retrospective validation of a metagenomic sequencing protocol for combined detection of RNA and DNA viruses using respiratory samples from pediatric patients. *J Mol Diagn.* (2020) 22:196–207. doi: 10.1016/j.jmoldx.2019.10.007

286. Prachayangprecha S, Schapendonk CM, Koopmans MP, Osterhaus AD, Schurch AC, Pas SD, et al. Exploring the potential of next-generation sequencing in detection of respiratory viruses. *J Clin Microbiol.* (2014) 52:3722–30. doi: 10.1128/JCM.01641-14

287. Yadav H, Jain S, Nagpal R, Marotta F. Increased fecal viral content associated with obesity in mice. *World J Diabetes.* (2016) 7:316–20. doi: 10.4239/wjd.v7.i15.316

288. Tan VPK, Ngim CF, Lee EZ, Ramadas A, Pong LY, Ng JI, et al. The association between obesity and dengue virus (DENV) infection in hospitalised patients. *PLoS ONE.* (2018) 13:e0200698. doi: 10.1371/journal.pone.0200698

289. Vangipuram SD, Yu M, Tian J, Stanhope KL, Pasarica M, Havel PJ, et al. Adipogenic human adenovirus-36 reduces leptin expression and secretion and increases glucose uptake by fat cells. *Int J Obes.* (2007) 31:87–96. doi: 10.1038/sj.ijo.0803366

290. Mukhopadhya I, Segal JP, Carding SR, Hart AL, Hold GL. The gut virome: the 'missing link' between gut bacteria and host immunity? *Therap Adv Gastroenterol.* (2019) 12:1756284819836620. doi: 10.1177/1756284819836620

291. Tian Y, Jennings J, Gong Y, Sang Y. Viral infections and interferons in the development of obesity. *Biomolecules.* (2019) 9:726. doi: 10.3390/biom9110726

292. Russell CD, Unger SA, Walton M, Schwarze J. The human immune response to respiratory syncytial virus infection. *Clin Microbiol Rev.* (2017) 30:481–502. doi: 10.1128/CMR.00090-16

293. Jaddoe VWV, Felix JF, Andersen AN, Charles MA, Chatzi L, Corpeleijn E, et al. The LifeCycle project-EU child cohort network: a federated analysis infrastructure and harmonized data of more than 250,000 children and parents. *Eur J Epidemiol.* (2020) 35:709–24. doi: 10.1007/s10654-020-00662-z

294. Piersigilli F, Lam TT, Vernocchi P, Quagliariello A, Putignani L, Aghai ZH, et al. Identification of new biomarkers of bronchopulmonary dysplasia using metabolomics. *Metabolomics.* (2019) 15:20. doi: 10.1007/s11306-019-1482-9

295. Sahni M, Yeboah B, Das P, Shah D, Ponnalagu D, Singh H, et al. Novel biomarkers of bronchopulmonary dysplasia and bronchopulmonary dysplasia-associated pulmonary hypertension. *J Perinatol.* (2020) 40:1634–43. doi: 10.1038/s41372-020-00788-8

296. Askenazi DJ, Koralkar R, Patil N, Halloran B, Ambalavanan N, Griffin R. Acute kidney injury urine biomarkers in very low-birth-weight infants. *Clin J Am Soc Nephrol.* (2016) 11:1527–35. doi: 10.2215/CJN.13381215

297. Baumert M, Surmiak P, Wiecek A, Walencka Z. Serum NGAL and copeptin levels as predictors of acute kidney injury in asphyxiated neonates. *Clin Exp Nephrol.* (2017) 21:658–64. doi: 10.1007/s10157-016-1320-6

298. Jung YH, Han D, Shin SH, Kim EK, Kim HS. Proteomic identification of early urinary-biomarkers of acute kidney injury in preterm infants. *Sci Rep.* (2020) 10:4057. doi: 10.1038/s41598-020-60890-x

299. Watanabe IKM, Jara ZP, Volpini RA, Franco MDC, Jung FF, Casarini DE. Up-regulation of renal renin-angiotensin system and inflammatory mechanisms in the prenatal programming by low-protein diet: beneficial effect of the post-weaning losartan treatment. *J Dev Origins Health Dis.* (2018) 9:530–5. doi: 10.1017/S2040174418000296

300. Flynn ER, Alexander BT, Lee J, Hutchens ZM, Jr Maric-Bilkan C. High-fat/fructose feeding during prenatal and postnatal development in female rats increases susceptibility to renal and metabolic injury later in life. *Am J Physiol Regul Integr Comp Physiol.* (2013) 304:R278–85. doi: 10.1152/ajpregu.00433.2012

301. Wixey JA, Chand KK, Colditz PB, Bjorkman ST. Review: neuroinflammation in intrauterine growth restriction. *Placenta.* (2017) 54:117–24. doi: 10.1016/j.placenta.2016.11.012

302. Bangma JT, Hartwell H, Santos HP, O'Shea TM, Fry RC. Placental programming, perinatal inflammation, and neurodevelopment impairment among those born extremely preterm. *Pediatr Res.* (2021) 89:326–35. doi: 10.1038/s41390-020-01236-1

303. Leviton A, Fichorova RN, O'Shea TM, Kuban K, Paneth N, Dammann O, et al. Two-hit model of brain damage in the very preterm newborn: small for gestational age and postnatal systemic inflammation. *Pediatr Res.* (2013) 73:362–70. doi: 10.1038/pr.2012.188

304. Leviton A, Allred EN, Fichorova RN, Kuban KC, Michael O'Shea T, Dammann O. Systemic inflammation on postnatal days 21 and 28 and indicators of brain dysfunction 2years later among children born before the 28th week of gestation. *Early Hum Dev.* (2016) 93:25–32. doi: 10.1016/j.earlhumdev.2015.11.004

305. Kuban KC, Joseph RM, O'Shea TM, Heeren T, Fichorova RN, Douglass L, et al. Circulating inflammatory-associated proteins in the first month of life and cognitive impairment at age 10 years in children born extremely preterm. *J Pediatr.* (2017) 180:116–23.e111. doi: 10.1016/j.jpeds.2016.09.054

306. Guo W, Guan X, Pan X, Sun X, Wang F, Ji Y, et al. Post-natal inhibition of NF-kappaB activation prevents renal damage caused by prenatal LPS exposure. *PLoS ONE.* (2016) 11:e0153434. doi: 10.1371/journal.pone.0153434

307. Nüsken E, Fink G, Lechner F, Voggel J, Wohlfarth M, Sprenger L, et al. Altered molecular signatures during kidney development after intrauterine growth restriction of different origins. *J Mol Med.* (2020) 98:395–407. doi: 10.1007/s00109-020-01875-1

308. Rounioja S, Rasanen J, Glumoff V, Ojaniemi M, Makikallio K, Hallman M. Intra-amniotic lipopolysaccharide leads to fetal cardiac dysfunction. A mouse model for fetal inflammatory response. *Cardiovasc Res.* (2003) 60:156–64. doi: 10.1016/S0008-6363(03)00338-9

Opposing Effects of TGFβ and BMP in the Pulmonary Vasculature in Congenital Diaphragmatic Hernia

Daphne S. Mous[1], Marjon J. Buscop-van Kempen[1,2], Rene M. H. Wijnen[1], Dick Tibboel[1], Rory E. Morty[3,4] and Robbert J. Rottier[1,2]*

[1] Department of Pediatric Surgery, Erasmus Medical Center – Sophia Children's Hospital, Rotterdam, Netherlands, [2] Department of Cell Biology, Erasmus Medical Center, Rotterdam, Netherlands, [3] Department of Lung Development and Remodelling, Max Planck Institute for Heart and Lung Research, Bad Nauheim, Germany, [4] Department of Internal Medicine (Pulmonology), University of Giessen and Marburg Lung Center (UGMLC), Giessen, Germany

*Correspondence:
Robbert J. Rottier
r.rottier@erasmusmc.nl

Background: Pulmonary hypertension is the major cause of morbidity and mortality in congenital diaphragmatic hernia (CDH). Mutations in several genes that encode signaling molecules of the transforming growth factor β (TGFβ) and bone morphogenetic protein (BMP) pathways have previously been associated with CDH. Since studies on the activation of these pathways in CDH are scarce, and have yielded inconsistent conclusions, the downstream activity of both pathways was assessed in the nitrofen-CDH rat model.

Methods and Results: Pregnant Sprague-Dawley rats were treated with nitrofen at embryonic day (E) 9.5 to induce CDH in offspring. At E21, lungs were screened for the expression of key factors of both signaling pathways, at both the mRNA transcript and protein levels. Subsequently, paying particular attention to the pulmonary vasculature, increased phosphorylation of SMAD2, and decreased phosphorylation of Smad5 was noted in the muscular walls of small pulmonary vessels, by immunohistochemistry. This was accompanied by increased proliferation of constituent cells of the smooth muscle layer of these vessels.

Conclusions: Increased activation of the TGFβ pathway and decreased activation of the BMP pathway in the pulmonary vasculature of rats with experimentally-induced CDH, suggesting that the deregulated of these important signaling pathways may underlie the development of pulmonary hypertension in CDH.

Keywords: lung, vasculature, BMP, TGF, congenital diagraphma hernia

INTRODUCTION

Congenital diaphragmatic hernia (CDH) is a severe developmental anomaly characterized by a diaphragmatic defect. The concomitant pulmonary hypertension (PH) that develops in affected lungs can cause severe problems in the newborn, and is responsible for the high morbidity and mortality in these patients. Although the muscularization of the pulmonary vessels has been demonstrated to be increased in CDH (1), the pathophysiological basis of PH in these patients remains largely unclarified. Mutations in different genes involved in the transforming growth factor β (TGFβ) and bone morphogenetic protein (BMP) pathways have been described in both adult and pediatric patients with familial, heritable, and idiopathic pulmonary arterial hypertension (PAH). Of these genes, the BMP receptor 2 (BMPR2) is most commonly affected (2).

TGFβ is a negative regulator of airway branching in early lung development. However, TGFβ signaling is also active in the vascular and airway smooth muscle and alveolar and airway epithelium during late lung development. Both up- and down-regulation of TGFβ signaling impairs the alveolarization process (3, 4), depending on the period of study during gestation. Both TGFβ and BMP are documented to influence the proliferation of endothelial and smooth muscle cells, and control apoptosis and extracellular matrix secretion and deposition (5).

Studies on the TGFβ pathway in CDH have not yielded consistent conclusions. Decreased expression of TGFβ1 was found at the mRNA level in the hearts of the nitrofen-exposed rat pups with CDH (6), where increased expression of TGFβ1 in affected lungs was evident by immunohistochemistry (7). In contrast, other studies have reported no perturbations to TGFβ expression and activity—assessed by the phosphorylation of SMAD2/3—in both human samples as well as tissues harvested from the nitrofen-CDH rat model (8). A study performed in pregnant women carrying CDH fetuses revealed decreased TGFβ levels in the amniotic fluid, but no differences in expression of TGFβ in the lungs of these children after birth (9). The expression of both TGFβ receptor (TGFBR) 1 and 2 as well as endoglin, an auxiliary receptor of TGFβ, were found to be decreased in nitrofen-CDH rat pups (10).

In contrast to the TGFβ pathway, conclusions drawn in several reports on components of the BMP pathway in CDH are consistent. Reduced expression of BMPR2 (11, 12) and BMP4 (12, 13) was found in the lungs of different animal models of CDH. Furthermore, the expression of apelin, a target gene of BMPR2 which can have a hypotensive function, is reported to be decreased in nitrofen-CDH rat pups (14); whilst expression of activin receptor-like kinase 1 (ALK1), another receptor of the BMP signaling pathway, was upregulated in the same animal model (15). However, Corbett et al. did not report any differences in downstream signaling of BMPR (16), and did not find any mutations in the BMPR2 gene in CDH patients (17). All findings reported to date addressing the TGFβ and BMP pathways in CDH is summarized in **Supplementary Table 1** and an overview of both pathways is displayed in **Figure 1**.

Investigations conducted to date have focused largely on the expression of receptors in both the TGFβ and BMP pathways, but little is known about the actual activation of these pathways. Therefore, we hypothesized that the analysis of downstream mediators would identify changes in TGFβ and BMP signaling pathways in the lungs of rats in which CDH was induced by nitrofen exposure.

MATERIALS AND METHODS
Animal Model
Pregnant Sprague-Dawley rats received either 100 mg nitrofen dissolved in 1 ml olive oil or just 1 ml olive oil by gavage on gestational age day E9.5. Nitrofen induces CDH in ~70% of the offspring, while all pups have pulmonary hypertension (18, 19). At embryonic day (E) 21, pups were delivered by cesarean section and euthanized by lethal injection of pentobarbital. Lung tissue of the CDH and control pups were isolated and processed for paraffin embedding (left lobes) or immediately snap frozen (right lobes) for protein and RNA analysis. All animal experiments were approved by an independent animal ethical committee and were conducted according to national guidelines.

Quantitative Real-Time Polymerase Chain Reaction (qPCR)
RNA isolation, cDNA synthesis and subsequent qPCR analysis on right lung lobes was performed as previously (20). The gene-specific primers used are available upon request.

Immunohistochemistry and Immunofluorescence Staining
Immunohistochemistry (IHC) was performed on 5-μm paraffin sections of the left lobe according to standard protocols, using the Envision™ detection system (Dako Cytomatic, Glostrup, Denmark) (20). Primary antibody used for IHC was ZEB2 [1:400, (21)]. Primary antibodies used for IF were smooth muscle actin (α-SMA; MS-113-P1; 1:500, Thermo Scientific, Fremont, CA, USA), phosphorylated SMAD 2 (pSMAD2; 1:250, Cell Signaling, Danvers, MA, USA), phosphorylated SMAD 1/5/8 (pSMAD1/5/8; 1:500, Kerafast, Boston, MA, USA), and KI-67 (1:100, Abcam, Cambridge, UK). Secondary antibodies against mouse (α-SMA) and rabbit (pSMAD2, pSMAD1/5/8, and KI-67) were used. Negative controls were performed by omitting the primary antibody. Antigen retrieval with citric acid buffer (pH 6.0) was used. Negative controls were performed by omitting the primary antibody.

Immunoblotting
Snap-frozen right lung lobes were homogenized on ice in Carin buffer (20 mM Tris pH 8.0, 137 mM NaCl, 10 mM EDTA, 1% NP40, 10% glycerol), containing protease inhibitor Complete (Roche, Basel, Switzerland). Samples were centrifuged at 14,200 r.p.m. for 15 min and protein concentration in the supernatant was measured using the Bradford method. Subsequently 50 μg of protein per lane was loaded onto an SDS-PAGE and transferred to nitrocellulose membranes using wet blotting. Antigens were detected with TGFβ (1:1,000, Abcam), pSMAD2 (1:1,000, Cell Signaling), SMAD2 (1:1,000, Cell Signaling), pSMAD5 (1:1,000, Abcam), SMAD5 (1:1,000, Cell Signaling), and Zeb2 [1:1,000, (21)]. Cofilin (1:400, Abcam) and β-actin (1:1,000, Cell Signaling) were used for loading control.

Statistical Analyses
Data are presented as percentages, means (SD) for normally distributed variables. Univariate analyses were performed using independent samples t-tests for normally distributed variables. The analyses were performed using SPSS 21.0 for Windows (Armonk, NY, USA: IBM Corp.). All statistical tests were two-sided and used a significance level of 0.05.

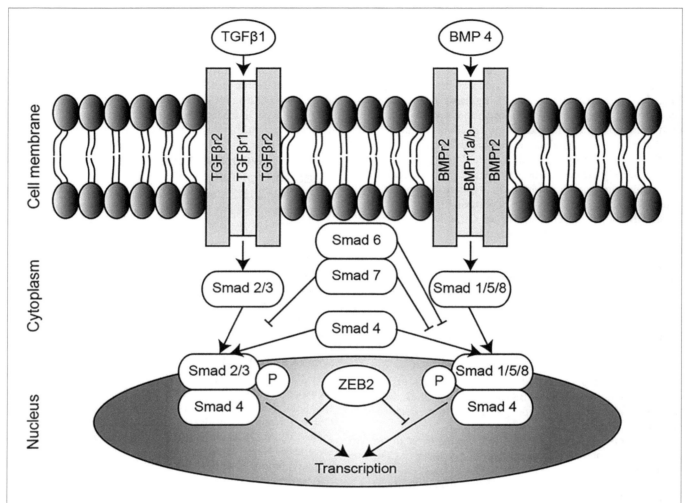

FIGURE 1 | Overview of TGFβ/BMP pathway. Overview of the TGFβ and BMP pathways. TGFβ, transforming growth factor β; BMP, bone morphogenetic protein; ZEB2, zinc finger E-box binding homeobox 2; P, phosphorylation.

RESULTS

TGFβ Activation Is Upregulated in CDH

The expression of key signaling factors in the TGFβ pathway was assessed in whole lung homogenates at the mRNA level, where an increase in the abundance of mRNA transcript encoding both *Tgfbr1* and *Tgfbr2* receptors, but no difference in the abundance of the ligand *Tgfb1* mRNA transcript was noted. The abundance of mRNA transcripts encoding both the receptor-activated SMADs, *Smad2*, and *Smad3*, as well as the co-SMAD, *Smad4*, which together form a signaling complex for translocation into the cell nucleus, was increased in CDH (**Figure 2A**). No differences were found in expression of the TGFβ1 ligand at the protein level (**Figure 2B**). For the activation of the TGFβ pathway, receptor-activated SMADs must be phosphorylated. The degree of phosphorylation of SMAD2 was not different in whole lung homogenates of CDH pups compared to controls (**Figure 2C**). Since the abnormalities in the pulmonary vasculature are key pathological hallmarks of CDH, changes in SMAD phosphorylation were assessed in the small pulmonary vessels (25–50 μm) using immunofluorescence staining. This approach revealed an increased number of smooth muscle actin (SMA)-positive cells in the small vessels of CDH pups expressing phosphorylated SMAD2 (pSMAD2), which points to an increased activation of this pathway in the pulmonary vasculature (**Figure 2D**).

BMP Activation Is Reduced in CDH

In contrast to the TGFβ receptors, a decrease in *Bmpr1b* mRNA transcript abundance was noted in CDH, while no differences in the abundance of the well-studied *Bmpr2* were noted, comparing both groups at mRNA level in whole lung homogenates. Activin receptor-like kinase 1 (*Alk1*), another receptor in the BMP/TGFβ pathway which mediates the signal of *Bmp9* and *Bmp10*, was slightly increased in CDH. *Bmp4*, one of the important ligands in this pathway, and the receptor-activated *Smad1* and *Smad5* showed an increase in CDH (**Figure 3A**). Western blot on whole lung homogenates showed a decreased

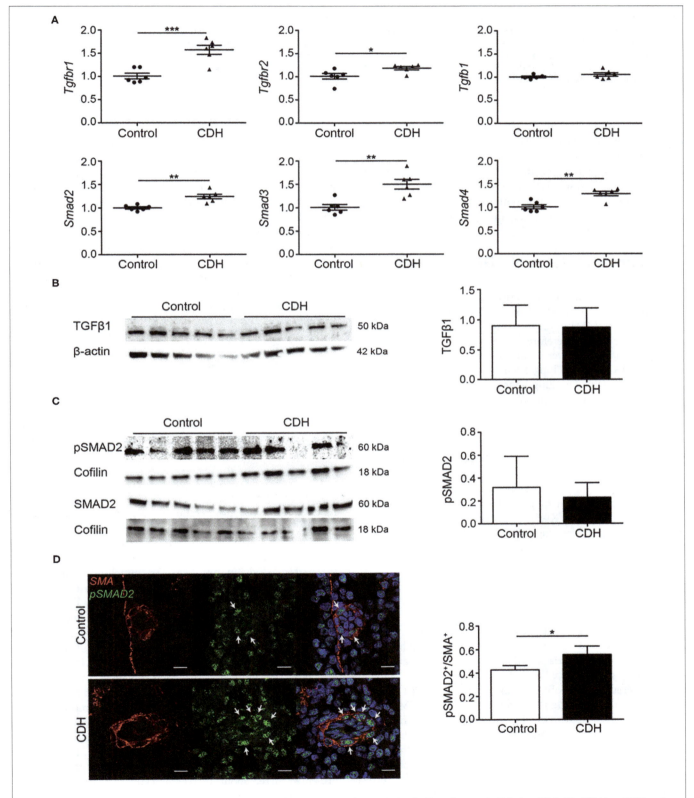

FIGURE 2 | TGFβ activation is upregulated in experimental CDH. (A) Quantitative PCR revealed a significant increase in *Tgfbr1* and *Tgfbr2* in CDH ($p < 0.001$ and $p = 0.033$, respectively), but no difference in *Tgfb1* mRNA transcript abundance compared to control. The abundance of *Smad2*, *Smad3*, and *Smad4* mRNA

(Continued)

FIGURE 2 | transcripts were all significantly higher in CDH ($p = 0.001$, $p = 0.002$, and $p = 0.002$, respectively; $n = 6$ for both groups). **(B)** Western blot on whole lung homogenates revealed no differences in TGFβ1 abundance between control and CDH, when normalized to total protein amount using β-actin as a loading control ($n = 5$ for both groups). **(C)** The abundance of pSMAD2 was related to the total SMAD2 protein levels, which was not different between control and CDH in whole lung homogenates, where Cofilin was used as a loading control ($n = 5$ for both groups). **(D)** Representative images of immunofluorescence staining indicate an increase in the ratio of pSMAD2/SMA double-positive cells in small pulmonary vessels in CDH ($p = 0.049$; $n = 3$ samples for both groups). Six vessels per sample were counted. Scale bars represent 10 μm. *$p < 0.05$, **$p < 0.01$, ***$p < 0.001$. Error bars represent SD.

expression of SMAD5 in CDH with no differences in relative phosphorylation (**Figure 3B**). However, when focusing on the important pulmonary vasculature, the number of SMA positive cells expressing phosphorylated SMAD1/5/8 was reduced in CDH on immunofluorescence staining, indicating a decreased activation of this pathway in the pulmonary vasculature (**Figure 3C**).

Downstream Effects of TGFβ and BMP Signaling

Both the TGFβ and BMP pathways can be inhibited by the inhibitory SMADs, SMAD6, and SMAD7. These proteins compete with SMAD4 in the formation of heteromeric signaling complexes and can, therefore, prevent transcription of target genes. No differences were noted in the expression of *Smad6* at the mRNA level, but lung *Smad7* transcript abundance was increased in CDH. The lung abundance of mRNA transcripts encoding *Zeb2*, a transcriptional corepressor of the activated pathway, were increases in CDH at the mRNA level (**Figure 4A**). However, no significant differences in protein levels of ZEB2 were noted by western blot analysis of whole lung homogenates (**Figure 4B**), and no changes in the expression of ZEB2 were noted in the small vessels using immunohistochemistry (**Figure 4C**). Since increased activation of the TGFβ pathway can induce proliferation of pulmonary artery smooth muscle cells, the expression of KI-67, a marker for proliferation, was used to identify proliferating cells in the vascular wall. In small pulmonary vessels in CDH, more SMA-positive cells expressed KI-67 (**Figures 4D,E**).

DISCUSSION

In this report, upregulated activation of the TGFβ pathway and downregulated activation of the BMP pathway in small pulmonary vessels in the nitrofen-CDH rat model are demonstrated at the cellular level.

No differences were observed in the ligand TGFβ1 and the degree of phosphorylation of both SMAD2 and SMAD5 at the protein level in whole lung homogenates. Although the total amount of SMAD5 and pSMAD5 was less in whole lung homogenates of CDH pups, no changes were noted in the degree of phosphorylation in total lung extracts. At the cellular level, however, the smooth muscle layer of the small pulmonary vessels of nitrofen-CDH pups revealed increased abundance of pSMAD2 and decreased abundance of pSMAD1/5/8, indicative of more active TGFβ signaling and reduced BMP signaling, respectively.

The latter is in line with Makenga and colleagues who reported decreased pSMAD1/5/8 in CDH lung homogenates. Moreover, the differences observed in the small pulmonary arteries in CDH lungs may also reflect the fact that the perivascular cells in CDH lungs are more differentiated compared to perivascular cells in control lungs (22).

Phosphorylation of the receptor-activated SMADs is necessary for the activation of downstream mediators and, therefore, plays an important role in pathway activation. The increased expression of the inhibitory *Smad7* and corepressor *Zeb2* at the mRNA level is in line with SMAD7 being a direct target of ZEB2 and may point to increased production of these inhibitors in order to inhibit the increased activity of the TGFβ pathway (23). The absence of any observed changes in *Smad6*, which only inhibits the BMP pathway, strengthens this idea. However, the expression of ZEB2 at the protein level in whole lung homogenates exhibited a trend toward an increase, and no differences were noted by immunostaining of the pulmonary vessels, indicating a discrepancy between RNA and protein expression. The latter could, in part, explain differences between several reports on TGFβ and BMP signaling in CDH. Moreover, the usage of specific parts of the lung or isolated lung cells may also lead to differences or even opposing results between different reports. Both TGFβ and BMP can regulate proliferation of vascular cells and previous studies have reported increased proliferation of pulmonary artery smooth muscle cells from patients with PAH in response to TGFβ1 (24, 25). The increased proliferation of constituent cells of the smooth muscle layer of small pulmonary vessels was noted in the present study in nitrofen-CDH pup lungs, which might indicate an abnormal response of these cells to the increased TGFβ activity.

TGFβ is a target of retinoic acid (RA) (26), and increased activity of the TGFβ pathway with higher levels of pSMAD2 has been described in RA-deficient foreguts, and in a mouse model with RA deficiency. In that study, lung agenesis was observed both by decreasing RA levels as well as by increasing TGFβ levels, indicating the interaction between both pathways early in development (27). Furthermore, a study in rats with alveolar hypoplasia caused by caloric restriction exhibited improvement of alveolar formation after treatment with RA, accompanied by a decrease in TGFβ activity at postnatal day 21 (28). These findings strengthen the results presented here, about increased TGFβ activity in nitrofen-exposed rats, where nitrofen has been reported to disrupt the retinoid signaling pathway (29). Since a reduction in retinol and retinol binding protein (RBP) has been found in human

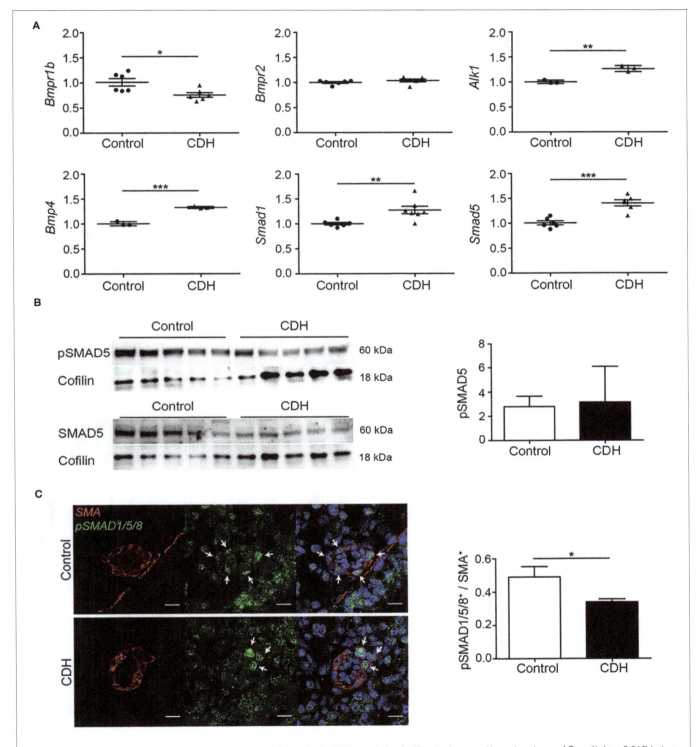

FIGURE 3 | BMP activation is reduced in experimental CDH. (A) Quantitative PCR revealed a significantly decreased lung abundance of Bmpr1b ($p = 0.016$) but no differences in Bmpr2, and increased abundance of Alk1 ($p = 0.003$) mRNA transcripts in CDH compared to control. The abundance of Bmp4, Smad1, and Smad5 mRNA transcripts was significantly higher in CDH [$p < 0.001$, $p = 0.009$, and $p < 0.001$, respectively; $n = 3$ (Alk1 and Bmp4) or 6 (rest) for both groups]. (B) The lung abundance of pSMAD5 was related to the total SMAD5 protein abundance, which was not different between control and CDH samples, where Cofilin was used as a loading control ($n = 5$ for both groups). (C) Representative images of immunofluorescence staining indicate a decrease in the ratio of pSMAD1/5/8/ SMA double-positive cells in small pulmonary vessels in CDH lungs ($p = 0.016$; $n = 3$ samples for both groups). Six vessels per sample were counted. Scale bars represent 10 μm. *$p < 0.05$, **$p < 0.01$, ***$p < 0.001$. Error bars represent SD.

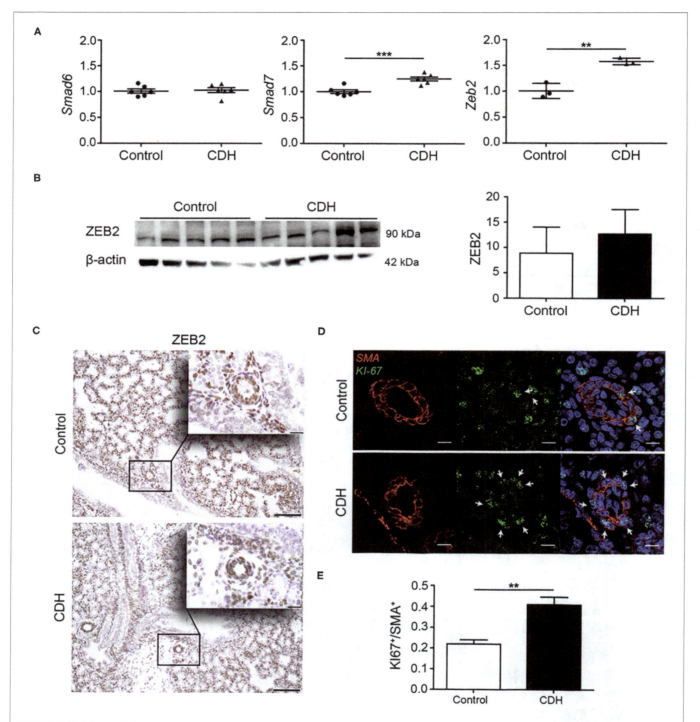

FIGURE 4 | Modulators of TGFβ signaling are upregulated in CDH. (A) Quantitative PCR revealed no difference in the abundance of the inhibitory *Smad6* mRNA transcript, but increased abundance of inhibitory *Smad7* and *Zeb2* mRNA transcripts [$p < 0.001$ and $p = 0.003$, respectively; $n = 3$ (*Zeb2*) or 6 (*Smad6*, *Smad7*) per group; y-axis indicated fold-change]. (B) Western blot analyses of whole lung homogenates revealed no significant differences in ZEB2 protein abundance comparing CDH and control groups, where β-actin was used as a loading control, and as a reference for quantification ($n = 5$ for both groups). (C) Representative images of immunohistochemistry staining show no differences in expression of ZEB2 in the small vessels of all lungs ($n = 3$ samples for both groups). Scale bars represent 100 μm (low power) and 20 μm (high power). **$p < 0.01$, ***$p < 0.001$. Error bars represent SD. (D) Increased proliferation of the muscular vessel wall in CDH. Representative images of immunofluorescence staining revealed an increase in KI-67/SMA double-positive cells in small pulmonary vessels in CDH ($p = 0.001$; $n = 3$ samples for both groups). (E) Quantification of proliferative SMA+ cells. Four vessels per sample were counted. Scale bars represent 10 μm. **$p < 0.01$, ***$p < 0.001$. Error bars represent SD.

newborns with CDH (30, 31), and several key components of the RA pathway are affected in human and experimental CDH (32), the increased activity of the TGFβ pathway might play an important role in the development of the lungs in CDH.

Studies available in the literature have reported conflicting trends in expression of different signaling factors in CDH, which might be explained by the differences in the gestation of the animals under study. In the present study, some variability between samples was also noted, suggesting that small differences in gestational age may have an appreciable impact on trends in the expression of signaling molecules under study.

We initially analyzed the TGF-β and BMP pathways in whole lungs, and given our previous report on vascular abnormalities in CDH (22), we focused on the activation of the TGF-β and BMP pathways in the vasculature, using immunofluorescence staining, showing a clearly difference in phosphorylation of SMAD2 and SMAD5.

In conclusion, increased phosphorylation of SMAD2 and decreased phosphorylation of SMAD5 was noted in the in the vessel walls of small pulmonary vessels of nitrofen-CDH pups. These data indicate increased activation of the TGFβ pathway and decreased activation of the BMP pathway in the pulmonary vasculature of these animals at day 21 of gestation, possibly leading to increased proliferation of the muscularized vessel wall. Since the different factors in these pathways are differently expressed during gestation and might differ from the human situation, further research must be conducted at different developmental stages, and most importantly, in material of human patients.

AUTHOR CONTRIBUTIONS

DT, RM, and RR: conceptualization and writing—original draft. DM, MB-vK, RM, and RR: data curation. DM, MB-vK, and RR: formal analysis and methodology. RM and RR: funding acquisition and supervision. DM and MB-vK: investigation and validation. DT and RW: resources. DM, MB-vK, RW, DT, RM, and RR: writing—review and editing. All authors contributed to the article and approved the submitted version.

ACKNOWLEDGMENTS

This manuscript was in part included in the dissertation of DSM, and is archived online at Erasmus University Rotterdam's institutional repository (33).

REFERENCES

1. Sluiter I, van der Horst I, van der Voorn P, Boerema-de Munck A, Buscop-van Kempen M, de Krijger R, et al. Premature differentiation of vascular smooth muscle cells in human congenital diaphragmatic hernia. *Exp Mol Pathol.* (2013) 94:195–202. doi: 10.1016/j.yexmp.2012.09.010

2. Ma L, Chung WK. The role of genetics in pulmonary arterial hypertension. *J Pathol.* (2017) 241:273–80. doi: 10.1002/path.4833

3. Alejandre-Alcazar MA, Michiels-Corsten M, Vicencio AG, Reiss I, Ryu J, de Krijger RR, et al. TGF-beta signaling is dynamically regulated during the alveolarization of rodent and human lungs. *Dev Dyn.* (2008) 237:259–69. doi: 10.1002/dvdy.21403

4. Chen H, Sun J, Buckley S, Chen C, Warburton D, Wang XF, et al. Abnormal mouse lung alveolarization caused by Smad3 deficiency is a developmental antecedent of centrilobular emphysema. *Am J Physiol Lung Cell Mol Physiol.* (2005) 288:L683–91. doi: 10.1152/ajplung.00298.2004

5. Eickelberg O, Morty RE. Transforming growth factor beta/bone morphogenic protein signaling in pulmonary arterial hypertension: remodeling revisited. *Trends Cardiovasc Med.* (2007) 17:263–9. doi: 10.1016/j.tcm.2007.09.003

6. Teramoto H, Shinkai M, Puri P. Altered expression of angiotensin II receptor subtypes and transforming growth factor-beta in the heart of nitrofen-induced diaphragmatic hernia in rats. *Pediatr Surg Int.* (2005) 21:148–52. doi: 10.1007/s00383-004-1311-7

7. Xu C, Liu W, Chen Z, Wang Y, Xiong Z, Ji Y. Effect of prenatal tetrandrine administration on transforming growth factor-beta1 level in the lung of nitrofen-induced congenital diaphragmatic hernia rat model. *J Pediatr Surg.* (2009) 44:1611–20. doi: 10.1016/j.jpedsurg.2008.09.021

8. Vuckovic A, Herber-Jonat S, Flemmer AW, Ruehl IM, Votino C, Segers V, et al. Increased TGF-beta: a drawback of tracheal occlusion in human and experimental congenital diaphragmatic hernia? *Am J Physiol Lung Cell Mol Physiol.* (2016) 310:L311–27. doi: 10.1152/ajplung.00122.2015

9. Candilera V, Bouche C, Schleef J, Pederiva F. Lung growth factors in the amniotic fluid of normal pregnancies and with congenital diaphragmatic hernia. *J Matern Fetal Neonatal Med.* (2016) 29:2104–8. doi: 10.3109/14767058.2015.1076387

10. Zimmer J, Takahashi T, Hofmann AD, Puri P. Decreased Endoglin expression in the pulmonary vasculature of nitrofen-induced congenital diaphragmatic hernia rat model. *Pediatr Surg Int.* (2017) 33:263–8. doi: 10.1007/s00383-016-4004-0

11. Gosemann JH, Friedmacher F, Fujiwara N, Alvarez LA, Corcionivoschi N, Puri P. Disruption of the bone morphogenetic protein receptor 2 pathway in nitrofen-induced congenital diaphragmatic hernia. *Birth Defects Res B Dev Reprod Toxicol.* (2013) 98:304–9. doi: 10.1002/bdrb.21065

12. Makanga M, Dewachter C, Maruyama H, Vuckovic A, Rondelet B, Naeije R, et al. Downregulated bone morphogenetic protein signaling in nitrofen-induced congenital diaphragmatic hernia. *Pediatr Surg Int.* (2013) 29:823–34. doi: 10.1007/s00383-013-3340-6

13. Emmerton-Coughlin HM, Martin KK, Chiu JS, Zhao L, Scott LA, Regnault TR, et al. BMP4 and LGL1 are down regulated in an ovine model of congenital diaphragmatic hernia. *Front Surg.* (2014) 1:44. doi: 10.3389/fsurg.2014.00044

14. Hofmann AD, Friedmacher F, Takahashi H, Hunziker M, Gosemann JH, Puri P. Decreased apelin and apelin-receptor expression in the pulmonary vasculature of nitrofen-induced congenital diaphragmatic hernia. *Pediatr Surg Int.* (2014) 30:197–203. doi: 10.1007/s00383-013-3450-1

15. Hofmann AD, Zimmer J, Takahashi T, Gosemann JH, Puri P. The role of activin receptor-like kinase 1 signaling in the pulmonary vasculature of experimental diaphragmatic hernia. *Eur J Pediatr Surg.* (2016) 26:106–11. doi: 10.1055/s-0035-1566105

16. Corbett HJ, Connell MG, Fernig DG, Losty PD, Jesudason EC. ANG-1 TIE-2 and BMPR signalling defects are not seen in the nitrofen model of pulmonary hypertension and congenital diaphragmatic hernia. *PLoS ONE.* (2012) 7:e35364. doi: 10.1371/journal.pone.0035364

17. Chiu JS, Ma L, Wynn J, Krishnan U, Rosenzweig EB, Aspelund G, et al. Mutations in BMPR2 are not present in patients with pulmonary hypertension associated with congenital diaphragmatic hernia. *J Pediatr Surg.* (2017) 52:1747–50. doi: 10.1016/j.jpedsurg.2017.01.007

18. Mous DS, Kool HM, Burgisser PE, Buscop-van Kempen MJ, Nagata K, Boerema-de Munck A, et al. Treatment of rat congenital diaphragmatic hernia with sildenafil and NS-304, selexipag's active compound, at

the pseudoglandular stage improves lung vasculature. *Am J Physiol Lung Cell Mol Physiol.* (2018) 315:L276–85. doi: 10.1152/ajplung.00392.2017

19. Mous DS, Kool HM, Buscop-van Kempen MJ, Koning AH, Dzyubachyk O, Wijnen RM, et al. Clinically relevant timing of antenatal sildenafil treatment reduces pulmonary vascular remodeling in congenital diaphragmatic hernia. *Am J Physiol Lung Cell Mol Physiol.* (2016) 311:L734–42. doi: 10.1152/ajplung.00180.2016

20. Rajatapiti P, van der Horst IW, de Rooij JD, Tran MG, Maxwell PH, Tibboel D, et al. Expression of hypoxia-inducible factors in normal human lung development. *Pediatr Dev Pathol.* (2008) 11:193–9. doi: 10.2350/07-04-0257.1

21. Seuntjens E, Nityanandam A, Miquelajauregui A, Debruyn J, Stryjewska A, Goebbels S, et al. Sip1 regulates sequential fate decisions by feedback signaling from postmitotic neurons to progenitors. *Nat Neurosci.* (2009) 12:1373–80. doi: 10.1038/nn.2409

22. Kool HM, Burgisser PE, Edel GG, de Kleer I, Boerema-de Munck A, de Laat I, et al. Inhibition of retinoic acid signaling induces aberrant pericyte coverage and differentiation resulting in vascular defects in congenital diaphragmatic hernia. *Am J Physiol Lung Cell Mol Physiol.* (2019) 317:L317–31. doi: 10.1152/ajplung.00104.2018

23. Weng Q, Chen Y, Wang H, Xu X, Yang B, He Q, et al. Dual-mode modulation of Smad signaling by Smad-interacting protein Sip1 is required for myelination in the central nervous system. *Neuron.* (2012) 73:713–28. doi: 10.1016/j.neuron.2011.12.021

24. Morrell NW, Yang X, Upton PD, Jourdan KB, Morgan N, Sheares KK, et al. Altered growth responses of pulmonary artery smooth muscle cells from patients with primary pulmonary hypertension to transforming growth factor-beta(1) and bone morphogenetic proteins. *Circulation.* (2001) 104:790–5. doi: 10.1161/hc3201.094152

25. Thomas M, Docx C, Holmes AM, Beach S, Duggan N, England K, et al. Activin-like kinase 5 (ALK5) mediates abnormal proliferation of vascular smooth muscle cells from patients with familial pulmonary arterial hypertension and is involved in the progression of experimental pulmonary arterial hypertension induced by monocrotaline. *Am J Pathol.* (2009) 174:380–9. doi: 10.2353/ajpath.2009.080565

26. Balmer JE, Blomhoff R. Gene expression regulation by retinoic acid. *J Lipid Res.* (2002) 43:1773–808. doi: 10.1194/jlr.R100015-JLR200

27. Chen F, Desai TJ, Qian J, Niederreither K, Lu J, Cardoso WV. Inhibition of Tgf beta signaling by endogenous retinoic acid is essential for primary lung bud induction. *Development.* (2007) 134:2969–79. doi: 10.1242/dev.006221

28. Londhe VA, Maisonet TM, Lopez B, Shin BC, Huynh J, Devaskar SU. Retinoic acid rescues alveolar hypoplasia in the calorie-restricted developing rat lung. *Am J Respir Cell Mol Biol.* (2013) 48:179–87. doi: 10.1165/rcmb.2012-0229OC

29. Beurskens N, Klaassens M, Rottier R, de Klein A, Tibboel D. Linking animal models to human congenital diaphragmatic hernia. *Birth Defects Res A Clin Mol Teratol.* (2007) 79:565–72. doi: 10.1002/bdra.20370

30. Beurskens LW, Tibboel D, Lindemans J, Duvekot JJ, Cohen-Overbeek TE, Veenma DC, et al. Retinol status of newborn infants is associated with congenital diaphragmatic hernia. *Pediatrics.* (2010) 126:712–20. doi: 10.1542/peds.2010-0521

31. Major D, Cadenas M, Fournier L, Leclerc S, Lefebvre M, Cloutier R. Retinol status of newborn infants with congenital diaphragmatic hernia. *Pediatr Surg Int.* (1998) 13:547–9. doi: 10.1007/s003830050399

32. Coste K, Beurskens LW, Blanc P, Gallot D, Delabaere A, Blanchon L, et al. Metabolic disturbances of the vitamin A pathway in human diaphragmatic hernia. *Am J Physiol Lung Cell Mol Physiol.* (2015) 308:L147–57. doi: 10.1152/ajplung.00108.2014

33. Mous DS. *Pulmonary Vascular Defects in Congenital Diaphragmatic Hernia: the Quest for Early Factors and Intervention.* Dissertation. Rotterdam: Erasmus University (2017).

3

An Experimental Model of Bronchopulmonary Dysplasia Features Long-Term Retinal and Pulmonary Defects but not Sustained Lung Inflammation

Lakshanie C. Wickramasinghe[1], Peter van Wijngaarden[2,3], Chad Johnson[4], Evelyn Tsantikos[1] and Margaret L. Hibbs[1]*

[1] Leukocyte Signalling Laboratory, Department of Immunology and Pathology, Central Clinical School, Monash University, Melbourne, VIC, Australia, [2] Department of Surgery - Ophthalmology, University of Melbourne, Melbourne, VIC, Australia, [3] Centre for Eye Research Australia, Royal Victorian Eye and Ear Hospital, East Melbourne, VIC, Australia, [4] Monash Micro Imaging, Alfred Research Alliance, Monash University, Melbourne, VIC, Australia

*Correspondence:
Margaret L. Hibbs
margaret.hibbs@monash.edu

Bronchopulmonary dysplasia (BPD) is a severe lung disease that affects preterm infants receiving oxygen therapy. No standardized, clinically-relevant BPD model exists, hampering efforts to understand and treat this disease. This study aimed to evaluate and confirm a candidate model of acute and chronic BPD, based on exposure of neonatal mice to a high oxygen environment during key lung developmental stages affected in preterm infants with BPD. Neonatal C57BL/6 mouse pups were exposed to 75% oxygen from postnatal day (PN)-1 for 5, 8, or 14 days, and their lungs were examined at PN14 and PN40. While all mice showed some degree of lung damage, mice exposed to hyperoxia for 8 or 14 days exhibited the greatest septal wall thickening and airspace enlargement. Furthermore, when assessed at PN40, mice exposed for 8 or 14 days to supplemental oxygen exhibited augmented septal wall thickness and emphysema, with the severity increased with the longer exposure, which translated into a decline in respiratory function at PN80 in the 14-day model. In addition to this, mice exposed to hyperoxia for 8 days showed significant expansion of alveolar epithelial type II cells as well as the greatest fibrosis when assessed at PN40 suggesting a healing response, which was not seen in mice exposed to high oxygen for a longer period. While evidence of lung inflammation was apparent at PN14, chronic inflammation was absent from all three models. Finally, exposure to high oxygen for 14 days also induced concurrent outer retinal degeneration. This study shows that early postnatal exposure to high oxygen generates hallmark acute and chronic pathologies in mice that highlights its use as a translational model of BPD.

Keywords: bronchopulmonary dysplasia, lung development, inflammation, animal model, supplemental oxygen, chronic obstructive pulmonary disease, retinopathy of prematurity, choroidal thinning

INTRODUCTION

Bronchopulmonary dysplasia (BPD) is the most common respiratory disorder affecting premature infants provided long-term oxygen therapy and respiratory support (1). Advancements in neonatal care have improved the survival of severely premature infants born earlier in gestation; however, the incidence of BPD has remained unchanged over the last decade (2). Surfactant therapy and corticosteroid treatments, in concert with less invasive respiratory support, have helped transform the lung phenotype observed in "old BPD" from extensive parenchymal fibrosis, interstitial edema and severe inflammation to a milder lung pathology observed in infants born today (3). The lung phenotype observed in infants that come into the neonatal intensive care unit (NICU) nowadays is characterized by impaired alveolar and vascular development and mild inflammation and fibrosis. Of greatest concern, is the capacity of this disease to progress into severe lung complications by adulthood, including reduced exercise capacity (4), childhood and adolescent asthma (5), and in serious cases, the development of chronic obstructive pulmonary disease (COPD) (6, 7).

Numerous high oxygen schemes have been used to model BPD in rodents. These models have contributed to our understanding of mechanisms responsible for the development of this condition, such as the role of oxidative stress and inflammation (8), and they have replicated some of the histological aberrations that occur within the human neonatal lung following the routine use of supplemental oxygen in the clinical setting (9). However, despite these findings, no single experimental model is used consistently. Previous models have used varying concentrations and durations of oxygen exposure. In most cases, there is no rationale for why a particular model was selected over others and whether concurrent changes in other tissues occur and disease persists into adulthood. Therefore, having a standardized experimental protocol of oxygen-induced BPD would limit the variability in data output between studies and most importantly, minimize discrepancies when trialing potential therapeutic candidates (10–12).

In previous studies, supraphysiological levels of oxygen (85–100%) have been administered over a long period of time (13, 14). Such high concentrations have been shown to increase the susceptibility to respiratory infections when recovering in room air (13). In addition, some mouse strains, such as FVB/N, are more susceptible to oxygen toxicity than others and therefore, sublethal oxygen concentrations can result in exaggerated lung pathology or in severe cases, death of mice in the litter (14). Even with the use of lower oxygen concentrations (40–65%), the length of oxygen exposure can also generate varying degrees of lung damage (15, 16). For instance, the use of oxygen concentrations as low as 40% administered over 7 days in the postnatal period has been shown to trigger a reduction in the total number of alveoli and an increase in respiratory resistance (15). Similarly, an oxygen concentration of 65% delivered over 1 month has also been shown to impair alveolar structure (16). In a 2015 review, it was noted that in a 30-month period alone, there were 41 publications that used different strategies to model BPD, highlighting the need to establish a model that would provide consistency and standardization across neonatal respiratory research studies (12). More recently, a comprehensive multi-model study tested oxygen concentrations of 40, 60, and 80% over 14 days, as well as a 24 h oscillating exposure that ranged from 85 to 40% (15). This study found that the use of 85% oxygen for 7 or 14 days from birth caused the most lung damage, inducing septal wall thickness and alveolar enlargement (15), which are two key features of "new" BPD. However, lung inflammation and fibrosis were not examined in this study, with the extent of both being an important distinguishing feature between the "old" form of BPD and "new" BPD. In addition, the long-term consequence of early life oxygen-induced injury in the adult period was not investigated, which is an essential component of any BPD model to aid in the understanding of the deleterious effect of oxygen therapy on long-term sequelae in the lung. Another important consideration is the capacity of a BPD model to induce concurrent retinal damage, given that in a clinical setting, retinopathy of prematurity (ROP) frequently presents as a co-morbidity of BPD (17). Therefore, an oxygen protocol modeling BPD that could also incite the development of other neonatal diseases that affect a preterm infant could enhance the clinical relevance of the model, as well as its pre-clinical utility.

The appearance of the alveolar deformities associated with BPD is largely connected with the interruption to normal lung development (8). This is almost certainly due to the fact that the majority of premature babies are born during the final two stages of lung organogenesis—the saccular and alveolar stages—the time at which they receive oxygen therapy. The saccular stage prepares the lung for life outside of the womb, with the formation of primitive alveoli called saccules and production of surfactants in cuboidal alveolar cells (18–20). Simultaneously, microvascular maturation in the parenchyma leads to the thinning of the double capillary layer into a single layer, necessary to meet the respiratory requirements of the growing fetus (18, 21, 22). In the final alveolar stage of organogenesis, the saccules undergo rapid subdivision (secondary septation) into smaller gas-exchange units called alveoli, expanding the gas-exchange surface area (23, 24). In mice, the saccular stage of lung development occurs in the first 5 days after birth, which is ordinarily complete in full-term infants (25). Thus, the fact that the last two lung developmental stages occur post-birth in mice renders mice an excellent experimental tool for BPD studies.

The purpose of this study was to validate whether acute high oxygen exposure received during key periods of lung development would lead to long-term pulmonary changes. Given that the aforementioned multi-model study only assessed lung damage at day 14, in this study, we have focused on evaluating different parameters of lung pathology that may arise in adulthood, and unlike other multi-model studies, the assessment of outer retinal changes as a common co-morbidity of BPD were also prioritized in this study. Herein, we demonstrate that prolonged oxygen exposure in early neonatal life leads to sustained alveolar deterioration in adulthood, as well as defects in retinal tissue, and therefore is a suitable model for early and later life studies of BPD and research into the long-term impact of oxygen toxicity to the eye.

MATERIALS AND METHODS

Experimental Models

C57BL/6 mice were used for this study and were purchased from Alfred Animal Services at the Alfred Research Alliance. Neonatal mice together with their dam, in litter sizes of 6–7 pups (to control for maternal nutrition), were exposed to 75% oxygen within 12 h of birth (defined as PN1) up to PN5, PN8, or PN14, and were cycled with 21% oxygen (room air) for 3 h per day to prevent oxygen toxicity to the dam (17). Following exposure, the mice were returned to room air and lungs were analyzed on PN14, PN40, and PN80. Neonatal pups and dams housed under room air conditions in the same experimental room, served as age-matched controls. All experiments were performed in accordance with National Health and Medical Research Council of Australia (NH&MRC) guidelines for animal experimentation, with ethics approval granted from the Alfred Research Alliance Animal Ethics Committee (experimental approval number: E/1746/2017/M).

Lung Histology and Immunohistochemistry

On PN14, PN40, and PN80, postmortem lungs were inflation-fixed with 10% neutral buffered formalin at 25 cm water pressure, embedded in paraffin and sectioned by microtome at 5 μm thickness prior to staining. Lung sections were stained with Hematoxylin and Eosin (H&E) or Picrosirius Red (PR). H&E stained sections were imaged using an Olympus BX-51 bright field microscope equipped with a DP-70 color camera and 10x and 40x objectives (Olympus Corporation, Tokyo, Japan). Quantitation of alveolar airspace diameter and septal wall thickness was determined using the mean linear intercept method and alveolar septal wall thickness technique, as previously described (17). Investigators were blinded to experimental groups. PR-stained sections were scanned using the Aperio ScanScope CS (Leica Biosystems, Wetzlar, Germany) whole slide scanner at 8x and 4x magnification. Images were uploaded into ImageJ Analysis software (1.37 (NIH, Bethesda, MD; http://imagej.nih.gov/ij) and analyzed using a published script (17) with minor modifications as follows. The script used a pre-defined color threshold (set by eye) to isolate the PR signal and created a binarized image, which was measured for area. A similar method was then used to threshold the background of the tissue, in order for the total tissue area within the image to be calculated. These results were used to calculate the % PR-stained area within the tissue.

For immunohistochemistry, deparaffinized sections underwent antigen-retrieval with DAKO Target Retrieval Solution (DAKO Corp, CA, USA). Sections were blocked for 30 min with 5% BSA and incubated for 3 h at room temperature with 1:500 dilution of anti-mouse CD45 (rabbit IgG, catalog; ab10558, Abcam, Cam, UK) to stain all immune cells. Control sections had primary antibody substituted with PBS. Staining was revealed by incubation with 1:500 HRP-conjugated secondary antibody (goat anti-rabbit IgG H+L, catalog; ab205718, Abcam, Cam, UK) for 1 h and color development with diaminobenzidine chromogen solution (Agilent, CA, USA). Slides were counterstained with hematoxylin. Cells expressing CD45 were labeled brown, while negative cells were stained blue. Four randomly selected microscopic fields (40x) of lung tissue per mouse were used to calculate the percentage of CD45 positive cells/total cells as described (17). On separate lung sections, type II alveolar epithelial cells (AEC-II) were detected by staining for Pro-SPC using a previously described method (26). AEC-II's were labeled with anti-mouse Pro-SPC (rabbit IgG, 1:500, catalog ab90716: Abcam, Cam, UK), followed by red fluorescent secondary antibody (AF568 donkey anti-rabbit IgG (H+L), 1:1,000, catalog ab175693; Abcam, Cam, UK). Control sections had secondary antibody only incubated to test for non-specific binding. Stained cells were imaged using a Nikon A1r inverted confocal microscope (Nikon Corporation, Tokyo, Japan). Two large scanned images at 20x magnification were taken at two randomly selected lung sites and analyzed using a bespoke ImageJ script (**Supplementary Table 1**). Briefly, quantitation of AEC-II numbers was conducted with the aid of a DAPI nuclear stain as well as the overall background fluorescence to segment a field of individual cells and create regions of interest (ROIs) for each fluorescent marker. These ROIs were then used to determine if each cell was positive for a specific color based on a user defined pixel intensity threshold for each channel set up at the start of the script.

Lung Function Assessment

At PN80, mice were anesthetized by intraperitoneal injection of 125 mg/kg of Ketamine and 10 mg/kg Xylazine (Centravet, FR). Following confirmation of deep anesthesia, mice underwent tracheostomy and a 19G cannula was inserted before being connected to an animal ventilator (Flexivent, SCIREQ, CA). Mice were mechanically ventilated (150 breaths/min, tidal volume 10 ml/kg) and a positive end-expiratory pressure (PEEP) was set at 3 cm H_2O. The flexiware software (v8.0.4) was used to perform respiratory system mechanics, as previously detailed (27). A negative pressure-driven forced expiratory (NPFE) maneuver was performed to generate the flow-volume loop used to calculate the forced expired volume over 0.1 s (FEV0.1) and forced vital capacity (FVC), which were used to determine the ratio between FEV0.1/FVC as a clinical measure of lung performance. Three independent measurements were taken for all perturbations for each mouse and the average was calculated.

Eye Histology

Paraffin-embedded eyes were sectioned at 3 μm thickness and every 20th section was stained with H&E. Four photomicrographs (x10) of each cross-section were captured across the full circumference of the eye and the average diameter (in μm) per section for each eye was determined to obtain choroidal thickness as previously described (17). Investigators were masked to the experimental groups.

Statistical Analysis

Values are presented as median ± IQR. Results from individual models were compared to the room air controls using the non-parametric unpaired T-test (Mann-Whitney) in GraphPad Prism software (version 4.03, SD, USA); $P < 0.05$ was considered statistically significant. Unmarked bars on figures indicate that no significance was achieved.

RESULTS

Body Weight Gain Is Affected in Mice Exposed to High Oxygen for Longer Periods

To define the best experimental model that most closely recapitulates BPD, we trialed three oxygen exposure protocols (**Supplementary Figures 1A–C**). For each of these, we used a moderate oxygen concentration of 75%, as we have previously reported that this concentration is sufficient to elicit both early and long-term damage in the neonatal lung and eye (17). Oxygen exposure in neonatal pups for 5 days had no effect on body weight gain at PN14 or PN40 as their weight was comparable to that of age-matched room air control mice (**Supplementary Figures 1D,E**). Conversely, neonatal mouse pups exposed to oxygen for 8 days had reduced body weight gain at PN14, which had normalized by PN40 (**Supplementary Figures 1D,E**). However, mice exposed to high oxygen for 14 days had reduced body weight gain at both PN14 and PN40 compared to mice exposed to high oxygen for shorter periods and age-matched room air controls, suggesting a more profound impact (**Supplementary Figures 1D,E**).

Prolonged Oxygen Exposure Leads to BPD-Like Damage in Neonatal Mice

In mice, the bulk of alveolarization in the lung is complete by PN14 (28), forming a suitable time-point for assessment of the major structural changes to the alveoli. We used two primary measurements, alveolar septal wall thickness and airspace size, to evaluate the structural damage induced in oxygen-exposed mouse lungs. Mice reared in room air from the day of birth, up to and including PN14, had normal alveolar structure, as shown by typical alveolar septal wall thickness and airspace diameter (**Figures 1A–C**). Exposure to 75% oxygen for the first 5 days of life (PN1-5) had minimal effect on the visual appearance of the lung. Morphometric measurement revealed a possible thickening of the septal wall compared to room air controls; however, this was not significant and there was no difference in airspace size between the oxygen-exposed and room air groups (**Figures 1A–C**). Extending the duration of oxygen exposure to 8 days (PN1-8) induced a change in parenchymal architecture, demonstrated by an increase in alveolar septal wall thickening and alveolar diameter (**Figures 1A–C**). Lengthening the oxygen exposure further to 14 days (PN1-14) gave rise to lungs with severe alveolar deformities, showing a marked increase in septal wall thickening and exaggerated alveolar size compared to room air controls. The airspace diameter in this group showed even greater enlargement compared to mice exposed to oxygen for 8 days (**Figures 1A–C**).

Prolonged Neonatal Oxygen Exposure Leads to the Development of Emphysema in Young Adult Mice

It is now well-appreciated that preterm infants diagnosed with BPD have an increased susceptibility to other lung diseases in later life, including COPD (6, 7). To examine the longer-term impact of neonatal oxygen exposure, the lungs of mice administered 75% oxygen for the first 5, 8, or 14 days of life, were examined at PN40. Mice that had been exposed from birth to 75% oxygen for 8 days (PN1-8), but not 5 days (PN1-5), showed modest yet significant increases in septal wall thickness and airspace size compared to age-matched room air controls at PN40 (**Figures 1D–F**). Interestingly, in the PN1-8 model, both the septal wall thickness and airspace size at PN40 were somewhat reduced compared to measurements at PN14, suggesting possible healing (**Figures 1C–F**). However, mice that had been exposed for their first 14 days of life to 75% oxygen demonstrated pronounced structural alternations in lung parenchyma, including a variable but highly significant increase in septal wall thickness and airspace diameter compared to mice exposed to oxygen for 8 days (**Figures 1D–F**). This finding demonstrates the capacity of the PN1-14 oxygen model to generate structural changes consistent with emphysema in adulthood (29).

Oxygen Exposure Did Not Induce Severe Parenchymal Fibrosis in Neonatal and Adult Lung

A phenotype of "old" BPD is the presence of extensive parenchymal fibrosis, however this trait is significantly milder in the lungs of infants with newly diagnosed BPD due to the changes in respiratory care implemented in the NICU over the last few decades (3, 30). Thus, contemporary experimental models should not feature severe parenchymal fibrosis. To determine the prevalence of fibrosis, the lungs of mice at PN14 were stained with Picrosirius Red (PR), a histological stain that renders collagen fibers red. Minimal collagen staining was observed in the extracellular matrix of the lungs of all mice at PN14, except mice exposed to 75% oxygen for 14 days (**Figures 2A,B**). While there was a significant increase in parenchymal fibrosis in mice exposed to high oxygen for 14 days, on average, only 1.94% of the lung tissue in this model was positive for PR (**Figures 2A,B**). When fibrosis was assessed at day 40, only mice exposed to 8 days of high oxygen demonstrated a significant increase in the proportion of lung tissue positive for PR compared to room air control mice, although changes were mild (**Figures 2C,D**). Thus, the concentration and window of oxygen exposure did not lead to the development of extensive fibrosis resembling old BPD in any of the three models tested in neonatal and adult life.

Eight Days of Oxygen Exposure in Neonatal Mice Stimulates Mild Expansion of Type II Alveolar Epithelial Cells in Adulthood

Hyperoxia has been associated with impaired AEC development, promoting an enlarged and simplified lung structure that is commonly observed in BPD (26, 31). To determine if the high

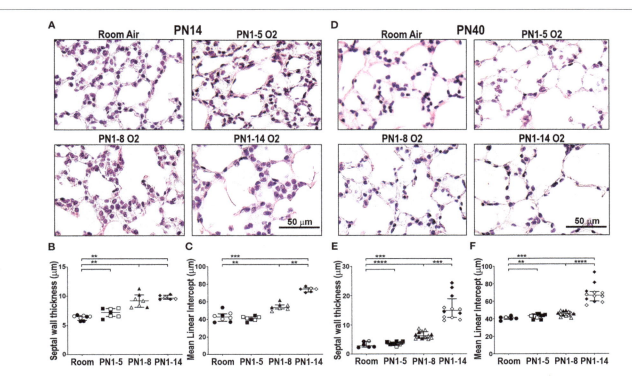

FIGURE 1 | Prolonged supplemental oxygen induces severe lung damage in neonatal mice that persists into young adulthood. C57BL/6 mice were housed in room air or treated from the day of birth with 75% O_2 for 5, 8, or 14 days, then analyzed at PN14 (A–C) or PN40 (D–F). (A) Representative photomicrographs of H&E-stained lung cross-sections at PN14. (B) Median alveolar septal wall thickness of mice in (A). (C) Alveolar airspace size by mean linear intercept length (μm) of mice in (A). (D) Representative photomicrographs of H&E-stained lung cross-sections at PN40. (E) Median alveolar septal wall thickness of mice in (D). (F) Alveolar airspace size by mean linear intercept length (μm) of mice in (D). Images in (A) and (D) were taken using a 40x objective using an Olympus BX-51 bright field microscope. Scale bar = 50 μm. For (B,C,E,F), data is median (μm) ± IQR. **$P < 0.01$, ***$P < 0.001$, ****$P < 0.0001$ by Mann-Whitney U-test (2-tailed). n ≥ 6 mice per group, with 1–2 L used to analyze each oxygen group in (A–C), and 2–3 L used to analyze each oxygen group in (D–F). Gender is represented by closed (male) and open symbols (female). PN, postnatal.

oxygen insult utilized in the three different models induced changes in the proportions of type II AECs in the lung parenchyma of adult mice, immunostaining of Pro-SPC was performed. At PN40, proportions of AEC-II in the lungs of mice exposed to high oxygen for 5 or 14 days were comparable with those in room air control mice, however surprisingly, there was a mild expansion of AEC-II in the lungs of mice exposed to 75% oxygen for 8 days (**Figures 3A,B**).

Neonatal Oxygen Exposure Induces Alveolar Inflammation in Early BPD

In order to investigate the effect of high oxygen exposure on lung inflammation in the neonate, immunohistochemical staining for CD45-expressing leukocytes was performed. In the normal developing lung at PN14, ∼20% of the cells present were CD45+ leukocytes, which were mostly found within the alveolar walls, around small vessels and occasionally also in the airspaces (**Figures 4A,B**). In all high oxygen-exposed models there was a variable increase in leukocytes in the lung, ∼10–15% more than in the room air control mice, which was significant in the PN1-5 and PN1-14 models (**Figures 4A,B**). Thus, an increase in lung inflammation is a feature of high oxygen exposure of neonatal mice.

Alveolar Inflammation Is Not a Feature of Adult Mice Exposed to an Oxygen Insult in Infancy

To determine if the high oxygen insult utilized in the three different models led to sustained inflammation in the lung parenchyma, immunostaining was performed on lung sections from 40-day-old mice. At PN40, proportions of CD45+ leukocytes in all high oxygen exposure models were comparable with the room air control mice (**Figures 4C,D**) indicating that lung inflammation observed at the early time period had resolved by adulthood.

Prolonged Oxygen Exposure Leads to Choroidal Thinning in Adulthood

The neonatal retina is highly susceptible to changes in oxygen tensions and it is a prominent co-morbidity of BPD. Survivors of this eye condition exhibit thinning of the outer retina (choroid). To evaluate the impact of neonatal high oxygen exposure on the thickness of the outer retina, H&E-stained eye sections from

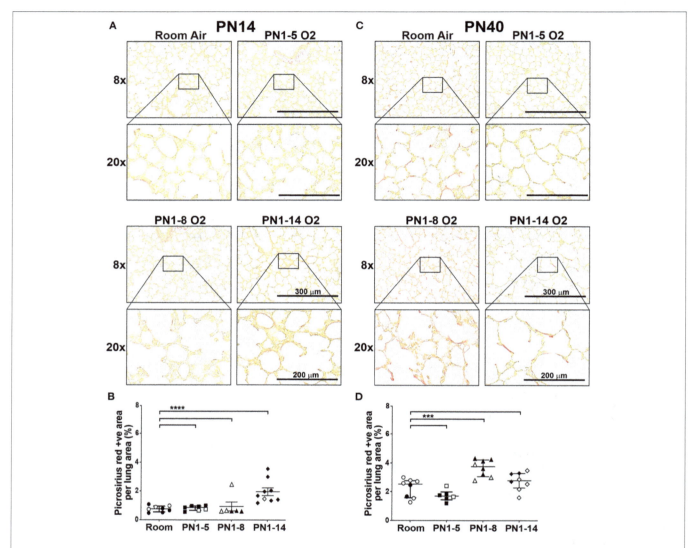

FIGURE 2 | Extensive fibrosis is not a feature of the lungs of neonatal or young adult mice exposed to prolonged supplemental oxygen in early life. C57BL/6 mice were housed in room air or treated from the day of birth with 75% O_2 for 5, 8, or 14 days, then analyzed at PN14 (A,B) or PN40 (C,D). (A) Representative images of PR-stained cross-sections of lungs at PN14. (B) Proportion of lung tissue of the mice in (A) stained with PR. (C) Representative images of PR-stained cross-sections of lungs at PN40. (D) Proportion of lung tissue of the mice in (C) stained with PR. For (A,C), images were taken with 8x and 20x objectives using Aperio ScanScope CS; scale bar = 300 and 200 μm, respectively. For (B,D), data is presented as median (μm) ± IQR. ***$P < 0.001$, ****$P < 0.0001$ by Mann-Whitney U-test (2-tailed). $n \geq 6$ mice per group, with 2–3 L used to analyze each oxygen group in (A,B), and 1–3 L used to analyze each oxygen group in (C,D). Gender is represented by closed (male) and open symbols (female). PN, postnatal.

40-day-old mice were examined. At PN40, there was a trending decrease in choroidal thickness in mice exposed to high oxygen for 5 ($p = 0.0513$) and 8 days ($p = 0.0728$) but it was significantly decreased in mice exposed to high oxygen for 14 days compared to room air control mice (**Figures 5A,B**). These results indicate that extended oxygen exposure in early infancy was sufficient to induce concurrent outer retinal changes in adulthood.

Lung Function Is Impaired in Mature Adult Mice Exposed to Hyperoxia in Infancy

A vital question arising from the above data is whether the structural deterioration observed in mice exposed to prolonged hyperoxia worsens structurally and functionally with age. At PN80, mature adult C57BL/6 mice that had been exposed from day of birth to 14 days of hyperoxia showed progressive alveolar hypoplasia, with larger and simplified alveoli, as indicated by increase in alveolar diameter, compared to those reared solely in room air conditions (**Figures 6A,B**). In patients with COPD, persistent airflow limitation is a clinical indicator of disease progression (32, 33). A significant increase in FEV0.1 and FVC was observed at PN80 in C57BL/6 mice that had received an oxygen insult during the first 14 days of neonatal development compared to room air control counterparts (**Figures 6C,D**). The ratio between FEV0.1/FVC, which is a clinical measure of COPD

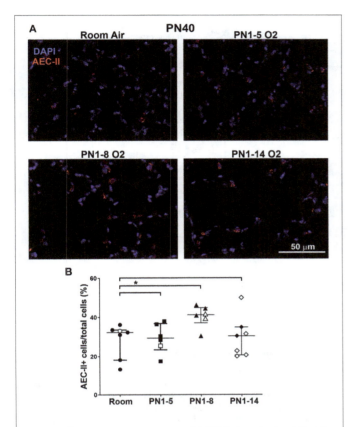

FIGURE 3 | Neonatal oxygen promotes mild AEC-II expansion in adulthood. **(A)** Representative immunofluorescent images of lungs from room air control mice or mice exposed to 75% oxygen for the indicated times. Staining was undertaken at PN40 with anti-Pro-SPC (red) to depict AEC-II. DAPI-stained nuclei appear blue. Scale bar = 50 μm. Images were taken with 20x glycerol objective using a Nikon A1r inverted confocal microscope, zoom setting 2. **(B)** Quantitation of proportions of AEC-II+ cells indicated as AEC-II+/total lung cells. Data is presented as median ± IQR. *$P < 0.05$ by Mann-Whitney U-test (2-tailed). $n \geq 6$ mice per group, with 2–4 L used in the analysis of each oxygen group. Gender is represented by closed (male) and open symbols (female). PN, postnatal.

in humans at FEV at 1 s, was significantly decreased (< 0.9) in oxygen exposed mice at PN80 (**Figure 6E**). These findings indicate that prolonged oxygen exposure in early infancy that induces BPD can progress into pulmonary function decline resembling COPD in adulthood.

DISCUSSION

There is an unresolved need for effective preventative and reparative treatments that can overcome the long-term respiratory burden faced by preterm infants that develop BPD. Over many years, the use of animal models has proven to be valuable for uncovering new disease mechanisms and new targets for therapy in a variety of human diseases. In BPD, a standardized experimental model is not used routinely and instead, many studies have used varying concentrations of oxygen, different lengths of oxygen exposures, contrasting initiation times, and additionally, insults to the mouse dam to promote an inflammatory environment, which only occurs in a small proportion of very low birth weight infants. Here, we investigated the long-term effect of 75% oxygen delivered at various developmental windows of lung organogenesis in the neonate, to best replicate the timing of injury in premature infants at risk of developing BPD and to assess the long-term repercussions of this early-life oxygen exposure on the lung but also to ocular structures such as the choroid. Importantly, all three models evaluated were initiated within 12 h of birth of the mouse.

Our findings show that two of the three models tested induced damage to the alveolar compartment in neonatal and adult mice, increasing in severity as the window of oxygen exposure lengthened. While both the PN1-8 and PN1-14 models yielded lung disease characteristics common to infants affected by BPD, the PN1-14 model yielded more exaggerated lung disease traits, particularly alveolar airspace enlargement at PN14 and PN40. At PN80, the PN1-14 model led to worsened emphysema, which was associated with a decline in respiratory mechanics, an important characteristic that is often overlooked. Therefore, our research supports that the delivery of 75% oxygen to mouse pups for 14 days is the optimal model for standardized use in BPD research, to investigate the early and long-term effects of neonatal hyperoxia.

In other hyperoxia models, prolonged exposure to high oxygen (85–100%) for 14 days or longer has been reported to result in the development of extensive fibrosis in the lung parenchyma (21, 34–36). This feature was prevalent in the early form of human BPD, that was encountered in the past (21). However, since the introduction of surfactant therapy, antenatal corticosteroids and advanced neonatal oxygen management, the BPD phenotype observed today no longer features severe pulmonary fibrosis (37). Thus, to accurately model contemporary BPD, it is important to understand whether mice delivered a high oxygen insult develop excessive parenchymal fibrosis, which is a feature that is not regularly considered in other studies. Despite a slight but significant increase in PR staining in the lung of mice exposed to high oxygen for 14 days, none of the models exhibited marked fibrosis in the extracellular matrix of the alveoli at the 14-day assessment timepoint. Interestingly, all mice showed mild increases in fibrosis between day 14 and 40, which likely reflects developmental remodeling of the extracellular matrix during lung alveolarization. However, mice that had been exposed to high oxygen for the first 8 days of life exhibited a significant increase in lung fibrosis at day 40 compared to room air controls that was not seen in the other models. While the reason for this is unknown, it is interesting that these mice were also the only group to show a significant increase in AEC-II numbers at day 40. This collectively implies a healing response, which is also suggested by a reduction in the thickness of septal walls and airspace size at PN40 compared to that seen at PN14. These features were not seen in mice given a prolonged oxygen insult, which may suggest that their lungs have become too damaged. Thus, we confirm that it is suitable to use a high

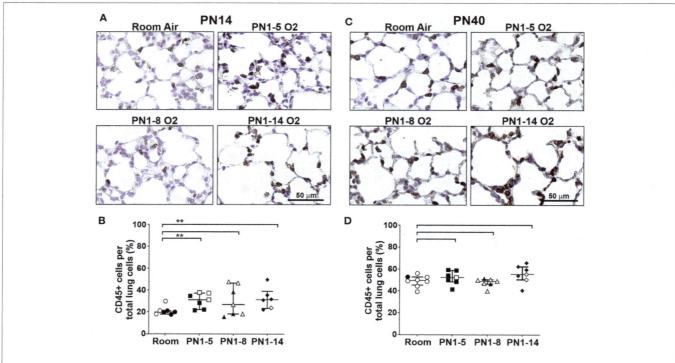

FIGURE 4 | Inflammation is present in the lungs of neonatal mice exposed at birth to supplemental oxygen but is moderated in young adult mice. C57BL/6 mice were housed in room air or treated from the day of birth with 75% O₂ for 5, 8, or 14 days, then their lungs were analyzed at PN14 (A,B) or PN40 (C,D) by staining with the pan-leukocyte cell surface marker CD45. (A) Representative images of lung paraffin sections stained at PN14, and (B) quantitation of the proportion of CD45+ immune cells per total alveolar cells. (C) Representative images of lung paraffin sections stained at PN40, and (D) quantitation of the proportion of CD45+ immune cells per total alveolar cells. In (A,C), sections were counter-stained with hematoxylin and CD45+ cells are indicated by brown staining; scale bar = 50 μm. Note that lungs were not perfused or flushed prior to fixation and extraction. Images were taken with 40x objective using an Olympus BX-51 bright field microscope. Data in (B,D) is presented as median ± IQR. **$P < 0.01$ by Mann-Whitney U-test (2-tailed). $n \geq 6$ mice per group, with 1–2 L used for analysis of each oxygen group in (A,B), and 2–3 L used for analysis of each oxygen group in (C,D). Gender is represented by closed (male) and open symbols (female). PN, postnatal.

oxygen concentration of 75% for up to 14 days in C57BL/6 mice to emulate the form of BPD that prevails in the neonatal clinic today.

Targeting oxygen exposure within the critical window of lung development in experimental models is an important consideration to maintain clinical relevance to human BPD. Importantly, the saccular and alveolar stages of lung development appear to be most impacted during oxygen administration in preterm infants in NICUs (38). The mouse represents an excellent system to model BPD, as the saccular stage of lung development, which is generally complete in full-term infants, occurs predominantly in the first 5 days of postnatal life of the mouse. In the first model tested, oxygen exposure was limited to this important developmental stage. This scheme did not induce major structural changes in the neonatal or adult lung, despite a hint of septal wall thickening at day 14. Previous studies have reported that this short window of exposure during the saccular stage of lung development was sufficient to elicit severe alveolar damage in 8–9-week-old adult mice (13, 39). This difference likely relates to the lower concentration of oxygen used in our model but may also be due to the housing environment or the assessment timepoint, since we examined mice at 40 days of age (13, 39). Thus, it is possible that lung defects may manifest later on if the damage progresses at a slower rate. In a study exposing neonatal pups to 40, 60, and 100% oxygen from PN1-4, only 100% oxygen led to lung dysmorphogenesis in C57BL/6 mice; however, outbred CD1 mice exhibited lung development changes in response to 60% oxygen as well (40), indicating that genetic background contributes to the response of the lungs to an oxygen insult. In the second model we tested, mice were exposed to high oxygen for 8 days, which encompasses the saccular stage and the start of the alveolar phase of lung development. Interestingly, this slightly longer insult led to the development of enlarged and simplified airspaces at both assessment timepoints, albeit lung damage at PN40 was moderate. There was also an expansion of AEC-II cells observed in the lungs of this model at PN40, which was not apparent in the PN1-5 and PN1-14 protocols at this timepoint. This was an unexpected finding as fewer AEC-II cells have previously been observed in adult mice recovering from neonatal oxygen exposure (41). However, in that study, newborn mice were exposed to 100% oxygen, which is a severe oxygen insult compared to the 75% oxygen concentration used in this study and one that is unlikely to be utilized in the NICU. Nevertheless, oxygen concentration and timing could influence the degree of activation/inhibition of different cell populations in the lung (41).

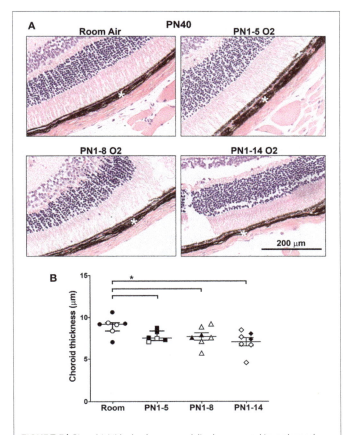

FIGURE 5 | Choroidal thinning in young adult mice exposed to prolonged oxygen in infancy. **(A)** Representative H&E photomicrographs of sections depicting choroid (white asterisk) at PN40 comparing C57BL/6 room air control mice and the indicated oxygen-exposed mice. Images were taken with 10x objective using Aperio ScanScope CS. Scale bar = 200 μm. **(B)** Quantitation of choroidal thickness (asterisk) of eye sections shown in **(A)**. All data are presented as median ± IQR and assessed using Mann-Whitney U-test (2-tailed); *$P < 0.05$. $n \geq 6$ mice per group, with 2 L used in the analysis of each oxygen group. Gender is represented by closed (male) and open symbols (female). PN, postnatal. The retinas were obtained from the same mice used to assess lung pathology in other figures. Outliers were removed using a ROUTS outlier test.

As expected, 14 days of high oxygen exposure generated the greatest degree of alveolar dysmorphogenesis in the neonatal lung, which manifested as severe pulmonary emphysema in the young and mature adult. The impact of this structural deterioration on lung mechanics was evident by the impaired respiratory function in mature adults exposed to this oxygen scheme. Taken together, these findings indicate that prolonged high oxygen exposure during the two final lung developmental stages in mice promotes lung injury that approximates that seen in preterm infants with BPD, and may even capture those infants that go onto to develop COPD in later life. This model will therefore also be useful to unravel mechanisms that underpin chronic lung conditions that have origins in early life. The ability of the 14-day exposure regime to generate long-term lung damage and functional decline within a relatively short time frame compared to current models in use (42, 43), also provides a unique advantage when trialing potential therapeutic interventions for BPD. For example, the efficacy of a select intervention to ameliorate or attenuate long-term damage can be determined in mice within 40 days of birth, making testing of therapeutics easily achievable. Another important consideration is the emerging influence of the lung and gut microbiome on the development of BPD. Given that selective pressures such as moisture, pH and nutrition can shape the local microbial niche (44), mice housed in different animal facilities are subsequently exposed to diverse environmental conditions. Therefore, these factors may also influence the severity of lung pathology generated in oxygen-exposed mice and could also account for the discrepancies observed between different research groups using the same oxygen models.

Inflammation is also recognized to contribute to the deterioration of the alveolar structure in the neonatal lung following a high oxygen insult (45). Airway sections obtained from preterm infants with BPD often show elevated levels of pro-inflammatory chemokines and cytokines, and can occur early in neonatal life before the presentation of clinical symptoms (46, 47). However, infants with BPD have demonstrated increased susceptibility to COPD, respiratory viral infections and asthma in later life compared to their non-BPD counterparts, which may involve the dysregulation of immune pathways in the lung during neonatal hyperoxia exposure (13). In a previous study, exposure to hyperoxia during the first 12 days of neonatal life led to persistent inflammation in the lungs of adult mice, implicating chronic inflammation in the lung of BPD survivors (48). To determine whether oxygen exposure at varying developmental windows would influence the immune profile in the adult lung, immunohistochemical staining for CD45+ leukocytes was conducted on lung tissue. All mice showed an increase in leukocytes in lung between day 14 and 40, which likely reflects the maturation of the immune system, which undergoes rapid development during the early postnatal period; however, alveolar inflammation at day 40 was not a feature of any of the three high oxygen regimes trialed in this study. This suggests that the structural changes apparent in adulthood are most likely the consequences of oxygen exposure during critical lung stages in infancy (49). Concurrently, there may also be changes occurring in other tissue components external to inflammation, such as modifications to extracellular matrix proteins (50).

A common clinical co-morbidity of infants diagnosed with BPD is ROP (51). The retinal vasculature is sensitive to the changes in oxygen tension and extreme hyperoxia/hypoxia can hinder the normal growth of the blood vessels in the retina which can lead to poor vision in later life (52). Adult survivors of ROP have been reported to exhibit late-onset vitreoretinal complications (53) and retinal detachment (54). In addition, a thinner choroid has been associated with reduced vision in individuals with a history of ROP, and has been speculated to be primary to the long-term changes in the inner retinal layers (55). Therefore, the degree of choroidal thinning was assessed across all three oxygen models and presents a unique aspect of this study. While only the 14-day exposure model showed a significant reduction in choroidal thickness, the other

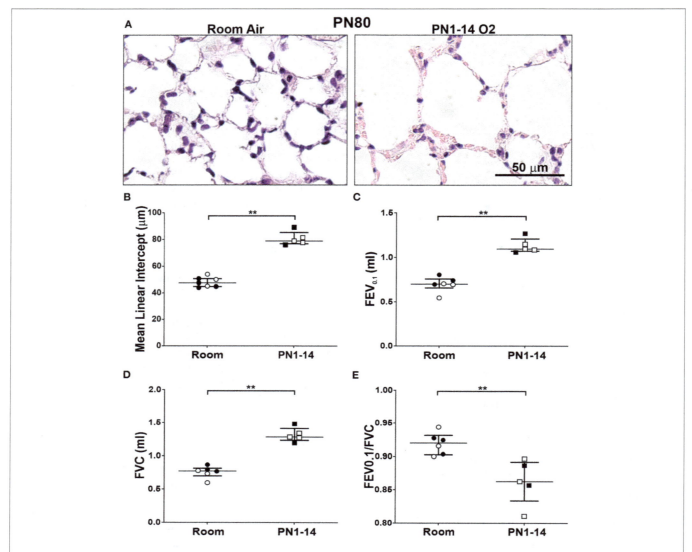

FIGURE 6 | Decline in lung function in mature adult mice exposed to prolonged supplemental oxygen in infancy. (A) Representative photomicrographs of H&E-stained lung cross-sections at PN80 comparing C57BL/6 room air control mice and PN1-14 oxygen-exposed mice. Images were taken with a 40x objective using an Olympus BX-51 bright field microscope. Scale bar = 50 μm. (B) Quantitation of airspace diameter (MLI) of lung sections shown in (A). Assessment of (C) FEV0.1, (D) FVC, and (E) FEV0.1/FVC ratio by negative pressure-driven forced expiration using the Flexivent. All data are presented as median ± IQR and assessed using Mann-Whitney U-test (2-tailed); **$P < 0.01$. $n = 5–6$ mice per group from 1 litter. Gender is represented by closed (male) and open symbols (female). PN, postnatal.

two models displayed trending degrees of vascular thinning. This demonstrates that an extended period of high oxygen exposure in neonatal life can also provoke long-term damage in organs outside of the lung and evaluation of other tissues implicated in BPD could enhance the clinical relevance and translatability of this model. However, the timing of the oxygen exposure soon after birth in the 14-day model employed in this study is considerably different to that used in the established model of ROP, known as the oxygen-induced retinopathy model. Due to differences in retinal development between mouse and man, high oxygen exposure in the oxygen-induced retinopathy model commences on postnatal day seven to mimic the vascular developmental stage in preterm infants (56). Therefore, the specific molecular changes underlying the vascular damage in the retina may be grossly different between the two oxygen schemes and should be considered closely before use in ocular research.

In the absence of a cure for BPD, there is a need to identify the mechanisms underlying this debilitating condition. Accordingly, the development of a benchmark model of BPD will allow for greater comparison of results amongst research groups and advances in the understanding of the disease. The current study describes a model of oxygen-induced BPD, comprised of a 14-day exposure to 75% oxygen, initiated within 12 h of birth, which was associated with features of contemporary BPD in neonatal mice. Moreover, the model was associated with the impaired development of alveoli in adult mice that resembled COPD encountered by adult survivors of BPD alongside outer retinal decay, which is a distinguishing feature of this model.

These findings provide a distinct advantage, suggesting that this model could be a key translational tool for the trialing of new treatments which may advance therapeutic strategies to improve the care and long-term outcome for vulnerable premature infants. We advocate that the standardized PN1-14 model described herein may facilitate studies into the early life impact of high oxygen-exposure but also expedite investigations into the lifelong effect of oxygen insults received during the neonatal period.

AUTHOR CONTRIBUTIONS

MH and LW conceived the study, designed research, and analyzed data. LW performed experiments. PW supplied an integral piece of equipment, provided critical intellectual content, and important manuscript revisions. CJ contributed a new analytic tool. ET provided valuable insight and made important intellectual contributions. LW and MH wrote the paper. All authors provided editorial comments and gave final approval for publication.

ACKNOWLEDGMENTS

The authors acknowledge the dedicated assistance of animal technicians for animal breeding and husbandry, and the Monash Histology Platform for support with histological studies. We are grateful to Ms. Suhashi M. Wickramasinghe (BSc, BOcc Therapy Hons) for comments on the manuscript.

SUPPLEMENTARY MATERIAL

Supplementary Figure 1 | Oxygen exposure models trialed in this study. Within 12 h of birth, neonatal C57BL/6 mice were exposed to **(A)** 75% O2 for 5 [PN1-5], **(B)** 8 [PN1-8], or **(C)** 14 days [PN1-14] with a daily 3-h period in room air (not shown in figure). Cohorts of mice were analyzed at PN14 or PN40, and for the PN1-14 model at PN80 (red arrows) alongside room air control mice. Body weights of room air control mice and oxygen-exposed mice at **(D)** PN14 or **(E)** PN40. **$P < 0.01$ and ***$P < 0.001$ by Mann-Whitney U-test (2-tailed). $n \geq 6$ mice per group, with 1–2 L used in the analysis of each oxygen group. Gender is represented by closed symbols (male) and open symbols (female). PN, postnatal.

Supplementary Table 1 | Custom imageJ script used for the quantitation of fluorescence positive cells.

REFERENCES

1. Baraldi E, Filippone M. Chronic lung disease after premature birth. *N Engl J Med.* (2007) 357:1946–55. doi: 10.1056/NEJMra 067279
2. Stoll B, Hansen N, Bell E, Walsh MC, Carlo WA, Shankaran S, et al. Human Development Neonatal Research NetworkTrends in care practices, morbidity, and mortality of extremely preterm neonates, 1993-2012. *JAMA.* (2015) 314:1039–51. doi: 10.1001/jama.2015.10244
3. Husain AN, Siddiqui NH, Stocker JT. Pathology of arrested acinar development in postsurfactant bronchopulmonary dysplasia. *Hum Pathol.* (1998) 29:710–7. doi: 10.1016/S0046-8177(98) 90280-5
4. Smith LJ, van Asperen PP, McKay KO, Selvadurai H, Fitzgerald DA. Reduced exercise capacity in children born very preterm. *Pediatrics.* (2008) 122:e287–93. doi: 10.1542/peds.2007-3657
5. Tarazona SP, Galan PS, Alguacil EB, Diego JA. Bronchopulmonary dysplasia as a risk factor for asthma in school children and adolescents: a systematic review. *Allergol Immunopathol.* (2018) 46:87–98. doi: 10.1016/j.aller.2017.02.004
6. Hilgendorff A, O'Reilly MA. Bronchopulmonary dysplasia early changes leading to long-term consequences. *Front Med.* (2015) 2:2. doi: 10.3389/fmed.2015.00002
7. Islam JY, Keller RL, Aschner JL, Hartert TV, Moore PE. Understanding the short-and long-term respiratory outcomes of prematurity and bronchopulmonary dysplasia. *Am J Respir Crit Care Med.* (2015) 192:134–56. doi: 10.1164/rccm.201412-2142PP
8. Hilgendorff A, Reiss I, Ehrhardt H, Eickelberg O, Alvira CM. Chronic lung disease in the preterm infant. lessons learned from animal models. *Am J Respir Cell Mol Biol.* (2014) 50:233–45. doi: 10.1165/rcmb.20 13-0014TR
9. Buczynski BW, Maduekwe ET, O'Reilly MA. The role of hyperoxia in the pathogenesis of experimental BPD. *Semin Perinatol.* (2013) 37:69–78. doi: 10.1053/j.semperi.2013.01.002
10. Dayanim S, Lopez B, Maisonet TM, Grewal S, Londhe VA. Caffeine induces alveolar apoptosis in the hyperoxia-exposed developing mouse lung. *Pediatr Res.* (2014) 75:395–402. doi: 10.1038/pr. 2013.233
11. Weichelt U, Cay R, Schmitz T, Strauss E, Sifringer M, Bührer C, et al. Prevention of hyperoxia-mediated pulmonary inflammation in neonatal rats by caffeine. *Europ Respir J.* (2013) 41:966–73. doi: 10.1183/09031936. 00012412

12. Silva DM, Nardiello C, Pozarska A, Morty RE. Recent advances in the mechanisms of lung alveolarization and the pathogenesis of bronchopulmonary dysplasia. *Am J Physiol Lung Cell Mol Physiol.* (2015) 309:L1239–L72. doi: 10.1152/ajplung.00268. 2015
13. O'Reilly MA, Yee M, Buczynski BW, Vitiello PF, Keng PC, Welle SL, et al. Neonatal oxygen increases sensitivity to influenza A virus infection in adult mice by suppressing epithelial expression of Ear1. *Am J Pathol.* (2012) 181:441–51. doi: 10.1016/j.ajpath.2012. 05.005
14. Warner BB, Stuart LA, Papes RA, Wispé JR. Functional and pathological effects of prolonged hyperoxia in neonatal mice. *Am J Physiol Lung Cell Mol Physiol.* (1998) 275:L110–L7. doi: 10.1152/ajplung.1998.275. 1.L110
15. Nardiello C, Mižíková I, Silva DM, Ruiz-Camp J, Mayer K, Vadász I, et al. Standardisation of oxygen exposure in the development of mouse models for bronchopulmonary dysplasia. *Dis Model Mech.* (2017) 10:185–96. doi: 10.1242/dmm.027086
16. Dauger S, Ferkdadji L, Saumon G, Vardon G, Peuchmaur M, Gaultier C, et al. Neonatal exposure to 65% oxygen durably impairs lung architecture and breathing pattern in adult mice. *Chest.* (2003) 123:530–8. doi: 10.1378/chest.123.2.530
17. Wickramasinghe LC, Lau M, Deliyanti D, Gottschalk TA, van Wijngaarden P, Talia D, et al. Lung and eye disease develop concurrently in supplemental oxygen-exposed neonatal mice. *Am J Pathol.* (2020) 190:1801–12. doi: 10.1016/j.ajpath.2020.05.016
18. Schittny JC. Development of the lung. *Cell Tissue Res.* (2017) 367:427–44. doi: 10.1007/s00441-016-2545-0
19. Kresch MJ, Christian C, Wu F, Hussain N. Ontogeny of apoptosis during lung development. *Pediatr Res.* (1998) 43:426–31. doi: 10.1203/00006450-199803000-00020
20. Solalígue DES, Rodríguez-Castillo JA, Ahlbrecht K, Morty RE. Recent advances in our understanding of the mechanisms of late lung development and bronchopulmonary dysplasia. *Am J Physiol Lung Cell Mol Physiol.* (2017) 313:L1101–53. doi: 10.1152/ajplung.00343.2017
21. Baker CD, Alvira CM. Disrupted lung development and bronchopulmonary dysplasia: opportunities for lung repair and regeneration. *Curr Opin Pediatr.* (2014) 26:306. doi: 10.1097/MOP.000000000 0000095
22. Mund SI, Stampanoni M, Schittny JC. Developmental alveolarization of the mouse lung. *Dev Dynam.* (2008) 237:2108–16. doi: 10.1002/dvdy.21633
23. Branchfield K, Li R, Lungova V, Verheyden JM, McCulley D,

Sun X. A three-dimensional study of alveologenesis in mouse lung. *Dev Biol.* (2016) 409:429–41. doi: 10.1016/j.ydbio.2015. 11.017

24. Gouveia L, Betsholtz C, Andrae J. Expression analysis of platelet-derived growth factor receptor alpha and its ligands in the developing mouse lung. *Physiol Rep.* (2017) 5:e13092. doi: 10.14814/phy2.13092

25. Domm W, Misra RS, O'Reilly MA. Affect of early life oxygen exposure on proper lung development and response to respiratory viral infections. *Front Med.* (2015) 2:55. doi: 10.3389/fmed.2015. 00055

26. Hou A, Fu J, Yang H, Zhu Y, Pan Y, Xu S, et al. Hyperoxia stimulates the transdifferentiation of type II alveolar epithelial cells in newborn rats. *Am J Physiol Lung Cell Mol Physiol.* (2015) 308:L861–L72. doi: 10.1152/ajplung.00099.2014

27. Nicola T, Hagood JS, James ML, MacEwen MW, Williams TA, Hewitt MM, et al. Loss of Thy-1 inhibits alveolar development in the newborn mouse lung. *Am J Physiol Lung Cell Mol Physiol.* (2009) 296:L738–L50. doi: 10.1152/ajplung.90603.2008

28. Pozarska A, Rodríguez-Castillo JA, Surate Solaligue DE, Ntokou A, Rath P, Mižíková I, et al. Stereological monitoring of mouse lung alveolarization from the early postnatal period to adulthood. *Am J Physiol Lung Cell Mol Physiol.* (2017) 312:L882–L95. doi: 10.1152/ajplung.00492.2016

29. Vlahovic G, Russell ML, Mercer RR, Crapo JD. Cellular and connective tissue changes in alveolar septal walls in emphysema. *Am J Respir Crit Care Med.* (1999) 160:2086–92. doi: 10.1164/ajrccm.160.6.9706031

30. Walkup LL, Tkach JA, Higano NS, Thomen RP, Fain SB, Merhar SL, et al. Quantitative magnetic resonance imaging of bronchopulmonary dysplasia in the neonatal intensive care unit environment. *Am J Respir Crit Care Med.* (2015) 192:1215–22. doi: 10.1164/rccm.201503-0552OC

31. Yee M, Buczynski BW, O'Reilly MA. Neonatal hyperoxia stimulates the expansion of alveolar epithelial type II cells. *Am J Respir Cell Mol Biol.* (2014) 50:757–66. doi: 10.1165/rcmb.2013-0207OC

32. Papandrinopoulou D, Tzouda V, Tsoukalas G. Lung compliance and chronic obstructive pulmonary disease. *Pulm Med.* (2012) 2012:542769. doi: 10.1155/2012/542769

33. Mikamo M, Shirai T, Mori K, Shishido Y, Akita T, Morita S, et al. Predictors of expiratory flow limitation measured by forced oscillation technique in COPD. *BMC Pulm Med.* (2014) 14:23. doi: 10.1186/1471-24 66-14-23

34. Velten M, Heyob KM, Rogers LK, Welty SE. Deficits in lung alveolarization and function after systemic maternal inflammation and neonatal hyperoxia exposure. *J Appl Physiol.* (2010) 108:1347–56. doi: 10.1152/japplphysiol.01392.2009

35. Deakins KM. Bronchopulmonary dysplasia. *Respir Care.* (2009) 54:1252–62.

36. Balany J, Bhandari V. Understanding the impact of infection, inflammation, and their persistence in the pathogenesis of bronchopulmonary dysplasia. *Front Med.* (2015) 2:90. doi: 10.3389/fmed.2015. 00090

37. Bland RD. Neonatal chronic lung disease in the post-surfactant era. *Neonatology.* (2005) 88:181–91. doi: 10.1159/000087581

38. Bourbon J, Boucherat O, Chailley-Heu B, Delacourt C. Control mechanisms of lung alveolar development and their disorders in bronchopulmonary dysplasia. *Pediatr Res.* (2005) 57:38–46. doi: 10.1203/01.PDR.0000159630.35883.BE

39. Yee M, Chess PR, McGrath-Morrow SA, Wang Z, Gelein R, Zhou R, et al. Neonatal oxygen adversely affects lung function in adult mice without altering surfactant composition or activity. *Am J Physiol Lung Cell Mol Physiol.* (2009) 297:L641–9. doi: 10.1152/ajplung.00023.2009

40. Leary S, Das P, Ponnalagu D, Singh H, Bhandari V. Genetic strain and sex differences in a hyperoxia-induced mouse model of varying severity of bronchopulmonary dysplasia. *Am J Pathol.* (2019) 189:999–1014. doi: 10.1016/j.ajpath.2019.01.014

41. Yee M, Vitiello PF, Roper JM, Staversky RJ, Wright TW, McGrath-Morrow SA, et al. Type II epithelial cells are critical target for hyperoxia-mediated impairment of postnatal lung development. *Am J Physiol Lung Cell Mol Physiol.* (2006) 291:L1101–L11. doi: 10.1152/ajplung.00126.2006

42. Woyda K, Koebrich S, Reiss I, Rudloff S, Pullamsetti S, Rühlmann A, et al. Inhibition of phosphodiesterase 4 enhances lung alveolarisation in neonatal mice exposed to hyperoxia. *European Respir J.* (2009) 33:861–70. doi: 10.1183/09031936.00109008

43. Tibboel J, Joza S, Reiss I, de Jongste JC, Post M. Amelioration of hyperoxia-induced lung injury using a sphingolipid-based intervention. *Europ Respir J.* (2013) 42:776–84. doi: 10.1183/09031936.00092212

44. Willis KA, Stewart JD, Ambalavanan N. Recent advances in understanding the ecology of the lung microbiota and deciphering the gut-lung axis. *Am J Physiol Lung Cell Mol Physiol.* (2020) 319:L710–L6. doi: 10.1152/ajplung.00360.2020

45. Speer C. Pulmonary inflammation and bronchopulmonary dysplasia. *J Perinatol.* (2006) 26:S57–62. doi: 10.1038/sj.jp.7211476

46. Kotecha S. Cytokines in chronic lung disease of prematurity. *Eur J Pediatr.* (1996) 155:S14–17. doi: 10.1007/BF01958074

47. Hjort MR, Brenyo AJ, Finkelstein JN, Frampton MW, LoMonaco MB, Stewart JC, et al. Alveolar epithelial cell-macrophage interactions affect oxygen-stimulated interleukin-8 release. *Inflammation.* (2003) 27:137–45. doi: 10.1023/A:1023817811850

48. Kumar VH, Lakshminrusimha S, Kishkurno S, Paturi BS, Gugino SF, Nielsen L, et al. Neonatal hyperoxia increases airway reactivity and inflammation in adult mice. *Pediatr Pulmonol.* (2016) 51:1131–41. doi: 10.1002/ppul.23430

49. Kumar VH, Wang H, Kishkurno S, Paturi BS, Nielsen L, Ryan RM. Long-term effects of neonatal hyperoxia in adult mice. *Anat Rec.* (2018) 301:717–26. doi: 10.1002/ar.23766

50. Kindermann A, Binder L, Baier J, Gündel B, Simm A, Haase R, et al. Severe but not moderate hyperoxia of newborn mice causes an emphysematous lung phenotype in adulthood without persisting oxidative stress and inflammation. *BMC Pulm Med.* (2019) 19:1–12. doi: 10.1186/s12890-019-0993-5

51. Kachurina D, Sadykova AZ, Tyan E, Tulebaeva ZS, Pirmakhanova A. The bronchopulmonary dysplasia in infants with retinopathy of prematurity. *Iran J Pediatr.* (2014) 24:S1.

52. Flynn JT, Bancalari E, Snyder ES, Goldberg RN, Feuer W, Cassady J, et al. A cohort study of transcutaneous oxygen tension and the incidence and severity of retinopathy of prematurity. *N Engl J Med.* (1992) 326:1050–4. doi: 10.1056/NEJM199204163261603

53. Tufail A, Singh A, Haynes R, Dodd C, McLeod D, Charteris D. Late onset vitreoretinal complications of regressed retinopathy of prematurity. *Br J Ophthalmol.* (2004) 88:243–6. doi: 10.1136/bjo.2003.022962

54. Terasaki H, Hirose T. Late-onset retinal detachment associated with regressed retinopathy of prematurity. *Jpn J Ophthalmol.* (2003) 47:492–7. doi: 10.1016/S0021-5155(03)00088-1

55. Wu W-C, Shih C-P, Wang N-K, Lien R, Chen Y-P, Chao A-N, et al. Choroidal thickness in patients with a history of retinopathy of prematurity. *JAMA Ophthalmol.* (2013) 131:1451–8. doi: 10.1001/jamaophthalmol.2013.5052

56. Smith LEH, Wesolowski E, McLellan A, Kostyk SK, D'Amato RJ, Sullivan R, et al., editors. Oxygen-induced retinopathy in the mouse. *Invest Ophthalmol Vis Sci.* (1994) 35:101–11.

4

Updates on Functional Characterization of Bronchopulmonary Dysplasia – The Contribution of Lung Function Testing

Anne Greenough [1,2]* and Anoop Pahuja[3]

[1] *Division of Asthma, Allergy and Lung Biology, MRC and Asthma UK Centre in Allergic Mechanisms of Asthma, King's College London, London, UK, [2] NIHR Biomedical Research Centre, Guy's and St. Thomas NHS Foundation Trust, London, UK, [3] Neonatal Intensive Care Centre, King's College Hospital NHS Foundation Trust, London, UK*

*Correspondence:
Anne Greenough,
NICU, King's College Hospital, 4th Floor Golden Jubilee Wing, Denmark Hill, London SE5 9RS, UK
anne.greenough@kcl.ac.uk

Bronchopulmonary dysplasia (BPD) is a chronic lung disease that predominantly affects prematurely born infants. Initially, BPD was described in infants who had suffered severe respiratory failure and required high pressure, mechanical ventilation with high concentrations of supplementary oxygen. Now, it also occurs in very prematurely born infants who initially had minimal or even no signs of lung disease. These differences impact the nature of the lung function abnormalities suffered by "BPD" infants, which are also influenced by the criteria used to diagnose BPD and the oxygen saturation level used to determine the supplementary oxygen requirement. Key also to interpreting lung function data in this population is whether appropriate lung function tests have been used and in an adequately sized population to make meaningful conclusions. It should also be emphasized that BPD is a poor predictor of long-term respiratory morbidity. Bearing in mind those caveats, studies have consistently demonstrated that infants who develop BPD have low compliance and functional residual capacities and raised resistances in the neonatal period. There is, however, no agreement with regard to which early lung function measurement predicts the development of BPD, likely reflecting different techniques were used in different populations in often underpowered studies. During infancy, lung function generally improves, but importantly airflow limitation persists and small airway function appears to decline. Improvements in lung function following administration of diuretics or bronchodilators have not translated into long-term improvements in respiratory outcomes. By contrast, early differences in lung function related to different ventilation modes have led to investigation and demonstration that prophylactic, neonatal high-frequency oscillation appears to protect small airway function.

Keywords: bronchopulmonary dysplasia, prematurity, resistance, compliance, diuretics, bronchodilators, corticosteroids

Introduction

Bronchopulmonary dysplasia (BPD) is a chronic lung disease that predominantly affects prematurely born infants, but can occur in those born at term if they are subjected to high-inflation pressures. Initially, BPD was described in prematurely born infants who often had suffered severe respiratory failure and required high pressure, mechanical ventilation with high concentrations of supplementary oxygen, often coined old BPD. Such infants were not routinely exposed to either antenatal corticosteroids or postnatal surfactant. BPD now also occurs in very prematurely born infants who initially had minimal or even no signs of lung disease, the so-called new BPD (1). At postmortem, infants with new rather than old BPD have less interstitial fibrosis, but an arrest in acinar development, resulting in fewer and larger alveoli (2). The chest radiograph (CXR) appearance of new BPD, that is small volume, hazy lung fields, is very different from the cystic abnormalities and interstitial fibrosis seen in "old" BPD. As a consequence, lung function abnormalities are likely to differ according to whether an infant is developing old or new BPD. The nature of the lung function abnormalities may also be influenced by the criteria used to diagnose BPD. These have included oxygen dependency at 28 days or 36 weeks post conceptional age (PCA) with or without radiological abnormalities. Nowadays, there is a consensus that infants should be diagnosed as having BPD if infants are oxygen dependent at 28 days after birth (3). They are then classified as suffering from mild, moderate, or severe BPD according to their respiratory support requirement at a later date (36 weeks PCA if born prematurely) (3) (**Table 1**). A further problem is that different levels of oxygen saturation have been used to determine the need for supplementary oxygen leading to wide variations in the occurrence of BPD (4). As a consequence, it is now recommended that an oxygen reduction test is used to determine whether supplementary oxygen is still required (5). Of note, lung function abnormalities as assessed by pulmonary function testing are not part of the current criteria to diagnose BPD, likely reflecting pulmonary function testing is not routinely available in all neonatal intensive care units (NICU).

Bearing in mind those caveats, an aim of this review is to describe lung function abnormalities in infants developing or with established BPD and how they change with increasing postnatal age during infancy. In addition, we will highlight if lung function testing in the NICU and during infancy gives added value. For example, do lung function test results so accurately predict BPD development that they could be used to identify infants who would benefit from intervention strategies or have improvements in lung function given an early indication of clinically efficacious interventions.

It, however, should be emphasized at the outset that a diagnosis of BPD is a poor predictor of ongoing pulmonary problems (6) and infants with and without BPD suffer respiratory morbidity at follow-up. In addition, certain randomized controlled trials (RCTs), which have demonstrated a reduction in BPD, have not been associated with improvements in long-term respiratory outcome (7) and equally interventions influencing long-term respiratory morbidity were not associated with a reduction in BPD (8, 9).

Appropriate Lung Function Tests

Key to interpreting lung function data is whether an appropriate test has been used and whether the test has been applied robustly. In infants with evolving or established BPD, the techniques have strengths and weaknesses. Dynamic lung compliance measurements do not require airway occlusions, which may be poorly tolerated in infants with respiratory distress. Esophageal pressure measurements, however, are required, which may not accurately reflect pleural pressure changes in prematurely born infants who have a floppy chest wall or in the presence of lung disease. Single breath mechanics do require airway occlusions and the underlying assumptions are invalid if the respiratory system cannot be described as single-compartment model. The high resistance of small endotracheal tubes (10) may invalidate attempts to detect small changes in resistance in intubated infants. Assessments of functional residual capacity (FRC) by gas dilution or washout, can be applied in ventilated infants, but may underestimate the FRC if insufficient time is allowed for complete equilibration (11). Nitrogen washout with pure oxygen is impractical for ventilated infants receiving a high-fractional inspired oxygen concentration and inappropriate for infants at risk of retinopathy of prematurity. Inert gases such as helium and sulfur hexafluoride (SF6) avoid these problems. As a relatively heavy gas with low diffusivity, SF6 has the additional advantage of being less susceptible than helium to leaks (12), especially those occurring around an uncuffed endotracheal tube. Certain centers, however, use shouldered tubes, which have been demonstrated to have minimal or no leak (13). The major strength of measuring lung volume using infant whole-body plethysmography is that the total lung volume can be measured and hence, if used in conjunction with a gas dilution technique, can provide an assessment of hyperinflation and gas trapping (14). Systems are commercially available, but depend on electronic manipulation to close the pressure flow loop, which can result in erroneous results (15). A further disadvantage is that plethysmographs are not suitable for cot side measurements. In addition, the accuracy of plethysmographic measurements is dependent on rapid equilibration of pressures during respiratory efforts against occlusions, so that pressure changes at the airway opening reflect those in the alveoli (16). In the presence of severe airway obstruction, this may not occur, resulting in a phase lag between airway pressure and box volume, usually resulting in overestimation of lung volume (11). As infants actively elevate their end expiratory level, all lung volume measurements should be made during quiet, non-rapid eye movement sleep (17). Respiratory impedance plethysmography (RIP) can provide information on respiratory rate and the degree of thoracoabdominal asynchrony. The interpretation of the results is dependent on sleep state and volume calibration is not possible in this population.

TABLE 1 | BPD severity modified from Jobe and Bancalari (3).

Infants <32 weeks of gestational age are assessed at 36 weeks PCA or at discharge home, whichever came first

Infants born at 32 weeks of gestation or greater are assessed at 56 days postnatal age or discharge home, whichever came first

The severity of BPD being graded in both groups accordingly

- mild BPD – breathing air
- moderate BPD – requirement for <30% supplementary oxygen
- severe BPD – requirement for more that 30% oxygen and/or positive pressure ventilation or nasal continuous positive airway pressure (CPAP)

Lung Function Abnormalities

Among infants with "old" BPD, increased resistance in the first week after birth and increased total respiratory and expiratory resistance with severe flow limitation, especially at low lung volumes at 28 days after birth was reported (18). More recent studies, which have included infants who usually have received surfactant, have demonstrated somewhat differing results. In a group of infants, the majority of whom had been given rescue surfactant, respiratory system resistance (Rrs) was abnormal at 10 days after birth, but then there was progressive improvement to normal values (19). In a series in which infants were given prophylactic surfactant and exposed to antenatal steroids, Rrs differed significantly between those who did and did not develop BPD on day three, but not at 14 days after birth (20).

Compliance is initially low in infants destined to develop BPD. In one series of ventilated infants, compliance of the respiratory system (Crs), using the single breath technique, was 50% of predicted at 10 days of age (19). Interestingly, there was a positive correlation ($r = 0.8$, $p < 0.001$) between those Crs results and maximal flow at FRC (V'_{max} FRC) using the forced expiratory volume technique at 2 years of age. In the presence of low-saccular compliance, the highly compliant distal bronchial tree is preferentially over distended resulting in marked distortion of both distal and central areas during mechanical ventilation (21). The authors (19), therefore, postulated that in infants with very low lung compliance in the neonatal period, cyclic bronchiolar stretching during positive pressure ventilation resulted in terminal airway ischemia and necrosis and subsequent fibrosis and smooth muscle hypertrophy. Compliance and lung volume abnormalities may persist over the neonatal period. Comparison of FRC results from 16 BPD infants (oxygen dependent for more than 28 days) and 8 infants without BPD demonstrated the BPD group had lower FRCs at both 14 and 28 days (22). Similarly, serial measurements of Crs and FRC in 74 infants, median gestational age 30 weeks, 35 of whom developed BPD (23 had moderate/severe BPD) demonstrated that those developing BPD, particularly moderate/severe BPD had significantly lower Crs and FRC results throughout the neonatal period compared to those who did not develop BPD (20). CXR thoracic areas and FRC measurements assessed in the first 72 h after birth in 53 infants, median gestational age of 28 weeks, also demonstrated lower FRCs in the BPD group, but the CXR thoracic areas were higher in the infants who subsequently developed BPD (oxygen dependency at 28 days) perhaps indicating gas trapping. The differences were particularly marked in infants who developed moderate/severe BPD (23). The reduced Crs in the neonatal period may be due to ongoing surfactant abnormalities, edema, and atelectasis. Similarly, the initial functional lung volume is likely reduced because of atelectasis.

During evolving BPD, there is gas trapping. FRC measured by plethysmography (FRCpleth) has been reported to be elevated in infants with BPD (24, 25) and in an early study FRCpleth was higher than FRC assessed by nitrogen washout (26). In established BPD, functional lung volume around term equivalent has been reported to still be significantly reduced compared, to data, from healthy term born infants both in an early (27) and in a more recent (24) study and associated with disturbed gas mixing

(28). Those results appear pertinent to the present population of prematurely born infants who develop BPD. In a subsequent study (29), approximately 50% of the infants were exposed to antenatal steroids and 100% of those who developed moderate or severe BPD received surfactant. At term corrected, the severe BPD group had lower FRC, less efficient gas mixing, and higher specific conductance than those with mild and moderate BPD or the prematurely born controls. The infants with mild or moderate BPD infants also differed from the controls (29). BPD infants have also been shown to have significant increases in FRC, residual volume (RV), and RV/total lung capacity, which were more marked in those with recurrent wheeze, suggestive of hyperinflation and air-trapping (24). In a follow-up of prematurely born infants all born at <29 weeks of gestational age, two-thirds of whom had BPD, the degree of gas trapping significantly correlated with days of wheeze (30).

Results from a small study suggest that single photon emission computed tomography (SPECT) may provide additional information about regional lung function in BPD infants (31). SPECT was used to measure the distribution of lung ventilation (V) and perfusion (Q) in 30 BPD infants at a median PCA of 37 weeks. An unsatisfactory V/Q match was not correlated with the time spent on supplemental oxygen or CPAP, but was significantly negatively correlated with the time spent on mechanical ventilation. Increasing severity of BPD, however, was not consistently associated with the degree of V/Q mismatch.

Other lung function abnormalities in infancy suggest impairment of alveolar development after very premature birth. Pulmonary diffusing capacity and alveolar volume were assessed at 11.6 months of age using a single breath hold maneuver at elevated lung volume in 39 BPD infants (oxygen requirement at 36 weeks) and 61 term born controls. The BPD patients had reduced pulmonary diffusing capacity when adjusted for body length or alveolar volume (32).

Longitudinal Assessment

Early studies assessing serial lung function highlighted that lung compliance and FRC improved with increasing age (19, 27), such that by 2 years of age they had reached the normal range (19). In addition, during the first 2 years after birth, a relative increase in FRC using a gas dilution technique was reported (19). More recently, results were apparently at variance as assessment of 55 sedated VLBW infants (29 with BPD, oxygen dependency at 36 weeks PCA) at 50, 70, and 100 weeks of PCA demonstrated significantly lower tidal volume, minute ventilation, compliance, and FRC results in the BPD infants (33). Those differences, however, were no longer statistically significant once the results were normalized for body weight, which was significantly lower in the BPD group (33).

Airflow limitation, however, appears to be a persisting problem. An early report highlighted that lower airway obstruction persisted in infants with BPD who had severe disease as indicated by requirement for a tracheostomy (34). Longitudinal assessment demonstrated that, in infants with severe BPD, abnormalities in forced vital capacity (FVC) took longer to improve them eventually reaching the normal range by 3 years of age, but there was no improvement in forced expiratory flow at 75% of vital capacity (FEF_{75}) over the study period (34). In another study, 70% of BPD infants assessed at 2 years had low flow rates below 40% of that predicted, whereas lung volumes, Crs, and Rrs results were in the normal range (19). More recent results in the present population of prematurely born infants confirm those results (25, 34). Assessment of 44 children with BPD (oxygen dependency at 28 days or 36 weeks PCA with CXR changes) highlighted that there were no improvements in V'_{max} FRC at 6, 12, and 24 months (35). In a longitudinal study, which examined infants at a PCA of 58 weeks and then 33 weeks later, the group mean lung volumes and flows tracked at or near their previous values, that is, there was a lack of catch up growth. There were, however, improvements in lung function in those with above average growth (25).

Serial lung function measurements in infants with BPD have shown a decline in small airway function (as evidenced by assessments of V'_{max} FRC) during the first year after birth (36). Similar changes in small airway function, however, have been reported in healthy, unsedated, prematurely born infants (37). Those findings emphasize the importance of using an appropriate control group when interpreting long-term effects of respiratory disease or management strategies in the neonatal period.

Prediction of BPD

Initial studies focused on compliance and resistance results with differing results. In certain studies, resistance, but not compliance, results were predictive of BPD development. One study, however, included only 20 infants who had required mechanical ventilation for at least 3 days; 8 developed BPD (supplementary oxygen for longer than 28 days) (38). In a study of 46 infants with a birth weight <1.0 kg, those who subsequently developed BPD had significantly higher Rrs, but not Crs, at 1 week and Rrs was significantly higher in those with evolving BPD throughout the neonatal period (39). In another study, Rrs but not Crs before surfactant therapy was associated with an increased risk of BPD. Areas under receiver operator characteristic (ROC) curves were reported and demonstrated that Rrs performed similarly to gestational age and birth weight (40).

By contrast, other studies have demonstrated compliance rather than resistance was predictive of BPD development. Dynamic compliance, assessed using flow measurements from a pneumotachograph related to mean airway pressures in 47 infants mean gestational age of 30 weeks in the first 3 days after birth, was significantly lower in those who developed BPD, which was diagnosed using radiological criteria (41). In a subsequent study, an occlusion technique was used to determine appropriate esophageal balloon placement and longitudinal assessment over the first month was made on 143 infants with a gestational age of 27–30 weeks. The model, which included gestational age and dynamic pulmonary compliance, had the highest positive predictive accuracy (100%) for BPD (the need for supplemental oxygen at 4 weeks of age), whereas the predictive value of total pulmonary resistance was minimal (42). In 39 ventilated infants with a mean gestational age 26–28 weeks, the predictive ability of the results of the interrupter technique was compared to respiratory mechanics results obtained during mechanical ventilation. Dynamic compliance of the respiratory system on day 1, birth weight and gestational age were all significantly lower in the BPD infants (BPD diagnosed if the infant developed lung disease in the first week after birth, was oxygen dependent at 28 days of age and developed characteristic chest x-ray changes), but there were no significant differences in the interrupter technique results. Dynamic compliance of the respiratory system was a better independent predictor of BPD development than gestational age or birth weight (43). More recently, among 52 prematurely born infants who were ventilated for more than 72 h and had received a single dose of porcine surfactant, initial compliance results did not differ between infants who went on to develop mild or severe BPD, but at days 7 and 10 the "severe" group had significantly poorer compliance results. BPD was diagnosed as a requirement of supplementary oxygen at 28 days to maintain oxygen saturation above 95%; the severity of BPD was determined by the CXR score. Compliance but not resistance on days 7 and 10 were predictive of severe BPD (44).

In other studies, neither compliance nor resistance results were predictive of BPD development (45, 46). In a study of 104 ventilator-dependent infants, with a mean gestational age 27–30 weeks, respiratory mechanics were measured using an airway occlusion technique between 6 and 48 h after birth and corrected for body length. Birth weight, but not respiratory system mechanics, predicted BPD development (supplemental oxygen requirement 28 days after birth) (45). In a series of 58 infants who had RDS, compliance and resistance results were assessed using a commercially available system. BPD was diagnosed as oxygen supplementation, respiratory distress, and an abnormal CXR at 28 days. Neither lung compliance nor pulmonary resistance on days 1–4 predicted BPD, but gestational age and a ventilatory index on day 3 (ventilator frequency × maximum inspiratory pressure) were predictive (46).

It is not possible to conclude from the above studies whether assessment of lung mechanics is helpful in predicting BPD development. The discrepancy in the results likely reflects that different techniques were used in different populations. Few of the above studies included a sample size calculation and thus there may have been both type I and II errors.

More recent studies have investigated whether assessment of FRC might be predictive of BPD. In 100 infants with a median gestational age 28 weeks and ventilated within 6 h of birth, FRCHe ≥19 ml/kg and a low gestational age in the first 48 h were more accurate predictors of BPD at 28 days than Crs or Rrs. Indeed, if only the 50 infants whose gestational age was ≤28 weeks of gestation were considered, a low FRC on day 2 was the best predictor of BPD development (47). Subsequently, the results of FRC and Crs on days 3 and 14 after birth were compared to a marker of inflammation, end-tidal carbon monoxide (ETCO). Seventy-eight infants with a median gestational age of 29 weeks were assessed; 39 developed BPD (oxygen dependency at 28 days); a sample size calculation was given. Gestational age, birth weight, ETCO, FRC, and Crs results on days 3 and 14 differed significantly between those who did and did not develop BPD. Multifactorial logistic analysis, however, demonstrated only birth weight and ETCO levels on day 14 were significant predictors of BPD with an area under the ROC curve of 0.97. Those ETCO results indicate ongoing inflammation in infants developing BPD (48).

Response to Therapies

Lung function tests have been used to assess the response to therapies in infants with evolving or established BPD. Variable and often conflicting results have been reported, which reflects the use of different techniques, some of which were inappropriate in this age group, lack of a sample size, or an inappropriate sample size based on too optimistic a view of the likely effect. A further problem in interpreting the results are that many of the studies were reported more than 20 years ago and, therefore, include infants not exposed to antenatal steroids or postnatal surfactant, which could have affected their response to the intervention. More importantly, reported changes in lung function results were not always accompanied by a change in clinical status or affected longer-term outcome.

Diuretics

Bronchopulmonary dysplasia infants often are poorly tolerant of fluid loads with excessive weight gain on standard fluid regimens. As a consequence, diuretics are frequently prescribed but have short- and long-term side-effects including electrolyte disturbance and nephrocalcinosis. It is, therefore, important to determine if they are having a positive effect. Early results demonstrated that administration of frusemide acutely increased lung compliance and reduced airway resistance (49, 50) was associated with a reduction in ventilator requirements (51) and transient improvements in blood gases (49). A systematic review, however, demonstrated that in prematurely born infants <3 weeks of age, frusemide administration had either inconsistent or no detectable effects (52). In addition, in 16 spontaneously breathing infants with postnatal ages ranging from 4 to 35 weeks, a single dose of frusemide was associated with improvement in pulmonary compliance but not blood gases or resistance. Furthermore, a 6- to 10-day course was associated with improvement in compliance and resistance (53), but better oxygenation was only achieved in 6 of the 16 infants.

Nebulized frusemide has been given with the hope that this would improve respiratory function while avoiding the systemic complications. In a study of eight ventilated infants with a mean postnatal age of 33 days, the effects of 0.1, 0.25, 0.5, and 1.0 mg/kg of nebulized frusemide were assessed. A dose of 1 mg/kg was associated with a 28% improvement in pulmonary resistance and a 51% improvement in pulmonary compliance at 1 h; the effects lasted for least 4 h. A systematic review demonstrated a significant improvement in tidal volume after 1 and 2 h, but no improvement in compliance at either time point (54).

Due to the side-effects of frusemide, infants who require chronic diuretic therapy are often changed to chlorothiazide and spironolactone. It had been suggested that the combination improved the outcome of babies with severe BPD (55). In a randomized, double blind, crossover trial, the effects of oral diuretics (chlorothiazide 20 mg/kg/dose and spironolactone 1.5 mg/kg/dose) given twice daily for a week were compared to placebo (56). The mean airway resistance, specific airway conductance, and dynamic compliance improved significantly, but only 10 infants were included in the study. In a further randomized trial (57), spironolactone and chlorothiazide were compared to placebo in 43 oxygen dependent BPD infants. Infants in the treatment group only had improvements in dynamic pulmonary compliance and airway resistance and, at 4 weeks after study entry, required less supplementary oxygen than the placebo group. There were, however, no significant differences in the pulmonary function test results after discontinuation of treatment, nor in the total number of days supplementary oxygen was required between the two groups. Orally administered diuretics (chlorothiazide and spironolactone) in combination with theophylline have been demonstrated to have an additive positive effect on dynamic compliance, but no effect on clinical outcomes were reported (58).

Bronchodilators

Inhaled bronchodilators have been reported to improve pulmonary resistance, dynamic compliance, and transcutaneous blood gases when administered to ventilated babies with BPD at approximately 1 month of age (59) and reduce airway resistance in infants with BPD at term (60–62). Intravenously administered salbutamol (30 µg/kg) in six infants aged between 54 and 105 days resulted in an improvement in respiratory system compliance and resistance using the occlusion technique, but there was no correlation between salbutamol serum concentration and pulmonary function changes (63). Comparison of the effectiveness of aerosol and intravenous delivery of salbutamol was made in eight ventilator-dependent infants in randomized order; there were similar improvements in pulmonary mechanics with the two delivery methods (64). In a comparison of different inhalation devices in infants during unassisted breathing as well as in a group of ventilated infants (65, 66), it was reported that both Crs and Rrs were sensitive indicators of a bronchodilator effect. Interpretation of those data is, however, limited because the studies were performed prior to standardization of the technique and intra-individual variability was not reported.

Synergism was reported between ipratropium bromide (IB) and salbutamol in improving pulmonary mechanics in ventilated infants for up to 1–2 h after administration (67). In 10, ventilator-dependent infants, mean age 25 days, various dose of IB (75, 125, and 175 µg) plus 0.04 mg salbutamol were compared to placebo. Rrs and Crs were measured by the single breath occlusion technique. The greatest decline in Rrs (mean 26%) was seen after 175 µg IB with salbutamol. The authors, therefore, concluded that muscarinic receptors contribute to the increased bronchomotor tone of infants with BPD (67). No synergy, however, was shown between metaproterenol and atropine with lung function returning to baseline after both treatments (68).

All of the above studies were undertaken more than 20 years ago, there were no sample size calculations and no long-term benefits reported. As a consequence, in the present population of premature infants, diuretics should only be given to treat incipient heart failure in infants with evolving or established BPD and stopped as soon as that problem ceases. Equally, bronchodilators should only be administered to treat troublesome wheeze and continued if the administration is associated with a reduction in respiratory support requirements. Administration should be via a metered dose inhaler and spacer rather than a nebulizer, as the nebulizing fluid can cause bronchoconstriction (69).

Dexamethasone

The efficacy of dexamethasone to prevent and treat BPD has been tested in many RCTs. Unfortunately, although systemically administered steroids have many positive effects, they have short- and long-term adverse effects. As a consequence, attention has been given to assessing the response to lower doses and inhaled steroids. A 1-week tapering course of dexamethasone starting at 0.5 mg/kg/day given at 7–14 days of age in ventilator dependent, VLBW infants increased pulmonary compliance and decreased the incidence of BPD at 36 weeks PCA (70). In a subsequent study, the effectiveness of that dose (total dose 2.35 mg/kg) compared to a lower dose (total dose 1 mg/kg) was compared. FRC using a nitrogen washout technique and Crs by an occlusion technique were measured in infants at a mean age of 11 days. The sample size was powered to detect that the increase in FRC in the lower dose group would be more than 10% smaller than in the higher dose group. No significant differences were shown (71). In a RCT, 10 days of dexamethasone were compared to 100 µg qds per day of budesonide in 40 infants with a median postnatal age 27 days. The study was powered to detect a difference of 7% in the inspired oxygen requirement 1 week after starting therapy. After 36 h, only the systemic group had significant reductions in the inspired oxygen concentration and Crs and at 1 week the systemic group had significantly better results than the inhaled group (72).

Respiratory Support

Lung function testing has been used to compare the acute and longer-term efficacy of respiratory support techniques. For example, in a randomized crossover study, proportional assist ventilation (PAV) and assist control ventilation (ACV) were examined in infants with evolving BPD. When on PAV the infants had superior respiratory muscle strength and a lower work of breathing and this was associated with better oxygenation (73). Follow-up studies assessing the efficacy of ventilation modes demonstrate the importance of which lung function technique was employed. In a follow-up study of an RCT, no advantage of HFO over conventional

ventilation (CMV) was reported with respect to lung function at 1 year corrected, but small airway function was only assessed by evaluation of gas trapping (74). In another study, V'_{max} FRC was assessed at 6 and 12 months in infants who developed BPD. Those who were initially supported by CMV showed the expected decline in small airway function, but this was not seen in those seen in the HRO group. As a consequence, at 12 months, the HFO group had superior lung function (75). The results of that non-randomized study suggested that HFO might protect small airway function. Follow-up at 11–14 years of children who had been entered into a neonatal RCT of prophylactic HFO has subsequently proved that hypothesis (9).

Conclusion and Future Directions

- Infants who develop BPD have low compliance and lung volumes and elevated resistances in the neonatal period.
- During infancy, lung function generally improves, but airflow limitation persists and small airway function declines.
- Improvements in lung function following administration of diuretics or bronchodilators have not translated into long-term improvements in respiratory outcomes, but assessment at follow-up has demonstrated neonatal high-frequency oscillation appears to protect small airway function.
- Further investigation should be undertaken to determine whether a lung function assessment accurately predicts chronic respiratory morbidity and hence prophylactic interventions can be appropriately targeted.
- Lung function assessment at follow-up should be incorporated into all neonatal RCTs, which are aimed at improving respiratory outcome.

Author Contributions

Both authors undertook a literature review and produced the manuscript.

References

1. Rojas MA, Gonzalez A, Bancalari E, Claure N, Poole C, Silva-Neto G. Changing trends in the epidemiology and pathogenesis of chronic lung disease. *J Pediatr* (1995) 126:605–10. doi:10.1016/S0022-3476(95)70362-4
2. Husain AN, Siddiqui NH, Stocker JT. Pathology of arrested acinar development in postsurfactant bronchopulmonary dysplasia. *Hum Pathol* (1998) 29:710–7. doi:10.1016/S0046-8177(98)90280-5
3. Jobe AH, Bancalari E. Bronchopulmonary dysplasia. *Am J Respir Crit Care Med* (2001) 163:1723–9. doi:10.1164/ajrccm.163.7.2011060
4. Ellsbury DL, Acarregui MJ, McGuiness GA, Klein JM. Variability in the use of supplemental oxygen for bronchopulmonary dysplasia. *J Pediatr* (2002) 149:247–9. doi:10.1067/mpd.2002.121933
5. Walsh MC, Yao Q, Gettner P, Hale E, Collins M, Hensman A, et al. Impact of a physiologic definition on bronchopulmonary dysplasia rates. *Pediatrics* (2004) 114:1305–11. doi:10.1542/peds.2004-0204
6. Parad RP, Davis JM, Lo J, Thomas M, Marlow N, Calvert S, et al. Prediction of respiratory outcome in extremely low gestational age infants. *Neonatology* (2015) 107:241–8. doi:10.1159/000369878
7. Ambalavanan N, Tyson JE, Kennedy KA, Hansen NI, Vohr BR, Wright LL, et al. Vitamin A supplementation for extremely low birth weight infants: outcome at 18 to 22 months. *Pediatrics* (2005) 115:e249–54. doi:10.1542/peds.2004-1812

8. Davis JM, Parad RB, Michele T, Allred E, Price A, Rosenfeld W, et al. Pulmonary outcome at one year corrected age in premature infants treated at birth with recombinant human CuZn superoxide dismutase. *Pediatrics* (2003) 111:469–76. doi:10.1542/peds.111.3.469
9. Zivanovic S, Peacock J, Alcazar-Paris M, Lo JW, Lunt A, Marlow N, et al. Late outcomes of a randomized trial of high frequency oscillation in neonates. *N Engl J Med* (2014) 370:1121–30. doi:10.1056/NEJMoa1309220
10. Manczur T, Greenough A, Nicholson GP, Rafferty GF. Resistance of pediatric and neonatal endotracheal tubes: influence of flow rate, size and shape. *Crit Care Med* (2000) 28:1595–8. doi:10.1097/00003246-200005000-00056
11. National Heart Lung and Blood Institute (NHLBI) Workshop . *Consensus Statement on Measurement of Lung Volumes in Humans* (2005). Available from: http://www.thoracic.org/adobe/lungvolume.pdf
12. Fox WW, Schwartz JG, Shaffer TH. Effects of endotracheal tube leaks on functional residual capacity determination in intubated neonates. *Pediatr Res* (1979) 13:60–4. doi:10.1203/00006450-197901000-00013
13. Hird M, Greenough A, Gamsu H. Gas trapping during high frequency positive pressure ventilation using conventional ventilators. *Early Hum Dev* (1990) 22:51–6. doi:10.1016/0378-3782(90)90025-E
14. Hulskamp G, Hoo AF, Ljungberg H, Lum S, Pillow JJ, Stocks J. Progressive decline in plethysmographic lung volumes in infants: physiology or technology? *Am J Respir Crit Care Med* (2003) 168:1003–9. doi:10.1164/rccm.200303-460OC

15. Broughton SJ, Sylvester KP, Page CM, Rafferty GF, Milner AD, Greenough A. Problems in the measurement of functional residual capacity. *Physiol Meas* (2006) **27**:99–107. doi:10.1088/0967-3334/27/2/001

16. Stocks J, Godfrey S, Beardsmore C, Bar-Yishay E, Castile R. Standards for infant respiratory function testing: plethysmographic measurements of lung volume and airway resistance. *Eur Respir J* (2001) **17**:302–12. doi:10.1183/09031936.01.17203020

17. Prechtl HFR. The behavioural states of the newborn infant (a review). *Brain Res* (1974) **76**:185–212. doi:10.1016/0006-8993(74)90454-5

18. Wolfson MR, Bhutani VK, Shaffer TH, Bowen FW Jr. Mechanics and energetics of breathing helium in infants with bronchopulmonary dysplasia. *J Pediatr* (1984) **104**:752–7. doi:10.1016/S0022-3476(84)80961-0

19. Baraldi E, Filippone M, Trevisanuto D, Zanardo V, Zacchello F. Pulmonary function until two years of life in infants with bronchopulmonary dysplasia. *Am J Respir Crit Care Med* (1997) **155**:149–55. doi:10.1164/ajrccm.155.1.9001304

20. May C, Kennedy C, Milner AD, Rafferty GF, Peacock JL, Greenough A. Lung function abnormalities in infants developing bronchopulmonary dysplasia. *Arch Dis Child* (2011) **96**:1014–9. doi:10.1136/adc.2011.212332

21. Abman SH, Groothius JR. Pathophysiology and treatment of bronchopulmonary dysplasia. *Pediatr Clin North Am* (1994) **41**:277–315.

22. Kavvadia V, Greenough A, Dimitriou G, Itakura Y. Lung volume measurements in infants with and without chronic lung disease. *Eur J Pediatr* (1998) **157**:336–9. doi:10.1007/s004310050823

23. May C, Prendergast M, Salman S, Rafferty GF, Greenough A. Chest radiograph thoracic areas and lung volumes in infants developing bronchopulmonary dysplasia. *Pediatr Pulmonol* (2009) **44**:80–5. doi:10.1002/ppul.20952

24. Robin B, Kim YJ, Huth J, Klocksieben J, Torres M, Tepper RS, et al. Pulmonary function in bronchopulmonary dysplasia. *Pediatr Pulmonol* (2004) **37**:236–42. doi:10.1002/ppul.10424

25. Filbrun AG, Popova AP, Linn MJ, McIntosh NA, Hershenson MB. Longitudinal measures of lung function in infants with bronchopulmonary dysplasia. *Pediatr Pulmonol* (2011) **46**:369–75. doi:10.1002/ppul.21378

26. Wauer RR, Maurer T, Nowotny T, Schmalisch G. Assessment of functional residual capacity using nitrogen washout and plethysmographic techniques in infants with and without bronchopulmonary dysplasia. *Intensive Care Med* (1998) **24**:469–75. doi:10.1007/s001340050598

27. Gerhardt T, Hehre D, Feller R, Reifenberg L, Bancalari E. Serial determination of pulmonary function in infants with chronic lung disease. *J Pediatr* (1987) **110**:448–56. doi:10.1016/S0022-3476(87)80516-4

28. Shao H, Sandberg K, Hjalmarson O. Impaired gas mixing and low lung volume in preterm infants with mild chronic lung disease. *Pediatr Res* (1998) **43**:536–41. doi:10.1203/00006450-199804000-00017

29. Hjalmarson O, Sandberg KL. Lung function at term reflects severity of bronchopulmonary dysplasia. *J Pediatr* (2005) **146**:86–90. doi:10.1016/j.jpeds.2004.08.044

30. Broughton S, Thomas MR, Marston L, Calvert SA, Marlow N, Peacock JL, et al. Very prematurely born infants wheezing at follow up: lung function and risk factors. *Arch Dis Child* (2007) **92**:776–80. doi:10.1136/adc.2006.112623

31. Kjellberg M, Björkman K, Rohdin M, Sanchez-Crespo A, Jonsson B. Bronchopulmonary dysplasia: clinical grading in relation to ventilation/perfusion mismatch measured by single photon emission computed tomography. *Pediatr Pulmonol* (2013) **48**:1206–13. doi:10.1002/ppul.22751

32. Balinotti JE, Chakr VC, Tiller C, Kimmel R, Coates C, Kisling J, et al. Growth of lung parenchyma in infants and toddlers with chronic lung disease of infancy. *Am J Respir Crit Care Med* (2010) **181**:1093–7. doi:10.1164/rccm.200908-1190OC

33. Schmalish G, Wilitzki S, Roehr CC, Proquitte H, Buhrer C. Development of lung function in very low birth weight infants with or without bronchopulmonary dysplasia: longitudinal assessment during the first 15 months of corrected age. *BMC Pediatr* (2012) **12**:37. doi:10.1186/1471-2431-12-37

34. Mallory GB, Chaney H, Mutich RL, Motoyama EEK. Longitudinal changes in lung function during the first three years of premature infants with moderate to severe bronchopulmonary dysplasia. *Pediatr Pulmonol* (1991) **11**:8–14. doi:10.1002/ppul.1950110103

35. Fakhoury KF, Sellers C, O'Brian Smith E, Rama JA, Fan LL. Serial measurements of lung function in a cohort of young children with bronchopulmonary dysplasia. *Pediatrics* (2010) **125**:e1441–7. doi:10.1542/peds.2009-0668

36. Gappa M, Stocks J, Merkus P. Lung growth and development after preterm birth: further evidence. *Am J Respir Crit Care Med* (2003) **168**:399. doi:10.1164/ajrccm.168.3.955

37. Hoo AF, Dezateux C, Henschen M, Costeloe K, Stocks J. Development of airway function in infancy after preterm delivery. *J Pediatr* (2002) **141**:652–8. doi:10.1067/mpd.2002.128114

38. Goldman SL, Gerhardt T, Sonni R, Feller R, Hehre D, Tapia JL, et al. Early prediction of chronic lung disease by pulmonary function testing. *J Pediatr* (1983) **102**:613–7.

39. Lui K, Lloyd J, Ang E, Rynn M, Gupta JM. Early changes in respiratory compliance and resistance during the development of bronchopulmonary dysplasia in the era of surfactant therapy. *Pediatr Pulmonol* (2000) **30**:282–90. doi:10.1002/1099-0496(200010)30:4<282::AID-PPUL2>3.0.CO;2-D

40. Choukroun ML, Tayara N, Fayon M, Demarquez JL. Early respiratory system mechanics and the prediction of chronic lung disease in ventilated preterm neonates requiring surfactant treatment. *Biol Neonate* (2003) **83**:30–5. doi:10.1159/000067015

41. Graff MA, Novo RP, Diaz M, Smith C, Hiatt IM, Hegyi T. Compliance measurement in respiratory distress syndrome: the prediction of outcome. *Pediatr Pulmonol* (1986) **2**:332–6. doi:10.1002/ppul.1950020604

42. Bhutani VK, Abbasi S. Relative likelihood of bronchopulmonary dysplasia based on pulmonary mechanics measured in preterm neonates during the first week of life. *J Pediatr* (1992) **120**:605–13. doi:10.1016/S0022-3476(05)82491-6

43. Freezer NJ, Sly PD. Predictive value of measurements of respiratory mechanics in preterm infants with HMD. *Pediatr Pulmonol* (1993) **16**:116–23. doi:10.1002/ppul.1950160207

44. Tortorolo L, Vento G, Matassa PG, Zecca E, Romagnoli C. Early changes of pulmonary mechanics to predict the severity of bronchopulmonary dysplasia in ventilated preterm infants. *J Matern Fetal Neonatal Med* (2002) **12**:332–7. doi:10.1080/jmf.12.5.332.337

45. Kirpalani H, Schmidt B, Gaston S, Santos R, Wilkie R. Birthweight, early passive respiratory system mechanics, and ventilator requirements as predictors of outcome in premature infants with respiratory failure. *Pediatr Pulmonol* (1991) **10**:195–8. doi:10.1002/ppul.1950100311

46. Van Lierde S, Smith J, Devlieger H, Eggermont E. Pulmonary mechanics during respiratory distress syndrome in the prediction of outcome and differentiation of mild and severe bronchopulmonary dysplasia. *Pediatr Pulmonol* (1994) **17**:218–24. doi:10.1002/ppul.1950170403

47. Kavvadia V, Greenough A, Dimitriou G. Early prediction of chronic oxygen dependency by lung function test results. *Pediatr Pulmonol* (2000) **29**:19–26. doi:10.1002/(SICI)1099-0496(200001)29:1<19::AID-PPUL4>3.3.CO;2-M

48. May C, Patel S, Kennedy C, Pollina E, Rafferty GF, Peacock JL, et al. Prediction of bronchopulmonary dysplasia. *Arch Dis Child Fetal Neonatal Ed* (2011) **96**:F410–6. doi:10.1136/adc.2010.189597

49. Kao LC, Warburton D, Sargent CW, Platzker AC, Keens TG. Furosemide acutely decreases airways resistance in chronic bronchopulmonary dysplasia. *J Pediatr* (1983) **103**:624–9. doi:10.1016/S0022-3476(83)80602-7

50. Najak ZD, Harris EM, Lazzara A Jr, Pruitt AW. Pulmonary effects of furosemide in preterm infants with lung disease. *J Pediatr* (1983) **102**:758–63. doi:10.1016/S0022-3476(83)80253-4

51. McCann EM, Lewis K, Deming DD, Donovan MJ, Brady JP. Controlled trial of furosemide therapy in infants with chronic lung disease. *J Pediatr* (1985) **106**:957–62. doi:10.1016/S0022-3476(85)80252-3

52. Stewart A, Brion LP. Intravenous or enteral loop diuretics for preterm infants with (or developing) chronic lung disease. *Cochrane Database Syst Rev* (2011) **9**:CD001453. doi:10.1002/14651858.CD001453.pub2

53. Engelhardt B, Elliott S, Hazinski TA. Short- and long-term effects of furosemide on lung function in infants with bronchopulmonary dysplasia. *J Pediatr* (1986) **109**:1034–9. doi:10.1016/S0022-3476(86)80295-5

54. Brion LP, Primhak RA, Yong W. Aerosolized diuretics for preterm infants with (or developing) chronic lung disease. *Cochrane Database Syst Rev* (2006) **3**:CD001694.

55. Albersheim SG, Solimano AJ, Sharma AK, Smyth JA, Rotschild A, Wood BJ, et al. Randomized, double-blind, controlled trial of long-term diuretic therapy for bronchopulmonary dysplasia. *J Pediatr* (1989) **115**:615–20. doi:10.1016/S0022-3476(89)80297-5

56. Kao LC, Warburton D, Cheng MH, Cedeno C, Platzker AC, Keens TG. Effect of oral diuretics on pulmonary mechanics in infants with chronic bronchopulmonary dysplasia: results of a double-blind crossover sequential trial. *Pediatrics* (1984) **74**:37–44.

57. Kao LC, Durand DJ, McCrea RC, Birch M, Powers RJ, Nickerson BG. Randomized trial of long term diuretic therapy for infants with oxygen dependent bronchopulmonary dysplasia. *J Pediatr* (1994) **124**:772–81. doi:10.1016/S0022-3476(05)81373-3

58. Rooklin AR, Moomjian AS, Shutack JG, Schwartz JG, Fox WW. Theophylline therapy in bronchopulmonary dysplasia. *J Pediatr* (1979) **95**:882–8. doi:10.1016/S0022-3476(79)80459-X

59. Cabal LA, Larrazabal C, Ramanathan R, Durand M, Lewis D, Siassi B, et al. Effects of metaproterenol on pulmonary mechanics, oxygenation, and ventilation in infants with chronic lung disease. *J Pediatr* (1987) **110**:116–9. doi:10.1016/S0022-3476(87)80302-5

60. Kao LC, Warburton D, Platzker AC, Keens TG. Effects of isoproterenol inhalation on airway resistance in chronic bronchopulmonary dyplasia. *Pediatrics* (1984) **73**:509–14.

61. Motoyama EK, Fort MD, Klesh KW, Mutich RL, Guthrie RD. Early onset of airway reactivity in premature infants with bronchopulmonary dysplasia. *Am Rev Respir Dis* (1987) **136**:50–7. doi:10.1164/ajrccm/136.1.50

62. Wilkie RA, Bryan MH. Effect of bronchodilators on airway resistance in ventilator-dependent neonates with chronic lung disease. *J Pediatr* (1987) **111**:278–82. doi:10.1016/S0022-3476(87)80087-2

63. Kirpalani H, Koren G, Schmidt B, Tan Y, Santos R, Soldin S. Respiratory response and pharmacokinetics of intravenous salbutamol in infants with bronchopulmonary dysplasia. *Crit Care Med* (1990) **18**:1374–7. doi:10.1097/00003246-199012000-00013

64. Pfenninger J, Aebi C. Respiratory response to salbutamol (albuterol) in ventilator-dependent infants with chronic lung disease: pressurized aerosol delivery versus intravenous injection. *Intensive Care Med* (1993) **19**:251–5. doi:10.1007/BF01690544

65. Fok TF, Lam K, Ng PC, Leung TF, So HK, Cheung KL, et al. Delivery of salbutamol to nonventilated preterm infants by metered-dose inhaler, jet nebulizer, and ultrasonic nebulizer. *Eur Respir J* (1998) **12**:159–64. doi:10.1183/09031936.98.12010159

66. Fok TF, Lam K, Ng PC, So HK, Cheung KL, Wong W, et al. Randomised crossover trial of salbutamol aerosol delivered by metered dose inhaler, jet nebuliser, and ultrasonic nebuliser in chronic lung disease. *Arch Dis Child Fetal Neonatal Ed* (1998) **79**:100–4. doi:10.1136/fn.79.2.F100

67. Brundage KL, Mohsini KG, Froese AB, Fisher JT. Bronchodilator response to ipratropium bromide in infants with bronchopulmonary dysplasia. *Am Rev Respir Dis* (1990) **142**:1137–42. doi:10.1164/ajrccm/142.5.1137

68. Kao LC, Durand DJ, Nickerson BG. Effects of inhaled metaproterenol and atropine on the pulmonary mechanics of infants with bronchopulmonary dysplasia. *Pediatr Pulmonol* (1989) **6**:74–80. doi:10.1002/ppul.1950060204

69. Yuksel B, Greenough A. Nebulised sodium cromoglycate in preterm infants – protection against water challenge-induced bronchoconstriction. *Respir Med* (1993) **87**:37–42. doi:10.1016/S0954-6111(05)80311-7

70. Durand M, Sardesai S, McEvoy C. Effects of early dexamethasone therapy on pulmonary mechanics and chronic lung disease in very low birth weight infants: a randomized, controlled trial. *Pediatrics* (1995) **95**:584–90.

71. McEvoy C, Bowling S, Williamson K, McGaw P, Durand M. Randomized, double-blinded trial of low-dose dexamethasone: II. Functional residual capacity and pulmonary outcome in very low birth weight infants at risk for bronchopulmonary dysplasia. *Pediatr Pulmonol* (2004) **38**:55–63. doi:10.1002/ppul.20037

72. Dimitriou G, Greenough A, Giffin FJ, Kavadia V. Inhaled versus systemic steroids in chronic oxygen dependency of preterm infants. *Eur J Pediatr* (1997) **156**:51–5. doi:10.1007/s004310050552

73. Bhat P, Patel DS, Hannam S, Rafferty GF, Peacock JL, Milner AD, et al. Crossover study of proportional assist versus assist control ventilation. *Arch Dis Child Fetal Neonatal Ed* (2015) **100**:F35–8. doi:10.1136/archdischild-2013-305817

74. Thomas MR, Rafferty GF, Limb ES, Peacock JL, Calvert SA, Marlow N, et al. Pulmonary function at follow-up of very preterm infants from the United Kingdom oscillation study. *Am J Respir Crit Care Med* (2004) **169**:868–72. doi:10.1164/rccm.200310-1425OC

75. Hofhuis W, Huysman MW, van der Wiel EC, Holland WP, Hop WC, Brinkhorst G, et al. Worsening of V9maxFRC in infants with chronic lung disease in the first year of life: a more favorable outcome after high-frequency oscillation ventilation. *Am J Respir Crit Care Med* (2002) **166**:1539–43. doi:10.1164/rccm.2202046

Intrauterine Growth Restriction Promotes Postnatal Airway Hyperresponsiveness Independent of Allergic Disease

Jack O. Kalotas[1], Carolyn J. Wang[1], Peter B. Noble[1] and Kimberley C. W. Wang[1,2*]

[1] School of Human Sciences, The University of Western Australia, Crawley, WA, Australia, [2] Telethon Kids Institute, The University of Western Australia, Nedlands, WA, Australia

*Correspondence:
Kimberley C. W. Wang
kimberley.wang@uwa.edu.au

Introduction: Intrauterine growth restriction (IUGR) is associated with asthma. Murine models of IUGR have altered airway responsiveness in the absence of any inflammatory exposure. Given that a primary feature of asthma is airway inflammation, IUGR-affected individuals may develop more substantial respiratory impairment if subsequently exposed to an allergen. This study used a maternal hypoxia-induced mouse model of IUGR to determine the combined effects of IUGR and allergy on airway responsiveness.

Methods: Pregnant BALB/c mice were housed under hypoxic conditions (10.5% O_2) from gestational day (GD) 11-GD 17.5 (IUGR group; term = GD 21). Following hypoxic exposure, mice were returned to a normoxic environment (21% O_2). A second group of pregnant mice were housed under normoxic conditions throughout pregnancy (Control). All offspring were sensitized to ovalbumin (OVA) and assigned to one of four treatment groups: Control – normoxic and saline challenge; IUGR – hypoxic and saline challenge; Allergy – normoxic and OVA challenge; and IUGR + Allergy – hypoxic and OVA challenge. At 8 weeks of age, and 24 h post-aerosol challenge, mice were tracheostomised for methacholine challenge and assessment of lung mechanics by the forced oscillation technique, and lungs subsequently fixed for morphometry.

Results: IUGR offspring were lighter than Control at birth and in adulthood. Both Allergy and IUGR independently increased airway resistance after methacholine challenge. The IUGR group also exhibited an exaggerated increase in tissue damping and elastance after methacholine challenge compared with Control. However, there was no incremental effect on airway responsiveness in the combined IUGR + Allergy group. There was no impact of IUGR or Allergy on airway structure and no effect of sex on any outcome.

Conclusion: IUGR and aeroallergen independently increased bronchoconstrictor response, but when combined the pathophysiology was not worsened. Findings suggest that an association between IUGR and asthma is mediated by baseline airway responsiveness rather than susceptibility to allergen.

Keywords: airway hyperresponsiveness, allergy, intrauterine growth restriction, asthma, lung function

INTRODUCTION

Asthma is an obstructive airway disease that affects patient quality of life, manifesting as episodes of breathing difficulties. Airway hyperresponsiveness (AHR), a major functional impairment in asthma, results in disproportionate airway narrowing that produces airflow limitation (1). There are numerous potential causes of AHR. A relationship between AHR and allergy has been established; inflammation, orchestrated by T-helper 2 (Th2) cells, results in the release of bronchoactive mediators including histamine, leukotriene B4, prostaglandin D2 and cytokines along with the recruitment of immune cells (2, 3) which mediate excessive airway constriction. "Airway remodeling" that is either independent or co-dependent on inflammation (4), is also associated with AHR. Airway remodeling is a change in the structure (mass, thickness, or volume) of the airway wall (5), exerting a multitude of effects, including increased airway smooth muscle (ASM) force production (1), and reduced and more variable airway caliber (1, 6), all of which at least contribute to the onset of AHR.

The above changes to airway structure-function in asthma have conventionally been attributed to environmental exposures (e.g., allergic stimuli) accumulated through postnatal life. An alternative proposal is that airway abnormalities are the result of a developmental disorder and we particularly note the association between intrauterine growth restriction (IUGR) and asthma (7). After establishing a mouse model of hypoxia-induced IUGR, we demonstrated airway hyperresponsiveness in female offspring and hyporesponsiveness in males (8). Functional changes after IUGR were not associated with airway remodeling (8, 9), rather our data implicated a shift in inflammatory phenotype; an increase in macrophages in the bronchial alveolar lavage (BAL) fluid from both male and female offspring with males also demonstrating an increase in interleukin (IL)-2, IL-13, and eotaxin (10). Importantly, this shift in inflammatory phenotype was the result of a prenatal disruption that persisted into adult life and occurred without exposure to typical environmental triggers (10). Together these observations suggest that developmental changes in airway responsiveness that occur concomitantly with inflammation will alter the susceptibility to environmental influences and subsequent airway disease.

The present study was therefore principally focused on the evolution of AHR in asthma, which as discussed is impacted by structural and inflammatory pathologies and potentially developmental programming. We specifically examined the interaction between IUGR and allergy and hypothesized that persistent biological changes after IUGR worsens the response to allergy and this manifests as more severe bronchoconstriction to contractile stimulation i.e., AHR. To address this study hypothesis, we used our established mouse model of IUGR and exposed both male and female offspring to ovalbumin (OVA) sensitization and challenge.

MATERIALS AND METHODS

Maternal Hypoxia-Induced IUGR Mouse Model

This study was approved by The University of Western Australia Animal Ethics Committee (approval number RA/3/100/1570). All animals were housed in the Pre-Clinical Facility at The University of Western Australia on a 15:9 light:dark cycle. Thirty pregnant BALB/c mice (gestational day "GD" 7) were obtained from the Animal Resources Center (Murdoch, WA, Australia). Mice were exposed to 10.5% O_2 from GD 11 to GD 17.5 (hypoxic conditions; IUGR group) (8–12) which corresponds to the pseudoglandular-canalicular stage in fetal mouse lung development, and therefore peak airway development. At GD 17.5, the pregnant mice were removed from the hypoxic chamber and returned to normoxic conditions (21% O_2) for the remainder of the pregnancy. Another group of pregnant mice remained under normoxic conditions throughout the entire duration of pregnancy (Control group). Only litter sizes of ≤6 pups were included in the study since larger litters reduce body weight independently of maternal hypoxia and compromises milk availability to pups. Offspring were weaned and sexed at 3 weeks of age, with access to standard chow and water *ad libitum*. Weights of offspring were recorded at birth and before lung function assessment (8 weeks of age). A subset of offspring was used to determine the effects of IUGR on diaphragm function and structure in postnatal life (11).

Allergy Sensitization Protocol

An established mouse allergy protocol from our lab was used in this study (13). At 5 and 7 weeks of age, all IUGR and Control offspring received 0.2 mL intra-peritoneal (i.p.) injection containing 5 mg.mL^{-1} of OVA (Sigma, St. Louis, MO, U.S.A.) suspended in 50 mL of alum (Alu-gel-S, Serva, Heidelberg, Germany). At 8 weeks of age, half of the Control and IUGR offspring received 1% OVA aerosol (MPC aerosol medication nebulizer, Braintree Scientific, Inc., MA, U.S.A), whilst remaining offspring received a saline aerosol. This resulted in four experimental groups: Control (males, $n = 8$; females, $n = 10$), normal mice with saline aerosol; Allergy (males, $n = 8$; females, $n = 10$), normal mice with OVA aerosol; IUGR (males, $n = 8$; females, $n = 9$), IUGR mice with saline aerosol; and IUGR + Allergy (males, $n = 7$; females, $n = 8$), IUGR mice with OVA aerosol (**Figure 1**).

Lung Function Assessment

Twenty-four h after the aerosol challenge, offspring were anesthetized by i.p. injection of ketamine (0.4 mg.g^{-1} body weight) and xylazine (0.02 mg.g^{-1} body weight). Once under anesthesia, each mouse was tracheostomised, transferred to a FlexiVent system (FX module 1, flexiWare version 7.5, SCIREQ, Montreal, QC, Canada) and then ventilated at 250 breaths.min^{-1} (8, 13). Lung volume history was standardized *via* three slow inflation-deflation manoeuvers up to 20 cmH$_2$O transrespiratory pressure.

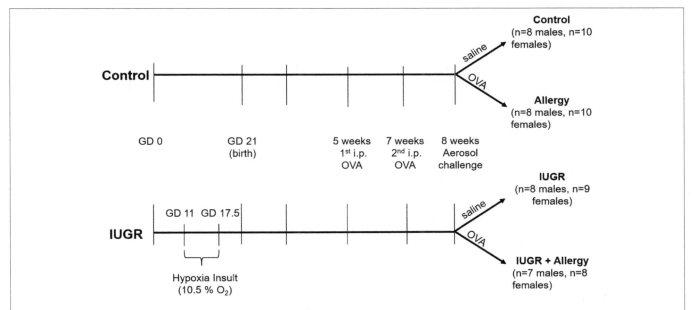

FIGURE 1 | Protocol for IUGR and allergy induction in mice. The superimposition of a maternal hypoxia-induced IUGR model and a well-established allergen protocol, produced 4 experimental groups; Control, Allergy, IUGR and IUGR + Allergy. GD, gestational day; OVA, ovalbumin; i.p., intra-peritoneal; IUGR, intrauterine growth restriction.

Respiratory impedance was measured by forced oscillation technique (FOT). Outcomes of airway resistance (R_{aw}), tissue damping (G), and tissue elastance (H) were derived from impedance using a constant phase model. Once the mouse was stabilized on the ventilator, FOT measurements were recorded once a min for 5 min to establish baseline respiratory mechanics. Mice were then challenged with 10 s aerosols of saline, followed by increasing doses of methacholine (MCh; β-methacholine chloride, Sigma-Aldrich, St. Louis, U.S.A; 0.1 mg.mL^{-1} to 30 mg.mL^{-1}) via the Aeroneb ultrasonic nebuliser (SCIREQ). After each challenge, measurements were again recorded every min for 5 min. Peak responses were used for analysis. After final MCh response was measured, 0.1 mL atropine (600 μg/mL) was delivered via i.p injection, to reverse airway constriction. Ten min after atropine administration, mice were euthanized with an overdose of ketamine and xylazine (13).

ELISA Assay

Following euthanasia, blood serum was collected via centrifugation of cardiac puncture samples to determine levels of OVA-specific immunoglobulin E (IgE), according to manufacturer's protocol (BioLegend, Inc.) (13).

Histology and Morphological Analysis

The analysis was only performed in IUGR mice (IUGR compared with IUGR + Allergy groups) since previous study have shown no effect of acute OVA exposure on airway dimensions (13). Lungs were inflation-fixed in situ at a transrespiratory pressure of 10 cmH$_2$O in 4% formaldehyde (8, 13). The left lung was embedded in paraffin wax and two 5 μm transverse sections were stained with Masson's Trichrome. The first section was acquired just below the transition from extra- to intraparenchymal bronchus [middle region in (14), and the second section marginally deeper into the lung toward the lower region in (14)] (14, 15). All airways within each section were measured. The perimeter of the basement membrane (P_{bm}) and areas of the ASM, inner and outer airway wall were measured by Stereo Investigator software (version 10.42.1, MBF Bioscience, United States of America). Airway measurements were averaged within each animal i.e., a case mean was calculated.

Data Analysis and Statistics

Data were normalized where necessary, to ensure assumptions of parametric tests were satisfied. An unpaired t-test was performed to assess differences in birth weight (unsexed) between IUGR and Control offspring. Body weights of offspring at 8 weeks of age were analyzed using a two-way ANOVA, examining the effects of sex and in utero treatment.

Lung function data were analyzed using two-way ANOVA, examining the effects of sex in three separate analyses; IUGR effect (Control compared with IUGR group), confirming the effect of IUGR on bronchoconstrictor response in saline exposed offspring only; Allergy effect (Control compared with Allergy group), confirming the effects of allergy on bronchoconstrictor response in Control offspring only; combined effect of IUGR and Allergy (IUGR compared with IUGR + Allergy group), examining the effects of allergy on bronchoconstrictor response in IUGR offspring. Outcomes (R_{aw}, G and H) were compared before and after methacholine challenge, and delta change in response to methacholine (e.g., ΔR_{aw}, G and H calculated from the difference between 30 mg.mL^{-1} MCh and saline).

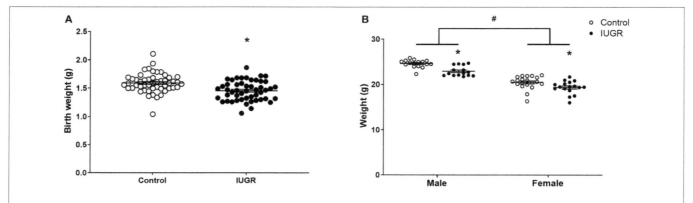

FIGURE 2 | Offspring body weights. Body weights of Control (n = 50) and IUGR (n = 50) offspring at birth (A) and at 8 weeks of age (Control male, n = 16; IUGR male, n = 15; Control female, n = 20; IUGR female, n = 17; B). Sample size of birth weight is larger than experimental sample size as the birth weight of all pups in each litter was recorded. Data are mean ± SEM. *Significant treatment effect (P < 0.05). #Significant sex effect (P < 0.05). IUGR, intrauterine growth restriction.

Data for OVA IgE levels were analyzed by separate two-way ANOVAs; Control compared with IUGR groups for male and female mice; Control compared with Allergy groups for male and female mice; IUGR compared with IUGR + Allergy groups for male and female mice. Airway dimensions were also analyzed by two-way ANOVA; IUGR and IUGR + Allergy groups for male and female mice. P-value < 0.05 was considered statistically significant. Graphical and statistical analysis were conducted using PRISM (version 7, GraphPad Software, La Jolla, CA, U.S.A) and SigmaPlot (version 13, Systat Software, Inc., San Jose, CA, U.S.A).

RESULTS

Offspring Growth Outcomes

The IUGR offspring were lighter than Control offspring at birth ($P = 0.0001$, unsexed; **Figure 2A**). The IUGR offspring remained lighter in adulthood (8 weeks; $P < 0.0001$; **Figure 2B**) and at this age, males were heavier than females ($P < 0.0001$; **Figure 2B**). There was no effect of OVA exposure on body weight at 8 weeks of age (saline, 21.81 ± 1.79 g; OVA, 21.94 ± 2.05 g; $P = 0.701$).

Airway Resistance, Tissue Damping, and Elastance

IUGR Effect

To determine the effect of IUGR on bronchoconstrictor response, data were compared in mice exposed only to saline aerosol (i.e., Control and IUGR groups). Before MCh challenge, there was no difference in R_{aw} between Control or IUGR groups ($P = 0.118$) and male or female ($P = 0.275$) mice (**Figure 3A**). After MCh challenge, R_{aw} ($P = 0.018$; **Figure 3B**) and ΔR_{aw} ($P = 0.005$; **Figure 3C**) of IUGR mice were greater than Control. There was no difference in R_{aw} between males and females after MCh challenge ($P = 0.249$).

Before MCh challenge, G ($P = 0.205$; **Supplementary Figure 1A**) and H ($P = 0.205$; **Supplementary Figure 2A**) were similar between IUGR and Control groups. After MCh challenge, G ($P = 0.025$; **Supplementary Figure 1B**) and H ($P = 0.025$; **Supplementary Figure 2B**) of the IUGR group were greater than the Control group. There was no difference in Δ G ($P = 0.053$; **Supplementary Figure 1C**) but a greater Δ H in the IUGR mice compared with Control mice ($P = 0.007$; **Supplementary Figure 2C**). Sex did not affect G (before MCh, $P = 0.431$; after MCh, $P = 0.429$) or H (before MCh, $P = 0.542$; after MCh, $P = 0.976$).

Allergy Effect

Data were compared in Control and Allergy groups to examine OVA effect on R_{aw}. Before MCh challenge, there was no difference in R_{aw} between Control or Allergy groups ($P = 0.671$) or between males and females ($P = 0.109$; **Figure 4A**). Airway resistance ($P = 0.006$; **Figure 4B**) and ΔR_{aw} ($P = 0.004$; **Figure 4C**) of the Allergy group was greater than Control group after MCh challenge. Male mice also exhibited a greater ΔR_{aw} compared with females ($P = 0.016$).

Tissue damping of Allergy and Control groups were similar before ($P = 0.622$) and after ($P = 0.21$) MCh challenge (**Supplementary Figures 3A,B**). Tissue elastance was also similar between Allergy and Control groups before ($P = 0.837$) and after ($P = 0.065$) MCh challenge (**Supplementary Figures 4A,B**). Sex had no effect on G (before MCh, $P = 0.758$; after MCh, $P = 0.608$) or H (before MCh, $P = 0.787$; after MCh, $P = 0.89$).

Combined Effect of IUGR and Allergy

To determine the combined effect of IUGR and Allergy on bronchoconstrictor response, data were compared in IUGR mice that were exposed to either saline or OVA aerosol (i.e., IUGR and IUGR + Allergy groups). There was no difference in R_{aw} of IUGR mice exposed to either saline or OVA, both before ($P = 0.345$; **Figure 5A**) and after ($P = 0.149$; **Figure 5B**) MCh challenge, and ΔR_{aw} ($P = 0.153$; **Figure 5C**). There was also no difference between sexes, before ($P = 0.841$) or after ($P = 0.670$) MCh challenge in R_{aw}.

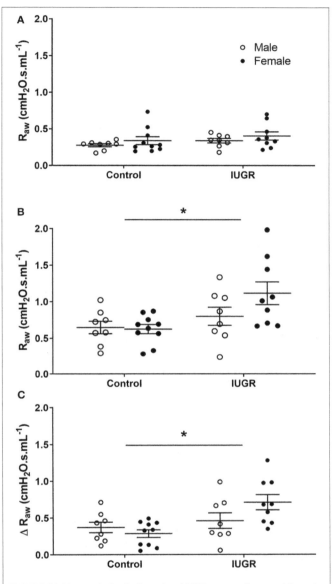

FIGURE 3 | Changes in R_{aw} in Control and IUGR groups. Airway resistance in Control male (n = 8) and female (n = 10), and IUGR male (n = 8) and female (n = 9) offspring before (A) and after (B) MCh challenge, and Δ R_{aw} (C). Data are mean ± SEM. *Significantly different from Control (P < 0.05). Males, open circles; Females, closed circles; R_{aw}, airway resistance; IUGR, intrauterine growth restriction; MCh, methacholine; Δ, net change after MCh challenge.

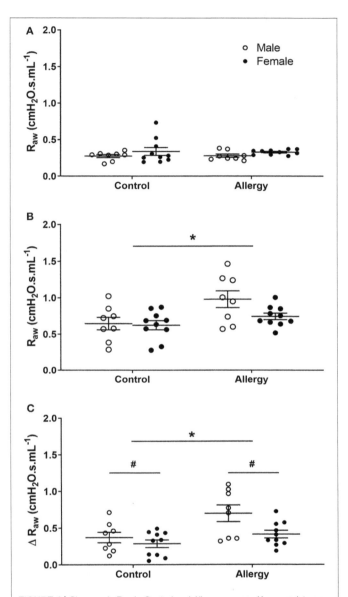

FIGURE 4 | Changes in R_{aw} in Control and Allergy groups. Airway resistance in Control male (n = 8) and female (n = 10), and Allergy male (n = 8) and female (n = 10) offspring before (A), and after (B) MCh challenge, and Δ R_{aw} (C). Data are mean ± SEM. *Significantly different from Control (P < 0.05). #Significantly different from males (P < 0.05). Males, open circles; Females, closed circles; R_{aw}, airway resistance; MCh, methacholine; Δ, net change after MCh challenge.

Tissue damping of the IUGR + Allergy group was similar to the IUGR group before (P = 0.345) and after (P = 0.149) MCh challenge (**Supplementary Figures 5A,B**). Tissue elastance of the IUGR + Allergy group was also similar to the IUGR group, both before (P = 0.578) and after (P = 0.225) MCh (**Supplementary Figures 6A,B**). There was no sex effect on G (before MCh, P = 0.62; after MCh, P = 0.395) or H (before MCh, P = 0.682; after MCh, P = 0.932).

OVA IgE Levels
Female offspring had higher OVA IgE levels than the male offspring in the IUGR group (P = 0.009; **Table 1**). There were no other differences between groups (P > 0.05).

Airway Morphometry of IUGR Offspring
Airway dimensions are provided in **Table 2** and representative images are shown in **Figure 6**. There were no differences in any of the airway wall parameters measured between IUGR and IUGR + Allergy groups (P > 0.05).

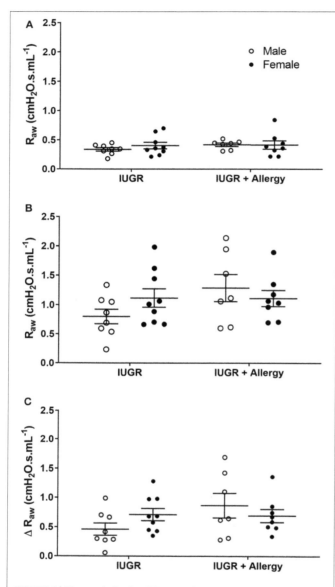

FIGURE 5 | Changes in R_{aw} in IUGR and IUGR + Allergy groups. Airway resistance in IUGR male (n = 8) and female (n = 9), and IUGR + Allergy male (n = 7) and female (n = 8) offspring before (A) and after (B) MCh challenge, and Δ R_{aw} (C). Data are mean ± SEM. Males, open circles; Females, closed circles; R_{aw}, airway resistance; IUGR, intrauterine growth restriction; MCh, methacholine; Δ, net change after MCh challenge.

DISCUSSION

Intrauterine growth restriction and low birth weight are associated with the development of asthma in childhood and adult life (7, 16, 17). Sex and age-dependent changes in AHR within IUGR mice have been documented (8), aligning well with human population studies that show differences in the prevalence of asthma between males and females in early life and adulthood (18–20). Allergy is a major risk factor for asthma (21) and may differentially impact individuals that were growth-restricted *in utero*. The present study used an established mouse model of maternal hypoxia-induced IUGR (8–12) to examine changes in airway responsiveness in IUGR offspring that were subsequently sensitized and challenged with an allergic stimulus i.e., OVA. Findings were unexpected in that the independent effects of IUGR and allergy in promoting AHR did not enhance bronchoconstriction when both abnormalities were combined.

The animal model of IUGR used in this study is robust; the reduction in body weight (at birth and 8 weeks of age) is comparable to that observed previously (8–12), affecting both male and female offspring (10, 11). An acute allergy exposure protocol was preferred as this produces an inflammatory-mediated increase in airway responsiveness (13, 22), without altering body weight (13, 23). Airway responsiveness was assessed from changes in resistance measured using FOT which showed an exaggerated response to MCh after OVA, consistent with AHR. An exaggerated increase in H was also observed, as has been previously documented (13, 22), although G was unchanged. Tissue damping response is at times affected by OVA (22), varying with aerosol deposition patterns (24).

The IUGR and OVA protocols have revealed several interesting biological phenomena, the first of which is apparent after pure sensitization, even prior to bronchial challenge. As discussed, IUGR offspring in the absence of sensitization exhibit sex-dependent changes in airway responsiveness (8). While adult female offspring are hyperresponsive after IUGR (8), males are hyporesponsive, an effect that may well be explained by reduced contractile capacity of the ASM layer (9). We here now observe that after OVA sensitization, male and female mice are both hyperresponsive, in that males switched from a hypo- to hyperresponsive phenotype, manifested by an exaggerated increase in resistance, damping and elastance. Why allergic sensitization modifies airway responsiveness in male offspring is unclear. It has been previously shown that IgE response to house dust mite and OVA sensitization in male and female placentally restricted lambs is increased compared with Control lambs (25), but the OVA-specific IgE levels were comparable between our male and female Control and IUGR mice. One possibility is that a normal response to OVA interacts with a primed basal immunity, previously documented in the offspring of male IUGR mice, specifically elevated IL-13 in BAL fluid (10). Interleukin-13 is produced by natural killer cells after OVA sensitization and is strongly correlated with the Th2-induced allergic cascade and exaggerated bronchoconstrictor response (26).

The primary aim of the study was to examine how a prenatal insult (IUGR) interacts with a common risk factor for asthma i.e., aeroallergen. It seemed reasonable to hypothesize that if IUGR and aeroallergen independently increase airway responsiveness, then combined the respiratory abnormality would worsen. Indeed, aeroallergen exaggerates bronchoconstriction in a mouse model of ASM thickening caused by localized expression of a growth factor (13). Results showed no additional effect (additive or synergistic) of IUGR and allergy on airway responsiveness. Previous studies examining the relationship between atopy and low birth weight report an attenuated allergic response in IUGR individuals (27–29), including a

TABLE 1 | OVA IgE levels.

	Male		Female		Male		Female	
	Control (n = 8)	Allergy (n = 8)	Control (n = 10)	Allergy (n = 10)	IUGR (n = 8)	IUGR + Allergy (n = 7)	IUGR (n = 9)	IUGR + Allergy (n = 8)
OVA IgE (ng/mL)	7.50 ± 2.27	4.87 ± 0.95	6.16 ± 1.13	5.67 ± 0.88	4.98 ± 1.49	3.07 ± 0.65	8.73 ± 1.82	8.33 ± 3.00[#]

Data are mean ± SEM.
[#]Indicates a significant effect of sex within treatment groups. IgE, immunoglobulin E; IUGR, intrauterine growth restriction; OVA, ovalbumin.

TABLE 2 | Airway dimensions in the IUGR offspring.

	Male		Female	
Structure	IUGR (n = 6)	IUGR + Allergy (n = 7)	IUGR (n = 9)	IUGR + Allergy (n = 8)
P_{bm} (μm)	1352.38 ± 129.28	1349.12 ± 79.64	1359.06 ± 214.62	1306.91 ± 81.53
Total airway wall ($\sqrt{area}/P_{bm}$)	0.147 ± 0.009	0.154 ± 0.005	0.150 ± 0.004	0.155 ± 0.007
Outer airway wall ($\sqrt{area}/P_{bm}$)	0.069 ± 0.004	0.068 ± 0.002	0.067 ± 0.002	0.069 ± 0.003
Inner airway wall ($\sqrt{area}/P_{bm}$)	0.129 ± 0.008	0.137 ± 0.004	0.134 ± 0.003	0.139 ± 0.006
Epithelium ($\sqrt{area}/P_{bm}$)	0.111 ± 0.006	0.119 ± 0.004	0.121 ± 0.004	0.121 ± 0.005
ASM ($\sqrt{area}/P_{bm}$)	0.056 ± 0.01	0.058 ± 0.002	0.056 ± 0.002	0.056 ± 0.003

Data are mean ± SEM. The sample size of IUGR male is reduced to 6 as two samples were damaged during tissue collection. ASM, airway smooth muscle; IUGR, intrauterine growth restriction; P_{bm}, perimeter of the basement membrane.

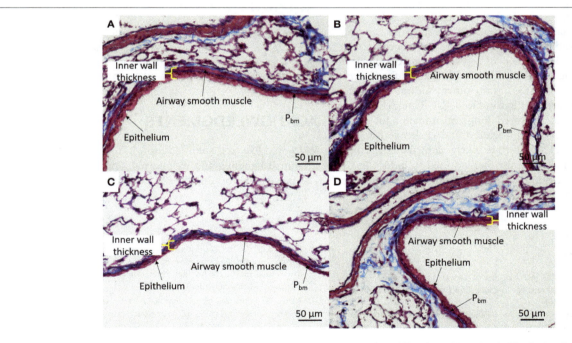

FIGURE 6 | Representative airway histology. IUGR male (A), IUGR + Allergy male (B), IUGR female (C), IUGR + Allergy female (D) offspring. P_{bm}, perimeter of the basement membrane.

reduced incidence of atopic dermatitis and food allergies (29). The relationship between low birth weight and asthma in childhood and adult life (7, 16, 17) may therefore reflect innate changes in airway responsiveness rather than a tendency to allergic disease.

We have previously reported no change in postnatal airway morphology after IUGR (8, 12) or acute exposure to OVA (13), including P_{bm} and the thickness of ASM and epithelial layers, and total airway wall thickness. In this study, we investigated whether the effects of IUGR and allergy interact to produce airway remodeling. Airway wall structure after IUGR was not affected by subsequent exposure to OVA. These data suggest that the increased bronchoconstrictor response observed in IUGR and OVA-induced allergic mice is independent of any change to airway wall structure.

A commonality between changes elicited by IUGR and OVA is airway inflammation; the former leading to increased lung macrophages at 2 and 8 weeks in mice (10) and in adult rats (30). The effects of macrophages are varied in asthma, exerting regulation through phagocytic, anti- and pro-inflammatory activities (31). It is conceivable that macrophage infiltration after IUGR favors excessive bronchoconstriction; macrophages are developed *in utero* and self-maintained throughout life *via* proliferation (32), and are activated by IL-13 (33) which appears in greater concentrations in IUGR male offspring (10). In patients with chronic obstructive pulmonary disease, a treatment-driven reduction in AHR was independently associated with a reduction in sputum macrophages as well as lymphocytes (34). At the same time, if anti-proliferative effects of macrophages dominate, an additional effect of IUGR could be to resist further abnormality following exposure to aeroallergen. Future research on how IUGR alters macrophage behavior is therefore warranted.

Other studies have also queried potential interactions between IUGR and allergen exposure. Landgraf et al. (35) used a gestational maternal undernutrition rat model of IUGR and reported an increase in airway responsiveness after OVA sensitization and challenge. However, in the study by Landgraf et al., IUGR alone did not appear to increase bronchoconstrictor response, although the method of assessing constriction from changes in perfusion pressure of excised lungs is quite indirect and may lack sensitivity (35). Two other studies which also used a maternal undernutrition-induced IUGR model in mice and rats demonstrate increased lung inflammation in IUGR offspring following OVA sensitization and challenge (36, 37). Differences in model parameters likely contribute to these disparate findings, including the method used to induce IUGR (hypoxia or undernutrition), duration of exposure and species. Despite these differences, animal models of IUGR seem to consistently report changes in airway biology that are of relevance to asthma.

We acknowledge that there are differences in mouse lung anatomy compared with human (38) which to some extent reduces the model's relevance to disease. However, the data generated allows us to form hypotheses on how prenatal and postnatal disorders interact and reveals new avenues for therapy. Airway responsiveness is modified by numerous exposures that do not necessarily share the same underlining mechanism. Given that airway biology can be modified by such a diverse range of factors, this could explain why not all treatments have the same efficacy on a given asthmatic patient. In addition to postnatal preventative measures for asthma, the prenatal window of susceptibility needs further consideration.

In summary, results indicate that while sensitized IUGR offspring are hyperresponsive to an inhaled bronchoconstrictor agonist, aeroallergen does not cause further functional disruption. These findings suggest that innate changes in bronchial reactivity are more likely to explain associations between IUGR and asthma, rather than an allergen driven inflammatory response within the lungs.

AUTHOR CONTRIBUTIONS

KW and PN: conceived and designed the experiments. JK, CW, and KW: performed the experiments. All authors analyzed the data, drafted and helped critically revise, read and approve the manuscript.

ACKNOWLEDGMENTS

We would like to thank Maddison R. Francis for her assistance in animal handling and monitoring, and Luke J. Berry for his assistance in performing the ELISA assay.

REFERENCES

1. Chapman DG, Irvin CG. Mechanisms of airway hyperresponsiveness in asthma: the past, present and yet to come. *Clin Exp Allergy.* (2015) 45:706–19. doi: 10.1111/cea.12506
2. Holgate ST, Peters-Golden M, Panettieri RA, Henderson WR. Roles of cysteinyl leukotrienes in airway inflammation, smooth muscle function, and remodeling. *J Allergy Clin Immunol.* (2003) 111:18–36. doi: 10.1067/mai.2003.25
3. Bradding P, Walls AF, Holgate ST. The role of the mast cell in the pathophysiology of asthma. *J Allergy Clin Immunol.* (2006) 117:1277–84. doi: 10.1016/j.jaci.2006.02.039
4. Elliot JG, Noble PB, Mauad T, Bai TR, Abramson MJ, McKay KO, et al. Inflammation-dependent and independent airway remodelling in asthma. *Respirology.* (2018) 23:1138–45. doi: 10.1111/resp. 13360
5. Fehrenbach H, Wagner C, Wegmann M. Airway remodeling in asthma: what really matters. *Cell Tissue Res.* (2017) 367:551–69. doi: 10.1007/s00441-016-2566-8

6. Dame Carroll JR, Magnussen JS, Berend N, Salome CM, King GG. Greater parallel heterogeneity of airway narrowing and airway closure in asthma measured by high-resolution CT. *Thorax.* (2015) 70:1163–70. doi: 10.1136/thoraxjnl-2014-206387
7. Källén B, Finnström O, Nygren KG, Otterblad Olausson P. Association between preterm birth and intrauterine growth retardation and child asthma. *Eur Respir J.* (2013) 41:671–6. doi: 10.1183/09031936.000 41912
8. Wang KCW, Larcombe AN, Berry LJ, Morton JS, Davidge ST, James AL, et al. Foetal growth restriction in mice modifies postnatal airway responsiveness in an age and sex-dependent manner. *Clin Sci.* (2018) 132:273–84. doi: 10.1042/CS20171554
9. Noble PB, Kowlessur D, Larcombe AN, Donovan GM, Wang KCW. Mechanical abnormalities of the airway wall in adult mice after intrauterine growth restriction. *Front Physiol.* (2019) 10:1073. doi: 10.3389/fphys.2019.01073
10. Looi K, Kicic A, Noble PB, Wang KCW. Intrauterine growth restriction predisposes to airway inflammation without disruption of epithelial integrity

10. in postnatal male mice. *J Dev Orig Health Dis.* (2021) 12:496–504. doi: 10.1017/S2040174420000744

11. Francis MR, Pinniger GJ, Noble PB, Wang KCW. Intrauterine growth restriction affects diaphragm function in adult female and male mice. *Pediatr Pulmonol.* (2020) 55:229–35. doi: 10.1002/ppul.24519

12. Wang KCW, Noble PB. Foetal growth restriction and asthma: airway smooth muscle thickness rather than just lung size? *Respirology.* (2020) 25:889–91. doi: 10.1111/resp.13851

13. Wang KCW, Le Cras TD, Larcombe AN, Zosky GR, Elliot JG, James AL, et al. Independent and combined effects of airway remodelling and allergy on airway responsiveness. *Clin Sci (Lond).* (2018) 132:327–38. doi: 10.1042/CS20171386

14. Sato S, Bartolák-Suki E, Parameswaran H, Hamakawa H, Suki B. Scale dependence of structure-function relationship in the emphysematous mouse lung. *Front Physiol.* (2015) 6:146. doi: 10.3389/fphys.2015.00146

15. Donovan GM, Wang KCW, Shamsuddin D, Mann TS, Henry PJ, Larcombe AN, et al. Pharmacological ablation of the airway smooth muscle layer-mathematical predictions of functional improvement in asthma. *Physiol Rep.* (2020) 8:e14451. doi: 10.14814/phy2.14451

16. Mu M, Ye S, Bai MJ, Liu GL, Tong Y, Wang SF, et al. Birth weight and subsequent risk of asthma: a systematic review and meta-analysis. *Heart Lung Circ.* (2014) 23:511–9. doi: 10.1016/j.hlc.2013.11.018

17. Xu XF, Li YJ, Sheng YJ, Liu JL, Tang LF, Chen ZM. Effect of low birth weight on childhood asthma: a meta-analysis. *BMC Pediatr.* (2014) 14:275. doi: 10.1186/1471-2431-14-275

18. de Marco R, Locatelli F, Sunyer J, Burney P. Differences in incidence of reported asthma related to age in men and women. A retrospective analysis of the data of the European Respiratory Health Survey. *Am J Respir Crit Care Med.* (2000) 162:68–74. doi: 10.1164/ajrccm.162.1.9907008

19. Ernst P, Ghezzo H, Becklake MR. Risk factors for bronchial hyperresponsiveness in late childhood and early adolescence. *Eur Respir J.* (2002) 20:635–9. doi: 10.1183/09031936.02.00962002

20. Manfreda J, Sears MR, Becklake MR, Chan-Yeung M, Dimich-Ward H, Siersted HC, et al. Geographic and gender variability in the prevalence of bronchial responsiveness in Canada. *Chest.* (2004) 125:1657–64. doi: 10.1378/chest.125.5.1657

21. Nelson HS. The importance of allergens in the development of asthma and the persistence of symptoms. *J Allergy Clin Immunol.* (2000) 105(6 Pt 2):S628–32. doi: 10.1067/mai.2000.106154

22. Zosky GR, Larcombe AN, White OJ, Burchell JT, Janosi TZ, Hantos Z, et al. Ovalbumin-sensitized mice are good models for airway hyperresponsiveness but not acute physiological responses to allergen inhalation. *Clin Exp Allergy.* (2008) 38:829–38. doi: 10.1111/j.1365-2222.2007.02884.x

23. Kim DI, Song MK, Lee K. Comparison of asthma phenotypes in OVA-induced mice challenged *via* inhaled and intranasal routes. *BMC Pulm Med.* (2019) 19:241. doi: 10.1186/s12890-019-1001-9

24. Zosky GR, von Garnier C, Stumbles PA, Holt PG, Sly PD, Turner DJ. The pattern of methacholine responsiveness in mice is dependent on antigen challenge dose. *Respir Res.* (2004) 5:15. doi: 10.1186/1465-9921-5-15

25. Wooldridge AL, Bischof RJ, Meeusen EN, Liu H, Heinemann GK, Hunter DS, et al. Placental restriction of fetal growth reduces cutaneous responses to antigen after sensitization in sheep. *Am J Physiol Regul Integr Comp Physiol.* (2014) 306:441–6. doi: 10.1152/ajpregu.00432.2013

26. Chen Z, Wang L. Ovalbumin induces natural killer cells to secrete Th2 cytokines IL-5 and IL-13 in a mouse model of asthma. *Mol Med Rep.* (2019) 19:3210–6. doi: 10.3892/mmr.2019.9966

27. Grieger JA, Clifton VL, Tuck AR, Wooldridge AL, Robertson SA, Gatford KL. In utero programming of allergic susceptibility. *Int Arch Allergy Immunol.* (2016) 169:80–92. doi: 10.1159/000443961

28. Lundholm C, Ortqvist AK, Lichtenstein P, Cnattingius S, Almqvist C. Impaired fetal growth decreases the risk of childhood atopic eczema: a Swedish twin study. *Clin Exp Allergy.* (2010) 40:1044–53. doi: 10.1111/j.1365-2222.2010.03519.x

29. Wooldridge AL, McMillan M, Kaur M, Giles LC, Marshall HS, Gatford KL. Relationship between birth weight or fetal growth rate and postnatal allergy: a systematic review. *J Allergy Clin Immunol.* (2019) 144:1703–13. doi: 10.1016/j.jaci.2019.08.032

30. Wang KCW, Morton JS, Davidge ST, Larcombe AN, James AL, Donovan GM, et al. Increased heterogeneity of airway calibre in adult rats after hypoxia-induced intrauterine growth restriction. *Respirology.* (2017) 22:1329–35. doi: 10.1111/resp.13071

31. van der Veen TA, de Groot LES, Melgert BN. The different faces of the macrophage in asthma. *Curr Opin Pulm Med.* (2020) 26:62–8. doi: 10.1097/MCP.0000000000000647

32. Guilliams M, De Kleer I, Henri S, Post S, Vanhoutte L, De Prijck S, et al. Alveolar macrophages develop from fetal monocytes that differentiate into long-lived cells in the first week of life *via* GM-CSF. *J Exp Med.* (2013) 210:1977–92. doi: 10.1084/jem.20131199

33. Martinez-Nunez RT, Louafi F, Sanchez-Elsner T. The interleukin 13 (IL-13) pathway in human macrophages is modulated by microRNA-155 *via* direct targeting of interleukin 13 receptor alpha1 (IL13Ralpha1). *J Biol Chem.* (2011) 286:1786–94. doi: 10.1074/jbc.M110.169367

34. van den Berge M, Vonk JM, Gosman M, Lapperre TS, Snoeck-Stroband JB, Sterk PJ, et al. Clinical and inflammatory determinants of bronchial hyperresponsiveness in COPD. *Eur Respir J.* (2012) 40:1098–105. doi: 10.1183/09031936.00169711

35. Landgraf MA, Landgraf RG, Jancar S, Fortes ZB. Influence of age on the development of immunological lung response in intrauterine undernourishment. *Nutrition.* (2008) 24:262–9. doi: 10.1016/j.nut.2007.12.005

36. Xing Y, Wei H, Xiao X, Chen Z, Liu H, Tong X, et al. Methylated Vnn1 at promoter regions induces asthma occurrence *via* the PI3K/Akt/NFκB-mediated inflammation in IUGR mice. *Biol Open.* (2020) 9:bio049106. doi: 10.1242/bio.049106

37. Xu XF, Hu QY, Liang LF, Wu L, Gu WZ, Tang LL, et al. Epigenetics of hyper-responsiveness to allergen challenge following intrauterine growth retardation rat. *Respir Res.* (2014) 15:137. doi: 10.1186/s12931-014-0137-7

38. Irvin CG, Bates JH. Measuring the lung function in the mouse: the challenge of size. *Respir Res.* (2003) 4:4. doi: 10.1186/rr199

6

Stem Cells and their Mediators – Next Generation Therapy for Bronchopulmonary Dysplasia

Marius A. Möbius[1,2,3] and Bernard Thébaud[3,4]*

[1] Department of Neonatology and Pediatric Critical Care Medicine, Medical Faculty, University Hospital Carl Gustav Carus, Technische Universität Dresden, Dresden, Germany, [2] DFG Research Center and Cluster of Excellence for Regenerative Therapies (CRTD), Technische Universität Dresden, Dresden, Germany, [3] Regenerative Medicine Program, Sprott Centre for Stem Cell Research, Ottawa Hospital Research Institute, University of Ottawa, Ottawa, ON, Canada, [4] Division of Neonatology, Department of Pediatrics, Children's Hospital of Eastern Ontario, University of Ottawa, Ottawa, ON, Canada

*Correspondence:
Bernard Thébaud,
Sprott Centre for Stem Cell Research,
Ottawa Hospital Research Institute,
CCW 6120, 501 Smyth Road,
Ottawa, ON K1H 8L6, Canada
bthebaud@ohri.ca

Bronchopulmonary dysplasia (BPD) remains a major complication of premature birth. Despite great achievements in perinatal medicine over the past decades, there is no treatment for BPD. Recent insights into the biology of stem/progenitor cells have ignited the hope of regenerating damaged organs. Animal experiments revealed promising lung protection/regeneration with stem/progenitor cells in experimental models of BPD and led to first clinical studies in infants. However, these therapies are still experimental and knowledge on the exact mechanisms of action of these cells is limited. Furthermore, heterogeneity of the therapeutic cell populations and missing potency assays currently limit our ability to predict a cell product's efficacy. Here, we review the therapeutic potential of mesenchymal stromal, endothelial progenitor, and amniotic epithelial cells for BPD. Current knowledge on the mechanisms behind the beneficial effects of stem cells is briefly summarized. Finally, we discuss the obstacles constraining their transition from bench-to-bedside and present potential approaches to overcome them.

Keywords: bronchopulmonary dysplasia, lung, stem cells, mesenchymal stromal cells, endothelial progenitor cells, current good manufacturing practice, potency assay

Introduction

The proper ventilation and oxygenation of a premature newborn is the foremost task in neonatology. But from the first breath of a premature newborn in the delivery room to the spontaneous or mechanical ventilation on the Neonatal Intensive Care Unit, the immature lung is always exposed to a non-physiological substance; it is not prepared for at this age: air, containing at least five times the oxygen concentration of the amniotic fluid (1). The abrupt confrontation of the immature lung to

---

Abbreviations: AEC, amnion epithelial cell; ARDS, acute respiratory distress syndrome; ATP, adenosine triphosphate; BMDAC, bone marrow-derived angiogenic cell; BOEC, blood outgrowth endothelial cell; BOS, bronchiolitis obliterans syndrome; BPD, bronchopulmonary dysplasia; CD, cluster of differentiation; CDH, congenital diaphragmatic hernia; CdM, conditioned media; cGMP, current good manufacturing practice; COPD, chronic obstructive pulmonary disease; CPC, circulating progenitor cell; ECFC, endothelial colony forming cell; EPC, endothelial progenitor cell; EpCam, epithelial cell adhesion molecule; FBS, fetal bovine serum; FiO_2 fraction of inspired oxygen; GvHD, graft-versus-host disease; IPF, idiopathic pulmonary fibrosis; MSC, mesenchymal stromal cell; PCR, polymerase chain reaction; PDGFR, platelet-derived growth factor receptor; SCID, severe combined immunodeficiency; SSEA, stage-specific embryonic antigen; TGF, transforming growth factor; VEGF, vascular endothelial growth factor.

this and other hostile extrauterine conditions leads to the chronic lung disease of prematurity or bronchopulmonary dysplasia (BPD).

Despite advances in the management of premature infants, respiratory complications still account for approximately one-quarter of all NICU deaths (2). BPD, characterized by impaired lung growth, remains the most common complication of premature birth (3, 4). Currently, there is no effective treatment for BPD and all present approaches remain either supportive, present major adverse effects (steriods) or show only small benefits (vitamin A, caffeine).

Cell-based therapies may open a completely new chapter in the therapy of BPD. Over the past years, animal studies using stem and progenitor cells as therapeutics showed very promising results, which have lead to first trials in human (5). This review summarizes our current knowledge about the therapeutic potential of these genuine facilitators of lung growth and regeneration.

Stem Cells – Origin of Growth, Repair, and Disease

Stem or progenitor cells reside in virtually all tissues at all stages of development. They are generally defined by the ability to (**I**) undergo self-renewal and (**II**) give rise to more differentiated cells. The extent to which these cells can differentiate is called potency. Stem cells harbor the potential to differentiate into placental and embryonic tissue (*totipotent* stem cells of the morula stage) and along the various embryonic germ layers (*pluripotent*, embryonic stem cells). They further give raise to several adult cell types (*multipotent*, i.e., hematopoietic stem cells). Conversely, progenitor cells are thought to give raise to only one specific adult cell type (*unipotent*, i.e., type 2 alveolar epithelial cells).

Toti-, pluri-, and multipotent stem cells enable early development of the embryonal structures and subsequent organ differentiation until the beginning of the fetal period approximately 8 weeks *post conceptionem*. After this period, derivates of these cells can be found as resident stem or progenitor cells in virtually all fetal and adult tissues deriving from all three germ layers, including the bone marrow (6), gut (7), brain (8), and lung (9).

Their major task is the facilitation of growth and of tissue regeneration and maintenance, e.g., providing new, differentiated cells after cell loss due to normal usage or injury while remaining in a proliferative, lesser differentiated state on their own (self-renewal). This happens to various extends. Some tissues – such as the gut or bone marrow – contain stem cells with high proliferative and regenerative capacity, while others – such as the brain and the heart – grow until adulthood, but have only limited regenerative potential once damaged.

The lung is a complex organ deriving from endodermal and mesodermal origin and harbors several endodermal (epithelial) and mesodermal (mesenchymal and endothelial) stem and progenitor cell types (10), each of them with different capabilities to differentiate and proliferate. As of now, over 40 different lung cell types have been described; numerous of them exert more or less characteristics of stem cells (9–11).

Since enabling growth and regeneration is the main role of stem or progenitor cells in non-embryonic tissues, organ failure would suggest a pathology of the organ resident stem cell population(s). Indeed, several events before (prolonged rupture of the membranes, oligohydramnios, severe intrauterine growth restriction, congenital diaphragmatic hernia/CDH) or after birth (mechanical ventilation, oxygen) may impair stem cell function. Lung diseases with abnormal growth of lung compartments, such as the bronchiolitis obliterans syndrome (BOS) following lung transplantation (12) or lung hypoplasia following CDH (13), can be linked to dysfunction of the resident progenitor cells.

In BPD, qualitative or quantitative impairment of resident mesenchymal and endothelial stem or progenitor cells seems to contribute to the disease pathogenesis or to the incapacity of the lung to repair itself (11). Less is known about the pathogenic role of stem or progenitor cells in the endodermal, epithelial lung compartments, such as the bronchioalveolar stem cells (BASCs) (14).

Conversely, exogenous stem cells or their products derived from the mesenchymal (14–26), epithelial (27–29), or endothelial (30, 31) compartment of easily accessible tissue, such as the bone marrow, placenta, or the umbilical cord prevent or restore lung damage in animal models of BPD. Most of these data have been generated in neonatal rodents exposed to hyperoxia, a model which will be discussed below. Newer models combining several factors contributing to BPD [such as antenatal hypoxia, inflammation, and mechanical ventilation (32, 33)] will be useful to assess the pathophysiology of BPD and therapeutic benefit of cell therapies more completely. Various cell therapies have been proposed (34), and the following paragraphs will focus on the most extensively explored therapeutic stem cells for BPD: mesenchymal stromal cells (MSCs), endothelial progenitor cells (EPCs, including endothelial colony forming cells, ECFCs), as well as amnion epithelial cells (AECs).

MSCs as Therapeutic Cells

Mesenchymal stem or stromal cells (MSCs) are the most promising cells in regenerative medicine. Their therapeutic potential is currently investigated in virtually every disease one can think of. As of February 2015, PubMed lists over 37,500 references for these cells; almost double the number from 2012 (35).

First described in hematopoietic tissues by Friedenstein and his colleagues in 1970 (36), MSCs have been identified in adult organs deriving from the mesodermal germ layer, including the bone marrow and adipose tissue. Furthermore, they can be found in fetal-restricted mesodermal derivates like the umbilical cord stroma and cord blood as well as in the placenta and the amniotic fluid [comprehensively reviewed by Hass and colleagues (37)]. Interestingly, MSCs have also been identified in tissues deriving from the (ectodermal) neural crest, such as the mandibula (38).

Cord-derived MSCs from the Wharton's Jelly are of particular interest for the treatment of neonatal diseases. Indeed, the umbilical cord stroma is

- readily available at birth and thus clinically relevant
- with 100 million births worldwide a large source of stem cells

- safe and painless to the mother and her child as cells are harvested after delivery from otherwise discarded tissue and thus devoid of ethical dilemma
- importantly, these cells hold superior healing capabilities compared to adult bone marrow cells (39).

As implied by their multiple residence tissues, MSCs represent a very heterogeneous cell population (40, 41). MSCs from one source exert different properties than MSCs from another (37, 42). Some cells within the MSC population are true stem cells with the potential to undergo complete self-renewal and some are not. Therefore, the global population of MSCs should be identified as "mesenchymal stromal cells" rather than "mesenchymal stem cells" (35).

The minimal criteria to define a MSC (41) are widely accepted, but relatively loose and include the following four:

- The ability of the cell to adhere and grow on plain, uncoated, tissue culture treated plastic surfaces, e.g., the ability to secrete large amounts of extracellular matrix.
- The presence of CD73, CD90 (thymocyte antigen *thy-1*), and CD105 (*endoglin 1*) on the cell's surface.
- The absence of the surface markers CD34, CD45, CD14/CD11b, CD19/CD79α, and HLA-DR, which label various cell lines from the hematopoetic lineage.
- The ability of the cells to differentiate along adipogenic, osteogenic, and chondrogenic lineages when stimulated *in vitro*.

These criteria were initially created to define MSCs derived from the bone marrow, where they need to be distinguished from the hematopoietic stem and progenitor cells giving rise to the blood cell lines. But as mentioned above, MSCs can also be found in other organs and tissues where they need to be distinguished from resident, mature fibroblasts, endothelial cells, and other non-hematopoetic cell types. Therefore, additional criteria for defining potentially therapeutic MSCs from, i.e., the umbilical cord or the adipose tissue, are required and currently under development. Several additional surface markers including CD10, CD29, CD106, CD146, CD166 or CD200 (42), and CD271 (43) have been proposed.

Bone marrow-derived MSCs exert a robust differentiation potential along osteogenic, chondrogenic, and adipogenic lineages. Conversely, some MSC populations can be differentiated into epithelial (44, 45), endothelial (46), and neural cells (47) while lacking the ability to differentiate along certain other, i.e., chondrogenic lineages (35). Therefore, criteria for a characterization by trilineage differentiation may need to be revised as well.

Functional tests, such as the assessment of the cell's immune-regulatory properties (48) and their secretome (49) following specific stimuli, gain importance and will open a new avenue for a functional, rather than a morphological description of potentially therapeutic MSC products. Nevertheless, a single, striking marker or feature to define an MSC has not yet been found; neither is there a valid test to assess the "stemness" or "therapeutic potential" of such a cell, a major problem, which will be discussed below.

Lung-Resident MSCs and the Development of BPD

Our current understanding of normal alveolar growth and the cellular and extracellular mechanisms behind its regulation suggest a crucial role of tissue-resident lung stem cells from mesenchymal, endothelial, and epithelial origin in this complex process (50, 51). Therefore, damage to the resident lung stem or progenitor cells – by inflammation, hyperoxia, malnutrition, shear stress, or other influences – may results in a loss or severe impairment of endogenous growth and regeneration potential.

The lung-resident MSC may play a critical role as regulator of lung development, coordinating epithelial and endothelial growth (52). When these cells become damaged in preterm infants, lung development gets out of sync leading to BPD. The properties of human neonatal and fetal lung MSCs are currently under investigation. While resident lung MSCs are by far not as well described as, i.e., BM-MSCs or adipose tissue-derived MSCs, pioneering work by Dr. Hershenson's group found that the presence of MSCs in the tracheal aspirates of ventilated preterm infants predicted BPD (53–55).

These cells express less platelet-derived growth factor-receptor alpha (PDGFR-α) as compared to MSCs from babies without BPD (56). Furthermore, they present a profound autocrine production of transforming growth factor beta 1 (TGF-1) (57) and increased β-catenin signaling (58). The disruption of these pathways controlling the myofibroblastic differentiation (PDGFR-α, TGF-β1, and β-catenin) leads to disrupted formation of alveolar tips and interstitial lung fibrosis (58, 59). Moreover, the function of specific lung-resident stem cells with mesenchymal, endothelial, and epithelial differentiation potential (lung side population cells) (60) is disrupted in murine hyperoxia-induced lung injury (61).

Therefore, these findings suggest that damage to endogenous MSCs may contribute to the disease pathogenesis of BPD. Conversely, exogenous MSCs show consistent therapeutic benefits in experimental neonatal lung injury models. How these exogenous MSCs affect resident lung MSCs is unknown.

Therapeutic Benefits of Exogenous MSCs

The beneficial effects of exogenous MSCs have best been described in hyperoxia-induced rodent models mimicking BPD (33, 62, 63). Rodents are convenient because they are born at the saccular stage of lung development, which corresponds to the lung developmental stage of a human infant born at 26–28 weeks of gestation (62). To summarize the models in brief, term born rodents are exposed to hyperoxia (FiO$_2$ 0.60–0.95) for 1–2 weeks; rats or mice subsequently develop structural lung changes consistent with pathological findings of human infants that died with BPD (64). Alveolar simplification, capillary rarefaction, and leakage with extravascular fibrin and plasma protein accumulation, lung fibrosis with increased collagen and disordered elastin deposition, pulmonary hypertension, as well as influx of inflammatory cells can be observed (33, 62, 63).

A second model using prematurely delivered baboons model at 125 days and mechanically ventilated for 2 weeks offers unique opportunities to test promising (stem cell-based) therapies in a model close to the clinical setting (65). Due to the close relationship to man, long-term effects of treatment on growth and development can easily be observed, giving valuable information for clinical applications in premature human infants.

Mesenchymal stromal cells have striking beneficial effects in the hyperoxia-induced model of BPD. In 2007, Tian et al. (26) reported that intravenous injection of bone marrow-derived MSCs ameliorates the oxygen-induced neonatal lung injury. Two papers published simultaneously by Aslam et al. (24) and van Haaften et al. (25) in 2009 demonstrated that MSCs derived from the bone marrow of healthy, adult rodents prevent oxygen-induced neonatal lung injury.

Both authors administered MSCs on postnatal day 4 before exposing the pups to hyperoxia to assess the preventive potential of the cells. Aslam and colleagues administered 5×10^4 cells (approximately 5×10^6 cells/kg bodyweight) intravenously, whereas van Haaften et al. used an intratracheal administration route and applied double the dose (1×10^7 MSCs/kg bodyweight). A significant decrease in alveolar wall thickness as well as an increase in vessel density and alveolar septation was observed in both studies. Furthermore, increased exercise capacity and reduced pulmonary hypertension was noted (18, 25).

Remarkably, very few of the injected cells were retained in the lung, indicating that cell engraftment contributes minimally – if at all – to the therapeutic benefit of MSCs. The intratracheal, intraperitoneal, or intravenous administration of cell free conditioned medium (CdM; concentrated tissue culture supernatant of MSCs) showed beneficial effects comparable to whole cell therapy. However, as no reliable methods to describe and normalize doses and composition of CdM have been utilized, a direct comparison of the two therapy regimens is inaccurate.

These experiments have been repeated several times with MSCs from the rat or human bone marrow (14, 17, 18, 21) or human cord blood (16, 22, 23, 66) and their respective conditioned media with similar results [reviewed by Fung et al. (67)]. Furthermore, recent pre-clinical studies by Chang and colleagues investigated the influences of the dose (22), timing (66), and administration route (23) of MSCs in a rat model of BPD. These studies favor an early, intratracheal administration of $0.5–5 \times 10^7$ MSCs/kg bodyweight.

MSCs and their CdM were also able to rescue hyperoxia-induced lung injury (16). Moreover, the beneficial effects of a treatment with these cells are not transient. Adult rats that received MSCs in their neonatal period before (16), during (17), or after exposure (16) to hyperoxia show persistent improvements in lung architecture, exercise capacity, and vascularization in long-term follow-up studies up to 6 months.

The exact mechanism behind the effects remains unclear. Secreted anti-inflammatory proteins, angiokines, and other lung protective substances including stanniocalcin-1 (19, 68), prostaglandin E2 (12), and TNF-stimulated gene/protein 6 (TSG-6) (69–71) are strongly suggested to account for the short-term effects and protect the lungs against the acute injury. These substances secreted by the MSCs blunt the immediate and oblique injury effects like the influx of inflammatory cells and their associated deleterious effects. This has not only been described in neonatal hyperoxic models but also in several other experimental studies using bleomycin (72), lipopolysaccharide (73), ovalbumin (74), or prolonged ventilation (75) to challenge the lung.

The pathophysiology of BPD is not limited to inflammation, despite a major contribution of this process to the development of the disease (76). BPD is a multi-factorial disease and the characteristic and life-impairing feature of BPD – compromised alveolar growth beyond the neonatal period – can best be explained by a persistent impairment of the mechanisms regulating lung growth and development, including the resident stem/progenitor cells.

The M&M's of Therapeutic Cells – Microvesicles and Mitochondria in Long-Term Effects of MSCs

As described above, very few cells engraft in the lung (25). The engrafted cells die rapidly and are not detectable with quantitative PCR methods or high-specific stainings after a few weeks when xenogeneic MSCs (=cells from a different species) were used (16). Authors using an allogeneic approach described a comparably low, but prolonged engraftment (up to 100 days) into the alveolar wall with potential transdifferentiation into surfactant-protein C producing cells (17, 25).

However, these events are very rare and do not contribute to the therapeutic effect of MSCs *in vivo* [reviewed by Kotton and Fine (77)]. Engraftment and transdifferentiation of MSCs may be considered as artifacts of the immunohistochemical detection method (78).

Microvesicles as Carriers of Therapeutic Agents

As discussed previously, secreted proteins mainly account for the short-term effects of transplanted MSCs or their CdM. But a long-term effect on the lung cells cannot be explained by just a single administration or secretion of cytokines. Extracellular vesicles, small microparticles containing nucleic acids, proteins, and lipids (79) may answer this question. Specific subtypes of these particles – so-called exosomes – are secreted by numerous cell types, including MSCs (80). They harbor the potential to reduce inflammation and blunt hypoxia-induced pulmonary hypertension (80) as well as to ameliorate endotoxin-induced lung injury (81).

Exosomes are, besides cytokines and other secreted proteins, the potential therapeutic components of conditioned medium. As reviewed comprehensively by Colombo et al. (79), exosomes can be taken up into the target cell by various mechanisms. Specific nucleic acids – so-called microRNA (82) – can transpose to the nucleus and silence specific genes for long periods (83) or interfere with the protein translation. These mechanisms could account for long-term beneficial effects on damaged lung cells in BPD.

Therapeutic Mitochondrial Transfer in Lung Disease

Another mechanism contributing to the long-term efficacy of MSCs may be the transfer of mitochondria from MSCs to damaged lung cells. Mitochondrial dysfunction plays a critical role in the development of experimental BPD in primates (84) and rodents (85–88).

In 2006, mitochondrial transfer from MSCs to other cells *in vitro* was described (89). Recent *in vivo* studies revealed that mitochondrial transfer plays a crucial role in animal models of lung injury. Intratracheally administered MSCs form microtubes and transpose mitochondria toward damaged alveolar type II cells, which leads to higher alveolar ATP-content and profound protection against lipopolysaccharide-induced acute lung injury (90). In chronic lung injury, therapeutic cells were able to reduce the alveolar damage as well as the interstitial fibrosis by mitochondrial transfer (91). Data supporting the role of mitochondrial transfer in neonatal chronic lung disease are pending.

Safe, Efficacious, Effective? MSCs in Clinical Studies

These promising laboratory studies have lead to early phase clinical trials exploring the feasibility and safety of MSCs in various pulmonary diseases (**Table 1**). Chang et al. recently completed the first phase I dose escalation study using allogeneic human umbilical cord blood-derived MSCs in 9 preterm infants at risk of developing BPD (5). They administered 1×10^7 or 2×10^7 MSCs derived from the cord blood of healthy-term infants intratracheally and observed no serious adverse events or acute toxicity of the cells. Currently, several follow-up studies evaluating the long-term effects of the administered cells are listed on www.clinicaltrials.gov, and a placebo-controlled phase II trial (NCT01828957) is recruiting patients.

Clinical studies with MSCs are warranted. Obviously, MSC therapy in the neonatal population requires extremely careful risk-benefit considerations. Lessons learned from large, placebo-controlled phase III clinical trials using MSCs in steroid-refractory graft-versus-host disease (GvHD) (93) suggest that despite very promising results in animal models and phase I and II studies (94) current MSC preparations have no predictable therapeutic effect. Therapy with MSCs is complex and influenced by more factors than other cellular therapies, such as blood transfusions or hematopoietic stem cells for bone marrow transplantation.

MSCs – a Pharmaceutical Product in the Making

A major problem for clinical trials is the heterogeneity of the cell population termed MSCs. The markers and features defining an MSC are still evolving. As outlined previously, the cells characteristics, such as surface marker-, protein- and gene expression vary with the source, isolation, culture and expansion methods and donor age (35). Virtually every laboratory established (and patented) its own protocols for isolation and culture of MSCs from various sources, which makes it difficult to compare even the results of pre-clinical studies (95).

For clinical trials, a defined, clinical-grade cell product is required. As of now, over 80% of the MSCs used in clinical studies are expanded in media containing fetal bovine serum (FBS) (42), a crude and undefined mixture of growth factors and various bovine proteins. Beyond the unknown influences of various FBS preparations on the therapeutic effect of MSCs, even the potential risk of a pathogen transmission (viruses, prions) makes cells cultured with FBS not optimal for a clinical therapy (96). Based on the MSCs source, many other products used during the isolation process – including enzymes and growth factors – also derive from animal origins. Ideally, a product suitable for administration to a critically ill patient should be produced under current good manufacturing practice (cGMP)-conditions using defined xenogenic free chemicals.

Furthermore, it is crucial to accurately monitor growth and aging of MSCs *in vitro*. It is known that MSCs age during *ex vivo* expansion and that this influences biological properties of the

TABLE 1 | MSCs in clinical trails for pulmonary diseases.

Condition	Phase	Design	Number of participants	Cell origin	NCT ID
Adult ARDS	I	Open	10	bm-msc (allo)	NCT02215811
	I	Randomized, double-blind	9	bm-msc (allo)	NCT01775774
	II	Randomized, placebo-controlled, double-blind	60	bm-msc (allo)	NCT02097641
	I	Randomized, placebo-controlled, double-blind	20	at-msc (allo)	NCT01902082
Air leakage after lung resection	I/II	Open	10	msc N/S (auto)	NCT02045745
Asthma	I/II	Open	20	cdm-uc (allo)	NCT02192736
BPD	I[‡] (5)	Open	9	ucb-msc (allo)	NCT01297205
	I	Open	12	ucb-msc (allo)	NCT02381366
	II	Randomized, placebo-controlled, double-blind	70	ucb-msc (allo)	NCT01828957
COPD	II[‡] (92)	Randomized, placebo-controlled, double-blind	62	bm-msc (allo)	NCT00683722
IPF	I	Open	18	bm-msc (auto)	NCT01919827
	I[‡]	Open	8	pla-msc (allo)	NCT01385644
	II	Randomized, open	60	at-msc (auto)	NCT02135380
BOS after lung transplantation	I	Open	9	bm-msc (allo)	NCT02181712
	I	Open	10	msc N/S (allo)	NCT01175655
Pulmonary emphysema	I/II	Randomized, open	30	bm-msc (allo)	NCT01849159

[‡] Completed trials are marked with a diesis.
pla-msc, placenta-derived MSCs; bm-msc, bone marrow-derived MSCs; ucb-msc, umbilical cord blood-derived MSCs; at-msc, adipose tissue-derived MSCs; cdm-uc, conditioned media from umbilical cord-derived MSCs; msc N/S, source of cells not specified; allo, allogenic cells; auto, autologous cells.

cells (97). Different methods to determine the age of MSCs have been utilized. Most investigators and companies producing MSCs determine the passage number, an easy but very inaccurate parameter influenced by many factors (98). Therefore, it is not possible to determine if insufficient clinical effects are caused by real therapy failure or just by the fact that senescent therapeutic cells have been administered. A better way than counting passages might be the implementation of cumulative population doubling measurements (99) and biochemical assays, such as telomere attrition or β-galactosidase activity (100).

Prolonged culture of MSCs may also lead to genetic instabilities (101, 102). The spontaneous malignant transformation of MSCs observed in long-term culture experiments (103) has been proven to be an *in vitro* contamination artifact (104). However, the risk of tumorigenicity in MSC-based therapies is still under discussion (99). A direct tumor formation seems unlikely, as MSCs do not engraft. Indeed, in rats receiving MSCs for BPD no tumor masses were seen 6 months after therapy with the cells (16). The risks of increased tumor formation by long-term immunosuppression (99) or the previously discussed stem cell-stimulating effects remain unclear. A first meta-analysis of clinical trials using MSCs showed no increased tumor risk in over 1000 patients after 3–60 months after treatment (105). But as with every drug, definitive data regarding these issues can only be acquired in large clinical trials.

While MSCs are immune-privileged and as such enable allogeneic cell therapy, autologous cell therapy has also been advocated for. Autologous therapy may be associated with lower ethical and technical boundaries than therapy with allogeneic cells. Conversely, the autologous approach is logistically more challenging as it requires the manipulation of a fetal tissue (cord blood, cord stroma . . .) *ex vivo*. Therefore, each product will need to be subjected to a rigorous sterility and quality testing, which takes time, financial, and human resources as opposed to a ready-to-use off-the-shelf allogeneic cell product. It is also not yet clear for which preterm infant an autologous cell product should be processed. Furthermore, the autologous approach may not always be possible (outborn) or potentially deleterious (severe chorioamnionitis). These considerations will mature over time as knowledge and manufacturing technologies advance, allowing us to rationally determine the best possible cell product.

The Quest for a "Potency Assay"

One fundamental problem hampering the widespread use of MSCs in clinical trials is the absence of valid assays to assess their quality or "therapeutic potential" prior to usage.

In applications were the anti-inflammatory effects of MSCs are predominant (like GvHD), tests assessing the immunosuppressive potential of the therapeutic cells may overcome this obstacle (100, 106). In brief, MSCs are co-cultured with mitogen-stimulated allogeneic lymphocytes. They suppress the induced proliferation of the inflammatory cells to various extends via paracrine effects following direct cell-cell interaction. A simple automated cell count assesses the "therapeutic potential" of the MSC-population in this setting. An even faster and easier method uses the interleukin-10 stimulated expression of a specific subtype of the HLA-receptor complex (HLA-G) on the surface of MSCs (107) to assess their

immunosuppressive potential. By now, it has not been validated if cells with higher anti-inflammatory potential *in vitro* lead to better therapeutic effects *in vivo* (100).

The situation for multi-factorial diseases affecting the lung – such as BPD – is, however, more complicated. As outlined previously, the mechanisms behind the beneficial effects of MSCs in BPD are complex and involve cytokines, the direct or paracrine interaction with resident cell types and maybe the transfer of mitochondria or exosomes. Therefore, the generation of such a simple functional assay is far ahead. *In vitro* approaches might involve the ability of MSCs to support the generation of alveolospheres out of murine alveolar type II cells in 3D organoid culture systems (108). The assessment of strain resistance in alveolar epithelial cells co-cultured with MSCs *in vitro* might be another interesting approach. Nevertheless, all these approaches remain far from an easy, fast, cheap, and reliable potency assay.

In summary, MSC therapies are promising and clinical conditions, such as BPD, urge for efficient treatment strategies. However, MSC therapies also represent a disruptive technology and for now, not a single trial investigated MSC products in man that met all current regulatory or cGMP criteria (95, 109). A safe and high-qualitative cell product to use in trials is still missing. As outlined recently in a position paper by Wuchter et al. (100), standardization and rigorous quality control of the production process is the *conditio sine qua non* for successful clinical testings using MSCs. If the product does not fulfill these criteria, how should we interpret the clinical results? Every disruptive technology is imperfect at the beginning and needs to evolve with experience and time. But it is imperative to do due diligence and obtain the best possible cell product before testing it in our most vulnerable patients.

No Vessels, No Lung Growth: Progenitor Cells from the Endothelial Lineage

Simplification of the pulmonary vasculature is a hallmark of BPD (110), and angiogenesis is crucial for normal postnatal alveolar development (111). Hyperoxia-induced lung injury can be attenuated by increasing the pulmonary supply of angiokines like VEGF in rodents (111, 112). Accordingly, if vascular growth factors and lung angiogenesis contribute to the integrity of the lung, then vascular progenitor cells are appealing candidate cells likely to be involved in the same mechanisms.

After their first description as circulating cells in the peripheral blood by Asahara et al. (113), endothelial progenitor cells have been shown to promote the repair of damaged blood vessels in various disease models [reviewed by Mund and colleagues (114)]. They are further investigated as biomarkers of cardiovascular diseases [reviewed by Sen et al. (115)]. EPCs harbor the potential to form tube-like structures on matrigel matrices *in vitro*, home to ischemic sites *in vivo*, and augment angiogenesis by paracrine effects (116).

However, the population termed EPCs is not homogeneous, and the exact origin and definition of these cells remain unclear. A direct relationship of EPC subsets to the myeloid progenitor line has been described (117). Two groups provided evidence for a hierarchy within circulating EPCs and identified a specific subset named blood outgrowth endothelial cells (BOEC) (118) or endothelial colony forming cells (ECFCs) (119). This population, further referred to as ECFCs, is thought to contain the therapeutically active progenitor cells of the endothelial lineage (117). In contrast to the global EPC population, ECFCs lack expression of CD133 and CD115, exert high-clonal proliferative potential and harbor the ability to form vessels *de novo* when transplanted into immunodeficient SCID-mice [recently reviewed by Basile and Yoder (116)].

Endothelial Progenitors in BPD

Using a mouse model of BPD, Balasubramaniam et al. described that hyperoxia-induced lung damage depletes circulating EPCs and bone marrow-derived angiogenic cells (BMDACs) (120). Administration of BMDACs from healthy mice rescues the alveolar and vascular structure after O_2 injury (31).

The role of circulating endothelial progenitors in the pathogenesis of BPD was further confirmed in studies with human infants. Borghesi and colleagues described that high numbers of ECFCs in the cord blood of preterm babies are associated with a lower risk to develop BPD (121). Interestingly, the blood counts of non-ECFC endothelial progenitors fail to predict or correlate to any disease associated with preterm birth (122), further substantiating the role of circulating ECFCs. Baker et al. also reported the association between low-ECFC counts and the development of BPD. They further showed that a decreased ratio between circulating progenitor cells with pronounced *in vitro* angiogenic potential (CPC) and those without (non-angiogenic, non-CPC) predicts the development of moderate or severe BPD (123). Moreover, ECFCs isolated from preterms are more prone to oxidative stress than cells from term infants (124). CdM from cord blood-derived ECFCs obtained from term infants promotes growth of the pulmonary vasculature, but fails to promote alveolar septation in bleomycin-induced lung injury (125).

The lung also harbors its own resident progenitor cells with vasculogenic capacity (30, 126, 127). Human fetal and neonatal rat lungs contain ECFCs with robust proliferative potential, secondary colony formation on replating, and *de novo* blood vessel formation. Exposure to hyperoxia *in vitro* and *in vivo* impedes ECFC function as exemplified by decreased proliferation, clonogenic, and angiogenic capacity. In experimental chronic hyperoxic lung injury in rats, administration of human cord blood-derived ECFCs restored resident lung ECFC colony- and capillary-like network-forming capabilities, lung function, alveolar and lung vascular growth, and attenuated pulmonary hypertension. At 10 months post-ECFC therapy improvement in lung structure, exercise capacity, and pulmonary hypertension persisted without signs of adverse effects (30). Comparable to MSCs, the benefit seems to be mediated by a paracrine effect since cell engraftment was minimal and CdM from ECFCs exerted similar therapeutic benefit to whole cell therapy.

Room for a Clinical Application?

As of February 2015, no clinical trials using endothelial progenitor cells or their CdM as therapeutic agents in BPD are listed on www.clinicaltrials.gov. In the past, Wang et al. conducted two clinical trials in adult patients suffering from idiopathic pulmonary hypertension (NCT00641836 and NCT00257413). They used a heterogeneous preparation of autologous endothelial progenitors and demonstrated safety and feasibility as well as significantly increased exercise capacity and reduced pulmonary blood pressures 12 weeks after intravenous administration (128). A Canadian phase I study using EPCs transfected with endothelial nitric oxide synthase (eNOS) in seven patients has recently been completed (NCT00469027); final results are pending.

EPCs for therapeutic purposes could be isolated from easily accessible peripheral blood or cord blood without the ethical problems raised by a bone marrow puncture to obtain BMSCs. With the SCID-mouse transplantation assay, an excellent and reliable method assessing the functional capacity of ECFCs is available (117). However, the relatively complicated isolation and expansion process requires sophisticated (and expensive) media as well as many manual steps including the individual lifting of emerging colonies (117, 119).

As of today, no large-scale production technique has been developed to reliably isolate the quantities of cells required for clinical studies. Compared to MSCs, less is known about the behavior of EPCs or ECFCs *in vivo* and *in vitro*. Nevertheless, given the importance of angiogenesis for a large variety of diseases, cell-based vascular therapies will rapidly develop as our understanding of EPC biology advances in parallel with our knowledge in bioengineering and cell manufacturing.

Not Stem Cells, Still Therapeutic: Amnion Epithelial Cells

Cells from the human amniotic epithelium (AECs) represent the third cell population that has been explored in experimental BPD. The amniotic membrane is widely used as an effective and low-immunogenic material to patch large skin defects (129). This tissue contains epithelial cells with distinct regenerative (130) and an anti-inflammatory potential (131) comparable to MSCs (132). AECs further possess the potential to differentiate along mesodermal, ectodermal, and endodermal lineages *in vitro* (130) and are considered "stem-like cells" (133).

In 2010, Moodley and colleagues described that i.v. injection of AECs abrogates lung fibrosis and inflammation in bleomycin-challenged immunodeficient mice. Furthermore, the cells homed and engrafted permanently into the damaged lung tissue, acquired the phenotype of alveolar type II cells, and started producing surfactant (133). In immunocompetent animals, similar effects without cell engraftment were observed (134). The potent anti-inflammatory and anti-fibrotic effects led to studies in fetal sheep with intraamniotic LPS-induced lung injury. Here, i.v. administration of AEC to the unborn lamb led to reduced lung inflammatory cytokines without significant improvements on lung structure (29).

In a study using *in utero* ventilation of fetal sheep to induce BPD-like changes in lung histology, Hodges et al. demonstrated significant improvements of the lung structure after combined i.v. and intratracheal administration of AEC during the ventilation procedure. Engraftment and transdifferentiation of AECs into alveolar type I and type II cells were noted. However, these rare events did not contribute to the overall impact of AECs in this animal model (28).

Currently, no clinical trials using AECs in pulmonary diseases are listed. However, AECs are investigated in a clinical trial for ocular limbal stem cell deficiency (135). Large quantities of the AECs can easily be produced from birth-associated tissues. But by now, no clear definitions and characterization regimen to define amniotic epithelial cells exist (136). Cells used in pre-clinical studies represent heterogenous populations, expressing a large variety of surface markers labeling pluripotent (SSEA-4), epithelial (cytokeratin-7, EpCam), and mesenchymal cells (CD73, CD90, CD166, among others) (29, 133). Nevertheless, first encouraging steps toward controlled, cGMP-conform isolation methods have been undertaken (137).

Conclusion

Cell therapies represent the next paradigm shift in medicine. Unlike previous therapeutic game-changers, such as small molecules and biologics, cells are part drug and part device, which can sense diverse signals, interact with their environment, integrate inputs to make decisions, and execute complex response behaviors (138). These unique attributes of stem cells have been harnessed for organ regeneration. In the developing lung, various cell types including MSCs, EPCs, and AECs harbor the fascinating potential to provide pleiotropic therapeutic agents to protect from and restore lung damage. These cells are thus ideally suited not only for the treatment of a multi-factorial disease, such as BPD, but also for other complications of extreme prematurity.

Phase I trials with MSCs have already started and while the time is ripe for carefully designed early phase clinical trials, more progress is required to better understand the mechanisms of action and to optimize cell products. As with all disruptive technology, there is a steep learning curve in the beginning and the first product may be imperfect. Early on, common reference standards of the isolation and manufacturing process should be established to ensure uniformly high quality, effective and practical cell products. This will be crucial not only to ensure success of stem cell clinical trials but also to interpret and compare these trials. Finally, establishment of registries of all treated patients are imperative to ensure long-term follow-up.

Three excellent reviews further addressing the obstacles of bench-to-bedside transition of current stem cell therapeutics have been written by D. Prockop, S. Prockop, and I. Bertonello (95), G. Daley (139) and M. Fischbach, J. Bluestone, and W. Lim (138).

Acknowledgments

The authors thank Prof. Dr. med. habil. Mario Rüdiger, Department of Neonatology and Pediatric Critical Care Medicine, University Hospital Carl Gustav Carus Dresden, Germany for his critical comments on the manuscript.

MM holds a merit scholarship from the German National Academic Foundation – Studienstiftung des deutschen Volkes. This work was further supported by a grant from the EFCNI (European Foundation for the Care of the Newborn Infant). BT holds a University of Ottawa Partnership Research Chair in Regenerative Medicine and is supported by the Canadian Health Research Institute (CIHR), Canadian Stem Cell Network, and the Canadian Lung Association.

References

1. Sjostedt S, Rooth G, Caligara F. The oxygen tension of the amniotic fluid. *Am J Obstet Gynecol* (1958) **76**:1226–30.
2. Jacob J, Kamitsuka M, Clark RH, Kelleher AS, Spitzer AR. Etiologies of nicu deaths. *Pediatrics* (2015) **135**:e59–65. doi:10.1542/peds.2014-2967
3. Stoll BJ, Hansen NI, Bell EF, Shankaran S, Laptook AR, Walsh MC, et al. Neonatal outcomes of extremely preterm infants from the nichd neonatal research network. *Pediatrics* (2010) **126**:443–56. doi:10.1542/peds. 2009-2959
4. Farstad T, Bratlid D, Medbo S, Markestad T. Bronchopulmonary dysplasia – prevalence, severity and predictive factors in a national cohort of extremely premature infants. *Acta Paediatr* (2011) **100**:53–8. doi:10.1111/j.1651-2227. 2010.01959.x
5. Chang YS, Ahn SY, Yoo HS, Sung SI, Choi SJ, Oh WI, et al. Mesenchymal stem cells for bronchopulmonary dysplasia: phase 1 dose-escalation clinical trial. *J Pediatr* (2014) **164**:966–72. doi:10.1016/j.jpeds.2013.12.011
6. Till JE, McCulloch EA. A direct measurement of the radiation sensitivity of normal mouse bone marrow cells. *Radiat Res* (1961) **14**:213–22. doi:10.2307/ 3570892
7. Stoffels GL, Preumont AM, De Reuck M. Cell differentiation in human gastric gland as revealed by nuclear binding of tritiated actinomycin. *Gut* (1979) **20**:693–7. doi:10.1136/gut.20.8.693
8. Temple S. Division and differentiation of isolated CNS blast cells in microculture. *Nature* (1989) **340**:471–3. doi:10.1038/340471a0
9. Wansleeben C, Barkauskas CE, Rock JR, Hogan BLM. Stem cells of the adult lung: their development and role in homeostasis, regeneration, and disease. *Wiley Interdiscip Rev Dev Biol* (2013) **2**:131–48. doi:10.1002/wdev.58
10. Kotton DN, Morrisey EE. Lung regeneration: mechanisms, applications and emerging stem cell populations. *Nat Med* (2014) **20**:822–32. doi:10.1038/nm. 3642
11. Collins JJP, Thebaud B. Progenitor cells of the distal lung and their potential role in neonatal lung disease. *Birth Defects Res A Clin Mol Teratol* (2014) **100**:217–26. doi:10.1002/bdra.23227
12. Walker NM, Badri LN, Wadhwa A, Wettlaufer S, Peters-Golden M, Lama VN. Prostaglandin e2 as an inhibitory modulator of fibrogenesis in human lung allografts. *Am J Respir Crit Care Med* (2012) **185**:77–84. doi:10.1164/rccm. 201105-0834OC
13. Jay PY, Bielinska M, Erlich JM, Mannisto S, Pu WT, Heikinheimo M, et al. Impaired mesenchymal cell function in gata4 mutant mice leads to diaphragmatic hernias and primary lung defects. *Dev Biol* (2007) **301**:602–14. doi:10. 1016/j.ydbio.2006.09.050
14. Tropea KA, Leder E, Aslam M, Lau AN, Raiser DM, Lee JH, et al. Bronchioalveolar stem cells increase after mesenchymal stromal cell treatment in a mouse model of bronchopulmonary dysplasia. *Am J Physiol Lung Cell Mol Physiol* (2012) **302**:L829–37. doi:10.1152/ajplung.00347.2011
15. Sdrimas K, Kourembanas S. Msc microvesicles for the treatment of lung disease: a new paradigm for cell-free therapy. *Antioxid Redox Signal* (2014) **21**:1905–15. doi:10.1089/ars.2013.5784
16. Pierro M, Ionescu L, Montemurro T, Vadivel A, Weissmann G, Oudit G, et al. Short-term, long-term and paracrine effect of human umbilical cord-derived stem cells in lung injury prevention and repair in experimental bronchopulmonary dysplasia. *Thorax* (2013) **68**:475–84. doi:10.1136/ thoraxjnl-2012-202323
17. Sutsko RP, Young KC, Ribeiro A, Torres E, Rodriguez M, Hehre D, et al. Long-term reparative effects of mesenchymal stem cell therapy following neonatal hyperoxia-induced lung injury. *Pediatr Res* (2013) **73**:46–53. doi:10.1038/pr. 2012.152
18. Hansmann G, Fernandez-Gonzalez A, Aslam M, Vitali SH, Martin T, Mitsialis SA, et al. Mesenchymal stem cell-mediated reversal of bronchopulmonary dysplasia and associated pulmonary hypertension. *Pulm Circ* (2012) **2**:170–81. doi:10.4103/2045-8932.97603

19. Waszak P, Alphonse R, Vadivel A, Ionescu L, Eaton F, Thebaud B. Preconditioning enhances the paracrine effect of mesenchymal stem cells in preventing oxygen-induced neonatal lung injury in rats. *Stem Cells Dev* (2012) **21**:2789–97. doi:10.1089/scd.2010.0566

20. Zhang H, Fang J, Su H, Yang M, Lai W, Mai Y, et al. Bone marrow mesenchymal stem cells attenuate lung inflammation of hyperoxic newborn rats. *Pediatr Transplant* (2012) **16**:589–98. doi:10.1111/j.1399-3046.2012.01709.x

21. Zhang X, Wang H, Shi Y, Peng W, Zhang S, Zhang W, et al. Role of bone marrow-derived mesenchymal stem cells in the prevention of hyperoxia-induced lung injury in newborn mice. *Cell Biol Int* (2012) **36**:589–94. doi:10.1042/CBI20110447

22. Chang YS, Choi SJ, Sung DK, Kim SY, Oh W, Yang YS, et al. Intratracheal transplantation of human umbilical cord blood-derived mesenchymal stem cells dose-dependently attenuates hyperoxia-induced lung injury in neonatal rats. *Cell Transplant* (2011) **20**:1843–54. doi:10.3727/096368911X565038

23. Chang YS, Oh W, Choi SJ, Sung DK, Kim SY, Choi EY, et al. Human umbilical cord blood-derived mesenchymal stem cells attenuate hyperoxia-induced lung injury in neonatal rats. *Cell Transplant* (2009) **18**:869–86. doi:10.3727/096368909X471189

24. Aslam M, Baveja R, Liang OD, Fernandez-Gonzalez A, Lee C, Mitsialis SA, et al. Bone marrow stromal cells attenuate lung injury in a murine model of neonatal chronic lung disease. *Am J Respir Crit Care Med* (2009) **180**:1122–30. doi:10.1164/rccm.200902-0242OC

25. van Haaften T, Byrne R, Bonnet S, Rochefort GY, Akabutu J, Bouchentouf M, et al. Airway delivery of mesenchymal stem cells prevents arrested alveolar growth in neonatal lung injury in rats. *Am J Respir Crit Care Med* (2009) **180**:1131–42. doi:10.1164/rccm.200902-0179OC

26. Tian ZF, DU J, Wang B, Hong XY, Feng ZC. [Intravenous infusion of rat bone marrow-derived mesenchymal stem cells ameliorates hyperoxia-induced lung injury in neonatal rats]. *Nan Fang Yi Ke Da Xue Xue Bao* (2007) **27**:1692–5.

27. Hodges RJ, Lim R, Jenkin G, Wallace EM. Amnion epithelial cells as a candidate therapy for acute and chronic lung injury. *Stem Cells Int* (2012) **2012**:709763. doi:10.1155/2012/709763

28. Hodges RJ, Jenkin G, Hooper SB, Allison B, Lim R, Dickinson H, et al. Human amnion epithelial cells reduce ventilation-induced preterm lung injury in fetal sheep. *Am J Obstet Gynecol* (2012) **206**:448.e8–15. doi:10.1016/j.ajog.2012.02.038

29. Vosdoganes P, Hodges RJ, Lim R, Westover AJ, Acharya RY, Wallace EM, et al. Human amnion epithelial cells as a treatment for inflammation-induced fetal lung injury in sheep. *Am J Obstet Gynecol* (2011) **205**:156.e26–33. doi:10.1016/j.ajog.2011.03.054

30. Alphonse RS, Vadivel A, Fung M, Shelley WC, Critser PJ, Ionescu L, et al. Existence, functional impairment, and lung repair potential of endothelial colony-forming cells in oxygen-induced arrested alveolar growth. *Circulation* (2014) **129**:2144–57. doi:10.1161/CIRCULATIONAHA.114.009124

31. Balasubramaniam V, Ryan SL, Seedorf GJ, Roth EV, Heumann TR, Yoder MC, et al. Bone marrow-derived angiogenic cells restore lung alveolar and vascular structure after neonatal hyperoxia in infant mice. *Am J Physiol Lung Cell Mol Physiol* (2010) **298**:L315–23. doi:10.1152/ajplung.00089.2009

32. Gortner L, Monz D, Mildau C, Shen J, Kasoha M, Laschke MW, et al. Bronchopulmonary dysplasia in a double-hit mouse model induced by intrauterine hypoxia and postnatal hyperoxia: closer to clinical features? *Ann Anat* (2013) **195**:351–8. doi:10.1016/j.aanat.2013.02.010

33. Berger J, Bhandari V. Animal models of bronchopulmonary dysplasia. The term mouse models. *Am J Physiol Lung Cell Mol Physiol* (2014) **307**:L936–47. doi:10.1152/ajplung.00159.2014

34. Monz D, Tutdibi E, Mildau C, Shen J, Kasoha M, Laschke MW, et al. Human umbilical cord blood mononuclear cells in a double-hit model of bronchopulmonary dysplasia in neonatal mice. *PLoS One* (2013) **8**:e74740. doi:10.1371/journal.pone.0074740

35. Keating A. Mesenchymal stromal cells: new directions. *Cell Stem Cell* (2012) **10**:709–16. doi:10.1016/j.stem.2012.05.015

36. Friedenstein AJ, Chailakhjan RK, Lalykina KS. The development of fibroblast colonies in monolayer cultures of guinea-pig bone marrow and spleen cells. *Cell Tissue Kinet* (1970) **3**:393–403.

37. Hass R, Kasper C, Bohm S, Jacobs R. Different populations and sources of human mesenchymal stem cells (MSC): a comparison of adult and neonatal tissue-derived MSC. *Cell Commun Signal* (2011) **9**:12. doi:10.1186/1478-811X-9-12

38. Yamaza T, Ren G, Akiyama K, Chen C, Shi Y, Shi S. Mouse mandible contains distinctive mesenchymal stem cells. *J Dent Res* (2011) **90**:317–24. doi:10.1177/0022034510387796

39. Yannarelli G, Dayan V, Pacienza N, Lee CJ, Medin J, Keating A. Human umbilical cord perivascular cells exhibit enhanced cardiomyocyte reprogramming and cardiac function after experimental acute myocardial infarction. *Cell Transplant* (2013) **22**:1651–66. doi:10.3727/096368912X657675

40. Prockop DJ. Repair of tissues by adult stem/progenitor cells (MSCs): controversies, myths, and changing paradigms. *Mol Ther* (2009) **17**:939–46. doi:10.1038/mt.2009.62

41. Dominici M, Le Blanc K, Mueller I, Slaper-Cortenbach I, Marini F, Krause D, et al. Minimal criteria for defining multipotent mesenchymal stromal cells. The international society for cellular therapy position statement. *Cytotherapy* (2006) **8**:315–7. doi:10.1080/14653240600855905

42. Mendicino M, Bailey AM, Wonnacott K, Puri RK, Bauer SR. MSC-based product characterization for clinical trials: an FDA perspective. *Cell Stem Cell* (2014) **14**:141–5. doi:10.1016/j.stem.2014.01.013

43. Jones EA, Kinsey SE, English A, Jones RA, Straszynski L, Meredith DM, et al. Isolation and characterization of bone marrow multipotential mesenchymal progenitor cells. *Arthritis Rheum* (2002) **46**:3349–60. doi:10.1002/art.10696

44. Sueblinvong V, Loi R, Eisenhauer PL, Bernstein IM, Suratt BT, Spees JL, et al. Derivation of lung epithelium from human cord blood-derived mesenchymal stem cells. *Am J Respir Crit Care Med* (2008) **177**:701–11. doi:10.1164/rccm.200706-859OC

45. Spees JL, Olson SD, Ylostalo J, Lynch PJ, Smith J, Perry A, et al. Differentiation, cell fusion, and nuclear fusion during ex vivo repair of epithelium by human adult stem cells from bone marrow stroma. *Proc Natl Acad Sci U S A* (2003) **100**:2397–402. doi:10.1073/pnas.0437997100

46. Yue WM, Liu W, Bi YW, He XP, Sun WY, Pang XY, et al. Mesenchymal stem cells differentiate into an endothelial phenotype, reduce neointimal formation, and enhance endothelial function in a rat vein grafting model. *Stem Cells Dev* (2008) **17**:785–93. doi:10.1089/scd.2007.0243

47. Ferroni L, Gardin C, Tocco I, Epis R, Casadei A, Vindigni V, et al. Potential for neural differentiation of mesenchymal stem cells. *Adv Biochem Eng Biotechnol* (2013) **129**:89–115. doi:10.1007/10_2012_152

48. Krampera M, Galipeau J, Shi Y, Tarte K, Sensebe L. Immunological characterization of multipotent mesenchymal stromal cells – the international society for cellular therapy (isct) working proposal. *Cytotherapy* (2013) **15**:1054–61. doi:10.1016/j.jcyt.2013.02.010

49. Makridakis M, Roubelakis MG, Vlahou A. Stem cells: insights into the secretome. *Biochim Biophys Acta* (2013) **1834**:2380–4. doi:10.1016/j.bbapap.2013.01.032

50. El Agha E, Bellusci S. Walking along the fibroblast growth factor 10 route: a key pathway to understand the control and regulation of epithelial and mesenchymal cell-lineage formation during lung development and repair after injury. *Scientifica (Cairo)* (2014) **2014**:538379. doi:10.1155/2014/538379

51. McGowan SE. Paracrine cellular and extracellular matrix interactions with mesenchymal progenitors during pulmonary alveolar septation. *Birth Defects Res A Clin Mol Teratol* (2014) **100**:227–39. doi:10.1002/bdra.23230

52. Collins JJP, Thebaud B. Lung mesenchymal stromal cells in development and disease: to serve and protect? *Antioxid Redox Signal* (2014) **21**:1849–62. doi:10.1089/ars.2013.5781

53. Bozyk PD, Popova AP, Bentley JK, Goldsmith AM, Linn MJ, Weiss DJ, et al. Mesenchymal stromal cells from neonatal tracheal aspirates demonstrate a pattern of lung-specific gene expression. *Stem Cells Dev* (2011) **20**:1995–2007. doi:10.1089/scd.2010.0494

54. Popova AP, Bozyk PD, Bentley JK, Linn MJ, Goldsmith AM, Schumacher RE, et al. Isolation of tracheal aspirate mesenchymal stromal cells predicts bronchopulmonary dysplasia. *Pediatrics* (2010) **126**:e1127–33. doi:10.1542/peds.2009-3445

55. Hennrick KT, Keeton AG, Nanua S, Kijek TG, Goldsmith AM, Sajjan US, et al. Lung cells from neonates show a mesenchymal stem cell phenotype. *Am J Respir Crit Care Med* (2007) **175**:1158–64. doi:10.1164/rccm.200607-941OC

56. Popova AP, Bentley JK, Cui TX, Richardson MN, Linn MJ, Lei J, et al. Reduced platelet-derived growth factor receptor expression is a primary feature of human bronchopulmonary dysplasia. *Am J Physiol Lung Cell Mol Physiol* (2014) **307**:L231–9. doi:10.1152/ajplung.00342.2013

57. Popova AP, Bozyk PD, Goldsmith AM, Linn MJ, Lei J, Bentley JK, et al. Autocrine production of tgf-beta1 promotes myofibroblastic differentiation of

57. neonatal lung mesenchymal stem cells. *Am J Physiol Lung Cell Mol Physiol* (2010) 298:L735-43. doi:10.1152/ajplung.00347.2009

58. Popova AP, Bentley JK, Anyanwu AC, Richardson MN, Linn MJ, Lei J, et al. Glycogen synthase kinase-3beta/beta-catenin signaling regulates neonatal lung mesenchymal stromal cell myofibroblastic differentiation. *Am J Physiol Lung Cell Mol Physiol* (2012) 303:L439-48. doi:10.1152/ajplung.00408.2011

59. Vicencio AG, Lee CG, Cho SJ, Eickelberg O, Chuu Y, Haddad GG, et al. Conditional overexpression of bioactive transforming growth factor-beta1 in neonatal mouse lung: a new model for bronchopulmonary dysplasia? *Am J Respir Cell Mol Biol* (2004) 31:650-6. doi:10.1165/rcmb.2004-0092OC

60. Majka SM, Beutz MA, Hagen M, Izzo AA, Voelkel N, Helm KM. Identification of novel resident pulmonary stem cells: form and function of the lung side population. *Stem Cells* (2005) 23:1073-81. doi:10.1634/stemcells.2005-0039

61. Irwin D, Helm K, Campbell N, Imamura M, Fagan K, Harral J, et al. Neonatal lung side population cells demonstrate endothelial potential and are altered in response to hyperoxia-induced lung simplification. *Am J Physiol Lung Cell Mol Physiol* (2007) 293:L941-51. doi:10.1152/ajplung.00054.2007

62. O'Reilly M, Thebaud B. Animal models of bronchopulmonary dysplasia. The term rat models. *Am J Physiol Lung Cell Mol Physiol* (2014) 307:L948-58. doi:10.1152/ajplung.00160.2014

63. Hilgendorff A, Reiss I, Ehrhardt H, Eickelberg O, Alvira CM. Chronic lung disease in the preterm infant. Lessons learned from animal models. *Am J Respir Cell Mol Biol* (2014) 50:233-45. doi:10.1165/rcmb.2013-0014TR

64. Coalson JJ. Pathology of bronchopulmonary dysplasia. *Semin Perinatol* (2006) 30:179-84. doi:10.1053/j.semperi.2006.05.004

65. Yoder BA, Coalson JJ. Animal models of bronchopulmonary dysplasia. The preterm baboon models. *Am J Physiol Lung Cell Mol Physiol* (2014) 307:L970-7. doi:10.1152/ajplung.00171.2014

66. Chang YS, Choi SJ, Ahn SY, Sung DK, Sung SI, Yoo HS, et al. Timing of umbilical cord blood derived mesenchymal stem cells transplantation determines therapeutic efficacy in the neonatal hyperoxic lung injury. *PLoS One* (2013) 8:e52419. doi:10.1371/journal.pone.0052419

67. Fung ME, Thebaud B. Stem cell-based therapy for neonatal lung disease: it is in the juice. *Pediatr Res* (2014) 75:2-7. doi:10.1038/pr.2013.176

68. Ohkouchi S, Block GJ, Katsha AM, Kanehira M, Ebina M, Kikuchi T, et al. Mesenchymal stromal cells protect cancer cells from ROS-induced apoptosis and enhance the Warburg effect by secreting STCL. *Mol Ther* (2012) 20:417-23. doi:10.1038/mt.2011.259

69. Tian W, Liu Y, Zhang B, Dai X, Li G, Li X, et al. Infusion of mesenchymal stem cells protects lung transplants from cold ischemia-reperfusion injury in mice. *Lung* (2015) 193:85-95. doi:10.1007/s00408-014-9654-x

70. Foskett AM, Bazhanov N, Ti X, Tiblow A, Bartosh TJ, Prockop DJ. Phase-directed therapy: Tsg-6 targeted to early inflammation improves bleomycin-injured lungs. *Am J Physiol Lung Cell Mol Physiol* (2014) 306:L120-31. doi:10.1152/ajplung.00240.2013

71. Wang N, Shao Y, Mei Y, Zhang L, Li Q, Li D, et al. Novel mechanism for mesenchymal stem cells in attenuating peritoneal adhesion: accumulating in the lung and secreting tumor necrosis factor alpha-stimulating gene-6. *Stem Cell Res Ther* (2012) 3:51. doi:10.1186/scrt142

72. Ortiz LA, Gambelli F, McBride C, Gaupp D, Baddoo M, Kaminski N, et al. Mesenchymal stem cell engraftment in lung is enhanced in response to bleomycin exposure and ameliorates its fibrotic effects. *Proc Natl Acad Sci U S A* (2003) 100:8407-11. doi:10.1073/pnas.1432929100

73. Ionescu L, Byrne RN, van Haaften T, Vadivel A, Alphonse RS, Rey-Parra GJ, et al. Stem cell conditioned medium improves acute lung injury in mice: in vivo evidence for stem cell paracrine action. *Am J Physiol Lung Cell Mol Physiol* (2012) 303:L967-77. doi:10.1152/ajplung.00144.2011

74. Ionescu LI, Alphonse RS, Arizmendi N, Morgan B, Abel M, Eaton F, et al. Airway delivery of soluble factors from plastic-adherent bone marrow cells prevents murine asthma. *Am J Respir Cell Mol Biol* (2012) 46:207-16. doi:10.1165/rcmb.2010-0391OC

75. Curley GF, Hayes M, Ansari B, Shaw G, Ryan A, Barry F, et al. Mesenchymal stem cells enhance recovery and repair following ventilator-induced lung injury in the rat. *Thorax* (2012) 67:496-501. doi:10.1136/thoraxjnl-2011-201059

76. Speer CP. Inflammation and bronchopulmonary dysplasia: a continuing story. *Semin Fetal Neonatal Med* (2006) 11:354-62. doi:10.1016/j.siny.2006.03.004

77. Kotton DN, Fine A. Lung stem cells. *Cell Tissue Res* (2008) 331:145-56. doi:10.1007/s00441-007-0479-2

78. Kotton DN, Fabian AJ, Mulligan RC. Failure of bone marrow to reconstitute lung epithelium. *Am J Respir Cell Mol Biol* (2005) 33:328-34. doi:10.1165/rcmb.2005-0175RC

79. Colombo M, Raposo G, Thery C. Biogenesis, secretion, and intercellular interactions of exo-somes and other extracellular vesicles. *Annu Rev Cell Dev Biol* (2014) 30:255-89. doi:10.1146/annurev-cellbio-101512-122326

80. Lee C, Mitsialis SA, Aslam M, Vitali SH, Vergadi E, Konstantinou G, et al. Exosomes mediate the cytoprotective action of mesenchymal stromal cells on hypoxia-induced pulmonary hypertension. *Circulation* (2012) 126:2601-11. doi:10.1161/CIRCULATIONAHA.112.114173

81. Zhu YG, Feng XM, Abbott J, Fang XH, Hao Q, Monsel A, et al. Human mesenchymal stem cell microvesicles for treatment of *Escherichia coli* endotoxin-induced acute lung injury in mice. *Stem Cells* (2014) 32:116-25. doi:10.1002/stem.1504

82. Valadi H, Ekstrom K, Bossios A, Sjostrand M, Lee JJ, Lotvall JO. Exosome-mediated transfer of mRNAs and microRNAs is a novel mechanism of genetic exchange between cells. *Nat Cell Biol* (2007) 9:654-9. doi:10.1038/ncb1596

83. Pegtel DM, Cosmopoulos K, Thorley-Lawson DA, van Eijndhoven MAJ, Hopmans ES, Lindenberg JL, et al. Functional delivery of viral mirnas via exosomes. *Proc Natl Acad Sci U S A* (2010) 107:6328-33. doi:10.1073/pnas.0914843107

84. Morton RL, Ikle D, White CW. Loss of lung mitochondrial aconitase activity due to hyperoxia in bronchopulmonary dysplasia in primates. *Am J Physiol* (1998) 274:L127-33.

85. Xu D, Guthrie JR, Mabry S, Sack TM, Truog WE. Mitochondrial aldehyde dehydrogenase attenuates hyperoxia-induced cell death through activation of erk/mapk and pi3k-akt pathways in lung epithelial cells. *Am J Physiol Lung Cell Mol Physiol* (2006) 291:L966-75. doi:10.1152/ajplung.00045.2006

86. Ratner V, Starkov A, Matsiukevich D, Polin RA, Ten VS. Mitochondrial dysfunction contributes to alveolar developmental arrest in hyperoxia-exposed mice. *Am J Respir Cell Mol Biol* (2009) 40:511-8. doi:10.1165/rcmb.2008-0341RC

87. Ratner V, Sosunov SA, Niatsetskaya ZV, Utkina-Sosunova IV, Ten VS. Mechanical ventilation causes pulmonary mitochondrial dysfunction and delayed alveolarization in neonatal mice. *Am J Respir Cell Mol Biol* (2013) 49:943-50. doi:10.1165/rcmb.2012-0172OC

88. Vadivel A, Alphonse RS, Ionescu L, Machado DS, O'Reilly M, Eaton F, et al. Exogenous hydrogen sulfide (h2s) protects alveolar growth in experimental o2-induced neonatal lung injury. *PLoS One* (2014) 9:e90965. doi:10.1371/journal.pone.0090965

89. Spees JL, Olson SD, Whitney MJ, Prockop DJ. Mitochondrial transfer between cells can rescue aerobic respiration. *Proc Natl Acad Sci U S A* (2006) 103:1283-8. doi:10.1073/pnas.0510511103

90. Islam MN, Das SR, Emin MT, Wei M, Sun L, Westphalen K, et al. Mitochondrial transfer from bone-marrow-derived stromal cells to pulmonary alveoli protects against acute lung injury. *Nat Med* (2012) 18:759-65. doi:10.1038/nm.2736

91. Li X, Zhang Y, Yeung SC, Liang Y, Liang X, Ding Y, et al. Mitochondrial transfer of induced pluripotent stem cell-derived mesenchymal stem cells to airway epithelial cells attenuates cigarette smoke-induced damage. *Am J Respir Cell Mol Biol* (2014) 51:455-65. doi:10.1165/rcmb.2013-0529OC

92. Weiss DJ, Casaburi R, Flannery R, LeRoux-Williams M, Tashkin DP. A placebo-controlled, randomized trial of mesenchymal stem cells in copd. *Chest* (2013) 143:1590-8. doi:10.1378/chest.12-2094

93. Osiris Therapeutics, Inc. Osiris therapeutics announces preliminary results for prochymal PHASE III GvHD trials (2009). Available from: http://investor.osiris.com/releasedetail.cfm?releaseid=407404

94. Introna M, Rambaldi A. Mesenchymal stromal cells for prevention and treatment of graft-versus-host disease: successes and hurdles. *Curr Opin Organ Transplant* (2015) 20:72-8. doi:10.1097/MOT.0000000000000158

95. Prockop DJ, Prockop SE, Bertoncello I. Are clinical trials with mesenchymal stem/progenitor cells too far ahead of the science? Lessons from experimental hematology. *Stem Cells* (2014) 32:3055-61. doi:10.1002/stem.1806

96. Sensebe L, Bourin P, Tarte K. Good manufacturing practices production of mesenchymal stem/stromal cells. *Hum Gene Ther* (2011) 22:19-26. doi:10.1089/hum.2010.197

97. Wagner W, Ho AD, Zenke M. Different facets of aging in human mesenchymal stem cells. *Tissue Eng Part B Rev* (2010) 16:445-53. doi:10.1089/ten.TEB.2009.0825

98. Wagner W, Bork S, Lepperdinger G, Joussen S, Ma N, Strunk D, et al. How to track cellular aging of mesenchymal stromal cells? *Aging (Albany NY)* (2010) 2:224–30.

99. Barkholt L, Flory E, Jekerle V, Lucas-Samuel S, Ahnert P, Bisset L, et al. Risk of tumorigenicity in mesenchymal stromal cell-based therapies-bridging scientific observations and regulatory viewpoints. *Cytotherapy* (2013) 15:753–9. doi:10.1016/j.jcyt.2013.03.005

100. Wuchter P, Bieback K, Schrezenmeier H, Bornhäuser M, Müller LP, Bönig H, et al. Standardization of good manufacturing practice-compliant production of bone marrow-derived human mesenchymal stromal cells for immunotherapeutic applications. *Cytotherapy* (2015) 17:128–39. doi:10.1016/j.jcyt.2014.04.002

101. Ben-David U, Mayshar Y, Benvenisty N. Large-scale analysis reveals acquisition of lineage-specific chromosomal aberrations in human adult stem cells. *Cell Stem Cell* (2011) 9:97–102. doi:10.1016/j.stem.2011.06.013

102. Grigorian AS, Kruglyakov PV, Taminkina UA, Efimova OA, Pendina AA, Voskresenskaya AV, et al. Alterations of cytological and karyological profile of human mesenchymal stem cells during in vitro culturing. *Bull Exp Biol Med* (2010) 150:125–30. doi:10.1007/s10517-010-1086-x

103. Rubio D, Garcia S, De la Cueva T, Paz MF, Lloyd AC, Bernad A, et al. Human mesenchymal stem cell transformation is associated with a mesenchymal-epithelial transition. *Exp Cell Res* (2008) 314:691–8. doi:10.1016/j.yexcr.2007.11.017

104. Torsvik A, Rosland GV, Svendsen A, Molven A, Immervoll H, McCormack E, et al. Spontaneous malignant transformation of human mesenchymal stem cells reflects cross-contamination: putting the research field on track – letter. *Cancer Res* (2010) 70:6393–6. doi:10.1158/0008-5472.CAN-10-1305

105. Lalu MM, McLntyre L, Pugliese C, Fergusson D, Winston BW, Marshall JC, et al. Safety of cell therapy with mesenchymal stromal cells (safecell): a systematic review and meta-analysis of clinical trials. *PLoS One* (2012) 7:e47559. doi:10.1371/journal.pone.0047559

106. Menard C, Pacelli L, Bassi G, Dulong J, Bifari F, Bezier I, et al. Clinical-grade mesenchymal stromal cells produced under various good manufacturing practice processes differ in their immunomodulatory properties: standardization of immune quality controls. *Stem Cells Dev* (2013) 22:1789–801. doi:10.1089/scd.2012.0594

107. Rizzo R, Lanzoni G, Stignani M, Campioni D, Alviano F, Ricci F, et al. A simple method for identifying bone marrow mesenchymal stromal cells with a high immunosuppressive potential. *Cytotherapy* (2011) 13:523–7. doi:10.3109/14653249.2010.542460

108. Barkauskas CE, Cronce MJ, Rackley CR, Bowie EJ, Keene DR, Stripp BR, et al. Type 2 alveolar cells are stem cells in adult lung. *J Clin Invest* (2013) 123:3025–36. doi:10.1172/JCI68782

109. Tyndall A. Mesenchymal stem cell treatments in rheumatology: a glass half full? *Nat Rev Rheumatol* (2014) 10:117–24. doi:10.1038/nrrheum.2013.166

110. Bhatt AJ, Pryhuber GS, Huyck H, Watkins RH, Metlay LA, Maniscalco WM. Disrupted pulmonary vasculature and decreased vascular endothelial growth factor, flt-1, and tie-2 in human infants dying with bronchopulmonary dysplasia. *Am J Respir Crit Care Med* (2001) 164:1971–80. doi:10.1164/ajrccm.164.10.2101140

111. Thebaud B, Ladha F, Michelakis ED, Sawicka M, Thurston G, Eaton F, et al. Vascular endothelial growth factor gene therapy increases survival, promotes lung angiogenesis, and prevents alveolar damage in hyperoxia-induced lung injury: evidence that angiogenesis participates in alveolarization. *Circulation* (2005) 112:2477–86. doi:10.1161/CIRCULATIONAHA.105.541524

112. Kunig AM, Balasubramaniam V, Markham NE, Morgan D, Montgomery G, Grover TR, et al. Recombinant human vegf treatment enhances alveolarization after hyperoxic lung injury in neonatal rats. *Am J Physiol Lung Cell Mol Physiol* (2005) 289:L529–35. doi:10.1152/ajplung.00336.2004

113. Asahara T, Murohara T, Sullivan A, Silver M, van der Zee R, Li T, et al. Isolation of putative progenitor endothelial cells for angiogenesis. *Science* (1997) 275:964–7. doi:10.1126/science.275.5302.964

114. Mund JA, Ingram DA, Yoder MC, Case J. Endothelial progenitor cells and cardiovascular cell-based therapies. *Cytotherapy* (2009) 11:103–13. doi:10.1080/14653240802714827

115. Sen S, McDonald SP, Coates PTH, Bonder CS. Endothelial progenitor cells: novel biomarker and promising cell therapy for cardiovascular disease. *Clin Sci (Lond)* (2011) 120:263–83. doi:10.1042/CS20100429

116. Basile DP, Yoder MC. Circulating and tissue resident endothelial progenitor cells. *J Cell Physiol* (2014) 229:10–6. doi:10.1002/jcp.24423

117. Yoder MC, Mead LE, Prater D, Krier TR, Mroueh KN, Li F, et al. Redefining endothelial progenitor cells via clonal analysis and hematopoietic stem/progenitor cell principals. *Blood* (2007) 109:1801–9. doi:10.1182/blood-2006-08-043471

118. Lin Y, Weisdorf DJ, Solovey A, Hebbel RP. Origins of circulating endothelial cells and endothelial outgrowth from blood. *J Clin Invest* (2000) 105:71–7. doi:10.1172/JCI8071

119. Ingram DA, Mead LE, Tanaka H, Meade V, Fenoglio A, Mortell K, et al. Identification of a novel hierarchy of endothelial progenitor cells using human peripheral and umbilical cord blood. *Blood* (2004) 104:2752–60. doi:10.1182/blood-2004-04-1396

120. Balasubramaniam V, Mervis CF, Maxey AM, Markham NE, Abman SH. Hyperoxia reduces bone marrow, circulating, and lung endothelial progenitor cells in the developing lung: implications for the pathogenesis of bronchopulmonary dysplasia. *Am J Physiol Lung Cell Mol Physiol* (2007) 292:L1073–84. doi:10.1152/ajplung.00347.2006

121. Borghesi A, Massa M, Campanelli R, Bollani L, Tzialla C, Figar TA, et al. Circulating endothelial progenitor cells in preterm infants with bronchopulmonary dysplasia. *Am J Respir Crit Care Med* (2009) 180:540–6. doi:10.1164/rccm.200812-1949OC

122. Borghesi A, Cova C, Gazzolo D, Stronati M. Stem cell therapy for neonatal diseases associated with preterm birth. *J Clin Neonatol* (2013) 2:1–7. doi:10.4103/2249-4847.109230

123. Baker CD, Balasubramaniam V, Mourani PM, Sontag MK, Black CP, Ryan SL, et al. Cord blood angiogenic progenitor cells are decreased in bronchopulmonary dysplasia. *Eur Respir J* (2012) 40:1516–22. doi:10.1183/09031936.00017312

124. Baker CD, Ryan SL, Ingram DA, Seedorf GJ, Abman SH, Balasubramaniam V. Endothelial colony-forming cells from preterm infants are increased and more susceptible to hyperoxia. *Am J Respir Crit Care Med* (2009) 180:454–61. doi:10.1164/rccm.200901-0115OC

125. Baker CD, Seedorf GJ, Wisniewski BL, Black CP, Ryan SL, Balasubramaniam V, et al. Endothelial colony-forming cell conditioned media promote angiogenesis in vitro and prevent pulmonary hypertension in experimental bronchopulmonary dysplasia. *Am J Physiol Lung Cell Mol Physiol* (2013) 305:L73–81. doi:10.1152/ajplung.00400.2012

126. Schniedermann J, Rennecke M, Buttler K, Richter G, Stadler AM, Norgall S, et al. Mouse lung contains endothelial progenitors with high capacity to form blood and lymphatic vessels. *BMC Cell Biol* (2010) 11:50. doi:10.1186/1471-2121-11-50

127. Alvarez DF, Huang L, King JA, ElZarrad MK, Yoder MC, Stevens T. Lung microvascular endothelium is enriched with progenitor cells that exhibit vasculogenic capacity. *Am J Physiol Lung Cell Mol Physiol* (2008) 294:L419–30. doi:10.1152/ajplung.00314.2007

128. Wang XX, Zhang FR, Shang YP, Zhu JH, Xie XD, Tao QM, et al. Transplantation of autologous endothelial progenitor cells may be beneficial in patients with idiopathic pulmonary arterial hypertension: a pilot randomized controlled trial. *J Am Coll Cardiol* (2007) 49:1566–71. doi:10.1016/j.jacc.2006.12.037

129. Faulk WP, Matthews R, Stevens PJ, Bennett JP, Burgos H, Hsi BL. Human amnion as an adjunct in wound healing. *Lancet* (1980) 1:1156–8. doi:10.1016/S0140-6736(80)91617-7

130. Ilancheran S, Michalska A, Peh G, Wallace EM, Pera M, Manuelpillai U. Stem cells derived from human fetal membranes display multilineage differentiation potential. *Biol Reprod* (2007) 77:577–88. doi:10.1095/biolreprod.106.055244

131. Li H, Niederkorn JY, Neelam S, Mayhew E, Word RA, McCulley JP, et al. Immunosuppressive factors secreted by human amniotic epithelial cells. *Invest Ophthalmol Vis Sci* (2005) 46:900–7. doi:10.1167/iovs.04-0495

132. Wolbank S, Peterbauer A, Fahrner M, Hennerbichler S, van Griensven M, Stadler G, et al. Dose-dependent immunomodulatory effect of human stem cells from amniotic membrane: a comparison with human mesenchymal stem cells from adipose tissue. *Tissue Eng* (2007) 13:1173–83. doi:10.1089/ten.2006.0313

133. Moodley Y, Ilancheran S, Samuel C, Vaghjiani V, Atienza D, Williams ED, et al. Human amnion epithelial cell transplantation abrogates lung fibrosis and augments repair. *Am J Respir Crit Care Med* (2010) **182**:643–51. doi:10.1164/rccm.201001-0014OC

134. Murphy S, Lim R, Dickinson H, Acharya R, Rosli S, Jenkin G, et al. Human amnion epithelial cells prevent bleomycin-induced lung injury and preserve lung function. *Cell Transplant* (2011) **20**:909–23. doi:10.3727/096368910X543385

135. Zakaria N, Possemiers T, Dhubhghaill SN, Leysen I, Rozema J, Koppen C, et al. Results of a phase i/ii clinical trial: standardized, non-xenogenic, cultivated limbal stem cell transplantation. *J Transl Med* (2014) **12**:58. doi:10.1186/1479-5876-12-58

136. Parolini O, Alviano F, Bergwerf I, Boraschi D, De Bari C, De Waele P, et al. Toward cell therapy using placenta-derived cells: disease mechanisms, cell biology, preclinical studies, and regulatory aspects at the round table. *Stem Cells Dev* (2010) **19**:143–54. doi:10.1089/scd.2009.0404

137. Murphy S, Rosli S, Acharya R, Mathias L, Lim R, Wallace E, et al. Amnion epithelial cell isolation and characterization for clinical use. *Curr Protoc Stem Cell Biol* (2010) **Chapter** 1:Unit1E.6. doi:10.1002/9780470151808.sc01e06s13

138. Fischbach MA, Bluestone JA, Lim WA. Cell-based therapeutics: the next pillar of medicine. *Sci Transl Med* (2013) **5**:179s7. doi:10.1126/scitranslmed.3005568

139. Daley GQ. The promise and perils of stem cell therapeutics. *Cell Stem Cell* (2012) **10**:740–9. doi:10.1016/j.stem.2012.05.010

Sequential Exposure to Antenatal Microbial Triggers Attenuates Alveolar Growth and Pulmonary Vascular Development and Impacts Pulmonary Epithelial Stem/ Progenitor Cells

Helene Widowski [1,2,3], Niki L. Reynaert [4,5], Daan R. M. G. Ophelders [1,3],
Matthias C. Hütten [6,7], Peter G. J. Nikkels [8], Carmen A. H. Severens-Rijvers [9],
Jack P. M. Cleutjens [9,10], Matthew W. Kemp [11], John P. Newnham [11], Masatoshi Saito [11,12],
Haruo Usuda [11,12], Matthew S. Payne [11], Alan H. Jobe [11,13], Boris W. Kramer [1,3,14],
Tammo Delhaas [2,10] and Tim G. A. M. Wolfs [1,3]*

[1] Department of Pediatrics, Maastricht University Medical Center, Maastricht, Netherlands, [2] Department of BioMedical Engineering, Maastricht University Medical Center, Maastricht, Netherlands, [3] GROW School for Oncology and Developmental Biology, Maastricht University Medical Center, Maastricht, Netherlands, [4] Department of Respiratory Medicine, Maastricht University, Maastricht, Netherlands, [5] NUTRIM School of Nutrition and Translational Research in Metabolism, Maastricht University Medical Center, Maastricht, Netherlands, [6] Neonatology, Pediatrics Department, Faculty of Health, Medicine and Life Sciences, Maastricht University Medical Center, Maastricht, Netherlands, [7] University Children's Hospital Würzburg, University of Würzburg, Würzburg, Germany, [8] Department of Pathology, University Medical Center Utrecht, Utrecht, Netherlands, [9] Department of Pathology, Maastricht University Medical Center, Maastricht, Netherlands, [10] CARIM School for Cardiovascular Diseases, Maastricht University Medical Center, Maastricht, Netherlands, [11] Division of Obstetrics and Gynecology, The University of Western Australia, Crawley, WA, Australia, [12] Tohoku University Centre for Perinatal and Neonatal Medicine, Tohoku University Hospital, Sendai, Japan, [13] Perinatal Institute Cincinnati Children's Hospital Medical Center, Cincinnati, OH, United States, [14] School for Mental Health and Neuroscience, Maastricht University, Maastricht, Netherlands

*Correspondence:
Tim G. A. M. Wolfs
tim.wolfs@maastrichtuniversity.nl

Perinatal inflammatory stress is strongly associated with adverse pulmonary outcomes after preterm birth. Antenatal infections are an essential perinatal stress factor and contribute to preterm delivery, induction of lung inflammation and injury, pre-disposing preterm infants to bronchopulmonary dysplasia. Considering the polymicrobial nature of antenatal infection, which was reported to result in diverse effects and outcomes in preterm lungs, the aim was to examine the consequences of sequential inflammatory stimuli on endogenous epithelial stem/progenitor cells and vascular maturation, which are crucial drivers of lung development. Therefore, a translational ovine model of antenatal infection/inflammation with consecutive exposures to chronic and acute stimuli was used. Ovine fetuses were exposed intra-amniotically to *Ureaplasma parvum* 42 days (chronic stimulus) and/or to lipopolysaccharide 2 or 7 days (acute stimulus) prior to preterm delivery at 125 days of gestation. Pulmonary inflammation, endogenous epithelial stem cell populations, vascular modulators and morphology were investigated in preterm lungs. Pre-exposure to UP attenuated neutrophil infiltration in 7d LPS-exposed lungs and prevented reduction of SOX-9 expression and increased SP-B expression, which could indicate protective responses induced by re-exposure. Sequential exposures did not markedly impact stem/progenitors of the proximal airways (P63+ basal cells) compared to single exposure to LPS. In contrast, the alveolar size was increased solely in the UP+7d LPS group. In line, the most pronounced reduction of AEC2 and proliferating cells (Ki67+) was detected in these sequentially UP + 7d LPS-exposed lambs. A similar sensitization effect of UP pre-exposure was reflected by the vessel density and expression of vascular markers VEGFR-2 and Ang-1 that were significantly reduced after UP exposure prior to 2d LPS, when compared to UP and LPS exposure alone. Strikingly, while morphological changes of alveoli and vessels were seen after sequential microbial exposure, improved lung function was observed in UP, 7d LPS, and UP+7d LPS-exposed lambs. In conclusion, although sequential exposures did not markedly further impact epithelial stem/progenitor cell populations, re-exposure to an inflammatory stimulus resulted in disturbed alveolarization and abnormal pulmonary vascular development. Whether these negative effects on lung development can be rescued by the potentially protective responses observed, should be examined at later time points.

Keywords: polymicrobial infection, vascular disturbances, adverse pulmonary outcomes, endogenous pulmonary stem cells, bronchopulmonary dysplasia, preterm birth, antenatal inflammation

INTRODUCTION

Perinatal inflammatory stress, including sepsis and mechanical ventilation are strongly associated with adverse pulmonary outcomes after preterm birth (1, 2). One of the most frequently occurring complications after perinatal insults and preterm birth is bronchopulmonary dysplasia (BPD), a chronic respiratory disorder of the premature infant. BPD results from a demand of respiratory support and supplemental oxygen after preterm birth and histologically manifests as a delay in alveolar growth and an impairment in vascular maturation (3, 4). Antenatal infections are an essential factor of perinatal stress and associated with preterm delivery and induction of lung inflammation and injury, thereby pre-disposing to BPD (5, 6).

Recently, we showed that timing of antenatal infection/inflammation and its duration of determine the extent and location of adverse effects in the preterm lungs (7). More precisely, we reported attenuated levels of endogenous stem/progenitor populations and their potential consequences, including altered surfactant protein expression and reduced alveolar differentiation in the course of antenatal inflammation (7).

Antenatal infection is often of polymicrobial nature, with *Ureaplasma* (UP) species being the most frequently cultivated bacteria in human amniotic fluid samples (8). Conceivably, potential interactions between various consecutive inflammatory stimuli might modulate the inflammatory response and either lead to a milder outcome, including a treatable surfactant deficiency, or more severe adverse pulmonary outcome (BPD) in the preterm infant. This concept is supported by earlier findings in different preterm organ systems, showing that sequentially occurring antenatal inflammatory insults of varying exposure time points and durations, cause either preconditioning or sensitization to a consecutive inflammatory hit (9–11). With respect to the lungs, *in utero* sequential exposure to antenatal

bacteria and bacteria-derived endotoxins resulted in increased inflammation, along with exacerbation of vascular disturbances in very preterm ovine lungs (12). Conversely, in fetuses of higher gestational age (GA), Kallapur et al. showed that chronic UP exposure pre-conditioned the immature lungs and thereby led to a decreased pro-inflammatory response to a subsequent endotoxin hit (13). The GA of the fetus and the duration of each antenatal insult have been shown to modulate the responsiveness of the lung tissue to inflammation and determine the extent of developmental changes.

Considering the increasing importance of aberrant vascular development in neonatal lung diseases (14), and recent findings of endogenous epithelial stem/progenitor cells playing a key role in the adverse pulmonary development (7, 15), our aim was to examine the consequences of sequential inflammatory stimuli on inflammatory read outs and on these crucial developmental aspects. For this purpose, we used a translational ovine model of antenatal infection/inflammation with consecutive exposures to a chronic and an acute stimulus. Ovine fetuses were exposed intra-amniotically (IA) to live *Ureaplasma parvum* 42 days (chronic stimulus) and/or to lipopolysaccharide (LPS) 2 or 7 days (acute stimulus) prior to preterm delivery at 124 days of gestational age (dGA). LPS exposure occurred at two different time points, since historical data report increased inflammatory and injurious pattern, upon treatment at respectively, 2 and 7 days before preterm delivery in the preterm ovine lungs (16, 17).

MATERIALS AND METHODS
Study Approval
Animal experiments were approved by the animal ethics committee of the University of Western Australia (Perth, Australia).

Animal Experiments and Tissue Sampling

Procedures of the animal experiments and group allocations were published previously (10) and are presented in **Figure 1**. Study groups included 42 day exposure to UP (UP group), LPS exposure 2 or 7 days prior to preterm delivery (2d LPS, 7d LPS groups) and combined 42 days pre-exposure to UP and LPS exposure 2 or 7 days before preterm delivery at 125d GA (UP + 2d LPS, UP + 7d LPS groups). The 125d of GA in sheep correspond to the human gestation at ∼31 weeks representing a moderate preterm neonate with a developing lung at the interface of the canalicular and saccular phase (18, 19).

Briefly, ultrasound-guided intra-amniotic injections were used to administer live UP serovar 3 strain HPA5 (Concentration: 2×10^5 color-changing units CCU) and/or LPS (Concentration: 10 mg, *Escherichia coli* 055:B5; Sigma-Aldrich, St. Louis, MO) at pre-defined time points to 28 time-mated Merino ewes. Therefore, stock cultures of UP were diluted first in sterile culture medium and further in sterile saline (1:100). Sterile saline was also used for the dissolution of LPS and served as a comparable injection in control animals. After surgical delivery of the fetus, both, the ewe and the fetus were euthanized.

Pulmonary pressure volume assessment was conducted after euthanasia. Hereto, an endotracheal tube was introduced into the trachea and the thoracic cavity was opened to allow expansion of the lungs. The inflation of the lungs was achieved with air to a maximum pressure of 40 cm H_2O. Lung deflation volumes were recorded at decreasing pressures starting at 40 cm H_2O. Lung volumes were corrected for the body weight of the fetus (20).

Lung tissue sampling included inflation-fixation of the right upper lobe (RUL) for 24 h with 10% buffered formalin and snap freezing of the right lower lobe (RLL). The whole left lung was used to obtain bronchial lavage fluid.

Histology and Immunohistochemistry

RUL paraffin-embedded lung sections of 4 μm thickness were used for (immuno)histochemical analysis. Tissue sections were stained with hematoxylin and eosin (H&E) for histological evaluation. In addition, the following cellular markers were visualized: CD45 for hematopoietic cells (1:500, MCA2220GA, Biorad, Hercules, CA), PU.1 for differentiating monocytes (1:400, Santa Cruz Biotechnology, H0503), myeloperoxidase for neutrophils (MPO, 1:500, A-0398, Dako, Santa Clara, CA), tumor protein 63 for basal cells (P63, 1:8000, ab124762, Abcam), keratin 14 for differentiating basal cells (KRT-14, 1:1000, 905301, Biolegend, San Diego, CA), thyroid transcription factor-1 for Club and alveolar epithelial type (AEC) 2 cells (TTF-1, 1:8000, WRAB-1231, Seven Hills Bioreagents, Cincinnati, OH) and Ki67 for proliferation (1:1000, 15580, Abcam, Cambridge, UK) (7, 12, 16, 21). Immunohistochemical protocols were performed as previously published, while the PU.1 protocol was modified for optimal signal emission. Briefly, lung sections were deparaffinized in xylol and decreasing ethanol series. Blocking of endogenous peroxidase activity was achieved by incubating in 0.3% H_2O_2 in 1xPBS for 20 min. For antigen retrieval, lung sections were boiled 5 min in citrate buffer (pH 6.0). To prevent aspecific binding of antibodies, sections were incubated with 5% bovine serum albumin in 1xPBS for 30 min. The primary antibody, PU.1 in 0.1% BSA/1xPBS, was added and incubated over night at 4°C. Next, sections were incubated for 1 h with biotin-labeled secondary Swine-anti-Rabbit antibody (1:200, E0353, Dako) in 0.1% BSA/1xPBS. Vectastain ABC Elite kit (PK-6100, Bio-connect) was used for the enhancement of the anti-body specific signal for 30 min. Tissue visualization was performed with diaminobenzidine staining for 90 s, followed by a counterstaining with hematoxylin for 20 s. Sections were dehydrated and coverslipped.

Immunohistochemical Analyses

Methods for the analyses of immunohistochemical experiments have been published previously (7). Results for P63+, KRT-14+ and TTF-1+ cells were presented as cells per bronchus ring of

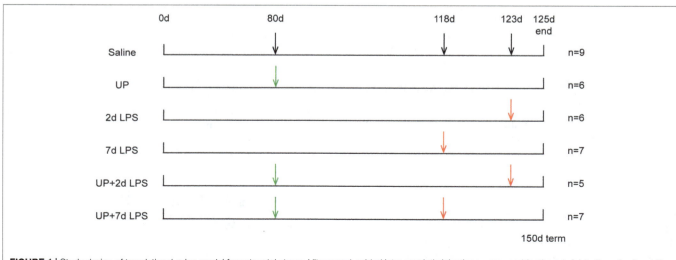

FIGURE 1 | Study design of translational ovine model for antenatal stress. Ultrasound-guided intra-amniotic injections were used for the administration of saline, UP and LPS. Lambs were delivered preterm at 125d GA (150d term).

proximal or distal airways, respectively. TTF-1+ and Ki67+ cells in alveoli were depicted as cells per high power field (HPF).

A magnification of 200x was used for PU.1 quantification and five randomly chosen pictures of alveoli (area of interest) were taken with a light microscope (Leica DM2000, Rijswijk, the Netherlands) and the Leica Application Suite 3.7.0 software (Leica Microsystem, Wetzlar, Germany). Alveolar region included the alveolar walls, alveolar airspaces and perivascular space. Analyses are presented as cells per HPF.

The wall-to-lumen ratio was determined on H&E sections, whereby vessels accompanying terminal bronchioles and an external diameter of <50 μm were investigated at a magnification of 400x. Five randomly chosen vessels were used and the wall-to-lumen ratio was calculated as media wall thickness divided by the radius of the vessel lumen (12).

Mean linear intercepts (MLI) and vessel density were also examined on H&E sections. Hereby, five and 10 images were taken randomly throughout the alveolar region, respectively for the MLI and the vessel quantification. In both cases bronchi and vessels (>50 μm external diameter) were excluded.

For the MLI assessment the ImageJ software (ImageJ 1.52i software, Bethesda, MD, USA) was used and images were superimposed with a 50 × 50 μm transparent grid. On five horizontal lines the intersections of the alveolar wall with the grid lines were counted. The MLI was determined according to the formula MLI = 2 × (L_{tot}/L_x), whereby, L_{tot} is the total length of all five lines and L_x is the total amount of intersections counted (22). Results are presented as micrometer of alveolar size.

With regard to the vessel quantification, all vessels, which were not accompanying a bronchus and had an external diameter <50 μm were counted (23). Surface area of alveolar tissue was determined with the Leica QWin Pro V3.5.1 software (Leica Microsystem) and results are displayed as vessels per square millimeter.

For all immunohistochemical stainings, as well as lung gas volumes, wall-to-lumen ratio, MLI and vessel quantification, the control values were presented as median and depicted as dotted line in all figures. Additionally, individual control values are provided in the **Supplementary Table 1**.

RNA Extraction and Real-Time PCR

Snap frozen RLL tissue was used for RNA isolation, transcribed and amplified for the following genes (12, 21, 24): interleukin (IL)−6, IL-8, SRY-related HMG-box (SOX)−2, SOX-9, surfactant proteins (SP) -A, -B, -C, -D, aquaporin (Aqp) 5, vascular endothelial growth factor (VEGF) -a, VEGF receptor (VEGFR)−2, Angiopoeitin (Ang)−1, tyrosine-protein kinase receptor (Tie)-2, ribosomal protein S15 (RPS15), Glyceraldehyde 3-phosphate dehydrogenase (GAPDH) and Human 14-3-3 protein zeta/delta (YWHAZ). Due to limited availability of lung tissue, mRNA analysis could not be performed for all animals (some experimental groups miss 1-2 animals). RT-PCR data were converted with the LinReg software and normalized to the Geomean of the housekeeping genes RPS15, GAPDH and YWHAZ. Mean fold changes were calculated with the saline control values set at one. For all RT-PCR results the control

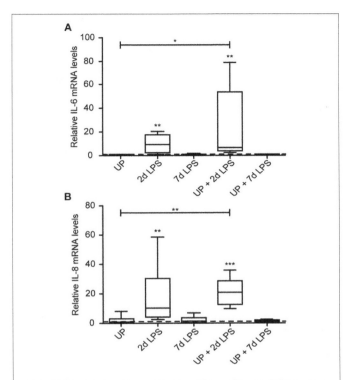

FIGURE 2 | Cytokine and chemokine expression are increased after exposure to 2d LPS and UP + 2d LPS in preterm ovine lung tissue. Fold changes in mRNA levels for IL-6 **(A)** and IL-8 **(B)** are depicted against saline. The median saline value is represented as dotted line. *$p < 0.05$, **$p < 0.01$, ***$p < 0.001$ compared to saline and UP.

values were presented as median and depicted as dotted line in all figures.

Statistical Analysis

A non-parametric analysis of variance (ANOVA) followed by the *post-hoc* analysis Dunn's Multiple Comparison Test and a significance threshold of $p < 0.05$ were used to determine the statistical significance of the results (17). Results are displayed as median and interquartile range (IQR). *P*-values between 0.05 and 0.1 were interpreted as biologically relevant, as described previously (17). Significant changes toward the control groups were presented with asterisks, while differences between the experimental groups were shown with bars and asterisks.

RESULTS

LPS Exposure Increases Pulmonary Inflammation, Which Is Not Further Modulated by Pre-exposure to UP

Single exposure to LPS resulted in increased immune activation when compared to control lambs, which was most pronounced in the 2d LPS-exposed lambs (**Figure 2**). In UP-exposed lambs, signs of increased inflammation were restricted to increased neutrophil infiltration. UP exposure prior to LPS exposure did not affect the observed increased expression of IL-6 and IL-8 after treatment with LPS alone.

With regard to immune cell infiltration, the increased number of CD45+ immune cells reported in 2d LPS-exposed animals (**Figure 3A**), was also not affected by prior exposure to UP. Further, single and sequential inflammatory insults did not change the numbers of differentiating macrophages in the pulmonary tissue (**Figure 3B**). In addition, pre-exposure to UP did not significantly affect the increased number of neutrophils observed in the 2d LPS groups (**Figure 3C**). However, UP + 7d LPS showed that neutrophil numbers were attenuated to values similar to baseline levels (**Figures 3D–F**).

Pre-exposure to UP Normalizes SOX-9 Expression, but Does Not Impact Stem/Progenitor Cell Responses, After an Initial Insult With LPS

Reduced numbers of endogenous stem/progenitor cell populations of the proximal airways have been reported after intra-amniotic exposure to LPS (7). Here, after sequential insults with UP and LPS no further reduction in P63+ and KRT-14+ cell numbers, as well as SOX-2 mRNA levels, were observed (**Figure 4**).

In distal airways, UP and 7d LPS exposure alone decreased SOX-9 mRNA significantly (**Figure 5A**), while pre-exposure to UP in 7d LPS-exposed animals prevented a decrease in SOX-9 mRNA levels by a 3-fold increase in its expression. Club cell numbers were decreased in UP, 2d and 7d LPS groups, as well as in the UP + 2d LPS and UP + 7d LPS animals (**Figures 5B,D–F**). The number of AEC2 was significantly decreased in UP-infected animals, as well as in UP + 2d LPS and UP + 7d LPS animals compared to control (**Figures 5C,G–I**). Sequential exposure to UP and LPS did not further affect Club cells. In contrast, the most significant reduction in AEC2 numbers was observed in UP + 7d LPS-exposed animals.

Prenatal Inflammation Affects Vascular Growth and Angiogenesis After Single Insults and UP Pre-exposure Sensitizes Vascular Disturbances to a Second Inflammatory Insult, Resulting in a Lower Vascular Density

Vascular remodeling is a common hallmark of BPD and has been found in models of pre- and postnatal inflammation. Here we assessed if single as well as sequential exposure induce vascular changes in preterm ovine lungs.

Vascular development and angiogenesis were influenced by prenatal inflammation as evidenced by a significant drop in mRNA levels of VEGFa after single exposure to UP or LPS (**Figure 6A**). Pre-exposure to UP similarly decreased mRNA levels of VEGFa in the UP + 2d LPS group, whereas the mRNA levels were normalized to control in the combined UP + 7d LPS group. VEGFR-2 mRNA levels were significantly reduced in 7d LPS and UP + 7d LPS-exposed animals (**Figure 6B**).

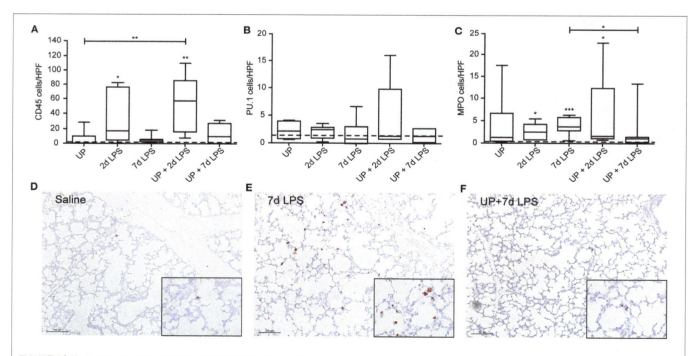

FIGURE 3 | Single and sequential exposure induce immune cell infiltrations in the lung tissue, whereas neutrophil numbers are attenuated after UP + 7d LPS exposure. CD45+ immune cells **(A)**, PU.1+ macrophages **(B)** and MPO+ neutrophils **(C)** were quantified in alveoli and are presented as cells per HPF. The median saline value is represented as dotted line. Representative images are shown for MPO in saline **(D)**, 7d LPS **(E)** and UP + 7d LPS **(F)** groups. Image magnification is 200x, scale bar 100 μm. *$p < 0.05$, **$p < 0.01$, ***$p < 0.001$ compared to saline, UP and 7d LPS.

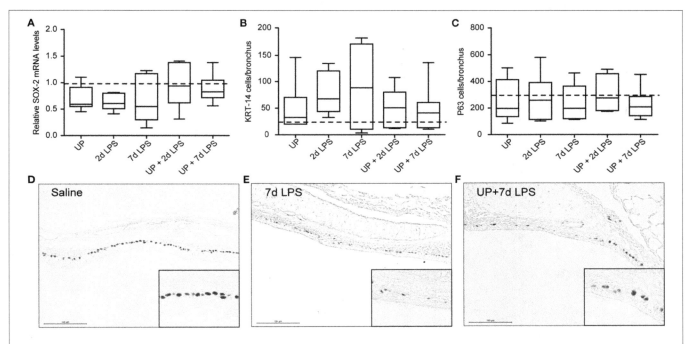

FIGURE 4 | No further changes are observed in basal cells of the proximal airways after single and sequential antenatal inflammation. (A) SOX-2 fold changes in mRNA levels are depicted against saline. P63+ (C) and KRT-14+ (B) basal cells were quantified in proximal airways and are presented as cells per bronchus. The median saline value is represented as dotted line. Representative images are shown for P63 in saline (D), 7d LPS (E) and UP + 7d LPS (F) groups. Image magnification is 200x, scale bar 100 μm.

Although mRNA levels of VEGFR-2 were unaffected in the 2d LPS group, they were significantly lower in the UP + 2d LPS group compared to control, UP and 2d LPS-exposed animals. Ang-1 mRNA levels were not changed by single exposure to chronic or acute triggers, but showed a significant drop in both sequential exposure groups (**Figure 6C**). Tie-2 mRNA levels were increased in UP and 7d LPS groups and were unaffected after sequential exposure (**Figure 6D**).

These changes on mRNA level of the studied vascular and angiogenic markers prompted us to determine vessel density in the alveolar walls. While UP exposure alone did not alter the density of vessels, 2d LPS exposure decreased the number of vessels significantly by half compared to the control (**Figure 6E**). Pre-exposure to UP before (2 and 7d) LPS attenuated the vascular density even more prominently than LPS exposure alone.

Although changes in vascular and angiogenic markers were detected and the density of vessel reduced after prenatal inflammation, no alterations were measured in the wall-to-lumen ratio of the vessels by single or sequential inflammatory insults (**Figure 6F**).

Developmental Alterations Found in Alveoli Are Most Prominent in UP + 7d LPS Exposed Lambs

Given the AEC2 alterations, we further assessed the alveolar development after sequential antenatal inflammation in terms of proliferation (Ki67) and differentiation (Aqp5) in the alveolar walls (**Figure 7**).

7d LPS and UP + 7d LPS exposure resulted in a significant drop to half of the amount of proliferating cells compared to the control group (**Figure 7A**). AEC1 were significantly decreased by half in the UP + 2d LPS group compared to control levels (**Figure 7B**). Additionally, while 7d LPS exposure decreased Aqp5 mRNA levels, sequential exposure did not result in a significant drop. With regard to the MLI, UP, and LPS exposure alone did not impact alveolar growth, whereas the exposure to UP followed by LPS 7 days before delivery increased the MLI. This result is consistent with the more significant decreased proliferation in the UP + 7d LPS group and the lower number of AEC2 in the same group when compared to single exposure with LPS (**Figure 7C**).

Sequential Exposure to UP and LPS Has Additional Impact on mRNA Levels of Surfactant Proteins Compared to Single Inflammatory Insults, but Does Not Affect Lung Mechanics

As stem/progenitor cell numbers dropped in the distal lung compartments and sensitization of vascular signaling was observed, we further assessed the effects of sequential antenatal insults on functional parameters, including surfactant synthesis and lung mechanics (static lung compliance).

While chronic UP exposure did not alter surfactant mRNA levels, we did see that 2d, 7d LPS groups, as well as pre-exposure with UP + 2d and +7d LPS caused an increase in

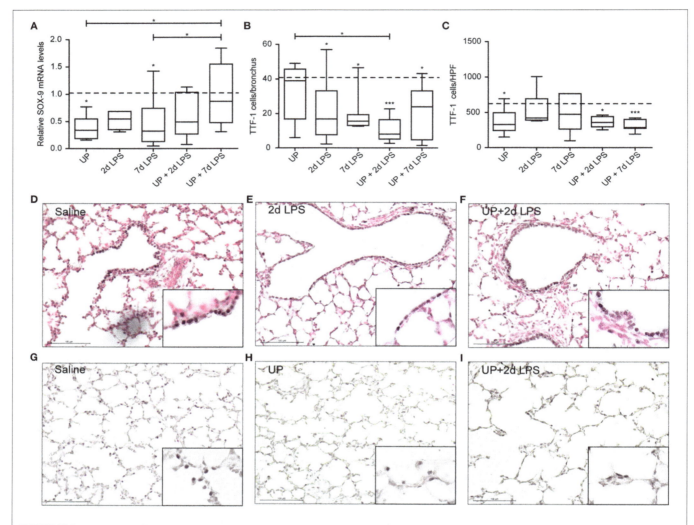

FIGURE 5 | Pre-exposure to UP before the 7d LPS exposure normalizes SOX-9 expression but does not further impact stem/progenitor populations of the distal lung. (A) SOX-9 fold changes in mRNA levels are depicted against saline. TTF1+ (B) Club cells were quantified in distal airways and presented as cells per bronchus, while TTF-1+ (C) AEC2 were counted in alveoli and are presented as cells per HPF. The median saline value is represented as dotted line. Representative images are shown for Club cells in saline (D), 2d LPS (E) and UP + 2d LPS (F) groups, and for AEC2 in saline (G), UP (H) and UP+2d LPS (I) animals. Image magnification is 200x, scale bar 100 μm. *$p < 0.05$, ***$p < 0.001$ compared to saline, UP and 7d LPS.

mRNA levels of SP-A compared to controls and UP exposure (**Figure 8A**). UP pre-exposure pre-conditioned to 2d and 7d LPS exposure and thereby significantly increased mRNA levels of SP-B, whereas UP, 2d or 7d LPS groups did not result in mRNA changes (**Figure 8B**).

mRNA levels of SP-C were significantly increased in UP + 7d LPS groups, as were mRNA levels for single 7d LPS exposure (**Figure 8C**).

UP + 2d LPS exposure increased mRNA levels for SP-D compared to control and UP alone (**Figure 8D**). In contrast, UP + 7d LPS groups showed normalized SP-D mRNA levels compared to 7d LPS exposure alone.

Lung gas volumes were significantly increased at applied pressures of 0 cmH$_2$O (data not shown) and 40 cmH$_2$O in 7d LPS (10-fold) and UP + 7d LPS groups (4-fold) (**Figure 8E**). UP + 2d LPS exposure resulted in significantly lower lung gas volumes compared to UP alone.

DISCUSSION

There is increasing evidence that structural and functional abnormalities of the developing lungs that are provoked during pregnancy by inflammatory triggers, can contribute to postnatal lung pathology (25, 26). However, the mechanisms underlying these antenatal alterations remain largely unknown.

As an essential driver of lung development, endogenous epithelial stem/progenitor cells might play a role in prenatal maldevelopment of the lungs following inflammatory stressors (15, 27). Previously, we demonstrated fewer endogenous stem/progenitor populations as well as potential consequences

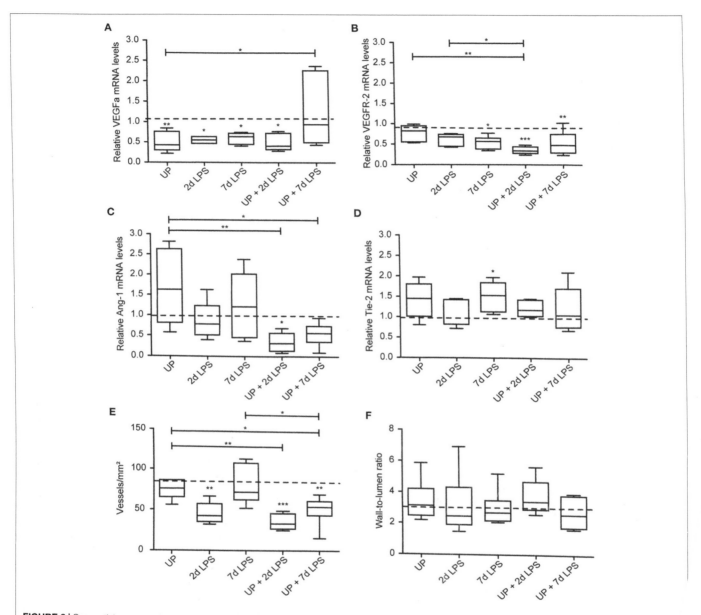

FIGURE 6 | Sequential exposure to UP sensitizes vascular marker VEGFR-2 and Ang-1 to secondary LPS exposure and reduces the vascular density in alveolar tissue. VEGFa (A), VEGFR-2 (B), Ang-1 (C) and Tie-2 (D) fold changes in mRNA levels are depicted against saline. (E) Vascular quantification (for vessels <50 μm diameter) was performed and corrected for surface area of alveolar tissue. (F) Wall-to-lumen ratio was measured and calculated from small vessels (<50 μm diameter). The median saline value is represented as dotted line. $*p < 0.05$, $**p < 0.01$, $***p < 0.001$ compared to saline, UP and 2d LPS.

thereof, including reduced alveolar differentiation, in the course of antenatal inflammation. Importantly, distinct stem cell changes in fetal ovine lungs were influenced by the timing and duration of a single chronic or acute inflammatory insult (7).

Clinically, perinatal organ development is frequently affected by multiple and repetitive inflammatory triggers, including infections, hypoxia, sepsis and mechanical ventilation, with serious consequences for the fetus/neonate. Clinical and preclinical studies have associated prenatal polymicrobial infections with a diversity of clinical outcomes (28, 29). This diversity in outcomes is difficult to estimate and therefore treatment of preterm infants might start too late to avoid se postnatal problems. Apart from the microorganisms inv investigating the effect of multiple inflammatory events pregnancy is of great importance to understand their infl and impact on prenatal lung development. Prenatal inf but also different maternal stressors and the event of b inevitable incidences that induce inflammation and that consequently has to cope with (30).

A prerequisite of studying multiple stressors is determine the effects of the single components, whicl reported recently (7). In the current study, we ext

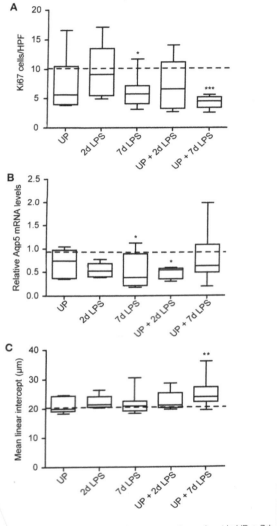

Developmental alveolar alterations are most prominent in UP + 7d lambs. (A) Ki67+ cells were quantified in alveoli and shown as 'B) Aqp5 fold changes in mRNA levels are depicted against LI was determined in alveolar tissue and represents the crometer. The median saline value is represented as dotted < 0.01, ***p < 0.001 compared to saline.

investigating the effect of multiple sequential development processes in the preterm lungs the clinical relevance of this pre-clinical additionally examined consequences of nmatory events with respect to alveolar ry vascular development in relation to l populations, mediators of vascular gical changes.
the strongest reduction of AEC2 +) was detected in lambs that UP and 7d LPS. In line with veolar growth was exclusively indicated by increased MLI. ure to inflammatory stimuli

did not result in significant morphological abnormalities, it negatively impacted epithelial stem/progenitor cell populations. These combined findings indicate that single inflammatory hits already negatively affect epithelial stem/progenitor cell populations including their function and numbers, a process that can be further aggravated when sequential inflammatory hits exert their negative effects synergistically. In this study, SOX-9 expression levels in the different experimental groups are of particular interest. SOX-9 expression is restricted to progenitor cells and disappears after proliferation and differentiation into different AEC2 subtypes (31, 32). The acquired single hit exposure data, which showed a reduction of SOX-9 expression in both the UP and LPS group, might potentially be responsible for reduced proliferation and reduced number of TTF-1+ AEC2 in developing alveoli. Of interest, consecutive hits with UP and (7d) LPS prevented a decrease in SOX-9 mRNA, while it caused the most pronounced reduction of TTF-1+ AEC2 and the number of proliferating cells, which was accompanied by an increased MLI. This finding potentially reflects a compensatory function for SOX-9 expression to counteract the reduced number of AEC2 with the pre-exposure to UP. It might be a timing effect that this compensatory function of SOX-9 did not initiate sufficient proliferation and differentiation yet to reverse the reduced number of AEC2. Such protective effects of SOX-9 have previously been observed in an acute lung injury (ALI) model, where SOX-9 was activated in the post-ALI phase and assumed to promote recovery of the damaged lungs (33). This scenario is currently investigated in ongoing postnatal studies. On the other hand, there are multiple transcription factors and developmental pathways involved in the complex process of distal lung development, which themselves potentially attenuated proliferation and growth of alveoli (34, 35). In this study, we also examined the pulmonary vasculature, due to its increasing importance in the development of BPD (36). Sequential inflammatory exposures negatively affected the growth and expansion of pulmonary vessels indicating that UP exposure primarily sensitizes animals that were subsequently exposed to 2d LPS. Consistent with this morphological observation, the pro-angiogenic and vascular factors, Ang-1 and VEGFR-2, were reduced by single inflammatory triggers and pre-exposure to UP sensitized these markers to a secondary insult with LPS. Moreover, VEGFa was decreased in all treatment groups, including this UP + 2d LPS group, which is further indicative for impaired vascularization. These current vascular changes after antenatal stress confirm and extend findings in a previous sequential hit study that was conducted at an earlier gestational age (94d GA in lambs, corresponding to extreme preterm infants in the canalicular stage of lung development) (12). These vascular disturbances, comprising decreased VEGFR-2 and Ang-1 mRNA levels after sequential exposure, seemed not affected by the GA of the fetuses, as comparable results were found in 94d and 125d GA fetuses. In addition, in both studies these disturbances were not associated with vascular remodeling in the preterm lungs (7, 12). Clinically, reduced and dysmorphic capillary networks have been reported in various BPD cohorts (37). Combined, the antenatal angiogenic data point toward a disturbed capillary network, which might be at the origin of postnatal

Sequential Exposure to Antenatal Microbial Triggers Attenuates Alveolar Growth and Pulmonary Vascular... 81

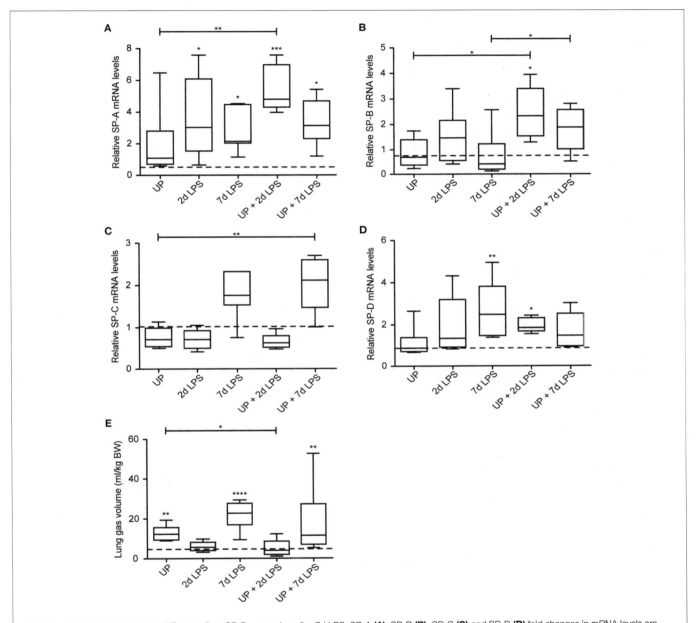

FIGURE 8 | Sequential exposure to UP normalizes SP-B expression after 7d LPS. SP-A (A), SP-B (B), SP-C (C) and SP-D (D) fold changes in mRNA levels are depicted against saline. (E) Lung gas volumes of a pressure of 40 cm H_2O are corrected for the bodyweight of the fetus and shown as ml/kg. The median saline value is represented as dotted line. *$p < 0.05$, **$p < 0.01$, ***$p < 0.001$, ****$p < 0.0001$ compared to saline, UP and 7d LPS.

adverse vascular development, an aspect that warrants further investigation (36).

In contrast to the attenuated alveolar growth and reduced vasculature, we observed a protective effect of sequential exposure with regard to surfactant synthesis, in particular SP-A and SP-B. Hereby increased SP-A and SP-B expression was found in UP + 2d LPS and UP + 7d LPS exposed animals, respectively, changes that were not as prominent in animals exposed to a single inflammatory trigger.

Our findings on SP-B expression are largely recapitulated by the observed inflammatory changes; Significant inflammatory changes were restricted to the number of neutrophils, which were attenuated in the 7d LPS group when they were pre-exposed to UP. It is tempting to speculate that this immune modulatory effect of UP, which has been described earlier by Kallapur et al. (13), might be involved in the protective effects on SP-B.

The essential role of SP-B in the survival of preterm infants at birth has been emphasized by various clinical studies (38). Chang et al. showed that a deficiency in SP-B through gene polymorphisms increased the risk to develop severe/lethal respiratory distress in preterm neonates (39, 40). Additionally, 75% of preterm infants with need for ventilation have been shown to have surfactant deficiencies in tracheal aspirates with 80% reduction in SP-B (41, 42). This key role of SP-B is attributed to its important function in the stabilization of the monolayer lipid films of surfactant, as well as in the absorption of lipids to the air/liquid interface (43, 44). Therefore, the increased SP-B mRNA levels, found after sequential insults with UP and LPS, might be an attempt to counteract the inflammation-driven changes, including decreased AEC2 numbers.

Besides this potentially protective effect of SP-B, also the increased expression of SP-A in UP pre-exposed animals (prior to 2d LPS) might indicate a beneficial effect. In the clinical situation and pre-clinical models, a deficiency in SP-A has been associated with an increased risk of BPD development in preterm neonates (24–29 week of GA) and immature baboons that received ventilation (45, 46). Additionally a reduced amount of SP-A mRNA has been reported in premature baboons with a BPD phenotype (47). These findings reveal a strong association between reduced SP-A proteins and BPD development. Through its important role in lung host defense, SP-A has been shown in vitro to promote increased ureaplasmacidal phagocytosis of UP isolates (from the BAL of premature infants with BPD) by murine macrophages (RAW 264.7) (48). Moreover, in in vivo studies, SP-A deficient mouse strains have been shown to display more excessive pulmonary inflammation after intra-tracheal UP administration compared to wild type controls. In these deficient SP-A mice also the clearance of UP occurred at a later time point (49). Taken together, the increased expression of SP-A after sequential exposure of UP and LPS could be interpreted as a means to eliminate UP from the preterm lungs.

Interestingly, these combined changes of increased SP-B and SP-A expression that suggest a protective effect by prior UP infection, did not overlap with improved lung function that was found to be significant in UP, 7d LPS, and UP + 7d LPS-exposed lambs. Moreover, this improved lung function was paralleled at the studied time points by detrimental alterations of stem/progenitor cells. This apparent lack of uniformity might be caused by a timing effect, but it most likely provides supporting evidence for the concept that perinatal inflammation improves lung function at the expense of inducing peripheral lung abnormalities, including decreased number of large and simplified alveoli, and abnormal pulmonary vascular development, predisposing to adverse postnatal pulmonary outcomes.

Besides the effects of consecutive inflammatory insults on lung development, also other immature organ systems are affected. The impact of multiple insults has been investigated in the preterm brain and gastrointestinal system. In particular, inflammation in the brain was less pronounced in LPS-exposed lambs when they were pre-exposed to UP. Additionally, the protective effect of UP was associated with reduced epigenetic changes (10). Sequential exposure of UP and LPS in utero did not amplify injury in the gastrointestinal and the enteric nervous system, that was caused by single exposure to UP or LPS (11). Taken together, these studies reflect the diversity in organ responses and outcomes after exposure to different infectious triggers (50). Additionally, also timing and duration of antenatal inflammatory triggers play a crucial role in the susceptibility of other organs and cells. Close monitoring of antenatal infection and inflammation is necessary for optimal risk classification of postnatal organ outcomes (10).

Regardless, these observed in utero alterations in essential cell populations, developmental factors and pulmonary morphology might render the preterm lungs more susceptible to sequential postnatal insults. Previously, it was shown that postnatal hits, including mechanical ventilation and oxygen supplementation, resulted in a decreased differentiation and proliferation potential in isolated lung endogenous stem cells (51). Postnatal cohort studies, using BPD and RDS samples, have also shown that preterm birth combined with common clinical practices, like oxygen supplementation and ventilation, resulted in decreased AEC2 and Club cell numbers, positive for TTF-1 (52, 53). Similarly, vascular abnormalities are a key hallmark of BPD and have been shown to be driven by perinatal insults (14, 36, 37). In a hyperoxia-induced BPD rat model, a lower capillary density was associated with reduced expression of VEGF and VEGFR-2 (54). Reduced and disorganized capillary development has further been reported in baboon models for BPD after interventional series of ventilation and supplemental oxygen (55).

The ovine pre-clinical model, which resembles the human in utero situation very closely, enables investigation of developmental disturbances in a prenatal inflammatory setting. The relatively long gestation of sheep, in which developmental stages occur similar as in humans, enables the precise interference in these stages (18, 19). In addition, microbial exposure can be exactly timed and thereby clinical inflammatory settings (chronic and acute) can be mimicked accurately. Another benefit of this study was the use of clinically relevant microorganisms, such as UP. Although LPS is not a living microorganism and specific microorganism-related responses might be missed, this Escherichia coli-derived endotoxin is a potent inducer of inflammation and therefore used to mimic clinical situations of acute inflammation. LPS responses are well-defined and accordingly less heterogenicity in responses is detected (56, 57).

Besides the advantages of the model and study, there are also some limitations. In the current study epithelial stem/progenitor populations have been investigated with the use of basic stem cells markers (P63, KRT-14, and TTF-1). However, the observed disturbances might be unique and restricted to a specific subpopulation. Additional examination with more extended techniques, such as cell sorting by FACS and single cell sequencing, would be informative to better define and understand the response of such subpopulations of stem/progenitor cells in the context of prenatal inflammation. Furthermore, considering the observed disturbances in vascular modulators, future investigations should include examination of endothelial stem/progenitor cell alterations. Moreover, fixed time points of intra-amniotic exposure to Ureaplasma or LPS were used, which did not enable us to dissect the effects of prenatal inflammation on extremely, moderate and late preterm organs. Importantly, the postnatal consequences of the observed in utero stem/progenitor cell changes are currently addressed in a postnatal follow up study.

Consistent with previous findings from our group and others, endogenous epithelial stem/progenitor cell populations are attenuated by perinatal inflammatory triggers (7, 58). Additionally, single inflammatory hits during pregnancy are also known to impair vascular growth (59). In the current study, we extended these findings by investigating the effects of sequential antenatal insults on alveolar growth and vascular maturation. We showed that exposure to a single inflammatory trigger already negatively impacts epithelial stem/progenitor cell populations including their function and numbers. This process was further aggravated by re-exposure to an inflammatory stimulus, resulting in disturbed alveolarization and abnormal pulmonary vascular development. The question whether these negative effects on lung development can be rescued by the potentially protective responses observed, will be addressed in an ongoing postnatal study.

Collectively, our data indicate that the type, timing and duration of antenatal stress determine the pulmonary outcome during pregnancy in the context of antenatal infections. Importantly, responses within the lungs can vary between lung compartment and cell types. Unraveling and linking the impact of antenatal and postnatal insults on the preterm lungs is of great importance to expand our understanding of the complex and multifactorial nature of BPD.

AUTHOR CONTRIBUTIONS

HW, NR, and TW conceived and designed the research questions. MK, JN, MS, HU, MP, AJ, and BK designed and performed the *in vivo* study. HW conducted experiments, acquired and analyzed data. HW, NR, BK, TD, and TW contributed to the interpretation of results and drafted the manuscript. HW, NR, DO, MH, PN, CS-R, BK, TD, and TW edited and revised the manuscript. HW, NR, DO, MH, PN, CS-R, JC, MK, JN, MS, HU, MP, AJ, BK, TD, and TW read and approved final version of manuscript. All authors contributed to the article and approved the submitted version.

ACKNOWLEDGMENTS

We thank Nico Kloosterboer, Lilian Kessels, Kimberly Massy a Anaïs van Leeuwen for their excellent technical assistance.

REFERENCES

1. Malleske DT, Chorna O, Maitre NL. Pulmonary sequelae and functional limitations in children and adults with bronchopulmonary dysplasia. *Paediatr Respir Rev.* (2018) 26:55–9. doi: 10.1016/j.prrv.2017.07.002
2. Kallapur SG, Jobe AH. Perinatal events and their influence on lung development and injury. In: *The Newborn Lung.* Elsevier (2019). p. 31–64. doi: 10.1016/B978-0-323-54605-8.00002-7
3. Jobe AH. The new bronchopulmonary dysplasia. *Curr Opin Pediatr.* (2011) 23:167–72. doi: 10.1097/MOP.0b013e3283423e6b
4. Yee M, Domm W, Gelein R, Bentley KL, Kottmann RM, Sime PJ, et al. Alternative progenitor lineages regenerate the adult lung depleted of alveolar epithelial type 2 cells. *Am J Respir Cell Mol Biol.* (2017) 56:453–64. doi: 10.1165/rcmb.2016-0150OC
5. Mandell EW, Abman SH. Fetal vascular origins of bronchopulmonary dysplasia. *J Pediatr.* (2017) 185:7–10 e11. doi: 10.1016/j.jpeds.2017.03.024
6. Taglauer E, Abman SH, Keller RL. Recent advances in antenatal factors predisposing to bronchopulmonary dysplasia. *Semin Perinatol.* (2018) 42:413–24. doi: 10.1053/j.semperi.2018.09.002
7. Widowski H, Ophelders D, van Leeuwen A, Nikkels PGJ, Severens-Rijvers CAH, LaPointe VLS, et al. Chorioamnionitis induces changes in ovine pulmonary endogenous epithelial stem/progenitor cells in utero. *Pediatr Res.* (2020) 1–11. doi: 10.1038/s41390-020-01204-9
8. Yoon BH, Romero R, Lim JH, Shim SS, Hong JS, Shim JY, et al. The clinical significance of detecting Ureaplasma urealyticum by the polymerase chain reaction in the amniotic fluid of patients with preterm labor. *Am J Obstet Gynecol.* (2003) 189:919–24. doi: 10.1067/S0002-9378(03)00839-1
9. Kallapur SG, Presicce P, Rueda CM, Jobe AH, Chougnet CA. Fetal immune response to chorioamnionitis. *Semin Reprod Med.* (2014) 32:56–67. doi: 10.1055/s-0033-1361823
10. Gussenhoven R, Ophelders D, Kemp MW, Payne MS, Spiller OB, Beeton ML, et al. The paradoxical effects of chronic intra-amniotic *Ureaplasma parvum* exposure on ovine fetal brain development. *Dev Neurosci.* (2017) 39:472–86. doi: 10.1159/000479021
11. Heymans C, de Lange IH, Hutten MC, Lenaerts K, de Ruijter NJE, Kessels L, et al. Chronic intra-uterine *Ureaplasma parvum* infection induces injury of the enteric nervous system in ovine fetuses. *Front Immunol.* (2020) 11:189. doi: 10.3389/fimmu.2020.00189
12. Willems MG, Kemp MW, Fast LA, Wagemaker NM, Janssen LE, Newnham JP, et al. Pulmonary vascular changes in extremely preterm sheep after intra-amniotic exposure to *Ureaplasma parvum* and lipopolysaccharide. *PLoS ONE.* (2017) 12:e0180114. doi: 10.1371/journal.pone.0180114
13. Kallapur SG, Kramer BW, Knox CL, Berry CA, Collins JJ, Kemp MW, et al. Chronic fetal exposure to *Ureaplasma parvum* suppresses innate immune responses in sheep. *J Immunol.* (2011) 187:2688–95. doi: 10.4049/jimmunol.1100779
14. Alvira CM. Aberrant pulmonary vascular growth and remodeling in bronchopulmonary dysplasia. *Front Med (Lausanne).* (2016) 3:21. doi: 10.3389/fmed.2016.00021
15. Collins JJ, Thébaud BJBDRPAC, Teratology M. Progenitor cells of the distal lung and their potential role in neonatal lung disease. *Birth Defects Res A Clin Mol Teratol.* (2014) 100:217–26. doi: 10.1002/bdra.23227
16. Collins JJ, Kuypers E, Nitsos I, Jane Pillow J, Polglase GR, Kemp MW, et al. LPS-induced chorioamnionitis and antenatal corticosteroids modulate Shh signaling in the ovine fetal lung. *Am J Physiol Lung Cell Mol Physiol.* (2012) 303:L778–87. doi: 10.1152/ajplung.00280.2011
17. Willems MG, Ophelders DR, Nikiforou M, Jellema RK, Butz A, Delhaas T, et al. Systemic interleukin-2 administration improves lung function and modulates chorioamnionitis-induced pulmonary inflammation in the ovine fetus. *Am J Physiol Lung Cell Mol Physiol.* (2016) 310:L1–7. doi: 10.1152/ajplung.00289.2015
18. Pringle KC. Human fetal lung development and related animal models. *Clin Obstet Gynecol.* (1986) 29:502–13. doi: 10.1097/00003081-198609000-00006
19. Kramer BW. Chorioamnionitis - new ideas from experimental models. *Neonatology.* (2011) 99:320–5. doi: 10.1159/000326620
20. Jobe AH, Newnham JP, Willet KE, Moss TJ, Gore Ervin M, Padbury JF, et al. Endotoxin-induced lung maturation in preterm lambs is not mediated by cortisol. *Am J Respir Crit Care Med.* (2000) 162:1656–61. doi: 10.1164/ajrccm.162.5.2003044

21. Kuypers E, Collins JJ, Kramer BW, Ofman G, Nitsos I, Pillow JJ, et al. Intra-amniotic LPS and antenatal betamethasone: inflammation and maturation in preterm lamb lungs. *Am J Physiol Lung Cell Mol Physiol.* (2012) 302:L380–9. doi: 10.1152/ajplung.00338.2011

22. Tschanz SA, Makanya AN, Haenni B, Burri PH. Effects of neonatal high-dose short-term glucocorticoid treatment on the lung: a morphologic and morphometric study in the rat. *Pediatr Res.* (2003) 53:72–80. doi: 10.1203/00006450-200301000-00014

23. Moreira A, Winter C, Joy J, Winter L, Jones M, Noronha M, et al. Intranasal delivery of human umbilical cord Wharton's jelly mesenchymal stromal cells restores lung alveolarization and vascularization in experimental bronchopulmonary dysplasia. *Stem Cells Transl Med.* (2020) 9:221–34. doi: 10.1002/sctm.18-0273

24. Atik A, Sozo F, Orgeig S, Suri L, Hanita T, Harding R, et al. Long-term pulmonary effects of intrauterine exposure to endotoxin following preterm birth in sheep. *Reprod Sci.* (2012) 19:1352–64. doi: 10.1177/1933719112450327

25. Gras-Le Guen C, Denis C, Franco-Montoya M-L, Jarry A, Delacourt C, Potel G, et al. Antenatal infection in the rabbit impairs post-natal growth and lung alveolarisation. *Eur Respir J.* (2008) 32:1520–8. doi: 10.1183/09031936.00023708

26. Kramer BW, Kallapur S, Newnham J, Jobe AH. Prenatal inflammation and lung development. *Semin Fetal Neonatal Med.* (2009) 14:2–7. doi: 10.1016/j.siny.2008.08.011

27. Leibel S, Post M. Endogenous and exogenous stem/progenitor cells in the lung and their role in the pathogenesis and treatment of pediatric lung disease. *Front Pediatr.* (2016) 4:36. doi: 10.3389/fped.2016.00036

28. Pammi M, Zhong D, Johnson Y, Revell P, Versalovic J. Polymicrobial bloodstream infections in the neonatal intensive care unit are associated with increased mortality: a case-control study. *BMC Infect Dis.* (2014) 14:390. doi: 10.1186/1471-2334-14-390

29. Yoneda N, Yoneda S, Niimi H, Ueno T, Hayashi S, Ito M, et al. Polymicrobial amniotic fluid infection with mycoplasma/ureaplasma and other bacteria induces severe intra-amniotic inflammation associated with poor perinatal prognosis in preterm labor. *Am J Reprod Immunol.* (2016) 75:112–25. doi: 10.1111/aji.12456

30. Mulder EJ, Robles de Medina PG, Huizink AC, Van den Bergh BR, Buitelaar JK, Visser GH. Prenatal maternal stress: effects on pregnancy and the (unborn) child. *Early Hum Dev.* (2002) 70:3–14. doi: 10.1016/S0378-3782(02)00075-0

31. Herriges M, Morrisey EE. Lung development: orchestrating the generation and regeneration of a complex organ. *Development.* (2014) 141:502–13. doi: 10.1242/dev.098186

32. Frank DB, Penkala IJ, Zepp JA, Sivakumar A, Linares-Saldana R, Zacharias WJ, et al. Early lineage specification defines alveolar epithelial ontogeny in the murine lung. *Proc Natl Acad Sci U S A.* (2019) 116:4362–71. doi: 10.1073/pnas.1813952116

33. Li L, Zhang H, Min D, Zhang R, Wu J, Qu H, et al. Sox9 activation is essential for the recovery of lung function after acute lung injury. *Cell Physiol Biochem.* (2015) 37:1113–22. doi: 10.1159/000430236

34. Okubo T, Knoepfler PS, Eisenman RN, Hogan BL. Nmyc plays an essential role during lung development as a dosage-sensitive regulator of progenitor cell proliferation and differentiation. *Development.* (2005) 132:1363–74. doi: 10.1242/dev.01678

35. Rawlins EL, Clark CP, Xue Y, Hogan BL. The Id2+ distal tip lung epithelium contains individual multipotent embryonic progenitor cells. *Development.* (2009) 136:3741–5. doi: 10.1242/dev.037317

36. Thebaud B, Abman SH. Bronchopulmonary dysplasia: where have all the vessels gone? Roles of angiogenic growth factors in chronic lung disease. *Am J Respir Crit Care Med.* (2007) 175:978–85. doi: 10.1164/rccm.200611-1660PP

37. Bhatt AJ, Pryhuber GS, Huyck H, Watkins RH, Metlay LA, Maniscalco WM. Disrupted pulmonary vasculature and decreased vascular endothelial growth factor, Flt-1, and TIE-2 in human infants dying with bronchopulmonary dysplasia. *Am J Respir Crit Care Med.* (2001) 164:1971–80. doi: 10.1164/ajrccm.164.10.2101140

38. Fehrholz M, Hutten M, Kramer BW, Speer CP, Kunzmann S. Amplification of steroid-mediated SP-B expression by physiological levels of caffeine. *Am J Physiol Lung Cell Mol Physiol.* (2014) 306:L101–9. doi: 10.1152/ajplung.00257.2013

39. Nogee LM, Garnier G, Dietz HC, Singer L, Murphy AM, deMello DE, et al. A mutation in the surfactant protein B gene responsible for fatal neonatal respiratory disease in multiple kindreds. *J Clin Invest.* (1994) 93:1860–3. doi: 10.1172/JCI117173

40. Chang HY, Li F, Li FS, Zheng CZ, Lei YZ, Wang J. Genetic polymorphisms of SP-A, SP-B, and SP-D and risk of respiratory distress syndrome in preterm neonates. *Med Sci Monit.* (2016) 22:5091–100. doi: 10.12659/MSM.898553

41. Merrill JD, Ballard RA, Cnaan A, Hibbs AM, Godinez RI, Godinez MH, et al. Dysfunction of pulmonary surfactant in chronically ventilated premature infants. *Pediatr Res.* (2004) 56:918–26. doi: 10.1203/01.PDR.0000145565.45490.D9

42. Ballard PL, Keller RL, Truog WE, Chapin C, Horneman H, Segal MR, et al. Surfactant status and respiratory outcome in premature infants receiving late surfactant treatment. *Pediatr Res.* (2019) 85:305–11. doi: 10.1038/s41390-018-0144-3

43. Veldhuizen EJ, Haagsman HP. Role of pulmonary surfactant components in surface film formation and dynamics. *Biochim Biophys Acta.* (2000) 1467:255–70. doi: 10.1016/S0005-2736(00)00256-X

44. Nkadi PO, Merritt TA, Pillers DA. An overview of pulmonary surfactant in the neonate: genetics, metabolism, and the role of surfactant in health and disease. *Mol Genet Metab.* (2009) 97:95–101. doi: 10.1016/j.ymgme.2009.01.015

45. Hallman M, Merritt TA, Akino T, Bry K. Surfactant protein A, phosphatidylcholine, and surfactant inhibitors in epithelial lining fluid. Correlation with surface activity, severity of respiratory distress syndrome, and outcome in small premature infants. *Am Rev Respir Dis.* (1991) 144:1376–84. doi: 10.1164/ajrccm/144.6.1376

46. Awasthi S, Coalson JJ, Crouch E, Yang F, King RJ. Surfactant proteins A and D in premature baboons with chronic lung injury (Bronchopulmonary dysplasia). Evidence for an inhibition of secretion. *Am J Respir Crit Care Med.* (1999) 160:942–9. doi: 10.1164/ajrccm.160.3.9806061

47. Coalson JJ, King RJ, Yang F, Winter V, Whitsett JA, Delemos RA, et al. SP-A deficiency in primate model of bronchopulmonary dysplasia with infection. *In situ* mRNA and immunostains. *Am J Respir Crit Care Med.* (1995) 151:854–66. doi: 10.1164/ajrccm/151.3_Pt_1.854

48. Okogbule-Wonodi AC, Chesko KL, Famuyide ME, Viscardi RM. Surfactant protein-A enhances ureaplasmacidal activity *in vitro*. *Innate Immun.* (2011) 17:145–51. doi: 10.1177/1753425909360552

49. Famuyide ME, Hasday JD, Carter HC, Chesko KL, He JR, Viscardi RM. Surfactant protein-A limits Ureaplasma-mediated lung inflammation in a murine pneumonia model. *Pediatr Res.* (2009) 66:162–7. doi: 10.1203/PDR.0b013e3181aabd66

50. Gantert M, Been JV, Gavilanes AW, Garnier Y, Zimmermann LJ, Kramer BW. Chorioamnionitis: a multiorgan disease of the fetus? *J Perinatol.* (2010) 30:S21–30. doi: 10.1038/jp.2010.96

51. Moreira AG, Siddiqui SK, Macias R, Johnson-Pais TL, Wilson D, Gelfond JAL, et al. Oxygen and mechanical ventilation impede the functional properties of resident lung mesenchymal stromal cells. *PLoS ONE.* (2020) 15:e0229521. doi: 10.1371/journal.pone.0229521

52. Stahlman MT, Gray ME, Whitsett JA. Expression of thyroid transcription factor-1 (TTF-1) in fetal and neonatal human lung. *J Histochem Cytochem.* (1996) 44:673–8. doi: 10.1177/44.7.8675988

53. Das I, Das RN, Paul B, Mandal B, Mukherjee S, Chatterjee U. A study of spectrum of pulmonary pathology and expression of thyroid transcription factor-1 during neonatal period. *Indian J Pathol Microbiol.* (2018) 61:334. doi: 10.4103/IJPM.IJPM_650_17

54. Thebaud B, Ladha F, Michelakis ED, Sawicka M, Thurston G, Eaton F, et al. Vascular endothelial growth factor gene therapy increases survival, promotes lung angiogenesis, and prevents alveolar damage in hyperoxia-induced lung injury: evidence that angiogenesis participates in alveolarization. *Circulation.* (2005) 112:2477–86. doi: 10.1161/CIRCULATIONAHA.105.541524

55. Coalson JJ, Winter VT, Siler-Khodr T, Yoder BA. Neonatal chronic lung disease in extremely immature baboons. *Am J Respir Crit Care Med.* (1999) 160:1333–46. doi: 10.1164/ajrccm.160.4.9810071

56. Raetz CR, Whitfield C. Lipopolysaccharide endotoxins. *Annu Rev Biochem.* (2002) 71:635–700. doi: 10.1146/annurev.biochem.71.110601.135414

57. Gilman-Sachs A, Dambaeva S, Salazar Garcia MD, Hussein Y, Kwak-Kim J, Beaman K. Inflammation induced preterm labor and birth. *J Reprod Immunol.* (2018) 129:53–8. doi: 10.1016/j.jri.2018.06.029

58. Möbius MA, Thébaud BJC. Bronchopulmonary dysplasia: where have all the stem cells gone?: origin and (potential) function of resident lung stem cells. *Chest.* (2017) 152:1043–52. doi: 10.1016/j.chest.2017. 04.173

59. Kallapur SG, Bachurski CJ, Le Cras TD, Joshi SN, Ikegami M, Jobe AH. Vascular changes after intra-amniotic endotoxin in preterm lamb lungs. *Am J Physiol Lung Cell Mol Physiol.* (2004) 287:L1178–85. doi: 10.1152/ajplung.00049.2004

The Future of Bronchopulmonary Dysplasia: Emerging Pathophysiological Concepts and Potential New Avenues of Treatment

Jennifer J. P. Collins[1]*, Dick Tibboel[1], Ismé M. de Kleer[2], Irwin K. M. Reiss[3] and Robbert J. Rottier[1]

[1] *Department of Pediatric Surgery, Sophia Children's Hospital, Erasmus University Medical Centre, Rotterdam, Netherlands,* [2] *Division of Pediatric Pulmonology, Department of Pediatrics, Sophia Children's Hospital, Erasmus University Medical Centre, Rotterdam, Netherlands,* [3] *Division of Neonatology, Department of Pediatrics, Sophia Children's Hospital, Erasmus University Medical Centre, Rotterdam, Netherlands*

*Correspondence:
Jennifer J. P. Collins
j.dewolf-collins@erasmusmc.nl

Yearly more than 15 million babies are born premature (<37 weeks gestational age), accounting for more than 1 in 10 births worldwide. Lung injury caused by maternal chorioamnionitis or preeclampsia, postnatal ventilation, hyperoxia, or inflammation can lead to the development of bronchopulmonary dysplasia (BPD), one of the most common adverse outcomes in these preterm neonates. BPD patients have an arrest in alveolar and microvascular development and more frequently develop asthma and early-onset emphysema as they age. Understanding how the alveoli develop, and repair, and regenerate after injury is critical for the development of therapies, as unfortunately there is still no cure for BPD. In this review, we aim to provide an overview of emerging new concepts in the understanding of perinatal lung development and injury from a molecular and cellular point of view and how this is paving the way for new therapeutic options to prevent or treat BPD, as well as a reflection on current treatment procedures.

Keywords: bronchopulmonary dysplasia, chronic lung disease of prematurity, respiratory distress syndrome, preterm birth, lung development, chronic lung disease

INTRODUCTION

Yearly over 15 million babies are born premature (<37 weeks gestational age), accounting for more than 1 in 10 births worldwide, of which approximately 2.4 million babies are born before 32 weeks of postmenstrual age (PMA) (1). Bronchopulmonary dysplasia (BPD) is the most common adverse outcome in very preterm neonates with an incidence of 5–68%, depending on the cohort and definition used, which increases significantly with declining gestational age (2, 3). BPD develops as a result of lung injury caused by maternal pre-eclampsia, chorioamnionitis, postnatal ventilation, hyperoxia, and/or inflammation, leading to an arrest in alveolar and microvascular development and pulmonary hypertension, although the relative contribution of the different pathogenic factors for the individual patient is hard to identify (4). Originally, BPD ("old" BPD) was defined based on lung injury resulting from mechanical ventilation and oxygen supplementation, and was seen mostly in premature infants born at 26–30 weeks PMA (5–7). The introduction of major interventions such as maternal corticosteroids (8, 9) and surfactant replacement therapy (10–12) resulted in a changed disease phenotype that was seen in preterm infants that could survive at younger gestational ages (24 to 26 weeks PMA). As a result, "new" BPD, defined as the requirement of supplemental oxygen at 36 weeks PMA or treatment with supplemental oxygen for more than 28 days (4), was characterized based on impaired alveolar and capillary development of the immature lungs (13). It is now becoming clear that BPD survivors continue to have respiratory morbidity after they leave the neonatal intensive care unit (NICU) [see comprehensive review by Islam et al. (14)], underlining that BPD really is a disease of disrupted lung development. Understanding how the alveoli and underlying capillary network develop and how these mechanisms are disrupted in BPD is critical for developing efficient therapies, which currently are lacking. Moreover, the nature of lung injury and consequently BPD is perpetually changing as treatment strategies evolve in an attempt to prevent injury to the premature lungs. Combined with increasing insight into the pathophysiology of BPD, this has started a discussion on yet a newer definition of what BPD is, basing it more on biomarkers, pulmonary hypertension and the underlying vascular basis of BPD (15–17). In this review, we provide an overview of emerging new pathophysiological concepts in the understanding of perinatal lung development and injury from a molecular and cellular point of view and how this is paving the way for new therapeutic options to prevent or treat BPD, as well as a reflection on how this compares with current treatment procedures.

Overview of Lung Development

To understand BPD pathophysiology, it is important to understand how the lung normally develops. Despite the large body of knowledge concerning the morphogenesis of the lung (18, 19), research on the intercellular communications that regulate growth, migration, and differentiation during lung development is still unfolding. Among the best characterized growth factors and their signaling components in early lung development are fibroblast growth factor (FGF), transforming growth factor β (TGFβ), bone morphogenetic protein (BMP), sonic hedgehog (SHH), wingless-type MMTV integration site family (WNT), vascular endothelial growth factor (VEGF), and retinoic acid signaling pathways [reviewed by Hogan and Morrissey (20) and Kool et al. (21)]. Far less is known about the molecular and cellular processes that direct saccular and alveolar development, the very stages that are clinically relevant after preterm birth and BPD pathogenesis. VEGF, which is expressed by alveolar epithelial type II cells in response to hypoxia-induced factor (HIF), is crucial in directing pulmonary microvascular development and alveolar development (22). Moreover, VEGF plays an important role in BPD pathogenesis as BPD patients express little or no VEGF in their lung epithelium, and lack expression of VEGF receptors in pulmonary microvascular endothelium (23). Multiple studies have demonstrated that platelet derived growth factor (PDGF) and FGF signaling is crucial for myofibroblast differentiation and subsequent onset of secondary septation (24–29). WNT, BMP, and TGFβ signaling components have also been implicated to play a role in fibroblast differentiation during alveolarization (30–32). Additionally, correct deposition of extracellular matrix (ECM) proteins by myofibroblasts, like elastin and collagen, plays a crucial role during secondary septation (33, 34). These and other ECM components may exert their role in lung development by functioning as a scaffold for the growth factors to coordinate the growth interactions of cells (35).

BPD IN 2017

Current Understanding of Perinatal Risk Factors

Because BPD is still very much a functional diagnosis, which is made when preterm infants have already been exposed to a wide variety of perinatal stressors [**Figure 1**; (36)], it is hard to pinpoint exactly which exposure is more detrimental for lung development. Most of these insights have been obtained through decades of work on animal models [reviewed by Jobe (37)] and correlations found through epidemiological research. Already before preterm birth, intrauterine conditions can have a profound impact on lung development and susceptibility to BPD. Risk factors established by statistical correlation are first and foremost maternal risk factors associated with preterm birth, such as

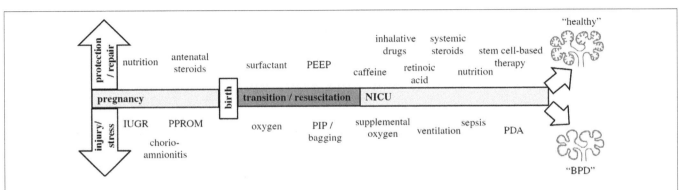

FIGURE 1 | **The pathogenesis of bronchopulmonary dysplasia (BPD) is highly multifactorial in nature, with a wide variety of pre- and postnatal exposures influencing lung development**. Depending on the timing and combinations of exposures, BPD likely exists of multiple different pathophysiologies that manifest themselves in a similar way clinically. The top arrow represents exposures that may to a certain extent protect from BPD pathogenesis and promote repair, while the bottom arrow indicates exposures that injure the preterm lung and contribute to BPD pathogenesis. Figure reprinted from Hütten et al., originally published by Springer (36).

smoking and socioeconomic background (38). Intrauterine growth restriction increases the risk of BPD threefold in infants born before 29 weeks (2, 39), while chorioamnionitis and pre-eclampsia trigger the release of cytokines and growth factors that directly inhibit alveolar and microvascular development of the fetal lungs (2, 36, 40). Placental abnormalities, such as gestational hypertension, pre-eclampsia, and eclampsia, are emerging as an important antenatal risk factor for BPD. A French prospective cohort study found that placenta-mediated pregnancy complications with fetal consequences are associated with moderate to severe BPD in very preterm infants (41). The maternal administration of corticosteroids prior to preterm birth leads to thinning of the primary septa, which narrows the air blood barrier, stimulates the production of surfactant, which stabilizes the alveolar sacs and prevents collapse after exhalation, and stimulates the clearance of fetal lung fluid (42). Although this accelerated development improves neonatal outcome and survival of the infant, antenatal corticosteroids have the unwanted side effect of inhibiting secondary septation and impairing microvasculature development (28, 43–45).

Postnatally, inflammation is also considered to be an important risk factor for the development of BPD [reviewed in Ref (46)], either as a result of lung injury caused by invasive mechanical ventilation and supplemental oxygen or in the form of sepsis. Due to their lung immaturity and apnea of prematurity, preterm infants are also frequently exposed to hypoxia, which just like hyperoxia leads to impaired alveolar and microvascular development (47). Recently, the presence of oxygen-sensitive intrapulmonary bronchopulmonary anastomoses (IBA) was discovered in preterm infants with BPD and other infants with chronic lung diseases, which may stay patent in the setting of persistent hypoxia (16, 48–52). Thus, IBA may in itself lead to persistent hypoxemia and contribute to the pulmonary hypertension that is often seen in conjunction with BPD, and could therefore be a significant risk factor for BPD (16). Considering that not all infants that are born very or extremely preterm go on to develop BPD, multiple pre- and/or postnatal hits are probably needed for lung development to be significantly affected, especially since the incidence of BPD has not decreased despite advances in neonatal care (2).

Current Treatment Procedures

In this complex multifactorial setting, current therapies are aimed to not only support the survival of the preterm infant, but also to limit or prevent further damage as much as possible [see review by Jain and Bancalari (53)]. In this regard, the most direct approach is to prevent the need for aggressive, prolonged invasive ventilation. The first treatment of choice to prevent respiratory distress syndrome (RDS) is still antenatal maternal corticosteroid administration, followed by prophylactic surfactant therapy through endotracheal bolus administration after birth. The maternal administration of a single or repeated intramuscular injection of betamethasone or dexamethasone within a time window of 24 h to 7 days prior to preterm birth can significantly increase survival of the preterm infant and decrease the incidence and severity of RDS (9, 54). However, there is no consensus yet on how the use of antenatal steroids can be optimized by improving the timing

of administration and dosing (42). Similarly, there is discussion as to whether surfactant therapy should be prophylactic or only selectively administered upon diagnosed RDS, as a result of the increased use of non-invasive ventilation methods such as nasal continuous positive airway pressure (CPAP) (53, 55). Without the application of routine CPAP, prophylactic surfactant treatment reduces neonatal mortality. However, the routine application of CPAP reduces the risk of BPD and neonatal death, and in these infants selective administration of surfactant is more beneficial (55). The INSURE method (intubate-surfactant-extubate to CPAP) is therefore now the recommended technique to avoid lung injury (56).

An alternative method of surfactant administration that builds on this is less invasive surfactant administration (LISA), which circumvents the need of endotracheal intubation and mechanical ventilation all together while improving pulmonary outcome in extreme premature infants (57–59). A more high-tech approach that is now being tested in the NICU is surfactant administration through aerosolization, nebulization, or atomization (60–67). It has proven technically challenging to achieve sufficient delivery of surfactant in the distal lung compared to bolus administration of surfactant, although the recent development of vibrating membrane nebulizers seems promising (67). Switching from animal-derived surfactants to new generation synthetic surfactants, which are more resistant to inactivation and even anti-inflammatory in cell culture and animal studies, may be another step forward (11, 68–75). Several clinical trials are testing two promising synthetic surfactants to combat RDS in the NICU. A multicenter phase 2 study is comparing the safety and efficacy of CHF5633, a synthetic surfactant with surfactant protein (SP)-B and SP-C analogs, with poractant alfa in preterm infants with RDS (ClinicalTrials.gov identifier NCT02452476). In addition, two multicenter phase 2 studies are assessing the safety and efficacy of aerosolized lucinactant (also known as KL4 surfactant, Aerosurf, and Surfaxin) in preterm neonates 26 to 32 weeks PMA receiving nasal CPAP (ClinicalTrials.gov identifiers NCT02636868 and NCT02528318). Optimizing ventilation strategies and surfactant therapy are therefore seen as the most easily achievable targets in the prevention of BPD.

Besides ventilation strategies, surfactant therapy and corticosteroids, there are a few therapies that have a profound effect in the prevention of BPD. Prophylactic caffeine therapy is recommended to counter apnea of prematurity and is now common practice after it was shown to be effective in reducing BPD and subsequent neurodisability (56, 76–78). The protective effect of caffeine therapy appears greater when given earlier rather than later, although there is still discussion among experts as early therapy is also associated with slightly greater mortality in some studies (79–81). This effect has been attributed to infants receiving earlier extubation and subsequently shorter mechanical ventilation times, alleviating the injury burden on the developing premature lung (76, 79). Multiple recent animal studies have attempted to elucidate whether caffeine itself can promote or protect alveolar development directly, with mixed results. Using the hyperoxia model of experimental BPD, caffeine could protect against alveolar simplification and inflammation in rats (82, 83) and rabbits (84), but not in mice (85, 86). Potential mechanisms include its abilities to amplify glucocorticoid-mediated SP-B expression in alveolar type 2 cells (87, 88), to modulate connective tissue growth factor (CTGF) expression (89) and TGFβ pathway members (85), and to attenuate endoplasmic reticulum (ER) stress (82). Conflictingly, both up- and downregulation of alveolar apoptosis has been reported (82, 86). Caffeine is however primarily known as a methylxanthine, which is a non-selective phosphodiesterase (PDE) inhibitor (78). PDE inhibitors have potent immunomodulatory and vascular effects and are therefore still interesting targets for neonatal intensive care medicine. Animal studies using the neonatal rodent hyperoxia model of experimental BPD have shown promise for non-selective PDE inhibitor pentoxyfilline (90), PDE4 inhibitors rolipram, piclamilast, and cilomilast (91–93), and PDE5 inhibitor sildenafil (94), which were able to ameliorate pulmonary inflammation and hypertension and improve lung alveolarization. Inhaled nitric oxide (iNO) therapy, which has a complementary mode of action to PDE inhibitors by boosting cyclic guanosine monophosphate (cGMP) (95), has long been the subject of clinical trials after promising results in animal models of BPD. Although iNO decreases inflammatory mediators in tracheal aspirates of treated preterm infants (96), systematic reviews show no protective effect in the development of BPD (97). Interestingly, iNO therapy was effective in reducing BPD incidence when combined with vitamin A therapy (98). Supplementation with vitamin A improved alveolarization in neonatal rats and lambs (99, 100), while in clinical studies, supplementation with vitamin A in preterm infants significantly reduced the risk of BPD (101–103). Unfortunately, these studies have not lead to the adoption of vitamin A supplementation in clinical practice, as the treatment benefits were deemed too small and the intramuscular route of administration too cumbersome in tiny preterm infants (104, 105). Other administration routes must be investigated for these promising therapies to become commonplace in the clinic.

For all currently used therapies, there is still ground to be gained through clinical trials and evidence-based medicine to ascertain optimal dosing, timing, and administration methods for maximum efficiency. It is essential that risk stratification takes place within the trial design to identify the real potential advantage of the different interventions. Despite all efforts at reducing lung injury through current treatment procedures, the incidence of BPD has remained stable over the past two decades (2). This is in part explained by the increased survival of extremely preterm infants born between 22 and 26 weeks PMA but probably also reflects the highly multifactorial nature of BPD. Prematurity is often not the first complication leading to BPD pathogenesis, as infants have already been exposed to a disadvantageous intrauterine environment, either through severe intrauterine growth restriction resulting from severe pre-eclampsia or chorioamnionitis. This is then followed by various exposures and comorbidities in the NICU, which in a substantial portion of these extreme premature infants leads to BPD with a similar phenotype, even though the underlying pathogenesis might have been quite different. It should not be forgotten that an astonishing portion of these infants does not go on to develop BPD, despite experiencing similar exposures. A better understanding of the pathophysiology leading to BPD

is therefore crucial to create a better tailored treatment regimen for premature infants.

CURRENT UNDERSTANDING OF BPD PATHOPHYSIOLOGY, NEW PATHOPHYSIOLOGICAL CONCEPTS, AND POTENTIAL THERAPIES

Infants at greatest risk of developing BPD are born when their developing lungs are still transitioning from the canalicular to saccular phase. Given the complexity of lung development and the wide variety of perinatal insults leading to BPD, there is likely no single pathophysiology of BPD. Because of a paucity of histopathological data from preterm infants and BPD patients, our current understanding of BPD pathophysiology has mostly been generated from various small and large animal models looking at the effect of perinatal inflammation, oxygen toxicity, and mechanical ventilation on lung development [reviewed by Jobe (37)]. Although these simplified animal models of BPD only approximate the actual disease in humans, they have helped us immensely to better understand the pathophysiology of BPD. A number of recent reviews have generated a detailed overview of the various pathophysiological mechanisms implicated in BPD that have been uncovered through these models [see review by Niedermaier and Hilgendorff (106) and Hilgendorff and O'Reilly (107)], focusing on the role of perinatal infection and inflammation (46, 108, 109), pulmonary vascular development (17), the mesenchyme (110), the extracellular matrix (111), and oxygen (112) [**Figure 2** (107)]. For the remainder of this review, we will highlight new pathophysiological concepts that are promising avenues for potential future therapies for BPD. Because of the inherent intertwinement of the pathophysiological mechanisms and potential therapies, we have chosen to present these side by side for each pathophysiological concept.

Stem Cells in Development and for Therapy of BPD

In the past decade, the field of stem cell biology has advanced significantly, especially with respect to tissue resident stem cells in development and repair. A wide variety of lung epithelial stem/progenitor cells has been described but also multipotent mesenchymal stromal cells (MSCs) and endothelial colony forming cells (ECFCs) [reviewed in Ref (113)]. In the developing lung, where an extensive microvasculature is crucial for lung function, resident lung MSCs (L-MSCs) are a heterogeneous progenitor population, which orchestrate the formation of the alveolar microvasculature, repair/regeneration, and tissue maintenance [reviewed in Ref (114, 115)]. Already at the beginning of lung budding, a multipotent cardiopulmonary mesoderm progenitor has been described, based on expression of Wnt2, Gli1 and Isl1, giving rise to pulmonary vascular and airway smooth muscle, proximal vascular endothelium and pericyte-like cells (116). During pseudoglandular lung development early Tbx4$^+$ multipotent MSCs give rise to a wide variety of distinct mesenchymal cell populations including airway and vascular smooth muscle and early fibroblast-like cells (117), reminiscent of quintipotential

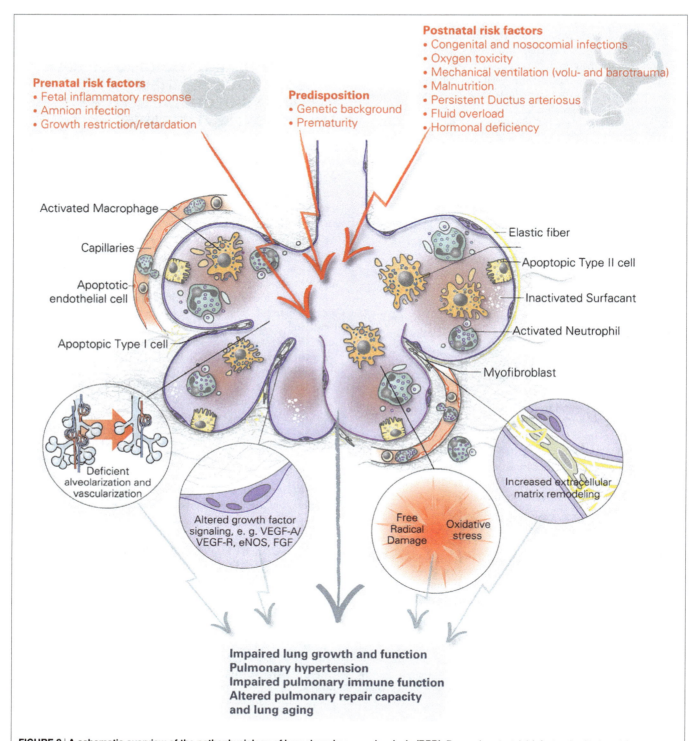

FIGURE 2 | A schematic overview of the pathophysiology of bronchopulmonary dysplasia (BPD). Pre- and postnatal risk factors lead to lung injury, resulting in apoptosis of distal lung cells, inflammation, extracellular matrix remodeling and altered growth factor signaling. These have long term effects on lung growth and function, including vascular and immune function, resulting in an increased disposition for chronic lung disorders. Figure reprinted from Hilgendorff and O'Reilly, originally published by Frontiers in Medicine (107).

MSCs in bone marrow (118). During saccular and alveolar lung development, $Pdgfr\alpha^+$, Shh^+, and $Fgf10^+$ L-MSCs give rise to myofibroblasts and lipofibroblasts, which are crucial for alveolar development (119–122). Importantly, $Pdgfr\alpha$ + L-MSCs are supportive of lung epithelial progenitor cells, which are unable to form colonies in their absence or in the presence of more differentiated myofibroblasts (123, 124). There is mounting evidence from both human patients and animal models that L-MSCs are perturbed in BPD, potentially actively contributing to BPD pathogenesis. The presence of L-MSCs in tracheal aspirates from ventilated preterm infants could predict the subsequent development of BPD (125). *In vitro*, these L-MSCs showed signs of dysfunction through reduced PDGFRα expression, a propensity toward myofibroblast differentiation and impaired migration capacity (126, 127). This is supported by a recent study in neonatal mice, where suppression of *Fgf10* expression left alveolar epithelial type 2 cells (AEC2) unable to regenerate after hyperoxia damage, leading to increased AEC1 differentiation (128). Combined with prior observations in parabronchial smooth muscle cells upon naphthalene injury (129), the secretion of FGF10 to stimulate epithelial repair may be one of the ways through which L-MSCs exert their regenerative capacities in the distal lung following injury (130).

Similarly, lung resident ECFCs, which are important for the development of the pulmonary microvasculature, were shown to be dysfunctional in a neonatal rat model of BPD (131). Moreover, the cord blood of preterm infants who go on to develop BPD contains lower numbers of circulating ECFCs, which are more vulnerable to hyperoxia-induced oxidative stress and dysfunction (132). Understanding how these resident progenitor populations are affected in BPD, but also how they normally mediate development, repair, and regeneration in the lung, will provide an insight into how we may mobilize these cells to actively engage in repair and normalize lung development.

Potential Therapies

Tapping into and stimulating the regenerative properties of L-MSCs and ECFCs through cell-based therapy may be a central way to ameliorate the lung injury leading to BPD pathogenesis. To this end, important lessons will come from exogenous stem cell therapy. In a neonatal rat hyperoxia model of BPD, intratracheal installation of either bone marrow or umbilical cord derived MSCs, or their conditioned media, could nearly completely repair experimental BPD, both on a histological and on a functional level (133, 134). The mode of action appears to be largely paracrine, as injection with MSC conditioned medium could promote alternatively activated (M2) macrophages (135). Exosomes, which are extracellular vesicles containing a cocktail of proteins, RNAs and even mitochondria, are secreted by a wide variety of cells including MSCs and likely play an active role in the paracrine therapeutic effects of MSCs (136). Their potential as a carrier of therapeutic paracrine factors makes them appealing and promising targets for cell-free MSC based therapy. However, several technical challenges must be overcome to ensure their safety, such as a robust reproducible isolation technique and their ability to facilitate infectious or damaging particles (137). The next decade will likely see large advances in the development of exogenous stem cell therapy for BPD and a vast array of other diseases, either by injecting stem cells themselves, their conditioned medium or through exosomes [see recent reviews by Möbius and Thébaud (138), O'Reilly and Thébaud (139), and Mitsialis and Kourembanas (136)].

Pulmonary Macrophages Contribute to Alveolar Development and Repair

Arguably the most important immune cells to participate in wound repair are alternatively activated macrophages. Besides peripheral blood derived macrophages, the pulmonary microenvironment contains three distinct resident pulmonary macrophage populations: alveolar macrophages, interstitial macrophages and primitive macrophages (140). Alveolar macrophages are the best-studied subset and are most abundantly present in the lung. They reside in the alveolar spaces where they phagocytose foreign particles and have a crucial role in the surfactant metabolism that facilitates alveolar function and gas exchange. Interstitial macrophages (IMF) reside on the other side of the epithelial barrier, among mesenchymal cells and capillaries. They have a distinct phenotype and behavior from alveolar macrophages and are geared more toward tissue repair and maintenance, antigen presentation and influencing dendritic cell functions to prevent allergy (140, 141). The third population, primitive macrophages, has only very recently been identified as a distinct subtype. These macrophages are the first to colonize the fetal lungs, and persist in adult lungs in the parenchyma of the peripheral alveoli. Because of their location in peripheral and perivascular spaces, which have been described as hotspots for alveolar regeneration, they are speculated to promote or be attracted to stem cell activity (140). The influx of these macrophages, which display an alternatively activated or M2 phenotype, and localization at the branching sites of the developing lung, suggest they potentially contribute to alveolar lung development (142). Conversely, if fetal lung macrophages are activated by an inflammatory stimulus, they actively inhibit expression of genes critical for lung development, leading to disrupted airway development and perinatal death in mice (143).

Potential Therapies

These insights provide new support for anti-inflammatory treatments. Furthermore, exogenous MSC therapy may be beneficial in regulating pulmonary macrophage activity. As cells with potent immunomodulatory capacities, MSCs can regulate macrophage function and polarization (144). Steady-state MSCs drive macrophages toward a wound healing or M2 phenotype through the production of IL-6 and inhibit differentiation toward dendritic cells (145, 146). However, in a proinflammatory environment MSCs stimulate macrophages toward a pro-inflammatory M1 phenotype (147). Using cell-based therapy to activate resident L-MSCs may therefore also be effective in promoting an M2 phenotype in pulmonary macrophages.

The Lung Microbiome: An Important Emerging Field of Interest

Although there has been a surge in interest in the microbiome thanks to the Human Microbiome Project, the lung was not included in this research project. Research interest in the lung microbiome is now however on the rise, uncovering that not only the upper but also the lower airways are colonized, with numbers of 10–100 bacterial cells per 1,000 human cells being reported (148). The six most commonly detected bacterial phyla are found throughout the body, but composition varies per organ. In the lung, composition varies between different areas, making consistent sampling of the same area extremely important when comparing between groups. The lungs of newborn infants are already colonized at birth with a variety of bacterial phyla, most predominately *Acinetobacter* (149). The composition of the lung microbiome changes and stabilizes in the first month of life, but is decidedly different in lungs of children and adult patients with lung disease (148, 149). Interestingly, amniotic fluid and the placenta harbor their own microbiota, suggesting that fetal tissues already get colonized *in utero*, potentially having an effect on early immune cell maturation (148).

Inflammation frequently occurs in preterm infants, both antenatal (chorioamnionitis) and postnatal (sepsis), and can strongly perturb lung development (150). In the neonatal period, the immune system is still immature, and evidence is mounting that host-microbial interactions are necessary for development and homeostatic control of the immune system (151). Recently, a strong correlation was found between decreased diversity of the lung microbiome at the time of birth in preterm infants and the development of BPD (149, 152). Other studies correlated prolonged antibiotics use during the first week of life and BPD (153, 154). The protective effect of bacterial exposure in early life on asthma and allergy development, the "hygiene hypothesis," is extensively studied, and a greater microbial diversity of commensal bacteria seems to underlie this protective effect (148). Beyond microbial diversity and exposure, the role of the lung microbiome in the regulation and maturation of the immature immune system and the developing neonatal lung is less clear. One route of how the lung microbiome might train the immature immune system is by inducing expression of programmed death ligand 1 (PD-L1) in pulmonary dendritic cells. Lack of microbial colonization, or blocking pulmonary PD-L1 during the first 2 weeks of life in mice, induced a disproportionate inflammatory response to allergens later in life (155).

An imbalanced microbiome, called dysbiosis, may further impact the inflammatory and tissue repair response to oxygen exposure, as beneficial bacteria are lost or overrun by other bacteria. An important emerging mechanism through which the microbiome can influence cell function is through the production of microbial metabolites, such as short chain fatty acids or tryptophane catabolites (156, 157). Tryptophane catabolites are produced via the enzyme indoleamine 2,3-dioxygenase 1 (IDO1) and function as agonists for the aryl hydrocarbon receptor (AhR). AhR activation leads to an immune suppressive response through the production of interleukin (IL) 22 and promotes development of regulatory T-cells (158). One genus of bacteria capable of metabolizing tryptophane into AhR agonists are Lactobacilli. The beneficial effects of tryptophane metabolites and Lactobacilli have been shown to inhibit inflammation and promote health in the gut, central nervous system and the lung (156, 157). Treatment of COPD patients with emphysema with the anti-inflammatory macrolide antibiotic azithromycin, resulted in increased levels of tryptophane catabolites in bronchoalveolar lavages, which decreased macrophage production of proinflammatory cytokines (156). In mice, intranasal administration of Lactobacilli was more potent in reducing allergic airway inflammation than intragastric

administration, possibly linked to an increase in regulatory T lymphocytes in the lungs (159). Interestingly, Lactobacilli were found to be significantly less abundant in the lungs of preterm infants who develop BPD compared to preterm infants who are BPD resistant (152). Within this cohort, Lactobacilli abundance was particularly low in infants born to mothers with chorioamnionitis. Coincidentally, azithromycin treatment could reduce the risk of BPD in preterm infants (160), particularly those colonized with *Ureaplasma* spp., which have been associated with chorioamnionitis and BPD (161, 162). The beneficial impact of the lung microbiome and specifically Lactobacilli on lung development is supported by a study in mice, where there was a positive correlation between microbial abundance and lung development (163). Injection of Lactobacilli into the lungs of germ-free mice could improve alveolar development (163).

Potential Therapies

In the near future, a potentially interesting avenue of therapy for the prevention or treatment of BPD may be the further exploration of the benefits of azithromycin. Following the bacterial lung microbiome, the lung virome and mycobiome are now slowly also becoming unraveled, which may provide further insights and treatment opportunities (148, 164, 165). Additionally, the benefits of pre- or probiotics to promote a healthy growth promoting lung microbiome should be investigated, and in particular the presence of Lactobacilli. D-Tryptophane was recently identified as a potent probiotic that could ameliorate allergic airway inflammation in a mouse model of allergic airway disease, and may therefore also be of interest in the setting of BPD (166). One possible way to achieve the same effect as tryptophane catabolites may be through the proton pump inhibitor omeprazole, which induces detoxification enzyme cytochrome P540 (CYP)1A1 possibly through an AhR-mediated process (167). AhR signaling is protective against hyperoxic injury in human fetal pulmonary microvascular cells and neonatal mice, likely because of its potent effects on the gene expression of immunomodulatory and developmental pathways (168). Combined pre- and postnatal omeprazole administration could attenuate hyperoxic lung injury in preterm rabbits even at low doses, making omeprazole an interesting potential therapeutic intervention to prevent BPD (167). Further studies are needed to validate its effects and to ascertain that it has no adverse effects on other developing organs.

Anti-inflammatory Agents

Bronchopulmonary dysplasia is primarily considered to be a developmental disease resulting from perinatal inflammation, and therefore specialists in the field have for the past decade called for a special focus on the development and improvement of anti-inflammatory therapies in BPD (169). Currently there are multiple anti-inflammatory therapies under investigation. Interleukin 1 receptor antagonist (IL1RA) is particularly promising, as it can prevent the development of experimental BPD when administered at a low dose in the neonatal rodent "double hit" model of BPD, consisting of hyperoxia and perinatal inflammation (170–172). In a sheep model for prenatal inflammation, intra-amniotic IL1RA could partially prevent the effects that lipopolysaccharide (LPS) had on lung maturation, measured as surfactant protein gene expression and lung compliance (173). Interestingly, preterm infants who go on to develop BPD have elevated levels of IL1RA in their tracheal aspirates (174). A more recent study in preterm ventilated baboon and human infants suggested however that an increased IL1β:IL1ra ratio on days 1 to 3 of life is more predictive of BPD (172). The same study provided compelling animal data that early IL1RA or glyburide therapy, which prevents the formation of the NLR family, pyrin domain containing 3 (NLRP3) inflammasome upstream of IL1β, can indeed ameliorate BPD development (172). IL1RA, also called anakinra or Kineret, and glyburide, also known as Diabeta, are both already approved by the Federal Drug Administration (FDA) for treatment in rheumatoid arthritis and type 2 diabetes, respectively, making them attractive treatment options. Future studies will have to show whether their use would also be safe in the neonatal setting.

Postnatal use of corticosteroids such as dexamethasone and hydrocortisone, which are potent anti-inflammatory compounds, can effectively reduce the incidence of BPD (175, 176). Despite this positive effect, there are significant adverse effects associated with systemic administration of corticosteroids. Short-term adverse effects include intestinal perforation, gastrointestinal bleeding, hypertension, hypertrophic cardiomyopathy, hyperglycemia, and growth failure, while follow-up studies pointed to adverse effects on neuronal development (175, 176). Experts in the field have therefore questioned whether the beneficial effects of reducing BPD and death can be weighed up to these significant adverse effects (175, 176), and are reluctant to recommend postnatal systemic corticosteroids for the prevention of BPD (177). A perhaps more compelling alternative would be to more specifically target the lung through intratracheal administration. Early results obtained with inhaled corticosteroids have been mixed (178, 179), likely due to its efficiency to reach the lung parenchyma. However, as more studies are being done, there is increasing evidence that inhaled corticosteroids prevent BPD and death when administered early, but long term follow-up studies are needed to assess the risk-benefit ratio (180–182). Recent *in vitro* studies in human fetal lungs attributed budenoside more potent anti-inflammatory effects than dexamethasone, swiftly decreasing gene expression of chemokines IL8 and CCL2 (MCP1) in whole lungs even in the presence of exogenous surfactant (183). Future validation studies should however closely monitor the combined effect of intratracheal corticosteroids and pre-existing pulmonary inflammation, as combined antenatal exposure of fetal sheep to LPS and corticosteroids had much stronger effects on lung inflammation and developmental pathways than either agent alone (184–187). Additionally, it will be important to validate with combined budenoside and surfactant treatment also has the potential to prevent BPD in premature infants that initially present with mild RDS and do not receive surfactant therapy (188).

Potential Therapies

As outlined above, IL1RA, glyburide, and inhaled budenoside are currently the most promising anti-inflammatory therapies that have the potential to prevent BPD in premature infants. However, more studies will have to look into the safety and potential long-term effects in human neonates.

Reactive Oxygen Species (ROS) and Mitochondrial Dysfunction

Although BPD pathogenesis has a very multifactorial nature, with oxygen exposure, mechanical ventilation and inflammation as some of the most widely accepted causes, one common pathway is shared by these insults: the generation of ROS. In animal models, exposure of neonatal animals to hyperoxia within a specific time period is sufficient to induce a pathophysiology similar to BPD (189). Underlying this pathophysiology is an exaggerated mitochondrial oxidant stress in response in newborn mice compared to adults, with an overall lower expression of antioxidant enzymes (190). The response to hyperoxia is developmentally regulated, leading specifically to the production of mitochondrial ROS-dependent NADPH oxidase 1 (NOX1) expression in neonatal animals (191). Expression of antioxidant enzymes is controlled by AhR, as AhR-deficient fetal human pulmonary microvascular cells displayed significantly attenuated antioxidant enzyme expression and increased hyperoxic injury (192). Deficiency of another key antioxidant enzyme, extracellular superoxide dismutase (EC-SOD), was sufficient to impair alveolar development and induce pulmonary hypertension in mice (193). This phenotype was worsened by additional oxidative stress caused by bleomycin exposure, which was also associated with decreased VEGF signaling (193). Further support for the hypothesis that ROS formation also plays a role in human BPD development has come from a genetic study in very low birth weight infants, which found an association between single nucleotide polymorphisms (SNPs) in antioxidant response genes and an increased or decreased risk for the development of BPD (194). The role of antioxidant enzymes in neonatal chronic lung disease is reviewed in depth by Berkelhamer and Farrow (195).

Mitochondria play a central role in oxygen metabolism, and mitochondrial abundance as measured by mitochondrial protein expression peaks around birth to facilitate the transition to the oxygen-rich world outside the womb (196, 197). Preterm infants are born before this peak, making them less prepared to deal with this shift in bioenergetics. Besides this mitochondrial immaturity, the exposures leading to chronic lung diseases have been linked to mitochondrial dysfunction (198, 199). Both hyperoxia exposure and mechanical ventilation of neonatal mice caused pulmonary mitochondrial dysfunction (200, 201). Moreover, direct inhibition of mitochondrial oxidative phosphorylation significantly impaired alveolar development, comparable to hyperoxia or mechanical ventilation. *In vitro* experiments indicate that elevated CO_2 levels, called hypercapnia, a common occurrence in BPD patients, also causes mitochondrial dysfunction (202). One potential mechanism through which mitochondrial dysfunction and ROS generation potentially lead to impaired alveolar development in hyperoxia exposed neonatal mice is through endoplasmic reticulum (ER) stress, which can cause apoptosis (82).

Potential Therapies

In animal studies, several potential treatments have been identified to decrease ROS generation. In neonatal mice, treatment with a specific mitochondrial antioxidant, (2-(2,2,6,6-tetramethylpiperidin-1-oxyl-4-ylamino)-2-oxoethyl)triphenylphosphonium chloride (mitoTEMPO), could protect against hyperoxia-induced lung injury (191). Another promising treatment compound is GYY4137, a slow-releasing H_2S donor, which could decrease ROS generation and thus protect and restore normal alveolar and microvascular development after neonatal hyperoxia injury in rats (203). Targeting the AhR would appear to be another promising approach considering it also has potent anti-inflammatory properties, as described above. Although omeprazole is generally seen as a potentiator of AhR activation, omeprazole treatment of hyperoxia-exposed newborn mice counterintuitively decreased functional AhR activation, worsening hyperoxic injury (204). Other approaches to promote AhR activation may however prove to be more effective. An entirely different approach in treating mitochondrial dysfunction may be through mitochondrial transfer, a process that has been reported as one of the therapeutic mechanisms of MSC therapy (205). In human BPD patients, most neonatal antioxidant trials have unfortunately not shown any benefit in the prevention of BPD, with the exception of vitamin A therapy (195). However, none of these antioxidant therapies were specifically targeted against mitochondrial ROS or dysfunction. More targeted approaches, as those outlined in the animal studies, may prove to be more promising.

Other Promising Therapeutic Options Based on Novel Pathophysiological Insights

Inflammation associated with BPD pathogenesis affects many molecular pathways, which by themselves can be interesting therapeutic targets. One of these is the ceramide pathway, which is upregulated in both hyperoxia and antenatal inflammation animal models (206–208) and also in other chronic lung diseases such as asthma, cystic fibrosis and COPD (209). Increased ceramide levels lead to increased apoptosis, both in epithelial cells of BPD patients and in animal models of BPD (208, 209). Intervention with a sphingosine-1-phosphate (S1P) analog in the mouse hyperoxia model of BPD could successfully ameliorate ceramide levels and hyperoxia-induced alveolar hypoplasia (208). In a more complex piglet model of lung injury by lavage, LPS instillation and injurious ventilation, tracheal installation with surfactant and D-myo-inositol-1,2,6-trisphosphate (IP3) could achieve a similar effect in reducing ceramide levels and improving oxygenation (210). In a different approach to decrease sensitivity to apoptosis in hyperoxia-exposed epithelial cells, inhibiting regulatory-associated protein of mechanistic target of rapamycin (RPTOR) could prevent hyperoxia-induced lung injury in neonatal mice (211). Based on these studies, selective pharmacological interventions which temporarily reduce apoptosis could be a promising way to prevent or repair neonatal lung injury and reduce BPD severity.

An intervention that has garnered attention in neonatal care is lactoferrin (LF), an iron-binding protein that is a normal component of human colostrum and milk (212). It has potent antimicrobial activity, can stimulate the innate immune system and promote epithelial proliferation and differentiation of the immature gut (213). Recent studies have identified LF supplementation as a promising agent for the reduction of late onset sepsis and necrotizing enterocolitis (214). Although the properties of LF may also be desirable for the prevention of BPD, to

date no study has been able to show a significant reduction in the development of BPD following LF supplementation (214).

A pathophysiological mechanism of BPD that is slowly gaining more attention is the link between pre-eclampsia and BPD. Pre-eclampsia a proven risk factor for BPD (41), and the underlying impact on the developing fetus may be three-fold. Firstly, maternal preeclampsia is a frequent cause of preterm birth before 28 weeks (215). Secondly, severe preeclampsia can lead to intrauterine growth restriction, which in itself is a strong risk factor for BPD (38, 39). Thirdly, the placental dysfunction that lies at the root of pre-eclampsia leads to an overproduction of soluble VEGF receptor 1 [also known as soluble fms-like tyrosine kinase-1 (sFlt-1)], which inhibits VEGF signaling (216, 217). This not only leads to increased sVEGFR-1 in maternal serum, but also in amniotic fluid (218). By giving pregnant rats intra-amniotic injections with sVEGFR-1, Steven Abman's group demonstrated a link between pre-eclampsia and BPD, as neonatal rats presented with impaired alveolar and microvascular development and right and left ventricular hypertrophy (40). Moreover, intrauterine exposure to excess sVEGFR-1 led to increased apoptosis of endothelial and mesenchymal cells in neonatal rat lungs. Placental dysfunction and subsequent overexpression of sVEGFR-1 may therefore be a potential therapeutic target to improve fetal outcome and prevent development of BPD. At the very least, the diagnosis of maternal pre-eclampsia should be considered as a serious predisposition for the development of BPD.

From a developmental biology perspective, developmental molecular pathways that are downregulated in BPD provide other potential targets for the amelioration of BPD pathogenesis. These include the Wnt signaling pathway (187, 219, 220), SHH signaling (185, 221–223), axonal guidance cues semaphorin 3 C and ephrin B2 (224, 225), Notch signaling (226, 227), and HIFs (228). In addition, a wealth of new molecular insights on mouse and human lung development has been and will be published in the upcoming years by the LungMAP consortium (1U01HL122638), funded by the National Heart, Lung, and Blood Institute (NHLBI) (http://www.lungmap.net) (229, 230). BPD is generally considered to be caused by environmental factors, but in recent years studies have uncovered that a genetic component may also be at play [reviewed in Ref (231, 232)]. Although associations are not conclusive, these studies suggest that genetic variants of genes in well-known lung development and repair pathways may predispose for severe BPD or mild/moderate BPD (232). microRNAs have emerged as both a pathophysiological mechanism and a tempting tool to target transcription of multiple of these developmental signaling pathways at once. Although multiple human and animal studies have reported an association between altered microRNA levels and BPD, valid concerns have been raised about the lack of a causal link between altered microRNA levels and BPD pathogenesis [reviewed in Ref (233)]. However, if such a causal link can be confirmed, as was recently seen in a study which demonstrated the regulation of alveolar septation by microRNA-489 (234), the use of specific microRNA antagonists or agonists may be considered as a potential therapy for BPD. Caution should however be exercised when directly modulating potent developmental pathways, either directly or through microRNA therapy. Further exploration of such therapeutic targets

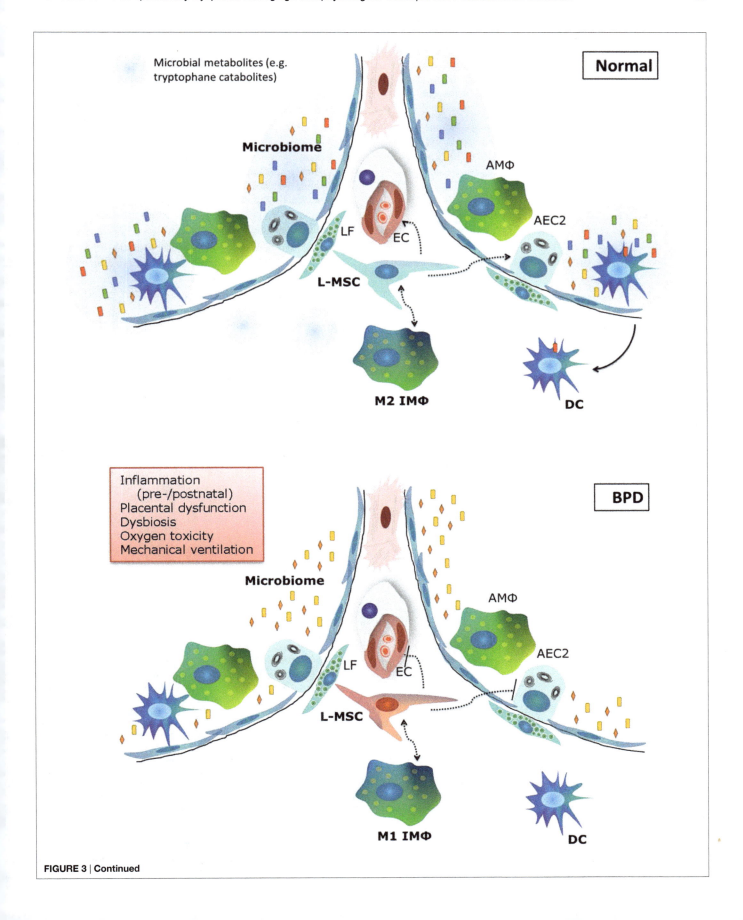

FIGURE 3 | Continued

FIGURE 3 | Continued

Summary of new pathophysiological concepts in bronchopulmonary dysplasia (BPD). In normal alveolar lung development, a diverse microbiome is necessary to train the pulmonary immune system and secrete metabolites that support lung development. Pulmonary M2 interstitial macrophages (M2 IMφ) are present and likely play an active role in lung development. L-MSCs support M2 IMφ, alveolar epithelial cells and the microvasculature. In BPD (bottom panel), pre- and postnatal risk factors lead to decreased microbiome diversity, a proinflammatory environment, dysfunctional L-MSCs, epithelial and endothelial injury and impaired repair. LF, lipofibroblast; EC, endothelial cell; AMΦ, alveolar macrophage; L-MSC, lung mesenchymal stromal cell; AEC2, alveolar epithelial cell type 2; M1/M2 IMΦ, type 1/2 interstitial macrophage; DC, dendritic cell.

should perhaps be combined with slow releasing microparticles or capsules to ensure a more physiological release and prevent pathological side effects.

Conclusion and Future Directions

The pathophysiology of BPD is extremely multifactorial, which is underlined by the emerging role of cell types that have only recently been acknowledged, such as the microbiome, macrophages, and tissue stem cells (**Figure 3**). Our knowledge on the pathophysiology is poised to move forward rapidly in the next decade, due to exciting new technological advances in the research field, and is opening avenues for the pursuit of therapeutic options. In addition, there is still promise for new and better applications of existing therapies, which have not yet fulfilled their promise in a clinical setting. In the next decade of BPD research, the most promising therapies and pathophysiological concepts that should be pursued for new therapeutic options are as follows:

- Animal models investigating the pathogenesis of BPD should identify different sub-pathophysiological processes that arise because of different combinations of pre-and postnatal exposures (e.g. pre-eclampsia, dysbiosis), as opposed to only looking at hyperoxia or inflammation models. Moreover, better appreciation of extrapulmonary issues related to BPD might be instructive, particularly neurodevelopmental outcome and retinopathy, which are frequent long-term outcomes resulting from BPD (235).

- Different routes of administration for effective therapies such as vitamin A and postnatal corticosteroids, in particular non-invasive intratracheal routes.
- Cell-based therapies, either through administration of stem cells and their products or by promoting the regenerative potential of resident lung stem cells.
- The commensal role of the pre- and postnatal (lung) microbiome in the normal and perturbed lung development, and its potential as a therapeutic target.
- The role of placental dysfunction in the pathogenesis of BPD, and its potential as a therapeutic target in the prevention of BPD.
- The role of the immune system not only as an adverse factor in BPD pathogenesis, but its importance in supporting normal lung development and repair.

AUTHOR CONTRIBUTIONS

Conception and outline of review: JC, DT, and RR. Writing of the manuscript: JC. Drafting of the manuscript: JC, DT, and RR. Critical revision of manuscript: JC, DT, IK, IR, and RR. Final approval of manuscript: JC, DT, IK, IR, and RR.

REFERENCES

1. March of Dimes, PMNCH, Save the Children, WHO. *Born Too Soon: The Global Action Report on Preterm Birth.* Geneva: World Health Organization (2012).
2. Jensen EA, Schmidt B. Epidemiology of bronchopulmonary dysplasia. *Birth Defects Res A Clin Mol Teratol* (2014) 100(3):145–57. doi:10.1002/bdra.23235
3. Stoll BJ, Hansen NI, Bell EF, Shankaran S, Laptook AR, Walsh MC, et al. Neonatal outcomes of extremely preterm infants from the NICHD Neonatal Research Network. *Pediatrics* (2010) 126(3):443–56. doi:10.1542/peds.2009-2959
4. Jobe AH, Bancalari E. Bronchopulmonary dysplasia. *Am J Respir Crit Care Med* (2001) 163(7):1723–9. doi:10.1164/ajrccm.163.7.2011060
5. O'Brodovich HM, Mellins RB. Bronchopulmonary dysplasia. Unresolved neonatal acute lung injury. *Am Rev Respir Dis* (1985) 132(3):694–709.
6. Coalson JJ. Pathology of new bronchopulmonary dysplasia. *Semin Neonatol* (2003) 8(1):73–81. doi:10.1016/S1084-2756(02)00193-8
7. Northway WH Jr, Rosan RC, Porter DY. Pulmonary disease following respirator therapy of hyaline-membrane disease. Bronchopulmonary dysplasia. *N Engl J Med* (1967) 276(7):357–68. doi:10.1056/NEJM19670216 2760701

8. Liggins GC, Howie RN. A controlled trial of antepartum glucocorticoid treatment for prevention of the respiratory distress syndrome in premature infants. *Pediatrics* (1972) 50(4):515–25.
9. Roberts D, Brown J, Medley N, Dalziel SR. Antenatal corticosteroids for accelerating fetal lung maturation for women at risk of preterm birth. *Cochrane Database Syst Rev* (2017) 3:CD004454. doi:10.1002/14651858. CD004454.pub3
10. Engle WA; American Academy of Pediatrics Committee on Fetus and Newborn. Surfactant-replacement therapy for respiratory distress in the preterm and term neonate. *Pediatrics* (2008) 121(2):419–32. doi:10.1542/peds.2007-3283
11. Curstedt T, Halliday HL, Speer CP. A unique story in neonatal research: the development of a porcine surfactant. *Neonatology* (2015) 107(4):321–9. doi:10.1159/000381117
12. Noack G, Berggren P, Curstedt T, Grossmann G, Herin P, Mortensson W, et al. Severe neonatal respiratory distress syndrome treated with the isolated phospholipid fraction of natural surfactant. *Acta Paediatr Scand* (1987) 76(5):697–705. doi:10.1111/j.1651-2227.1987.tb10552.x
13. Husain AN, Siddiqui NH, Stocker JT. Pathology of arrested acinar development in postsurfactant bronchopulmonary dysplasia. *Hum Pathol* (1998) 29(7):710–7. doi:10.1016/S0046-8177(98)90280-5

14. Islam JY, Keller RL, Aschner JL, Hartert TV, Moore PE. Understanding the short- and long-term respiratory outcomes of prematurity and bronchopulmonary dysplasia. *Am J Respir Crit Care Med* (2015) 192(2):134–56. doi:10.1164/rccm.201412-2142PP

15. Day CL, Ryan RM. Bronchopulmonary dysplasia: new becomes old again! *Pediatr Res* (2016) 81(1–2):210–3. doi:10.1038/pr.2016.201

16. Thebaud B. Impaired lung development and neonatal lung diseases: a never-ending (vascular) story. *J Pediatr* (2017) 180:11–3. doi:10.1016/j.jpeds.2016.10.030

17. Alvira CM. Aberrant pulmonary vascular growth and remodeling in bronchopulmonary dysplasia. *Front Med* (2016) 3:21. doi:10.3389/fmed.2016.00021

18. Burri PH. Structural aspects of postnatal lung development – alveolar formation and growth. *Biol Neonate* (2006) 89(4):313–22. doi:10.1159/000092868

19. Kitaoka H, Burri PH, Weibel ER. Development of the human fetal airway tree: analysis of the numerical density of airway endtips. *Anat Rec* (1996) 244(2):207–13. doi:10.1002/(SICI)1097-0185(199602)244:2<207::AID-AR8>3.0.CO;2-Y

20. Morrisey EE, Hogan BL. Preparing for the first breath: genetic and cellular mechanisms in lung development. *Dev Cell* (2010) 18(1):8–23. doi:10.1016/j.devcel.2009.12.010

21. Kool H, Mous D, Tibboel D, de Klein A, Rottier RJ. Pulmonary vascular development goes awry in congenital lung abnormalities. *Birth Defects Res C Embryo Today* (2014) 102(4):343–58. doi:10.1002/bdrc.21085

22. Thebaud B, Ladha F, Michelakis ED, Sawicka M, Thurston G, Eaton F, et al. Vascular endothelial growth factor gene therapy increases survival, promotes lung angiogenesis, and prevents alveolar damage in hyperoxia-induced lung injury: evidence that angiogenesis participates in alveolarization. *Circulation* (2005) 112(16):2477–86. doi:10.1161/CIRCULATIONAHA.105.541524

23. Bhatt AJ, Pryhuber GS, Huyck H, Watkins RH, Metlay LA, Maniscalco WM. Disrupted pulmonary vasculature and decreased vascular endothelial growth factor, Flt-1, and TIE-2 in human infants dying with bronchopulmonary dysplasia. *Am J Respir Crit Care Med* (2001) 164(10 Pt 1):1971–80. doi:10.1164/ajrccm.164.10.2101140

24. Weinstein M, Xu X, Ohyama K, Deng CX. FGFR-3 and FGFR-4 function cooperatively to direct alveogenesis in the murine lung. *Development* (1998) 125(18):3615–23.

25. Snyder JM, Jenkins-Moore M, Jackson SK, Goss KL, Dai HH, Bangsund PJ, et al. Alveolarization in retinoic acid receptor-beta-deficient mice. *Pediatr Res* (2005) 57(3):384–91. doi:10.1203/01.PDR.0000151315.81106.D3

26. Liebeskind A, Srinivasan S, Kaetzel D, Bruce M. Retinoic acid stimulates immature lung fibroblast growth via a PDGF-mediated autocrine mechanism. *Am J Physiol Lung Cell Mol Physiol* (2000) 279(1):L81–90.

27. Perl AK, Gale E. FGF signaling is required for myofibroblast differentiation during alveolar regeneration. *Am J Physiol Lung Cell Mol Physiol* (2009) 297(2):L299–308. doi:10.1152/ajplung.00008.2009

28. Bourbon J, Boucherat O, Chailley-Heu B, Delacourt C. Control mechanisms of lung alveolar development and their disorders in bronchopulmonary dysplasia. *Pediatr Res* (2005) 57(5 Pt 2):38R–46R. doi:10.1203/01.PDR.0000159630.35883.BE

29. Chao CM, Moiseenko A, Zimmer KP, Bellusci S. Alveologenesis: key cellular players and fibroblast growth factor 10 signaling. *Mol Cell Pediatr* (2016) 3(1):17. doi:10.1186/s40348-016-0045-7

30. Boucherat O, Franco-Montoya ML, Thibault C, Incitti R, Chailley-Heu B, Delacourt C, et al. Gene expression profiling in lung fibroblasts reveals new players in alveolarization. *Physiol Genomics* (2007) 32(1):128–41. doi:10.1152/physiolgenomics.00108.2007

31. Nakanishi H, Sugiura T, Streisand JB, Lonning SM, Roberts JD Jr. TGF-beta-neutralizing antibodies improve pulmonary alveologenesis and vasculogenesis in the injured newborn lung. *Am J Physiol Lung Cell Mol Physiol* (2007) 293(1):L151–61. doi:10.1152/ajplung.00389.2006

32. Alejandre-Alcazar MA, Shalamanov PD, Amarie OV, Sevilla-Perez J, Seeger W, Eickelberg O, et al. Temporal and spatial regulation of bone morphogenetic protein signaling in late lung development. *Dev Dyn* (2007) 236(10):2825–35. doi:10.1002/dvdy.21293

33. Burri PH. The postnatal growth of the rat lung. 3. Morphology. *Anat Rec* (1974) 180(1):77–98. doi:10.1002/ar.1091800109

34. Brody JS, Kaplan NB. Proliferation of alveolar interstitial cells during postnatal lung growth. Evidence for two distinct populations of pulmonary fibroblasts. *Am Rev Respir Dis* (1983) 127(6):763–70.

35. Neptune ER, Frischmeyer PA, Arking DE, Myers L, Bunton TE, Gayraud B, et al. Dysregulation of TGF-beta activation contributes to pathogenesis in Marfan syndrome. *Nat Genet* (2003) 33(3):407–11. doi:10.1038/ng1116

36. Hutten MC, Wolfs TG, Kramer BW. Can the preterm lung recover from perinatal stress? *Mol Cell Pediatr* (2016) 3(1):15. doi:10.1186/s40348-016-0043-9

37. Jobe AH. Animal models, learning lessons to prevent and treat neonatal chronic lung disease. *Front Med* (2015) 2:49. doi:10.3389/fmed.2015.00049

38. Behrman RE, Stith Butler A, editors. *Preterm Birth: Causes, Consequences and Prevention*. Washington: National Academies Press (2007).

39. Bose C, Van Marter LJ, Laughon M, O'Shea TM, Allred EN, Karna P, et al. Fetal growth restriction and chronic lung disease among infants born before the 28th week of gestation. *Pediatrics* (2009) 124(3):e450–8. doi:10.1542/peds.2008-3249

40. Tang JR, Karumanchi SA, Seedorf G, Markham N, Abman SH. Excess soluble vascular endothelial growth factor receptor-1 in amniotic fluid impairs lung growth in rats: linking preeclampsia with bronchopulmonary dysplasia. *Am J Physiol Lung Cell Mol Physiol* (2012) 302(1):L36–46. doi:10.1152/ajplung.00294.2011

41. Torchin H, Ancel PY, Goffinet F, Hascoet JM, Truffert P, Tran D, et al. Placental complications and bronchopulmonary dysplasia: EPIPAGE-2 cohort study. *Pediatrics* (2016) 137(3):e20152163. doi:10.1542/peds.2015-2163

42. Kemp MW, Newnham JP, Challis JG, Jobe AH, Stock SJ. The clinical use of corticosteroids in pregnancy. *Hum Reprod Update* (2016) 22(2):240–59. doi:10.1093/humupd/dmv047

43. Willet KE, McMenamin P, Pinkerton KE, Ikegami M, Jobe AH, Gurrin L, et al. Lung morphometry and collagen and elastin content: changes during normal development and after prenatal hormone exposure in sheep. *Pediatr Res* (1999) 45(5 Pt 1):615–25. doi:10.1203/00006450-199905010-00002

44. Willet KE, Jobe AH, Ikegami M, Kovar J, Sly PD. Lung morphometry after repetitive antenatal glucocorticoid treatment in preterm sheep. *Am J Respir Crit Care Med* (2001) 163(6):1437–44. doi:10.1164/ajrccm.163.6.2003098

45. Bunton TE, Plopper CG. Triamcinolone-induced structural alterations in the development of the lung of the fetal rhesus macaque. *Am J Obstet Gynecol* (1984) 148(2):203–15. doi:10.1016/S0002-9378(84)80177-5

46. Balany J, Bhandari V. Understanding the impact of infection, inflammation, and their persistence in the pathogenesis of bronchopulmonary dysplasia. *Front Med* (2015) 2:90. doi:10.3389/fmed.2015.00090

47. Ramani M, Bradley WE, Dell'Italia LJ, Ambalavanan N. Early exposure to hyperoxia or hypoxia adversely impacts cardiopulmonary development. *Am J Respir Cell Mol Biol* (2015) 52(5):594–602. doi:10.1165/rcmb.2013-0491OC

48. Bush D, Abman SH, Galambos C. Prominent intrapulmonary bronchopulmonary anastomoses and abnormal lung development in infants and children with down syndrome. *J Pediatr* (2017) 180: 156–62.e1. doi:10.1016/j.jpeds.2016.08.063

49. Ali N, Abman SH, Galambos C. Histologic evidence of intrapulmonary bronchopulmonary anastomotic pathways in neonates with meconium aspiration syndrome. *J Pediatr* (2015) 167(6):1445–7. doi:10.1016/j.jpeds.2015.08.049

50. Acker SN, Mandell EW, Sims-Lucas S, Gien J, Abman SH, Galambos C. Histologic identification of prominent intrapulmonary anastomotic vessels in severe congenital diaphragmatic hernia. *J Pediatr* (2015) 166(1):178–83. doi:10.1016/j.jpeds.2014.09.010

51. Galambos C, Sims-Lucas S, Abman SH. Three-dimensional reconstruction identifies misaligned pulmonary veins as intrapulmonary shunt vessels in alveolar capillary dysplasia. *J Pediatr* (2014) 164(1):192–5. doi:10.1016/j.jpeds.2013.08.035

52. Galambos C, Sims-Lucas S, Abman SH. Histologic evidence of intrapulmonary anastomoses by three-dimensional reconstruction in severe bronchopulmonary dysplasia. *Ann Am Thorac Soc* (2013) 10(5):474–81. doi:10.1513/AnnalsATS.201305-124OC

53. Jain D, Bancalari E. Bronchopulmonary dysplasia: clinical perspective. *Birth Defects Res A Clin Mol Teratol* (2014) 100(3):134–44. doi:10.1002/bdra.23229

54. Wapner R, Jobe AH. Controversy: antenatal steroids. *Clin Perinatol* (2011) 38(3):529–45. doi:10.1016/j.clp.2011.06.013

55. Rojas-Reyes MX, Morley CJ, Soll R. Prophylactic versus selective use of surfactant in preventing morbidity and mortality in preterm infants.

Cochrane Database Syst Rev (2012) 14(3):CD000510. doi:10.1002/14651858. CD000510.pub2

56. Sweet DG, Carnielli V, Greisen G, Hallman M, Ozek E, Plavka R, et al. European consensus guidelines on the management of respiratory distress syndrome – 2016 update. *Neonatology* (2016) 111(2):107–25. doi:10.1159/000448985

57. Gopel W, Kribs A, Ziegler A, Laux R, Hoehn T, Wieg C, et al. Avoidance of mechanical ventilation by surfactant treatment of spontaneously breathing preterm infants (AMV): an open-label, randomised, controlled trial. *Lancet* (2011) 378(9803):1627–34. doi:10.1016/S0140-6736(11)60986-0

58. Gopel W, Kribs A, Hartel C, Avenarius S, Teig N, Groneck P, et al. Less invasive surfactant administration is associated with improved pulmonary outcomes in spontaneously breathing preterm infants. *Acta Paediatr* (2015) 104(3):241–6. doi:10.1111/apa.12883

59. Isayama T, Iwami H, McDonald S, Beyene J. Association of noninvasive ventilation strategies with mortality and bronchopulmonary dysplasia among preterm infants: a systematic review and meta-analysis. *JAMA* (2016) 316(6):611–24. doi:10.1001/jama.2016.10708

60. Hutten MC, Kuypers E, Ophelders DR, Nikiforou M, Jellema RK, Niemarkt HJ, et al. Nebulization of poractant alfa via a vibrating membrane nebulizer in spontaneously breathing preterm lambs with binasal continuous positive pressure ventilation. *Pediatr Res* (2015) 78(6):664–9. doi:10.1038/pr.2015.165

61. Milesi I, Tingay DG, Zannin E, Bianco F, Tagliabue P, Mosca F, et al. Intratracheal atomized surfactant provides similar outcomes as bolus surfactant in preterm lambs with respiratory distress syndrome. *Pediatr Res* (2016) 80(1):92–100. doi:10.1038/pr.2016.39

62. Finer NN, Merritt TA, Bernstein G, Job L, Mazela J, Segal R. An open label, pilot study of Aerosurf(R) combined with nCPAP to prevent RDS in preterm neonates. *J Aerosol Med Pulm Drug Deliv* (2010) 23(5):303–9. doi:10.1089/jamp.2009.0758

63. Dijk PH, Heikamp A, Oetomo SB. Surfactant nebulization versus instillation during high frequency ventilation in surfactant-deficient rabbits. *Pediatr Res* (1998) 44(5):699–704. doi:10.1203/00006450-199811000-00012

64. Berggren E, Liljedahl M, Winbladh B, Andreasson B, Curstedt T, Robertson B, et al. Pilot study of nebulized surfactant therapy for neonatal respiratory distress syndrome. *Acta Paediatr* (2000) 89(4):460–4. doi:10.1111/j.1651-2227. 2000.tb00084.x

65. Jorch G, Hartl H, Roth B, Kribs A, Gortner L, Schaible T, et al. Surfactant aerosol treatment of respiratory distress syndrome in spontaneously breathing premature infants. *Pediatr Pulmonol* (1997) 24(3):222–4. doi:10.1002/(SICI)1099-0496(199709)24:3<222::AID-PPUL9>3.0.CO;2-O

66. Lampland AL, Wolfson MR, Mazela J, Henderson C, Gregory TJ, Meyers P, et al. Aerosolized KL4 surfactant improves short-term survival and gas exchange in spontaneously breathing newborn pigs with hydrochloric acid-induced acute lung injury. *Pediatr Pulmonol* (2014) 49(5):482–9. doi:10.1002/ppul.22844

67. Pillow JJ, Minocchieri S. Innovation in surfactant therapy II: surfactant administration by aerosolization. *Neonatology* (2012) 101(4):337–44. doi:10.1159/000337354

68. Seehase M, Collins JJ, Kuypers E, Jellema RK, Ophelders DR, Ospina OL, et al. New surfactant with SP-B and C analogs gives survival benefit after inactivation in preterm lambs. *PLoS One* (2012) 7(10):e47631. doi:10.1371/journal.pone.0047631

69. Glaser K, Fehrholz M, Henrich B, Claus H, Papsdorf M, Speer CP. Anti-inflammatory effects of the new generation synthetic surfactant CHF5633 on Ureaplasma-induced cytokine responses in human monocytes. *Expert Rev Anti Infect Ther* (2017) 15(2):181–9. doi:10.1080/14787210.2017. 1259067

70. Fehrholz M, Glaser K, Seidenspinner S, Ottensmeier B, Curstedt T, Speer CP, et al. Impact of the new generation reconstituted surfactant CHF5633 on human CD4+ lymphocytes. *PLoS One* (2016) 11(4):e0153578. doi:10.1371/journal.pone.0153578

71. Glaser K, Fehrholz M, Curstedt T, Kunzmann S, Speer CP. Effects of the new generation synthetic reconstituted surfactant CHF5633 on pro- and anti-inflammatory cytokine expression in native and LPS-stimulated adult CD14+ monocytes. *PLoS One* (2016) 11(1):e0146898. doi:10.1371/journal. pone.0146898

72. Glaser K, Fehrholz M, Papsdorf M, Curstedt T, Kunzmann S, Speer CP. The new generation synthetic reconstituted surfactant CHF5633 suppresses

LPS-induced cytokine responses in human neonatal monocytes. *Cytokine* (2016) 86:119–23. doi:10.1016/j.cyto.2016.08.004

73. Ardell S, Pfister RH, Soll R. Animal derived surfactant extract versus protein free synthetic surfactant for the prevention and treatment of respiratory distress syndrome. *Cochrane Database Syst Rev* (2015) 8:CD000144. doi:10.1002/14651858.CD000144.pub3

74. Sato A, Ikegami M. SP-B and SP-C containing new synthetic surfactant for treatment of extremely immature lamb lung. *PLoS One* (2012) 7(7):e39392. doi:10.1371/journal.pone.0039392

75. Jordan BK, Donn SM. Lucinactant for the prevention of respiratory distress syndrome in premature infants. *Expert Rev Clin Pharmacol* (2013) 6(2):115–21. doi:10.1586/ecp.12.80

76. Schmidt B, Roberts RS, Davis P, Doyle LW, Barrington KJ, Ohlsson A, et al. Caffeine therapy for apnea of prematurity. *N Engl J Med* (2006) 354(20):2112–21. doi:10.1056/NEJMoa054065

77. Schmidt B, Roberts RS, Davis P, Doyle LW, Barrington KJ, Ohlsson A, et al. Long-term effects of caffeine therapy for apnea of prematurity. *N Engl J Med* (2007) 357(19):1893–902. doi:10.1056/NEJMoa073679

78. Kreutzer K, Bassler D. Caffeine for apnea of prematurity: a neonatal success story. *Neonatology* (2014) 105(4):332–6. doi:10.1159/000360647

79. Kua KP, Lee SW. Systematic review and meta-analysis of clinical outcomes of early caffeine therapy in preterm neonates. *Br J Clin Pharmacol* (2017) 83(1):180–91. doi:10.1111/bcp.13089

80. Adzikah S, Maletzki J, Ruegger C, Bassler D. Association of early versus late caffeine administration on neonatal outcomes in very preterm neonates. *Acta Paediatr* (2017) 106(3):518. doi:10.1111/apa.13691

81. Schmidt B, Davis PG, Roberts RS. Timing of caffeine therapy in very low birth weight infants. *J Pediatr* (2014) 164(5):957–8. doi:10.1016/j. jpeds.2014.01.054

82. Teng RJ, Jing X, Michalkiewicz T, Afolayan AJ, Wu TJ, Konduri GG. Attenuation of endoplasmic reticulum stress by caffeine ameliorates hyperoxia-induced lung injury. *Am J Physiol Lung Cell Mol Physiol* (2017) 312(5):L586–98. doi:10.1152/ajplung.00405.2016

83. Weichelt U, Cay R, Schmitz T, Strauss E, Sifringer M, Buhrer C, et al. Prevention of hyperoxia-mediated pulmonary inflammation in neonatal rats by caffeine. *Eur Respir J* (2013) 41(4):966–73. doi:10.1183/09031936.00012412

84. Nagatomo T, Jimenez J, Richter J, De Baere S, Vanoirbeek J, Naulaers G, et al. Caffeine prevents hyperoxia-induced functional and structural lung damage in preterm rabbits. *Neonatology* (2016) 109(4):274–81. doi:10.1159/000442937

85. Rath P, Nardiello C, Solaligue DE, Agius R, Mizikova I, Huhn S, et al. Caffeine administration modulates TGF-beta signaling but does not attenuate blunted alveolarization in a hyperoxia-based mouse model of bronchopulmonary dysplasia. *Pediatr Res* (2017) 81:795–805. doi:10.1038/pr.2017.21

86. Dayanim S, Lopez B, Maisonet TM, Grewal S, Londhe VA. Caffeine induces alveolar apoptosis in the hyperoxia-exposed developing mouse lung. *Pediatr Res* (2014) 75(3):395–402. doi:10.1038/pr.2013.233

87. Fehrholz M, Hutten M, Kramer BW, Speer CP, Kunzmann S. Amplification of steroid-mediated SP-B expression by physiological levels of caffeine. *Am J Physiol Lung Cell Mol Physiol* (2014) 306(1):L101–9. doi:10.1152/ajplung. 00257.2013

88. Fehrholz M, Bersani I, Kramer BW, Speer CP, Kunzmann S. Synergistic effect of caffeine and glucocorticoids on expression of surfactant protein B (SP-B) mRNA. *PLoS One* (2012) 7(12):e51575. doi:10.1371/journal. pone.0051575

89. Fehrholz M, Glaser K, Speer CP, Seidenspinner S, Ottensmeier B, Kunzmann S. Caffeine modulates glucocorticoid-induced expression of CTGF in lung epithelial cells and fibroblasts. *Respir Res* (2017) 18(1):51. doi:10.1186/s12931-017-0535-8

90. ter Horst SA, Wagenaar GT, de Boer E, van Gastelen MA, Meijers JC, Biemond BJ, et al. Pentoxifylline reduces fibrin deposition and prolongs survival in neonatal hyperoxic lung injury. *J Appl Physiol (1985)* (2004) 97(5):2014–9. doi:10.1152/japplphysiol.00452.2004

91. de Visser YP, Walther FJ, Laghmani el H, Steendijk P, Middeldorp M, van der Laarse A, et al. Phosphodiesterase 4 inhibition attenuates persistent heart and lung injury by neonatal hyperoxia in rats. *Am J Physiol Lung Cell Mol Physiol* (2012) 302(1):L56–67. doi:10.1152/ajplung.00041.2011

92. de Visser YP, Walther FJ, Laghmani EH, van Wijngaarden S, Nieuwland K, Wagenaar GT. Phosphodiesterase-4 inhibition attenuates pulmonary inflam-

mation in neonatal lung injury. *Eur Respir J* (2008) 31(3):633–44. doi:10.1183/09031936.00071307

93. Woyda K, Koebrich S, Reiss I, Rudloff S, Pullamsetti SS, Ruhlmann A, et al. Inhibition of phosphodiesterase 4 enhances lung alveolarisation in neonatal mice exposed to hyperoxia. *Eur Respir J* (2009) 33(4):861–70. doi:10.1183/09031936.00109008

94. de Visser YP, Walther FJ, Laghmani el H, Boersma H, van der Laarse A, Wagenaar GT. Sildenafil attenuates pulmonary inflammation and fibrin deposition, mortality and right ventricular hypertrophy in neonatal hyperoxic lung injury. *Respir Res* (2009) 10:30. doi:10.1186/1465-9921-10-30

95. Montani D, Chaumais MC, Guignabert C, Gunther S, Girerd B, Jais X, et al. Targeted therapies in pulmonary arterial hypertension. *Pharmacol Ther* (2014) 141(2):172–91. doi:10.1016/j.pharmthera.2013.10.002

96. Laube M, Amann E, Uhlig U, Yang Y, Fuchs HW, Zemlin M, et al. Inflammatory mediators in tracheal aspirates of preterm infants participating in a randomized trial of inhaled nitric oxide. *PLoS One* (2017) 12(1):e0169352. doi:10.1371/journal.pone.0169352

97. Barrington KJ, Finer N, Pennaforte T. Inhaled nitric oxide for respiratory failure in preterm infants. *Cochrane Database Syst Rev* (2017) 1:CD000509. doi:10.1002/14651858.CD000509.pub5

98. Gadhia MM, Cutter GR, Abman SH, Kinsella JP. Effects of early inhaled nitric oxide therapy and vitamin A supplementation on the risk for bronchopulmonary dysplasia in premature newborns with respiratory failure. *J Pediatr* (2014) 164(4):744–8. doi:10.1016/j.jpeds.2013.11.040

99. Massaro GD, Massaro D. Postnatal treatment with retinoic acid increases the number of pulmonary alveoli in rats. *Am J Physiol* (1996) 270(2 Pt 1): L305–10.

100. Albertine KH, Dahl MJ, Gonzales LW, Wang ZM, Metcalfe D, Hyde DM, et al. Chronic lung disease in preterm lambs: effect of daily vitamin A treatment on alveolarization. *Am J Physiol Lung Cell Mol Physiol* (2010) 299(1):L59–72. doi:10.1152/ajplung.00380.2009

101. Tyson JE, Wright LL, Oh W, Kennedy KA, Mele L, Ehrenkranz RA, et al. Vitamin A supplementation for extremely-low-birth-weight infants. National Institute of Child Health and Human Development Neonatal Research Network. *N Engl J Med* (1999) 340(25):1962–8. doi:10.1056/NEJM199906243402505

102. Ambalavanan N, Tyson JE, Kennedy KA, Hansen NI, Vohr BR, Wright LL, et al. Vitamin A supplementation for extremely low birth weight infants: outcome at 18 to 22 months. *Pediatrics* (2005) 115(3):e249–54. doi:10.1542/peds.2004-1812

103. Moreira A, Caskey M, Fonseca R, Malloy M, Geary C. Impact of providing vitamin A to the routine pulmonary care of extremely low birth weight infants. *J Matern Fetal Neonatal Med* (2012) 25(1):84–8. doi:10.3109/14767058.2011.561893

104. Ambalavanan N, Kennedy K, Tyson J, Carlo WA. Survey of vitamin A supplementation for extremely-low-birth-weight infants: is clinical practice consistent with the evidence? *J Pediatr* (2004) 145(3):304–7. doi:10.1016/j.jpeds.2004.04.046

105. Kaplan HC, Tabangin ME, McClendon D, Meinzen-Derr J, Margolis PA, Donovan EF. Understanding variation in vitamin A supplementation among NICUs. *Pediatrics* (2010) 126(2):e367–73. doi:10.1542/peds.2009-3085

106. Niedermaier S, Hilgendorff A. Bronchopulmonary dysplasia – an overview about pathophysiologic concepts. *Mol Cell Pediatr* (2015) 2(1):2. doi:10.1186/s40348-015-0013-7

107. Hilgendorff A, O'Reilly MA. Bronchopulmonary dysplasia early changes leading to long-term consequences. *Front Med* (2015) 2:2. doi:10.3389/fmed.2015.00002

108. Shahzad T, Radajewski S, Chao CM, Bellusci S, Ehrhardt H. Pathogenesis of bronchopulmonary dysplasia: when inflammation meets organ development. *Mol Cell Pediatr* (2016) 3(1):23. doi:10.1186/s40348-016-0051-9

109. Kunzmann S, Collins JJ, Kuypers E, Kramer BW. Thrown off balance: the effect of antenatal inflammation on the developing lung and immune system. *Am J Obstet Gynecol* (2013) 208(6):429–37. doi:10.1016/j.ajog.2013.01.008

110. Chao CM, El Agha E, Tiozzo C, Minoo P, Bellusci S. A breath of fresh air on the mesenchyme: impact of impaired mesenchymal development on the pathogenesis of bronchopulmonary dysplasia. *Front Med* (2015) 2:27. doi:10.3389/fmed.2015.00027

111. Mizikova I, Morty RE. The extracellular matrix in bronchopulmonary dysplasia: target and source. *Front Med* (2015) 2:91. doi:10.3389/fmed.2015.00091

112. Domm W, Misra RS, O'Reilly MA. Affect of early life oxygen exposure on proper lung development and response to respiratory viral infections. *Front Med* (2015) 2:55. doi:10.3389/fmed.2015.00055

113. Collins JJ, Thebaud B. Progenitor cells of the distal lung and their potential role in neonatal lung disease. *Birth Defects Res A Clin Mol Teratol* (2014) 100(3):217–26. doi:10.1002/bdra.23227

114. Collins JJ, Thebaud B. Lung mesenchymal stromal cells in development and disease: to serve and protect? *Antioxid Redox Signal* (2014) 21(13):1849–62. doi:10.1089/ars.2013.5781

115. Mobius MA, Rudiger M. Mesenchymal stromal cells in the development and therapy of bronchopulmonary dysplasia. *Mol Cell Pediatr* (2016) 3(1):18. doi:10.1186/s40348-016-0046-6

116. Peng T, Tian Y, Boogerd CJ, Lu MM, Kadzik RS, Stewart KM, et al. Coordination of heart and lung co-development by a multipotent cardiopulmonary progenitor. *Nature* (2013) 500(7464):589–92. doi:10.1038/nature12358

117. Kumar ME, Bogard PE, Espinoza FH, Menke DB, Kingsley DM, Krasnow MA. Mesenchymal cells. Defining a mesenchymal progenitor niche at single-cell resolution. *Science* (2014) 346(6211):1258810. doi:10.1126/science.1258810

118. Sarugaser R, Hanoun L, Keating A, Stanford WL, Davies JE. Human mesenchymal stem cells self-renew and differentiate according to a deterministic hierarchy. *PLoS One* (2009) 4(8):e6498. doi:10.1371/journal.pone.0006498

119. Ntokou A, Klein F, Dontireddy D, Becker S, Bellusci S, Richardson WD, et al. Characterization of the platelet-derived growth factor receptor alpha-positive cell lineage during murine late lung development. *Am J Physiol Lung Cell Mol Physiol* (2015) 309(9):L942–58. doi:10.1152/ajplung.00272.2014

120. El Agha E, Herold S, Al Alam D, Quantius J, MacKenzie B, Carraro G, et al. Fgf10-positive cells represent a progenitor cell population during lung development and postnatally. *Development* (2014) 141(2):296–306. doi:10.1242/dev.099747

121. McGowan SE, McCoy DM. Platelet-derived growth factor-A and sonic hedgehog signaling direct lung fibroblast precursors during alveolar septal formation. *Am J Physiol Lung Cell Mol Physiol* (2013) 305(3):L229–39. doi:10.1152/ajplung.00011.2013

122. Liu L, Kugler MC, Loomis CA, Samdani R, Zhao Z, Chen GJ, et al. Hedgehog signaling in neonatal and adult lung. *Am J Respir Cell Mol Biol* (2013) 48(6):703–10. doi:10.1165/rcmb.2012-0347OC

123. McQualter JL, McCarty RC, Van der Velden J, O'Donoghue RJ, Asselin-Labat ML, Bozinovski S, et al. TGF-beta signaling in stromal cells acts upstream of FGF-10 to regulate epithelial stem cell growth in the adult lung. *Stem Cell Res* (2013) 11(3):1222–33. doi:10.1016/j.scr.2013.08.007

124. Barkauskas CE, Cronce MJ, Rackley CR, Bowie EJ, Keene DR, Stripp BR, et al. Type 2 alveolar cells are stem cells in adult lung. *J Clin Invest* (2013) 123(7):3025–36. doi:10.1172/JCI68782

125. Popova AP, Bozyk PD, Bentley JK, Linn MJ, Goldsmith AM, Schumacher RE, et al. Isolation of tracheal aspirate mesenchymal stromal cells predicts bronchopulmonary dysplasia. *Pediatrics* (2010) 126(5):e1127–33. doi:10.1542/peds.2009-3445

126. Popova AP, Bozyk PD, Goldsmith AM, Linn MJ, Lei J, Bentley JK, et al. Autocrine production of TGF-beta1 promotes myofibroblastic differentiation of neonatal lung mesenchymal stem cells. *Am J Physiol Lung Cell Mol Physiol* (2010) 298(6):L735–43. doi:10.1152/ajplung.00347.2009

127. Popova AP, Bentley JK, Cui TX, Richardson MN, Linn MJ, Lei J, et al. Reduced platelet-derived growth factor receptor expression is a primary feature of human bronchopulmonary dysplasia. *Am J Physiol Lung Cell Mol Physiol* (2014) 307(3):L231–9. doi:10.1152/ajplung.00342.2013

128. Chao CM, Yahya F, Moiseenko A, Tiozzo C, Shrestha A, Ahmadvand N, et al. Fgf10 deficiency is causative for lethality in a mouse model of bronchopulmonary dysplasia. *J Pathol* (2017) 241(1):91–103. doi:10.1002/path.4834

129. Volckaert T, Dill E, Campbell A, Tiozzo C, Majka S, Bellusci S, et al. Parabronchial smooth muscle constitutes an airway epithelial stem cell niche in the mouse lung after injury. *J Clin Invest* (2011) 121(11):4409–19. doi:10.1172/JCI58097

130. Volckaert T, De Langhe S. Lung epithelial stem cells and their niches: Fgf10 takes center stage. *Fibrogenesis Tissue Repair* (2014) 7:8. doi:10.1186/1755-1536-7-8

131. Alphonse RS, Vadivel A, Fung M, Shelley WC, Critser PJ, Ionescu L, et al. Existence, functional impairment, and lung repair potential of endothelial colony-forming cells in oxygen-induced arrested alveolar growth. *Circulation* (2014) 129(21):2144–57. doi:10.1161/CIRCULATIONAHA.114.009124

132. Bertagnolli M, Nuyt AM, Thebaud B, Luu TM. Endothelial progenitor cells as prognostic markers of preterm birth-associated complications. *Stem Cells Transl Med* (2017) 6(1):7–13. doi:10.5966/sctm.2016-0085

133. van Haaften T, Byrne R, Bonnet S, Rochefort GY, Akabutu J, Bouchentouf M, et al. Airway delivery of mesenchymal stem cells prevents arrested alveolar growth in neonatal lung injury in rats. *Am J Respir Crit Care Med* (2009) 180(11):1131–42. doi:10.1164/rccm.200902-0179OC

134. Pierro M, Ionescu L, Montemurro T, Vadivel A, Weissmann G, Oudit G, et al. Short-term, long-term and paracrine effect of human umbilical cord-derived stem cells in lung injury prevention and repair in experimental bronchopulmonary dysplasia. *Thorax* (2013) 68(5):475–84. doi:10.1136/thoraxjnl-2012-202323

135. Ionescu L, Byrne RN, van Haaften T, Vadivel A, Alphonse RS, Rey-Parra GJ, et al. Stem cell conditioned medium improves acute lung injury in mice: in vivo evidence for stem cell paracrine action. *Am J Physiol Lung Cell Mol Physiol* (2012) 303(11):L967–77. doi:10.1152/ajplung.00144.2011

136. Mitsialis SA, Kourembanas S. Stem cell-based therapies for the newborn lung and brain: possibilities and challenges. *Semin Perinatol* (2016) 40(3):138–51. doi:10.1053/j.semperi.2015.12.002

137. Thebaud B, Stewart DJ. Exosomes: cell garbage can, therapeutic carrier, or trojan horse? *Circulation* (2012) 126(22):2553–5. doi:10.1161/CIRCULATIONAHA.112.146738

138. Mobius MA, Thebaud B. Stem cells and their mediators – next generation therapy for bronchopulmonary dysplasia. *Front Med* (2015) 2:50. doi:10.3389/fmed.2015.00050

139. O'Reilly M, Thebaud B. Cell-based therapies for neonatal lung disease. *Cell Tissue Res* (2017) 367(3):737–45. doi:10.1007/s00441-016-2517-4

140. Tan SY, Krasnow MA. Developmental origin of lung macrophage diversity. *Development* (2016) 143(8):1318–27. doi:10.1242/dev.129122

141. Johansson A, Lundborg M, Skold CM, Lundahl J, Tornling G, Eklund A, et al. Functional, morphological, and phenotypical differences between rat alveolar and interstitial macrophages. *Am J Respir Cell Mol Biol* (1997) 16(5):582–8. doi:10.1165/ajrcmb.16.5.9160840

142. Jones CV, Williams TM, Walker KA, Dickinson H, Sakkal S, Rumballe BA, et al. M2 macrophage polarisation is associated with alveolar formation during postnatal lung development. *Respir Res* (2013) 14:41. doi:10.1186/1465-9921-14-41

143. Blackwell TS, Hipps AN, Yamamoto Y, Han W, Barham WJ, Ostrowski MC, et al. NF-kappaB signaling in fetal lung macrophages disrupts airway morphogenesis. *J Immunol* (2011) 187(5):2740–7. doi:10.4049/jimmunol.1101495

144. Eggenhofer E, Hoogduijn MJ. Mesenchymal stem cell-educated macrophages. *Transplant Res* (2012) 1(1):12. doi:10.1186/2047-1440-1-12

145. Melief SM, Geutskens SB, Fibbe WE, Roelofs H. Multipotent stromal cells skew monocytes towards an anti-inflammatory function: the link with key immunoregulatory molecules. *Haematologica* (2013) 98(9):e121–2. doi:10.3324/haematol.2012.078055

146. Melief SM, Geutskens SB, Fibbe WE, Roelofs H. Multipotent stromal cells skew monocytes towards an anti-inflammatory interleukin-10-producing phenotype by production of interleukin-6. *Haematologica* (2013) 98(6):888–95. doi:10.3324/haematol.2012.078055

147. Bernardo ME, Fibbe WE. Mesenchymal stromal cells: sensors and switchers of inflammation. *Cell Stem Cell* (2013) 13(4):392–402. doi:10.1016/j.stem.2013.09.006

148. Marsland BJ, Gollwitzer ES. Host-microorganism interactions in lung diseases. *Nat Rev Immunol* (2014) 14(12):827–35. doi:10.1038/nri3769

149. Lohmann P, Luna RA, Hollister EB, Devaraj S, Mistretta TA, Welty SE, et al. The airway microbiome of intubated premature infants: characteristics and changes that predict the development of bronchopulmonary dysplasia. *Pediatr Res* (2014) 76(3):294–301. doi:10.1038/pr.2014.85

150. Gantert M, Been JV, Gavilanes AW, Garnier Y, Zimmermann LJ, Kramer BW. Chorioamnionitis: a multiorgan disease of the fetus? *J Perinatol* (2010) 30(Suppl):S21–30. doi:10.1038/jp.2010.96

151. Surana NK, Kasper DL. Deciphering the tete-a-tete between the microbiota and the immune system. *J Clin Invest* (2014) 124(10):4197–203. doi:10.1172/JCI72332

152. Lal CV, Travers C, Aghai ZH, Eipers P, Jilling T, Halloran B, et al. The airway microbiome at birth. *Sci Rep* (2016) 6:31023. doi:10.1038/srep31023

153. Novitsky A, Tuttle D, Locke RG, Saiman L, Mackley A, Paul DA. Prolonged early antibiotic use and bronchopulmonary dysplasia in very low birth weight infants. *Am J Perinatol* (2015) 32(1):43–8. doi:10.1055/s-0034-1373844

154. Cantey JB, Huffman LW, Subramanian A, Marshall AS, Ballard AR, Lefevre C, et al. Antibiotic exposure and risk for death or bronchopulmonary dysplasia in very low birth weight infants. *J Pediatr* (2017) 181:289–93.e1. doi:10.1016/j.jpeds.2016.11.002

155. Gollwitzer ES, Saglani S, Trompette A, Yadava K, Sherburn R, McCoy KD, et al. Lung microbiota promotes tolerance to allergens in neonates via PD-L1. *Nat Med* (2014) 20(6):642–7. doi:10.1038/nm.3568

156. Segal LN, Clemente JC, Wu BG, Wikoff WR, Gao Z, Li Y, et al. Randomised, double-blind, placebo-controlled trial with azithromycin selects for anti-inflammatory microbial metabolites in the emphysematous lung. *Thorax* (2017) 72(1):13–22. doi:10.1136/thoraxjnl-2016-208599

157. Marsland BJ. Regulating inflammation with microbial metabolites. *Nat Med* (2016) 22(6):581–3. doi:10.1038/nm.4117

158. Zelante T, Iannitti RG, Cunha C, De Luca A, Giovannini G, Pieraccini G, et al. Tryptophan catabolites from microbiota engage aryl hydrocarbon receptor and balance mucosal reactivity via interleukin-22. *Immunity* (2013) 39(2):372–85. doi:10.1016/j.immuni.2013.08.003

159. Pellaton C, Nutten S, Thierry AC, Boudousquie C, Barbier N, Blanchard C, et al. Intragastric and intranasal administration of *Lactobacillus paracasei* NCC2461 modulates allergic airway inflammation in mice. *Int J Inflam* (2012) 2012:686739. doi:10.1155/2012/686739

160. Smith C, Egunsola O, Choonara I, Kotecha S, Jacqz-Aigrain E, Sammons H. Use and safety of azithromycin in neonates: a systematic review. *BMJ Open* (2015) 5(12):e008194. doi:10.1136/bmjopen-2015-008194

161. Ballard HO, Shook LA, Bernard P, Anstead MI, Kuhn R, Whitehead V, et al. Use of azithromycin for the prevention of bronchopulmonary dysplasia in preterm infants: a randomized, double-blind, placebo controlled trial. *Pediatr Pulmonol* (2011) 46(2):111–8. doi:10.1002/ppul.21352

162. Ozdemir R, Erdeve O, Dizdar EA, Oguz SS, Uras N, Saygan S, et al. Clarithromycin in preventing bronchopulmonary dysplasia in Ureaplasma urealyticum-positive preterm infants. *Pediatrics* (2011) 128(6):e1496–501. doi:10.1542/peds.2011-1350

163. Yun Y, Srinivas G, Kuenzel S, Linnenbrink M, Alnahas S, Bruce KD, et al. Environmentally determined differences in the murine lung microbiota and their relation to alveolar architecture. *PLoS One* (2014) 9(12):e113466. doi:10.1371/journal.pone.0113466

164. Mitchell AB, Oliver BG, Glanville AR. Translational aspects of the human respiratory virome. *Am J Respir Crit Care Med* (2016) 194(12):1458–64. doi:10.1164/rccm.201606-1278CI

165. Nguyen LD, Viscogliosi E, Delhaes L. The lung mycobiome: an emerging field of the human respiratory microbiome. *Front Microbiol* (2015) 6:89. doi:10.3389/fmicb.2015.00089

166. Kepert I, Fonseca J, Muller C, Milger K, Hochwind K, Kostric M, et al. D-tryptophan from probiotic bacteria influences the gut microbiome and allergic airway disease. *J Allergy Clin Immunol* (2017) 139(5):1525–35. doi:10.1016/j.jaci.2016.09.003

167. Richter J, Jimenez J, Nagatomo T, Toelen J, Brady P, Salaets T, et al. Proton-pump inhibitor omeprazole attenuates hyperoxia induced lung injury. *J Transl Med* (2016) 14(1):247. doi:10.1186/s12967-016-1009-3

168. Shivanna B, Maity S, Zhang S, Patel A, Jiang W, Wang L, et al. Gene expression profiling identifies cell proliferation and inflammation as the predominant pathways regulated by aryl hydrocarbon receptor in primary human fetal lung cells exposed to hyperoxia. *Toxicol Sci* (2016) 152(1):155–68. doi:10.1093/toxsci/kfw071

169. Walsh MC, Szefler S, Davis J, Allen M, Van Marter L, Abman S, et al. Summary proceedings from the bronchopulmonary dysplasia group. *Pediatrics* (2006) 117(3 Pt 2):S52–6. doi:10.1542/peds.2005-0620I

170. Nold MF, Mangan NE, Rudloff I, Cho SX, Shariatian N, Samarasinghe TD, et al. Interleukin-1 receptor antagonist prevents murine bronchopulmonary dysplasia induced by perinatal inflammation and

170. hyperoxia. *Proc Natl Acad Sci U S A* (2013) 110(35):14384–9. doi:10.1073/pnas. 1306859110

171. Rudloff I, Cho SX, Bui CB, McLean C, Veldman A, Berger PJ, et al. Refining anti-inflammatory therapy strategies for bronchopulmonary dysplasia. *J Cell Mol Med* (2016). doi:10.1111/jcmm.13044

172. Liao J, Kapadia VS, Brown LS, Cheong N, Longoria C, Mija D, et al. The NLRP3 inflammasome is critically involved in the development of bronchopulmonary dysplasia. *Nat Commun* (2015) 6:8977. doi:10.1038/ncomms9977

173. Kallapur SG, Nitsos I, Moss TJ, Polglase GR, Pillow JJ, Cheah FC, et al. IL-1 mediates pulmonary and systemic inflammatory responses to chorioamnionitis induced by lipopolysaccharide. *Am J Respir Crit Care Med* (2009) 179(10):955–61. doi:10.1164/rccm.200811-1728OC

174. Kakkera DK, Siddiq MM, Parton LA. Interleukin-1 balance in the lungs of preterm infants who develop bronchopulmonary dysplasia. *Biol Neonate* (2005) 87(2):82–90. doi:10.1159/000081504

175. Doyle LW, Ehrenkranz RA, Halliday HL. Early (< 8 days) postnatal corticosteroids for preventing chronic lung disease in preterm infants. *Cochrane Database Syst Rev* (2014) 5:CD001146. doi:10.1002/14651858.CD001146. pub4

176. Doyle LW, Ehrenkranz RA, Halliday HL. Late (> 7 days) postnatal corticosteroids for chronic lung disease in preterm infants. *Cochrane Database Syst Rev* (2014) 5:CD001145. doi:10.1002/14651858.CD001145.pub3

177. Onland W, De Jaegere AP, Offringa M, van Kaam A. Systemic corticosteroid regimens for prevention of bronchopulmonary dysplasia in preterm infants. *Cochrane Database Syst Rev* (2017) 1:CD010941. doi:10.1002/14651858. CD010941.pub2

178. Onland W, Offringa M, van Kaam A. Late (>/= 7 days) inhalation corticosteroids to reduce bronchopulmonary dysplasia in preterm infants. *Cochrane Database Syst Rev* (2012) 4:CD002311. doi:10.1002/14651858.CD002311. pub3

179. Bassler D, Plavka R, Shinwell ES, Hallman M, Jarreau PH, Carnielli V, et al. Early inhaled budesonide for the prevention of bronchopulmonary dysplasia. *N Engl J Med* (2015) 373(16):1497–506. doi:10.1056/NEJMoa1501917

180. Shah VS, Ohlsson A, Halliday HL, Dunn M. Early administration of inhaled corticosteroids for preventing chronic lung disease in very low birth weight preterm neonates. *Cochrane Database Syst Rev* (2017) 1:CD001969. doi:10.1002/14651858.CD001969.pub4

181. Bassler D. Inhaled budesonide for the prevention of bronchopulmonary dysplasia. *J Matern Fetal Neonatal Med* (2016):1–3. doi:10.1080/14767058. 2016.1248937

182. Shinwell ES, Portnov I, Meerpohl JJ, Karen T, Bassler D. Inhaled corticosteroids for bronchopulmonary dysplasia: a meta-analysis. *Pediatrics* (2016) 138(6):e20162511. doi:10.1542/peds.2016-2511

183. Barrette AM, Roberts JK, Chapin C, Egan EA, Segal MR, Oses-Prieto JA, et al. Antiinflammatory effects of budesonide in human fetal lung. *Am J Respir Cell Mol Biol* (2016) 55(5):623–32. doi:10.1165/rcmb.2016-0068OC

184. Kuypers E, Collins JJ, Kramer BW, Ofman G, Nitsos I, Pillow JJ, et al. Intra-amniotic LPS and antenatal betamethasone: inflammation and maturation in preterm lamb lungs. *Am J Physiol Lung Cell Mol Physiol* (2012) 302(4):L380–9. doi:10.1152/ajplung.00338.2011

185. Collins JJ, Kuypers E, Nitsos I, Pillow JJ, Polglase GR, Kemp MW, et al. LPS-induced chorioamnionitis and antenatal corticosteroids modulate Shh signaling in the ovine fetal lung. *Am J Physiol Lung Cell Mol Physiol* (2012) 303(9):L778–87. doi:10.1152/ajplung.00280.2011

186. Collins JJ, Kunzmann S, Kuypers E, Kemp MW, Speer CP, Newnham JP, et al. Antenatal glucocorticoids counteract LPS changes in TGF-beta pathway and caveolin-1 in ovine fetal lung. *Am J Physiol Lung Cell Mol Physiol* (2013) 304(6):L438–44. doi:10.1152/ajplung.00251.2012

187. Kuypers E, Willems MG, Collins JJ, Wolfs TG, Nitsos I, Jane Pillow J, et al. Altered canonical Wingless-Int signaling in the ovine fetal lung after exposure to intra-amniotic lipopolysaccharide and antenatal betamethasone. *Pediatr Res* (2014) 75(2):281–7. doi:10.1038/pr.2013.226

188. Bancalari E, Jain D, Jobe AH. Prevention of bronchopulmonary dysplasia: are intratracheal steroids with surfactant a magic bullet? *Am J Respir Crit Care Med* (2016) 193(1):12–3. doi:10.1164/rccm.201509-1830ED

189. Nardiello C, Mizikova I, Silva DM, Ruiz-Camp J, Mayer K, Vadasz I, et al. Standardisation of oxygen exposure in the development of mouse models for bronchopulmonary dysplasia. *Dis Model Mech* (2017) 10(2):185–96. doi:10.1242/dmm.027086

190. Berkelhamer SK, Kim GA, Radder JE, Wedgwood S, Czech L, Steinhorn RH, et al. Developmental differences in hyperoxia-induced oxidative stress and cellular responses in the murine lung. *Free Radic Biol Med* (2013) 61:51–60. doi:10.1016/j.freeradbiomed.2013.03.003

191. Datta A, Kim GA, Taylor JM, Gugino SF, Farrow KN, Schumacker PT, et al. Mouse lung development and NOX1 induction during hyperoxia are developmentally regulated and mitochondrial ROS dependent. *Am J Physiol Lung Cell Mol Physiol* (2015) 309(4):L369–77. doi:10.1152/ajplung.00176.2014

192. Zhang S, Patel A, Chu C, Jiang W, Wang L, Welty SE, et al. Aryl hydrocarbon receptor is necessary to protect fetal human pulmonary microvascular endothelial cells against hyperoxic injury: mechanistic roles of antioxidant enzymes and RelB. *Toxicol Appl Pharmacol* (2015) 286(2):92–101. doi:10.1016/j.taap.2015.03.023

193. Delaney C, Wright RH, Tang JR, Woods C, Villegas L, Sherlock L, et al. Lack of EC-SOD worsens alveolar and vascular development in a neonatal mouse model of bleomycin-induced bronchopulmonary dysplasia and pulmonary hypertension. *Pediatr Res* (2015) 78(6):634–40. doi:10.1038/pr.2015.166

194. Sampath V, Garland JS, Helbling D, Dimmock D, Mulrooney NP, Simpson PM, et al. Antioxidant response genes sequence variants and BPD susceptibility in VLBW infants. *Pediatr Res* (2015) 77(3):477–83. doi:10.1038/pr.2014.200

195. Berkelhamer SK, Farrow KN. Developmental regulation of antioxidant enzymes and their impact on neonatal lung disease. *Antioxid Redox Signal* (2014) 21(13):1837–48. doi:10.1089/ars.2013.5515

196. Gnanalingham MG, Mostyn A, Gardner DS, Stephenson T, Symonds ME. Developmental regulation of the lung in preparation for life after birth: hormonal and nutritional manipulation of local glucocorticoid action and uncoupling protein-2. *J Endocrinol* (2006) 188(3):375–86. doi:10.1677/joe.1.06530

197. Mostyn A, Wilson V, Dandrea J, Yakubu DP, Budge H, Alves-Guerra MC, et al. Ontogeny and nutritional manipulation of mitochondrial protein abundance in adipose tissue and the lungs of postnatal sheep. *Br J Nutr* (2003) 90(2):323–8. doi:10.1079/BJN2003912

198. Agrawal A, Mabalirajan U. Rejuvenating cellular respiration for optimizing respiratory function: targeting mitochondria. *Am J Physiol Lung Cell Mol Physiol* (2016) 310(2):L103–13. doi:10.1152/ajplung.00320.2015

199. Schumacker PT, Gillespie MN, Nakahira K, Choi AM, Crouser ED, Piantadosi CA, et al. Mitochondria in lung biology and pathology: more than just a powerhouse. *Am J Physiol Lung Cell Mol Physiol* (2014) 306(11):L962–74. doi:10.1152/ajplung.00073.2014

200. Ratner V, Starkov A, Matsiukevich D, Polin RA, Ten VS. Mitochondrial dysfunction contributes to alveolar developmental arrest in hyperoxia-exposed mice. *Am J Respir Cell Mol Biol* (2009) 40(5):511–8. doi:10.1165/rcmb.2008-0341RC

201. Ratner V, Sosunov SA, Niatsetskaya ZV, Utkina-Sosunova IV, Ten VS. Mechanical ventilation causes pulmonary mitochondrial dysfunction and delayed alveolarization in neonatal mice. *Am J Respir Cell Mol Biol* (2013) 49(6):943–50. doi:10.1165/rcmb.2012-0172OC

202. Vohwinkel CU, Lecuona E, Sun H, Sommer N, Vadasz I, Chandel NS, et al. Elevated CO(2) levels cause mitochondrial dysfunction and impair cell proliferation. *J Biol Chem* (2011) 286(43):37067–76. doi:10.1074/jbc. M111.290056

203. Vadivel A, Alphonse RS, Ionescu L, Machado DS, O'Reilly M, Eaton F, et al. Exogenous hydrogen sulfide (H2S) protects alveolar growth in experimental O2-induced neonatal lung injury. *PLoS One* (2014) 9(3):e90965. doi:10.1371/ journal.pone.0090965

204. Shivanna B, Zhang S, Patel A, Jiang W, Wang L, Welty SE, et al. Omeprazole attenuates pulmonary aryl hydrocarbon receptor activation and potentiates hyperoxia-induced developmental lung injury in newborn mice. *Toxicol Sci* (2015) 148(1):276–87. doi:10.1093/toxsci/kfv183

205. Islam MN, Das SR, Emin MT, Wei M, Sun L, Westphalen K, et al. Mitochondrial transfer from bone-marrow-derived stromal cells to pulmonary alveoli protects against acute lung injury. *Nat Med* (2012) 18(5):759–65. doi:10.1038/nm.2736

206. Kunzmann S, Collins JJ, Yang Y, Uhlig S, Kallapur SG, Speer CP, et al. Antenatal inflammation reduces expression of caveolin-1 and influences multiple signaling pathways in preterm fetal lungs. *Am J Respir Cell Mol Biol* (2011) 45(5):969–76. doi:10.1165/rcmb.2010-0519OC

207. Husari AW, Dbaibo GS, Bitar H, Khayat A, Panjarian S, Nasser M, et al. Apoptosis and the activity of ceramide, Bax and Bcl-2 in the lungs of neonatal rats exposed to limited and prolonged hyperoxia. *Respir Res* (2006) 7:100. doi:10.1186/1465-9921-7-100

208. Tibboel J, Joza S, Reiss I, de Jongste JC, Post M. Amelioration of hyperoxia-induced lung injury using a sphingolipid-based intervention. *Eur Respir J* (2013) 42(3):776–84. doi:10.1183/09031936.00092212

209. Tibboel J, Reiss I, de Jongste JC, Post M. Sphingolipids in lung growth and repair. *Chest* (2014) 145(1):120–8. doi:10.1378/chest.13-0967

210. Preuss S, Stadelmann S, Omam FD, Scheiermann J, Winoto-Morbach S, von Bismarck P, et al. Inositol-trisphosphate reduces alveolar apoptosis and pulmonary edema in neonatal lung injury. *Am J Respir Cell Mol Biol* (2012) 47(2):158–69. doi:10.1165/rcmb.2011-0262OC

211. Sureshbabu A, Syed M, Das P, Janer C, Pryhuber G, Rahman A, et al. Inhibition of regulatory-associated protein of mechanistic target of rapamycin prevents hyperoxia-induced lung injury by enhancing autophagy and reducing apoptosis in neonatal mice. *Am J Respir Cell Mol Biol* (2016) 55(5):722–35. doi:10.1165/rcmb.2015-0349OC

212. Valenti P, Antonini G. Lactoferrin: an important host defence against microbial and viral attack. *Cell Mol Life Sci* (2005) 62(22):2576–87. doi:10.1007/s00018-005-5372-0

213. Sharma D, Murki A, Murki S, Pratap OT. Use of lactoferrin in the newborn: where do we stand? *J Matern Fetal Neonatal Med* (2015) 28(15):1774–8. doi:10.3109/14767058.2014.968548

214. Sharma D, Shastri S, Sharma P. Role of lactoferrin in neonatal care: a systematic review. *J Matern Fetal Neonatal Med* (2016):1–13. doi:10.1080/14767058.2016.1220531

215. McElrath TF, Hecht JL, Dammann O, Boggess K, Onderdonk A, Markenson G, et al. Pregnancy disorders that lead to delivery before the 28th week of gestation: an epidemiologic approach to classification. *Am J Epidemiol* (2008) 168(9):980–9. doi:10.1093/aje/kwn202

216. Shibuya M. Structure and function of VEGF/VEGF-receptor system involved in angiogenesis. *Cell Struct Funct* (2001) 26(1):25–35. doi:10.1247/csf.26.25

217. Maynard SE, Min JY, Merchan J, Lim KH, Li J, Mondal S, et al. Excess placental soluble fms-like tyrosine kinase 1 (sFlt1) may contribute to endothelial dysfunction, hypertension, and proteinuria in preeclampsia. *J Clin Invest* (2003) 111(5):649–58. doi:10.1172/JCI17189

218. Vuorela P, Helske S, Hornig C, Alitalo K, Weich H, Halmesmaki E. Amniotic fluid – soluble vascular endothelial growth factor receptor-1 in preeclampsia. *Obstet Gynecol* (2000) 95(3):353–7. doi:10.1097/00006250-200003000-00008

219. Ota C, Baarsma HA, Wagner DE, Hilgendorff A, Konigshoff M. Linking bronchopulmonary dysplasia to adult chronic lung diseases: role of WNT signaling. *Mol Cell Pediatr* (2016) 3(1):34. doi:10.1186/s40348-016-0062-6

220. Frank DB, Peng T, Zepp JA, Snitow M, Vincent TL, Penkala IJ, et al. Emergence of a wave of Wnt signaling that regulates lung alveologenesis by controlling epithelial self-renewal and differentiation. *Cell Rep* (2016) 17(9):2312–25. doi:10.1016/j.celrep.2016.11.001

221. Peng T, Frank DB, Kadzik RS, Morley MP, Rathi KS, Wang T, et al. Hedgehog actively maintains adult lung quiescence and regulates repair and regeneration. *Nature* (2015) 526(7574):578–82. doi:10.1038/nature14984

222. Yang L, Liu C, Dang H, Fang F, Tan L, Zhao P, et al. Substance P attenuates hyperoxiainduced lung injury in neonatal rats. *Mol Med Rep* (2014) 9(2):595–9. doi:10.3892/mmr.2013.1809

223. Dang H, Wang S, Yang L, Fang F, Xu F. Upregulation of Shh and Ptc1 in hyperoxiainduced acute lung injury in neonatal rats. *Mol Med Rep* (2012) 6(2):297–302. doi:10.3892/mmr.2012.929

224. Vadivel A, Alphonse RS, Collins JJ, van Haaften T, O'Reilly M, Eaton F, et al. The axonal guidance cue semaphorin 3C contributes to alveolar growth and repair. *PLoS One* (2013) 8(6):e67225. doi:10.1371/journal.pone.0067225

225. Vadivel A, van Haaften T, Alphonse RS, Rey-Parra GJ, Ionescu L, Haromy A, et al. Critical role of the axonal guidance cue EphrinB2 in lung growth, angiogenesis, and repair. *Am J Respir Crit Care Med* (2012) 185(5):564–74. doi:10.1164/rccm.201103-0545OC

226. Sucre JM, Wilkinson D, Vijayaraj P, Paul M, Dunn B, Alva-Ornelas JA, et al. A three-dimensional human model of the fibroblast activation that accompanies bronchopulmonary dysplasia identifies Notch-mediated pathophysiology. *Am J Physiol Lung Cell Mol Physiol* (2016) 310(10):L889–98. doi:10.1152/ajplung.00446.2015

227. Tsao PN, Matsuoka C, Wei SC, Sato A, Sato S, Hasegawa K, et al. Epithelial Notch signaling regulates lung alveolar morphogenesis and airway epithelial integrity. *Proc Natl Acad Sci U S A* (2016) 113(29):8242–7. doi:10.1073/pnas.1511236113

228. Vadivel A, Alphonse RS, Etches N, van Haaften T, Collins JJ, O'Reilly M, et al. Hypoxia inducible factors promotes alveolar development and regeneration. *Am J Respir Cell Mol Biol* (2013) 50(1):96–105. doi:10.1165/rcmb.2012-0250OC

229. Du Y, Guo M, Whitsett JA, Xu Y. 'LungGENS': a web-based tool for mapping single-cell gene expression in the developing lung. *Thorax* (2015) 70(11):1092–4. doi:10.1136/thoraxjnl-2015-207035

230. Du Y, Kitzmiller JA, Sridharan A, Perl AK, Bridges JP, Misra RS, et al. Lung Gene Expression Analysis (LGEA): an integrative web portal for comprehensive gene expression data analysis in lung development. *Thorax* (2017) 72(5):481–4. doi:10.1136/thoraxjnl-2016-209598

231. Yu KH, Li J, Snyder M, Shaw GM, O'Brodovich HM. The genetic predisposition to bronchopulmonary dysplasia. *Curr Opin Pediatr* (2016) 28(3):318–23. doi:10.1097/MOP.0000000000000344

232. Lal CV, Ambalavanan N. Genetic predisposition to bronchopulmonary dysplasia. *Semin Perinatol* (2015) 39(8):584–91. doi:10.1053/j.semperi.2015.09.004

233. Nardiello C, Morty RE. MicroRNA in late lung development and bronchopulmonary dysplasia: the need to demonstrate causality. *Mol Cell Pediatr* (2016) 3(1):19. doi:10.1186/s40348-016-0047-5

234. Olave N, Lal CV, Halloran B, Pandit K, Cuna AC, Faye-Petersen OM, et al. Regulation of alveolar septation by microRNA-489. *Am J Physiol Lung Cell Mol Physiol* (2016) 310(5):L476–87. doi:10.1152/ajplung.00145.2015

235. Poon AW, Ma EX, Vadivel A, Jung S, Khoja Z, Stephens L, et al. Impact of bronchopulmonary dysplasia on brain and retina. *Biol Open* (2016) 5(4):475–83. doi:10.1242/bio.017665

Close Association Between Platelet Biogenesis and Alveolarization of the Developing Lung

Xueyu Chen[1], Junyan Zhong[1], Dongshan Han[1], Fang Yao[2], Jie Zhao[2], Gerry. T. M. Wagenaar[3], Chuanzhong Yang[2]* and Frans J. Walther[4,5]*

[1] Laboratory of Neonatology, Department of Neonatology, Affiliated Shenzhen Maternity and Child Healthcare Hospital, Southern Medical University, Shenzhen, China, [2] Department of Neonatology, Shenzhen Maternity and Child Healthcare Hospital, The First School of Clinical Medicine, Southern Medical University, Shenzhen, China, [3] Faculty of Science, VU University Amsterdam, Amsterdam, Netherlands, [4] Department of Pediatrics, David Geffen School of Medicine, University of California, Los Angeles, Los Angeles, CA, United States, [5] The Lundquist Institute for Biomedical Innovation at Harbor-UCLA Medical Center, Torrance, CA, United States

*Correspondence:
Chuanzhong Yang
yangczgd@163.com
Frans J. Walther
fjwalther@ucla.edu

Bronchopulmonary dysplasia (BPD) is a neonatal chronic lung disease characterized by an arrest in alveolar and vascular development. BPD is secondary to lung immaturity, ventilator-induced lung injury, and exposure to hyperoxia in extremely premature infants, leading to a lifelong impairment of lung function. Recent studies indicate that the lung plays an important role in platelet biogenesis. However, the dynamic change of platelet production during lung development and BPD pathogenesis remains to be elucidated. We investigated the dynamic change of platelet parameters in extremely premature infants during BPD development, and in newborn rats during their normal development from birth to adulthood. We further studied the effect of hyperoxia exposure on platelet production and concomitant pulmonary maldevelopment in an experimental BPD rat model induced by prolonged exposure to hyperoxia. We detected a physiological increase in platelet count from birth to 36 weeks postmenstrual age in extremely premature infants, but platelet counts in extremely premature infants who developed BPD were persistently lower than gestational age-matched controls. In line with clinical findings, exposure to hyperoxia significantly decreased the platelet count in neonatal rats. Lung morphometry analysis demonstrated that platelet counts stabilized with the completion of lung alveolarization in rats. Our findings indicate a close association between platelet biogenesis and alveolarization in the developing lung. This phenomenon might explain the reduced platelet count in extremely premature infants with BPD.

Keywords: lung development, neonatal lung injury, mean platelet volume, platelet distribution width, hyperoxia, platelet counts

INTRODUCTION

Bronchopulmonary dysplasia (BPD) is one of the most common complications of prematurity and can lead to chronic lung disease with long-term respiratory insufficiency (1). Despite advances in perinatal care, BPD continues to affect up to 40% of extremely premature infants (2). BPD is histologically characterized by arrested lung development as a result of a complex process in which lung immaturity, ventilator-induced lung injury, and exposure to hyperoxia play major roles (3). There is a growing body of knowledge about the various mechanisms underlying BPD pathogenesis

(4). However, therapeutic approaches based on these mechanisms are far from being effective in clinical practice, indicating that these mechanisms probably do not operate in isolation. As the pathogenesis of lung damage in infants with BPD is not completely understood, other possible causal factors need to be elucidated (5).

Recent studies elegantly unravel the close interplay between platelet biogenesis and lung development. Tsukiji et al. report that platelet-derived CLEC-2 signals activate platelets through spleen tyrosine kinase, inducing the release of TGF-β driving the differentiation of mesothelial cells into alveolar duct myofibroblasts that are critical to primary septum formation and elastogenesis in alveolarization of the lung (6). Rafii et al. demonstrated that activated platelets release stromal-cell-derived factor and stimulate the expression of SDF-1 receptors on pulmonary capillary endothelial cells, subsequently enhancing the proliferation of alveolar epithelial cells and neo-alveolarization (7). The lungs are a major site for platelet biogenesis in humans and rodents and contribute ~50% of the total platelet production (8–12).

Little is known about the dynamic changes in platelets during the complex process that leads to BPD in extremely premature infants. Besides, the impact of clinical oxygen supplementation exposure on platelet biogenesis is unclear. We hypothesize that platelets play an important role in normal lung development and that disturbed platelet biogenesis might contribute to disrupted lung development and BPD pathogenesis. In this study, we first investigated the dynamic change of platelet parameters in a cohort of extremely premature infants within the time window of BPD development, and in newborn rats during their normal development until young adults. We also used an experimental BPD rat model to evaluate the effect of hyperoxia exposure on platelet production and aberrant pulmonary development.

METHODS AND MATERIALS
Clinical Study
A retrospective study was performed at the Neonatal Intensive Care Unit (NICU) of the Shenzhen Maternity and Child Healthcare Hospital after approval by the Institutional Ethical Committee [SFYLS (2019)-119]. The acquirement of informed consent was waived given that no personal data were explicitly reported. Since premature infants with a younger gestational age have an increased chance to develop BPD, we only included extremely premature infants with a gestational age ≤28 weeks and/or a birth weight ≤1,000 grams. BPD was diagnosed as a requirement of supplemental oxygen at 36 weeks' postmenstrual age or discharge.

Platelet parameters were collected from complete blood counts (CBC) in the 1st week, 2nd week, 4th week, and 8th week after birth. CBC testing was performed on a Mindray 5390 analyzer (Shenzhen, China), using blood samples obtained from arterial and venipuncture or a central catheter.

Animal Study
All animal procedures in this study were approved by the Institutional Animal Care and Use Committee of Shenzhen Institutes of Advanced Technology of the Chinese Academy of Sciences. Newborn pups from 9 pregnant Wistar rats were randomized into 8 groups: an experimental BPD group ($N = 10$) and 7 control groups (raised in room air, $N = 10$ for each group) sacrificed on postnatal day 3, 6, 10, 20, 30, 60, and at adulthood (day 90). Experimental BPD was induced by hyperoxia exposure as previously reported (13). Briefly, newborn pups were raised in a Plexiglas chamber filled with 95% oxygen for 10 days. Pups were anesthetized at the designated day by intraperitoneal injection of pentobarbital (40 mg/kg). All blood samples were drawn from the abdominal aorta, mixed with EDTA and analyzed using a Mindray 5390 analyzer (Shenzhen, China) to acquire platelet parameters. Lung tissue was fixed *in situ* under constant pressure of 27 cmH$_2$O for 6 min with formalin as previously reported (13). Hereafter, the thorax was opened, the lungs were removed, fixed additionally in formalin for 24 h, embedded in paraffin and sectioned for hematoxylin and eosin (HE) staining.

Lung Morphometry
Mean linear intercept (MLI) was used to assess lung development status. At least 1,000 alveoli per animal were measured to calculate the MLI. Briefly, 10 non-overlapping photos of lung tissues were made with an Olympus CX43 microscope (Tokyo, Japan) at 200x magnification. Structures, including big vessels and airways, were excluded. The photos were applied for alveolar diameter analysis using a WZCamera S50 software (Shenzhen, China). Alveoli with an area of more than 100 μm^2 were analyzed and simulated to circles for calculation of the absolute alveolar diameter. Two independent researchers blinded to the hyperoxia exposure performed the analysis.

Statistics
Continuous parameters were displayed as mean ± standard deviation or median [interquartile range (IQR)], and analyzed

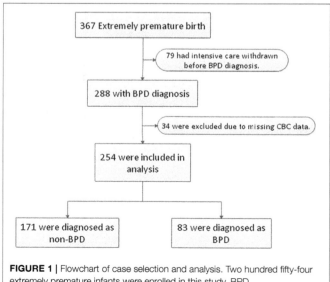

FIGURE 1 | Flowchart of case selection and analysis. Two hundred fifty-four extremely premature infants were enrolled in this study. BPD, bronchopulmonary dysplasia. CBC, complete blood counts.

Close Association Between Platelet Biogenesis and Alveolarization of the Developing Lung

TABLE 1 | Clinical characteristics of 254 extremely premature infants by BPD status.

	Control (*N* = 171)	BPD (*N* = 83)	$Z/t/\chi^2$	*P*-value
Gestational Age [Wk, M(Q1,Q3)]	27.1 (26.2, 27.6)	26.3 (25.5, 27.2)	−4.01	<0.001
Birth Weight [gr, M(Q1,Q3)]	930 (842, 1,060)	858 (720, 950)	−4.378	<0.001
Sex (male)	91	49	0.765	0.382
Gestational Diabetes Mellitus (GDM)	21	7	0.843	0.359
Gestational Hypertension (GH)	18	7	0.276	0.600
Antenatal steroid	134	66	0.094	0.760
PPROM	56	35	2.375	0.123
Twin	48	28	0.855	0.355
Delivery (C-section)	60	28	0.045	0.832
AS^{1min} [score, M(Q1,Q3)]	8 (5, 9)	6 (5, 8)	−2.049	0.040
AS^{5min} [score, M(Q1,Q3)]	10 (9, 10)	10 (9, 10)	−1.015	0.310
Surfactant	124	76	11.250	0.001
Early onset sepsis (EOS)	75	55	11.959	0.003
Intubation	83	64	21.826	<0.001
Duration of intubation (Days)	0 (0,1)	3.6 (0.8, 22)	−4.417	<0.001
Duration of CPAP (Days)	16 (7, 30)	23 (14, 41)	−3.664	<0.001
Duration of supplemental oxygen (Days)	24 (13, 41)	50 (32, 71)	−6.470	<0.001

CPAP, continuous positive airway pressure. Continuous parameters were displayed as median [interquartile range (IQR)], and analyzed by Mann-Whitney U-test. Categorical variables were displayed with numbers and analyzed by Chi-square test. The statistics were performed using SPSS statistical software version 24.0 (IBM Corporation, NY).

by student *t*-test or Mann-Whitney *U*-test, as appropriate. Categorical variables were displayed with numbers and percentages, and analyzed by Chi-square or Fisher's exact test correspondingly. The patients' data were analyzed using SPSS statistical software version 24.0 (IBM Corporation, NY), and the animals' data were analyzed using GraphPad Prism version 8 software package (San Diego, CA, USA). A *p* < 0.05 was considered statistically significant.

RESULTS

Clinical Characteristics of the Patients
A total of 367 inborn extremely premature infants were admitted to our NICU during the study period. Seventy-nine infants were excluded due to life-support withdrawal before the diagnosis of BPD. Thirty-four infants were excluded due to incomplete CBC data. The remaining 254 extremely premature infants were included in the analysis, of whom 225 (88.6%) were born before 28 weeks and 29 (11.4%) were born after 28 weeks with a birth weight lower than 1,000 grams. The diagnosis of BPD was made in 83 (32.7%) infants (**Figure 1**). The median gestational age was 27.0 (interquartile range: 26.1–27.5) weeks, the median body weight was 910.0 (interquartile range: 807.5, 1013.2) grams. The clinical characteristics of 254 infants by BPD diagnosis were summarized in **Table 1**.

Dynamic Change of Platelet Parameters During BPD Development
A total of 254 extremely premature infants were included in the analysis. BPD was diagnosed in 83 (32.7%) infants. Platelet counts (PLT) continuously increased during the first 8 weeks of postnatal

life, while mean platelet volume (MPV) and platelet distribution width (PDW) showed a tendency to decline. However, platelet counts at consecutive time-points of analysis were significantly lower in infants developing BPD compared to infants without BPD (196 ± 85 vs. 231 ± 103 × 10^9/L in the 1st week, 252 ± 112 vs. 293 ± 112 × 10^9/L in the 2nd week, 291 ± 136 vs. 339 ± 136 × 10^9/L in the 4th week, and 308 ± 134 vs. 382 ± 135 × 10^9/L in the 8th week). MPV showed striking changes over the first 2 weeks, with lower values in the 1st week and higher values in the 2nd week in BPD infants compared to infants without BPD (10.39 ± 1.10 vs. 10.85 ± 1.11 fl in the 1st week, 11.27 ± 1.07 vs. 10.97 ± 0.98 fl in the 2nd week. No significant differences in PDW were observed in the two groups (**Figure 2**). In addition, we observed increased PLT and decreased MPV and PDW with advancing postmenstrual age (PMA). BPD infants had lower PLT after PMA of 30–32 weeks than non-BPDs (**Figure 2**).

Rats With Hyperoxia-Induced BPD had Lower Platelet Counts
MLI, an indicator of alveolar size, was significantly higher in rat pups exposed to hyperoxia compared to their age-matched room air (RA) controls (52.1 ± 2.4 vs. 39.5 ± 1.3, *p* < 0.001, **Figures 3D–F**). Similar to our clinical findings shown above, PLT were significantly lower in hyperoxia-induced BPD rats compared to controls raised in room air (642 ± 19 vs. 725 ± 23, *p* = 0.0344). MPV and PDW were significantly higher in experimental BPD pups compared to the controls (8.93 ± 0.35 vs. 7.68 ± 0.17, *p* = 0.001 and 15.81 ± 0.09 vs. 15.43 ± 0.04, *p* < 0.001, respectively, **Figures 3A–C**).

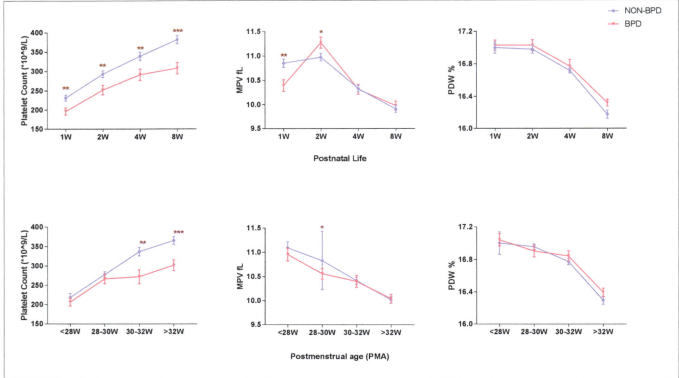

FIGURE 2 | Longitudinal change of platelet parameters defined by postnatal age and postmenstrual age in BPD infants (N = 83) and non-BPD infants (N = 171). PLT, platelet count, 10^9/L, (A). MPV, mean platelet volume, fL, (B). PDW, platelet distribution width, %, (C). Values are expressed as mean ± SD. *$p < 0.05$, **$p < 0.01$, ***$p < 0.001$, compared with age-matched non-BPDs using the student t-test.

Physiological Increase of Platelet Count Synchronized With Alveolarization in Rat Lung

In normal rat development, platelet counts increased from 246 ± 74 × 10^9/L on day 3 to near-adult level of 950 ± 66 × 10^9/L on postnatal day 20 (**Figure 4A**). The MPV and PDW persistently decreased to near-adult levels on postnatal day 20 (**Figures 4B,C**). Alveolarization of rat lung also advanced with age and was complete at around postnatal day 20, as indicated by the stabilization of the MLI (**Figure 4D**) and histology (**Figures 4E–J**).

To better depict the relationship between MLI and platelet parameters, we performed a correlation analysis on MLI and platelet indexes from 3, 6, 9, and 20 days old rats. A significant negative correlation ($r = -0.9959$, $p = 0.0041$) was observed between MLI and PLT. MPV and PDW showed a tendency toward positive correlations with MLI ($p = 0.0643$ and $p = 0.0642$, respectively, **Figure 5**).

DISCUSSION

In this study the dynamic change of longitudinal platelet parameters in premature infants and neonatal rats was investigated. We also evaluated the associations between platelet parameters and lung alveolarization in neonatal rats and found that platelet counts were significantly lower in clinical and experimental BPD. After birth, platelet counts showed a physiological increase in neonatal infants and rat pups while MPV and PDW showed a decrease. Histologically, we confirmed that platelet counts reached stable levels after completion of lung alveolarization in rats (at around postnatal day 20). Correlation analysis demonstrated that platelet counts in rats were significantly associated with the MLI, a marker of alveolar size.

As far as we know, this is the first time to demonstrate an association between platelet index and perinatal lung development. We found a persistent increase in PLT and an overall decrease of MPV and PDW during the first 8 weeks of life of extremely premature infants, which was partly supported by the study from Henry et al., who showed a stepwise increase in platelets during the first 3 months of life in newborn infants (14). Notably, the authors also showed that newborns with advancing gestational age had higher platelet levels at birth (14), suggesting that the platelet parameters are dynamically changing with development during early life. This study also showed a correlation between platelet indexes and lung alveolarization in rats. The lung is an important organ in platelet biogenesis. In humans and rodents around 50% of circulating platelets are generated in the lung (8, 10–12). In the lung, platelets arise in the vascular bed by shedding from megakaryocytes and proplatelets which embolize in the lungs. Shear stress, turbulence,

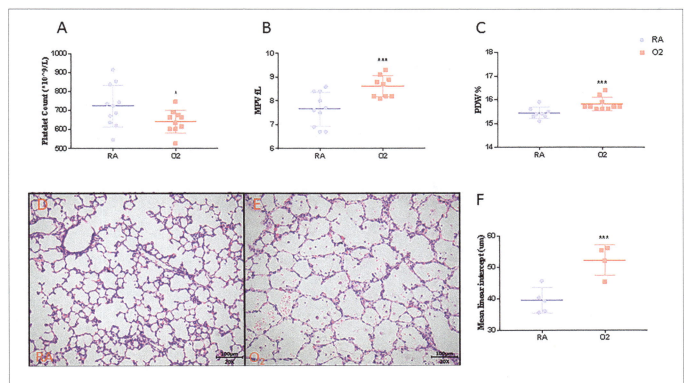

FIGURE 3 | Platelet parameters ($N = 9$–10, A–C), mean linear intercept (MLI, $N = 4$–5, F) and representative photos of rat pups exposed to room air (RA, D) or hyperoxia (O_2, E) at postnatal Day 10. Values are expressed as mean ± SD. *$p < 0.05$, ***$p < 0.001$, compared with age-matched RA controls using the student t-test. Magnification, 200 x.

and endothelial interaction in the pulmonary vascular bed play an important role in platelet biogenesis by activating shedding from megakaryocytes and pro-platelets (9). During lung development the size of the vascular bed increases, thereby increasing the capacity of platelet synthesis and secretion into the systemic circulation. This explains at least in part the gradual increase in PLT during normal postnatal lung development. Two elegant studies have demonstrated that platelets contribute to embryonic lung development (6) and lung regeneration after pneumonectomy (7), which may explain why the decrease of platelets led to blunted lung development in the current study.

This study showed that platelet counts are significantly lower in infants developing BPD and in rats with experimental BPD induced by hyperoxia. This finding is in line with a study by Okur et al. who reported a lower PLT and PMI in BPD infants during the first week of life (15), but is not supported by Go et al. who report that platelet parameters at birth were not associated with BPD after multivariate analysis (16). This difference might be due to the different timing of these studies. Common pulmonary diseases in adults, including asthma, chronic obstructive pulmonary disease, idiopathic pulmonary fibrosis, and pulmonary hypertension, are not associated with reduced platelet counts (9). This is probably caused by redundancy of the adult pulmonary vascular bed. Only in severe cases of acute respiratory distress syndrome thrombocytopenia was observed, caused by either increased platelet consumption or decreased platelet production (17). PLT largely depend on platelet synthesis and consumption, in which the lung plays an important role. We speculate that in BPD systemic PLT are low because (I) the production of platelets is decreased due to a reduced vascular bed caused by aberrant alveolar and vascular development and lung injury, and (II) increased platelet consumption in the injured lung exposed to hyperoxia.

Previous studies have shown that platelet production may be regulated by oxygen tension. Acute hypoxia in rodents led to a biphasic response with an initial increase, followed by a decrease in platelet counts after 1 week of hypoxia, which may be caused by hypoxia-induced hemoconcentration, platelet activation and vasoconstriction (9, 18, 19). Hyperoxia decreases platelet counts by inhibiting platelet production and enhancing platelet activation for thrombi formation and platelet consumption (20–22). Therefore, there may be a vicious cycle linking platelet production and blunted lung development in the BPD setting (**Figure 6**). However, platelet production and postnatal lung development are both evolving processes, so it is hard to speculate whether decreased platelet biogenesis contributes to BPD, or BPD leads to the reduction of platelets. Well-designed experimental studies are needed to elucidate this interaction.

The study by Henry et al. and our study found a transient increase of MPV in infants during their first 2 weeks of life and then a decrease, which is independent of gestational age at

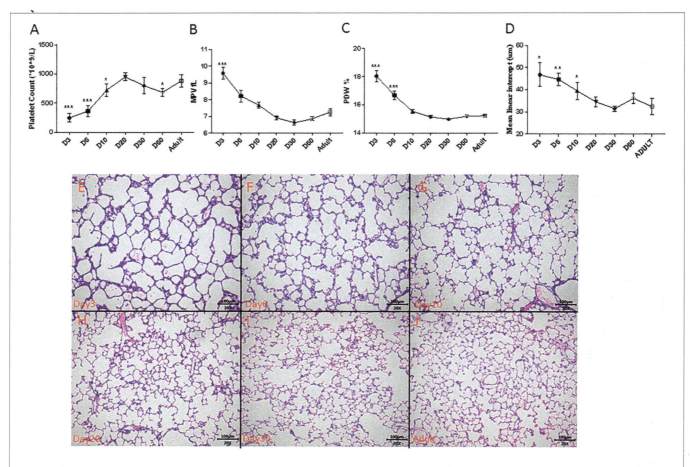

FIGURE 4 | Dynamic change of platelet parameters during lung alveolarization (N = 8–10, **A–C**), mean linear intercept (MLI, N = 3–5, **D**) and representative photos during rats' development **(E–J)** in normoxia. Values are expressed as mean ± SD. *p < 0.05, **p < 0.01, ***p < 0.001, compared with adults using one-way ANOVA. Magnification, 200x.

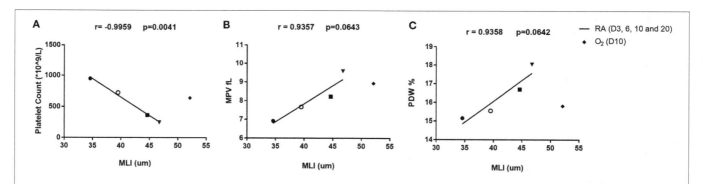

FIGURE 5 | Correlation analysis between platelet parameters and MLI in rats on day 3, 6, 10, and 20 after birth. Correlation between platelet count (PLT) and MLI **(A)**, mean platelet volume (MPV) and MLI **(B)**, platelet distribution width (PDW) and MLI **(C)**. The correlation was analyzed by Pearson correlation using GraphPad Prism version 8. Triangles (▼) indicate 3-day old rats. Squares (■) indicate 6-day old rats. Open circles (○) indicate 10-day old rats and solid circles (●) indicate 20-day old rats. Diamonds (♦) stand for rats exposed to hyperoxia for 10 days in a row. The hyperoxia data were only plotted in the figure but not included in the correlation analysis.

birth (14). However, these findings were inconsistent with the studies from Dani et al. and Cekmez et al. who reported that infants developing BPD had higher MPV levels at 1–3 days of life compared to those without BPD (23, 24). This discrepancy might be attributed to the different time points that platelet parameters were measured. MPV and PDW are both indicators of platelet

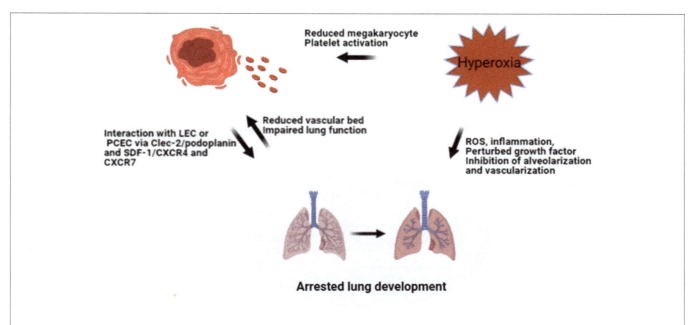

FIGURE 6 | Hypothesis on the interaction between hyperoxia, platelet biogenesis, and lung injury. Hyperoxia may reduce the number of megakaryocytes in the lung and increase platelet consumption by activating platelets, leading to decreased platelet count directly. Hyperoxia may also impair the developing lung by inhibiting alveolarization and vascularization, leading to BPD. The reduction of the vascular bed in BPD, together with impaired lung function might result in reduced shedding of megakaryocytes and pro-platelets trapped in pulmonary capillaries. Meanwhile, reduced PLT may hamper lung development by interacting with LEC and PCEC via ligands and receptors. ROS, reactive oxygen species; LEC, lymphatic endothelial cells; PCEC, pulmonary capillary endothelial cells; Clec-2, C-type lectin-like receptor-2; SDF-1, stromal-cell-derived factor-1; CXCR4 and CXCR7, receptors of SDF-1 on PCEC.

size, indicating platelets are being produced or activated. In the animal experiment, we observed an increase in MPV and PDW in oxygen-exposed rats, which might indicate more platelets are activated in these pups. In BPD infants, we also observed a lower platelet count and a higher MPV at postnatal week 2, which might indicate more platelets are activated in these infants. Besides, we also observed a physiological increase in MPV in these infants, the mechanism under this phenomenon still needs investigation. We speculate that platelet parameters in the first days after birth are prone to be affected by the neonatal transition and medical treatments. Therefore, the analysis of platelet parameters over the clinically defined time window of BPD may provide more reliable evidence.

There are several limitations to this study. The most relevant one is that the direct correlation between impaired platelet formation and arrested lung development was not studied. Besides, we could not evaluate the effect of hyperoxia itself on platelet parameters in extremely premature infants due to the complexity of their clinical condition. Moreover, platelet parameters in rats exposed to hyperoxia were only measured on day 10. It would be interesting to track the interaction between platelet parameters and lung development for a longer period.

In conclusion, clinical and experimental BPD are significantly associated with lower platelet levels. The physiological increase of platelet counts synchronizes with postnatal alveolarization in neonatal rats. Understanding the role of platelets in neonatal lung development may shed new light on BPD prevention in clinics.

ETHICS STATEMENT

The studies involving human participants were reviewed and approved by the Institutional Ethical Committee of Shenzhen Maternity and Child Healthcare Hospital. Written informed consent for participation was not provided by the participants' legal guardians/next of kin because: Acquirement of informed consent was waived given that no personal data were explicitly reported. The animal study was reviewed and approved by the Institutional Animal Care and Use Committee of Shenzhen Institutes of Advanced Technology of the Chinese Academy of Sciences.

AUTHOR CONTRIBUTIONS

CY, FW, and XC conceptualized and designed the study and wrote the first draft of the manuscripts. XC, JZho, and FY carried out the clinical data collection. XC and JZha performed the data analysis. GW, CY, and FW reviewed and revised the manuscripts. All authors read and approved the final manuscript.

ACKNOWLEDGMENTS

We kindly acknowledged Chun Chen for her help in data preparation.

REFERENCES

1. Hwang JS, Rehan VK. Recent advances in bronchopulmonary dysplasia: pathophysiology, prevention, and treatment. *Lung.* (2018) 196:129–38. doi: 10.1007/s00408-018-0084-z
2. Stoll BJ, Hansen NI, Bell EF, Walsh MC, Carlo WA, Shankaran S, et al. Trends in care practices, morbidity, and mortality of extremely preterm neonates, 1993-2012. *JAMA.* (2015) 314:1039–51. doi: 10.1097/01.aoa.0000482610.95044.1b
3. Bancalari E, Jain D. Bronchopulmonary dysplasia: 50 years after the original description. *Neonatology.* (2019) 115:384–91. doi: 10.1159/000497422
4. Morty RE. Recent advances in the pathogenesis of BPD. *Semin Perinatol.* (2018) 42:404–12. doi: 10.1053/j.semperi.2018.09.001
5. Naeem A, Ahmed I, Silveyra P. Bronchopulmonary dysplasia: an update on experimental therapeutics. *Europ Med J.* (2019) 4:20–9.
6. Tsukiji N, Inoue O, Morimoto M, Tatsumi N, Nagatomo H, Ueta K, et al. Platelets play an essential role in murine lung development through Clec-2/podoplanin interaction. *Blood.* (2018) 132:1167–79. doi: 10.1182/blood-2017-12-823369
7. Rafii S, Cao Z, Lis R, Siempos, II, Chavez D, et al. Platelet-derived SDF-1 primes the pulmonary capillary vascular niche to drive lung alveolar regeneration. *Nat Cell Biol.* (2015) 17:123–36. doi: 10.1038/ncb3096
8. Lefrancais E, Ortiz-Munoz G, Caudrillier A, Mallavia B, Liu F, Sayah DM, et al. The lung is a site of platelet biogenesis and a reservoir for haematopoietic progenitors. *Nature.* (2017) 544:105–9. doi: 10.1038/nature21706
9. Lefrançais E, Looney MR. Platelet biogenesis in the lung circulation. *Physiology.* (2019) 34:392–401. doi: 10.1152/physiol.00017.2019
10. Kaufman RM, Airo R, Pollack S, Crosby WH. Circulating megakaryocytes and platelet release in the lung. *Blood.* (1965) 26:720–31. doi: 10.1182/blood.V26.6.720.720
11. Levine RF, Eldor A, Shoff PK, Kirwin S, Tenza D, Cramer EM. Circulating megakaryocytes: delivery of large numbers of intact, mature megakaryocytes to the lungs. *Eur J Haematol.* (1993) 51:233–46. doi: 10.1111/j.1600-0609.1993.tb00637.x
12. Pedersen NT. Occurrence of megakaryocytes in various vessels and their retention in the pulmonary capillaries in man. *Scand J Haematol.* (1978) 21:369–75. doi: 10.1111/j.1600-0609.1978.tb00381.x
13. Chen X, Orriols M, Walther FJ, Laghmani EH, Hoogeboom AM, Hogen-Esch ACB, et al. Bone morphogenetic Protein 9 protects against neonatal hyperoxia-induced impairment of alveolarization and pulmonary inflammation. *Front Physiol.* (2017) 8:486. doi: 10.3389/fphys.2017.00486
14. Henry E, Christensen RD. Reference intervals in neonatal hematology. *Clin Perinatol.* (2015) 42:483–97. doi: 10.1016/j.clp.2015.04.005
15. Okur N, Buyuktiryaki M, Uras N, Oncel MY, Ertekin O, Canpolat FE, et al. Platelet mass index in very preterm infants: can it be used as a parameter for neonatal morbidities? *J Matern Fetal Neonatal Med.* (2016) 29:3218–22. doi: 10.3109/14767058.2015.1121475
16. Go H, Ohto H, Nollet KE, Takano S, Kashiwabara N, Chishiki M, et al. Using platelet parameters to anticipate morbidity and mortality among preterm neonates: a retrospective study. *Front Pediatrics.* (2020) 8:90. doi: 10.3389/fped.2020.00090
17. Wei Y, Tejera P, Wang Z, Zhang R, Chen F, Su L, et al. A missense genetic variant in LRRC16A/CARMIL1 improves acute respiratory distress syndrome survival by attenuating platelet count decline. *Am J Respir Critic Care Med.* (2017) 195:1353–61. doi: 10.1164/rccm.201605-0946OC
18. McDonald TP, Cottrell M, Clift R. Effects of short-term hypoxia on platelet counts of mice. *Blood.* (1978) 51:165–75. doi: 10.1182/blood.V51.1.165.bloodjournal511165
19. Jackson CW, Edwards CC. Biphasic thrombopoietic response to severe hypobaric hypoxia. *Br J Haematol.* (1977) 35:233–44. doi: 10.1111/j.1365-2141.1977.tb00580.x
20. Yang J, Yang M, Xu F, Li K, Lee SKM, Ng P-C, et al. Effects of oxygen-induced lung damage on megakaryocytopoiesis and platelet homeostasis in a rat model. *Pediatr Res.* (2003) 54:344–52. doi: 10.1203/01.PDR.0000079186.86219.29
21. Barazzone C, Tacchini-Cottier F, Vesin C, Rochat AF, Piguet PF. Hyperoxia induces platelet activation and lung sequestration: an event dependent on tumor necrosis factor-alpha and CD11a. *Am J Respir Cell Mol Biol.* (1996) 15:107–14. doi: 10.1165/ajrcmb.15.1.8679214
22. Passmore MR, Ki KK, Chan CHH, Lee T, Bouquet M, Wood ES, et al. The effect of hyperoxia on inflammation and platelet responses in an ex vivo extracorporeal membrane oxygenation circuit. *Artif Organs.* (2020) 44:1276–85. doi: 10.1111/aor.13771
23. Dani C, Poggi C, Barp J, Berti E, Fontanelli G. Mean platelet volume and risk of bronchopulmonary dysplasia and intraventricular hemorrhage in extremely preterm infants. *Am J Perinatol.* (2011) 28:551–6. doi: 10.1055/s-0031-1274503
24. Cekmez F, Tanju IA, Canpolat FE, Aydinoz S, Aydemir G, Karademir F, et al. Mean platelet volume in very preterm infants: a predictor of morbidities? *Eur Rev Med Pharmacol Sci.* (2013) 17:134–7.

10

The Extracellular Matrix in Bronchopulmonary Dysplasia: Target and Source

Ivana Mižíková[1,2] and Rory E. Morty[1,2]*

[1] Department of Lung Development and Remodelling, Max Planck Institute for Heart and Lung Research, Bad Nauheim, Germany, [2] Pulmonology, Department of Internal Medicine, University of Giessen and Marburg Lung Center, Giessen, Germany

*Correspondence:
Rory E. Morty
rory.morty@mpi-bn.mpg.de

Bronchopulmonary dysplasia (BPD) is a common complication of preterm birth that contributes significantly to morbidity and mortality in neonatal intensive care units. BPD results from life-saving interventions, such as mechanical ventilation and oxygen supplementation used to manage preterm infants with acute respiratory failure, which may be complicated by pulmonary infection. The pathogenic pathways driving BPD are not well-delineated but include disturbances to the coordinated action of gene expression, cell–cell communication, physical forces, and cell interactions with the extracellular matrix (ECM), which together guide normal lung development. Efforts to further delineate these pathways have been assisted by the use of animal models of BPD, which rely on infection, injurious mechanical ventilation, or oxygen supplementation, where histopathological features of BPD can be mimicked. Notable among these are perturbations to ECM structures, namely, the organization of the elastin and collagen networks in the developing lung. Dysregulated collagen deposition and disturbed elastin fiber organization are pathological hallmarks of clinical and experimental BPD. Strides have been made in understanding the disturbances to ECM production in the developing lung, but much still remains to be discovered about how ECM maturation and turnover are dysregulated in aberrantly developing lungs. This review aims to inform the reader about the state-of-the-art concerning the ECM in BPD, to highlight the gaps in our knowledge and current controversies, and to suggest directions for future work in this exciting and complex area of lung development (patho)biology.

Keywords: bronchopulmonary dysplasia, extracellular matrix, hyperoxia, mechanical ventilation, collagen, elastin, lung development

BRONCHOPULMONARY DYSPLASIA IN CONTEXT

The lung is the key organ of gas exchange in air-breathing mammals. This gas exchange structure is derived from the primitive foregut and proceeds through a phase of early (embryonic) development (1–3), when the conducting airways and conducting vessels are generated and organized (4). Early lung development initiates with the embryonic stage that occurs 4–7 weeks post-conception in humans [embryonic day (E)9–E12 in the mouse]. The embryonic stage is followed by the pseudoglandular stage, which occurs at 5–17 weeks post-conception in humans (E12–E17 in mice). The final stage of *early lung development* is the canalicular stage, occurring at 16–26 weeks post-conception in humans (E17–E18 in mice), at which point, the process of alveolarization begins, which is characterized by the thinning of the interstitial tissue (**Figure 1**). This marks the beginning of *late lung development*, where the distal airways then form saccular units in the saccular stage, which is evident in humans at 24–38 weeks post-conception [E18-post-natal day (P)4 in mice], and these saccular units are divided by secondary septa (the process of "secondary septation") during the alveolar stage, which is evident at 36 weeks post-conception to 36 months post-natal (and beyond) in humans (P4–P28 in mice). The objective of late lung development is the production of a large number of small alveoli, the principal gas exchange units of the lung. This process, which is poorly understood, creates a large surface area over which gas exchange takes place. Current knowledge on late lung development implicates transcription factors and epigenetic effects, which together regulate genetic programs driving lung development. These programs work in concert with contact- and growth factor-mediated cell–cell communication (5–7) to drive lung development. The development of the lung is also driven in part by physical forces from breathing motions and the production and remodeling of the extracellular matrix (ECM) scaffold.

Multiple diseases are complicated by disturbances to lung development. Notable among these is bronchopulmonary dysplasia (BPD), which affects prematurely born infants with acute respiratory failure that receive oxygen therapy, first described by William (Bill) Northway and colleagues in 1967 (10, 11). While oxygen supplementation is a life-saving intervention, the associated oxygen toxicity stunts the post-natal development of the lung. This damage to the developing lung is exacerbated by barotrauma and volutrauma caused by positive-pressure mechanical ventilation, and also by inflammation. Affected infants exhibit blunted lung maturation, and BPD represents a significant cause of morbidity and mortality in a neonatal intensive care setting (11–14). Longitudinal studies suggest that disease sequelae persist into adult life (15–17). Examinations of autopsy material from patients that have died with BPD have formed the basis of hypotheses about pathogenic processes at play that limit alveolarization. These observations include (i) severe disturbances to the development of the pulmonary vasculature (18), (ii) changes in the cellular structure and composition of the developing alveolar units, (iii) increased proteolysis in the alveolar compartments, (iv) increased inflammatory cell infiltration, (v) deregulated growth factor signaling, and (vi) perturbations to the ECM architecture of the developing lung: most notably, the abundance and organization of collagen and elastin fibers (19–22). These disturbances have also been noted in animal models of BPD (23, 24).

It is the objective of this review to highlight key observations made regarding changes to the ECM architecture of the lung – both in clinical BPD and in experimental animal models of BPD (referred to herein as "experimental BPD") – and to integrate these observations into a pathogenic pathway. Furthermore, attention will be paid to current controversies in the field, and also, to the key gaps in our knowledge, where urgent additional work is still to be undertaken.

EARLY STUDIES: THE ECM IN LUNG DEVELOPMENT AND BPD

The ECM represents a very complex network of structurally, mechanically, and biochemically heterogeneous components (25). The components include the classic "players": collagen and elastin, which constitute 50% (26) and 18% (27), respectively, of the lung ECM. This list continues to grow, with fibrillin (28) and fibulin (29) glycoproteins, and integrin receptors of ECM components (30) being more recent additions. The ECM serves as a scaffold that directs lung development, and the ECM structure itself is continuously remodeled as lung development proceeds (31, 32). As such, the production of ECM components, as well as the systems that regulate the deposition and stability of the ECM, must be considered. These systems include chaperones and enzymes that catalyze the post-translational processing of ECM components, as well as systems that destabilize and degrade the

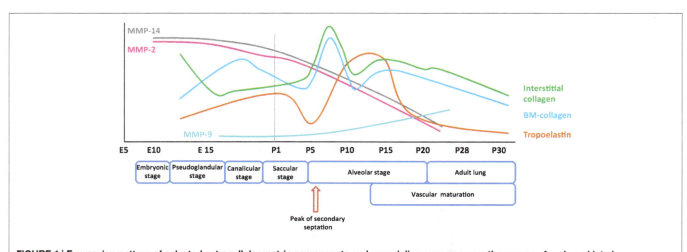

FIGURE 1 | Expression pattern of selected extracellular matrix components and remodeling enzymes over the course of early and late lung development in mice. The trends illustrated represent a synthesis of the data presented in several publications (8, 9), and span the embryonic and post-natal lung maturation period. Abbreviations: BM, basement membrane; E, embryonic day; MMP, matrix metalloproteinase; P, post-natal day.

The Extracellular Matrix in Bronchopulmonary Dysplasia: Target and Source

ECM to facilitate ECM renewal. The remodeling of collagen during lung development has been recognized since the early 1970s (33). Pioneering work by Ron Crystal's group identified the heterogeneity of fibrillar collagens in the lung during lung development (34–36). Observations on the dynamic remodeling of other collagen types, including basement membrane-type IV collagen then followed, in the context of early lung development (37, 38). Similarly, pioneering work by Janet Powell and Philip Whitney in the early 1980s described changes in lung elastin levels as post-natal lung development proceeded (39). Subsequent work by Ron Crystal (40) and Robert Rucker's (41) teams highlighted the dynamic expression of tropoelastin during the course of post-natal lung development. Building on these studies, early work demonstrating that lathyrogens could disturb normal lung development (42) highlighted the role of collagen and elastin in the post-natal maturation of the lung. Soon to follow these reports were key observations of perturbed ECM structures in disorders of lung development. Leading work by Donald Thibeault and William Truog, in particular, identified secondary collagen fibers in the developing parenchyma of neonates with BPD that were "disorganized, tortuous, and thickened" (20, 21). Similarly, elastin fibers exhibited an abnormal structure in infants with BPD, both in the parenchyma (43–45) and in the vasculature (46). These early studies firmly established a role for

proper lung ECM homeostasis in normal lung development, and described severe structural perturbations to the lung ECM that accompanied aberrant lung development. Clearly, it is important to note that it is sometimes difficult to establish whether the perturbations to ECM structure noted in clinical subjects with BPD are a cause of aberrant alveolarization, or a consequence of blunted lung development. This applies equally to pathological material from animals in which BPD has been modeled. Since these initial studies reported above, many strides have been made in our understanding of the production of the structural components of the ECM during post-natal lung development, which will be considered in detail below.

KEY STRUCTURAL COMPONENTS OF THE ECM: COLLAGEN AND ELASTIN

Collagen

Collagen is the most abundant protein within the interstitial ECM. In the lung, collagen fibers [represented predominantly by the fibrillar collagens, collagen type I and III produced by fibroblasts (**Table 1**)] are found in the bronchi, blood vessels, and the alveolar septa (35, 47, 48). The abundance of lung parenchymal collagen increases over the course of lung development. In mice,

TABLE 1 | Cellular localization and origin of individual components of extracellular matrix and extracellular matrix remodeling enzymes.

Extracellular matrix component	Origin/source				
	Epithelial cells	Fibroblasts	Endothelial cells	Smooth muscle cells	Inflammatory cells
Collagen		(51–53)			
EC-SOD	(54, 55)				
Elastin		(51, 53, 56)		(51, 57)	
Fibrillin-1		(58, 59)			
Fibronectin		(58, 60–62)	(60)	(60)	(60, 61)
Fibulin-5/DANCE		(63)		(64)	
Heparan sulfate	(65)	(66)			
Integrins	(67–71)	(69)	(70)	(70)	
LOX		(72, 73)		(72, 73)	
LOXL1		(72, 73)		(72, 73)	
LOXL2		(72, 73)		(72, 73)	
LTBP2		(58)			
MMP-1	(74)	(74)			
MMP-14/MT1-MMP	(74–76)	(75)	(76)		
MMP-2	(74, 75, 77, 78)	(75)	(74)		(77)
MMP-9	(74, 77–79)	(61)			(77, 79)
PLOD1	(80)	(80)	(80)	(80)	
PLOD2	(80)	(80)	(80)	(80)	
PLOD3	(80)	(80)	(80)	(80)	
Tenascin C	(81, 82)	(81–84)	(83, 84)	(83)	(81)
TGF-β	(78)	(61)			
TGM2/tTG	(85–87)	(52, 85, 86)	(85)	(85)	
TIMP-1	(75)	(75)			
TIMP-2	(74, 75)	(75)	(74)		

Numbers in parentheses indicate the citations reporting the identification of the extracellular matrix components or remodeling enzymes in the indicated lung cell types. The citations are not all inclusive, and represent only a selection of reports.
EC-SOD, extracellular superoxide dismutase 3; LOX, lysyl oxidase; LoxL1, lysyl oxidase-like 1; LoxL2, lysyl oxidase-like 2; LTBP2, latent TGF-β-binding protein 2; MMP, matrix metalloproteinase; MT1, membrane-type 1; PLOD, procollagen-lysine, 2-oxoglutarate 5-dioxygenase; TGF-β, transforming growth factor-β; TGM2, transglutaminase 2; TIMP, tissue inhibitor of metalloproteinase; tTG, tissue transglutaminase.

gene expression of fibrillar collagens *Col1a1* and *Col3a1*, as well as basement membrane collagens *Col4a1* and *Col4a2*, is reported to have peaked at P7 (**Figure 1**). By this time, the collagen had formed a delicate interstitial network of fibers that could aid the process of alveolar development (8). While *Col1a1*$^{-/-}$ mice, which lack collagen Iα_1, died *in utero* due to the rupture of major blood vessels, no abnormalities were noted in lung branching morphogenesis in these mice (49, 50). However, elevated levels of other fibrillar collagens, including collagen III and V levels, were noted in *Col1a1*$^{-/-}$ mouse embryos, suggesting a possible compensation for the loss of functional collagen I (50).

Alterations to the structure and integrity of collagen networks have been reported in several animal models of BPD and emphysema, which are diseases of the lung parenchyma that represent a failure of alveolar formation and the destruction of existing alveoli, respectively (21, 72, 88). Studies in various BPD animal models have revealed increased collagen production (**Table 2**), thickened collagen fibers, and increased rigidity of the lung (72, 88, 89) to be associated with experimental BPD. This is consistent with observations made in clinical subjects, where an increased number of collagen-positive cells, elevated levels of the fibrillar collagens, collagen I and collagen III were observed; and BPD patients revealed a specific increase in the collagen I/collagen III ratio (48, 90). Furthermore, elevated levels of collagen IV (91) have been noted in bronchoalveolar lavage (BAL) fluids from patients with BPD. These observations are supported by microscopic studies on patient tissues. Thibeault and colleagues (21) observed thickened and disorganized collagen fibers, and a generally damaged collagen network in the lungs of infants diagnosed with BPD after positive-pressure ventilation. It was proposed by those investigators that enlargement of alveoli due to ventilation leads to compression of surrounding ECM structures and damage to the collagen and elastin niche, disturbing the normal septation process. However, both adult rats (92) and newborn mice (93) exposed to sub-lethal normobaric hyperoxia up-regulated collagen I production, assessed by northern blot and immunoblot, respectively. In the case of newborn mice, the increased collagen I production was attributed to activation of the pro-fibrotic growth factor, transforming growth factor (TGF)-β, which stimulated collagen production and secretion by fibroblasts. Increased collagen deposition in the lung parenchyma of newborn mice has been confirmed in the hyperoxia-based mouse BPD model by picrosirius red staining (72, 94). Additionally, total lung collagen protein levels were increased by 63% after exposure of developing mouse pups to hyperoxia (89). Taken together, these reports make a strong case for dysregulated collagen expression in aberrant lung development associated with clinical and experimental BPD.

Collagen production under physiological and pathophysiological conditions is regulated by inter alia growth factors, such as TGF-β, where *in vitro* stimulation of primary lung fibroblasts drives *Col1a1* production (95, 116). This is significant, because elevated TGF-β levels were associated with BPD in preterm infants (115). TGF-β has also been causally implicated in the blunted alveolar development associated with hyperoxia exposure in the mouse hyperoxia model of BPD (117). The connection between TGF-β and collagen deposition in the developing lung is noteworthy. Over-expression of TGF-β driven by the *Scgb1a1*

(encoding surfactant-associated protein C, pro-SPC) promoter in a doxycycline-inducible system is sometimes used as an animal model of BPD. Over-expression of TGF-β in this model not only resulted in blunted alveolarization but also increased deposition of collagen in the developing septa (118). Furthermore, over-expression of TGF-β in the developing lung *in utero* caused pulmonary hypoplasia that was accompanied by thickening of the collagen fibers and excessive collagen deposition in the septa (119). Exactly how the blunted alveolarization connects with perturbed ECM generation, both of which are guided by TGF-β, remains to be clarified.

Failed alveolar septation in both clinical and experimental BPD is clearly accompanied by changes to collagen production and deposition in the lungs. Studies, to date, have addressed primarily the fibrillar collagens collagen I and collagen III, however, the remaining 26 other collagens have received little or no attention. It remains of interest to explore whether perturbations to the expression of those collagens might be associated with arrested alveolar development. Similarly, no studies, to date, have examined the regulation or activity of the procollagen processing proteases, bone morphogenetic protein 1 (BMP-1) and ADAM metallopeptidase with thrombospondin type 1 motif, 2 (ADAMTS2). Both enzymes are required for procollagen processing and assembly into fibrils, during lung development.

Elastin

Elastic fibers consist of extensively cross-linked elastin and fibrillin (28) microfibrils. These structures are associated with accessory molecules, including latent TGF-β-binding protein (LTBP), microfibril-associated proteins, fibulin, emilin, and microfibril-associated glycoprotein (MAGP) family members. Elastin fibers are located throughout the developing lung, in the developing conducting airways and alveolar ducts, the conducting vessels, and the developing septa. As illustrated in **Figure 1**, the expression of elastin in mice is dynamically regulated over the alveolarization period. Elastin expression dramatically increases at a time-point coincident with the "burst" of secondary septation that drives the formation of the alveoli. Elastin expression remains high throughout the secondary septation period [for example, in mice, over (P5–P15)] and rapidly decreases once alveolarization has been completed (8, 120). However, reactivation of elastin expression occurs in adult lungs under pathological conditions, such as emphysema and pulmonary fibrosis, where disorganized elastic fibers have been described (22, 120). The first hints that elastin plays a role in lung development included the observations that lung elastin levels were modulated as post-natal lung development proceeded (39). Additionally, the expression of tropoelastin, the "elastin monomer," was dynamically regulated over the course of post-natal lung development in rodents (40, 41). During lung alveolarization, elastin is specifically deposited in "foci" at the tips of developing septa, suggesting a role in the process of secondary septation, which generates the alveoli. The spatially regulated deposition of elastin that coincides with secondary septation has led to the idea that elastin is a driver of lung development (121–123).

Further support for a role for elastin in lung development has been obtained using elastin-deficient mice. Elastin deficiency

The Extracellular Matrix in Bronchopulmonary Dysplasia: Target and Source

TABLE 2 | Dysregulation of the expression of extracellular matrix components and remodeling enzymes in clinical bronchopulmonary dysplasia and experimental animal models.

ECM component	Expression in the disease/experimental condition		
	Bronchopulmonary dysplasia	Hyperoxia	Mechanical ventilation
Collagen	↑ (48, 91)	↓ (Fibroblasts, *in vitro*) (95) ↑ (Mouse) (72, 89, 93) ↑ (Rat) (92)	
EC-SOD		↓ (Mouse) (55)	
Elastin		↓ (Fibroblasts, *in vitro*) (95) ↓ (Mouse) (89, 96) ↑ (Mouse) (51, 72, 93, 97) ↑ (Rat) (98)	↑ (Mouse) (23, 99–101) ↑ (Lamb) (24, 102) ↑ (Rat) (103)
Fibrillin-1		↑ (Mouse) (51)	↑ (Mouse) (99) ↑ (Lamb) (24)
EMILIN-1		↑ (Mouse) (23, 72)	↓ (Mouse) (23)
Fibrillin-2		↑ (Mouse) (51)	↓ (Mouse) (23, 99)
Fibronectin	↑ (60, 62, 104, 105)	↑ (Mouse) (105) ↑ (Rabbit) (106)	
Fibulin-5/DANCE		↑ (Mouse) (51, 72)	↓ (Mouse) (23) ↑ (Rat) (103) ↑ (Lamb) (24)
Integrins		↑ (Mouse) (51)	
Lox	↑ (72)	↑ (Mouse) (51, 72, 89)	↑ (Mouse) (23) ↑ (Lamb) (24)
Loxl1	↑ (72)	↑ (Mouse) (72, 89)	↓ (Mouse) (23) ↑ (Lamb) (24) ↑ (Rat) (103)
Loxl2		↑ (Mouse) (72, 89)	
MMP-1		↑ (Rat) (92)	↓ (Baboon) (107)
MMP-16		↓ (Rat) (108)	
MMP-2	↓ (109)	↓ (Rat) (110) ↕ (Rat) (78) ↑ (Rat) (77) ↑ (Mice) (93)	
MMP-8	↑ (111, 112)		↓ (Baboon) (107)
MMP-9		↓ (Rat) (110) ↕ (Rat) (78) ↑ (Rat) (77) ↑ (Mice) (93)	↑ (Rat) (103) ↑ (Mouse) (100, 101) ↑ (Baboon) (107)
MMP-9:TIMP-1	↑ (113, 114)		↑ (Baboon) (107)
MT1-MMP		↑ (Rat) (78)	
PLOD1		↑ (Mouse) (80)	
PLOD2	↑ (80)	↑ (Mouse) (80)	
PLOD3		↑ (Mouse) (80)	
Tenascin C	↑ (83)	↓ (Fibroblasts, *in vitro*) (95)	↑ (Rat) (103)
TGF-β	↑ (115)	↑ (Mouse) (51) ↑ (Rat) (78, 92)	↑ (Lamb) (24)
TIMP-1	↓ (113)	↑ (Fibroblasts, *in vitro*) (95) ↑ (Rat) (78, 110)	
tTG	↑ (85)	↑ (Mouse) (85)	

Arrows indicate the direction of dysregulated expression: ↓, down-regulation; ↑, up-regulation; ↕, temporal regulation in either direction over time.
ECM, extracellular matrix; EC-SOD, extracellular superoxide dismutase 3; EMILIN-1, elastin microfibril interfacer 1; LOX, lysyl oxidase; LoxL1, lysyl oxidase-like 1; LoxL2, lysyl oxidase-like 2; LTBP2, latent TGF-β-binding protein 2; MMP, matrix metalloproteinase; MT1, membrane-type 1; PLOD, procollagen-lysine, 2-oxoglutarate 5-dioxygenase; TGF-β, transforming growth factor-β; TGM2, transglutaminase 2; TIMP, tissue inhibitor of metalloproteinase; tTG, tissue transglutaminase.

is accompanied by perinatal lethality, and $Eln^{-/-}$ mice exhibit arrested perinatal development of the terminal airway branches, and enlarged terminal air sacs (124). Elastin haploinsufficient ($Eln^{+/-}$) mice, which express 50% of the elastin seen in wild-type mice (125), exhibited normal lung development and normal alveolar structures, although there is some evidence that the elastin deposition in $Eln^{-/-}$ mice was abnormal (99). Modulating the dose of elastin to <50%, by expressing the human elastin gene in a transgenic homozygous-null $Eln^{-/-}$ mouse strain reduced elastin levels to 37% of wild-type mouse levels. While transgenic expression of human elastin rescued the perinatal lethality observed in $Eln^{-/-}$ mice, a pronounced blunting of alveolar development was noted (125). These data indicate that a baseline threshold of elastin abundance is required for normal lung development to proceed. All of these observations underscore important roles for the correct spatio-temporal production of elastin structures in the developing lung.

In the context of lung disease, abnormal elastin fiber structures have been observed in the parenchyma of aberrantly developing lungs from prematurely born ventilated neonates (126). Parallel trends have been observed in animal models of BPD, where in response to mechanical ventilation or perinatal exposure to hyperoxia, the normally organized deposition of elastin fibers into foci at the tips of developing septa is lost. Rather, elastin fibers are noted in the walls (not the tips) of the thickened developing septa and have been described to be "brush-like," "thickened," and "loose" (32, 102, 127–129).

The pathological mechanisms behind the disturbed production and deposition of elastin in aberrantly developing lungs remains to be clarified, however, much work in this area has been already done, and remains ongoing. There is a body of evidence that suggests that expression of the Eln gene is up-regulated by hyperoxia in animal models of BPD, as revealed by real-time reverse transcription (RT)-polymerase chain reaction (PCR) analysis of mRNA pools from lung homogenates (51, 72, 97). The cell types reported to produce elastin in the lung are listed in **Table 1**, which include fibroblasts and smooth muscle cells. How hyperoxia modulates Eln gene expression might be attributed to growth factor stimulation or inhibition of elastin synthesis. Both TGF-β (130, 131) and insulin-like growth factor (IGF) (132) stimulated Eln gene expression, whereas some forms of platelet-derived growth factor (PDGF) suppressed Eln gene expression (133). Furthermore, the stability of Eln mRNA was increased by TGF-β, without impacting mRNA synthesis by lung fibroblasts (134). This is important, since increased TGF-β signaling and levels of TGF-β ligands were associated with experimental (117) and clinical BPD (115). Apart from TGF-β, increased IGF levels were also associated with experimental (135) and clinical (136) BPD, whereas decreased levels of some forms of PDGF were associated with clinical BPD (137). Taken together, these data would suggest that the pro-elastogenic effects of TGF-β and IGF were promoted, while the anti-elastogenic activity of PDGF was blocked during arrested alveolarization associated with BPD. These effects may also explain the increased abundance of Eln mRNA in the lung in hyperoxia-based experimental animal models of BPD.

It might be argued that given the extraordinarily long half-life of elastin fibers in the lung [estimated to be several years in the mouse (138)], studies on gene expression are less meaningful than studies on elastin protein production and organization into elastic fibers. Experimental studies on alveolarization tend to examine elastin distribution by light microscopy [for example, with Hart's stain (72, 100, 101) or immunohistochemistry (51)], and infer elastin abundance from those studies. However, some studies have directly addressed insoluble elastin fiber abundance biochemically, where, in contrast to elevated mRNA levels, there appeared to be a paucity of insoluble elastin in affected lungs, assessed by lung desmosine or isodesmosine amounts (89, 96). The paucity of elastin was generally accompanied by the clearly disorganized structure and distribution of elastin fibers evident in the developing septa. This discord between elastin gene expression (which was increased) and the abundance of insoluble elastin (which was decreased) in injured developing lungs (together with perturbed elastin fiber structure and distribution) has several possible explanations, none of which have yet been experimentally tested. (i) The post-transcriptional regulation of Eln gene expression may be affected. For example, translation of mature Eln mRNA may be blocked by microRNA species generated in response to hyperoxia. Among the microRNA species that have been identified the target elastin are miR-29a/b/c (139) and miR-184, miR-194, miR-299, and miR-376b (http://www.mirbase.org). The possibility of microRNA regulation of elastin expression in the lung has not yet been addressed. Alternatively, the paucity of insoluble elastin in the background of increased Eln mRNA abundance might be attributed to (ii) defective post-translational maturation of elastin during fiber formation, or (iii) increased proteolytic degradation of elastin. Concerning post-translational maturation of elastin fibers, many accessory proteins have been identified that can associate with elastin fibers. These include the glycoproteins emilin (140), fibulin (29), LTBP (141), and MAGP family members (142). Discordant expression of these elastin fiber-associated proteins may result in unstable or malformed fiber structures. Indeed, Richard Bland has proposed that the uncoupling of elastin synthesis and assembly is a pathogenic contributor to disordered elastin fiber generation in BPD (23). Elastin fibers with abnormal physical properties may also result from the aberrant activity of the elastin maturation machinery, including the hydroxylation and cross-linking activities of lysyl hydroxylases and lysyl oxidases, respectively. These possibilities are discussed below. Alternatively, changes in the proteolytic capacity of injured, developing lungs may impact elastin fiber production or turnover, either directly (by proteolysis) or indirectly (by regulating the activity of mediators of elastin production). It is these lines of enquiry that are likely to further our understanding of *why* elastin organization is disturbed, and *what* impact this has on alveolarization in the developing lungs.

Some reports addressing the role of serine proteinases in the regulation of elastin production have already yielded exciting data. The group of Richard Bland has examined the utility of blocking serine peptidase activity in the context of BPD. Serine peptidase activity, such as that of neutrophil elastase, was elevated in the lung in clinical and experimental BPD. Mechanical ventilation of mouse pups with 40% O_2 increased elastin degradation and disturbed septal elastin fiber deposition in the mouse lung, which was prevented by intratracheal administration of the neutrophil elastase inhibitor elafin (100). Thus, inhibition of neutrophil elastase activity [and probably matrix metalloproteinase (MMP)-9 activity as well, since MMP-9 can also be inhibited by elafin] partially restored proper elastin structures and improved lung alveolarization in this model. Furthermore, inhibition of neutrophil elastase activity blunted inflammation and inhibited the generation of active TGF-β that was proposed to be released from the ECM by proteolysis. In support of this idea, transgenic over-expression of elafin in the vascular endothelium similarly protected mice against the aberrant alveolarization and perturbed elastin assembly caused by mechanical ventilation (101). Subsequent exciting work by Keith Tanswell's group has similarly reported that neutrophil elastase inhibition with sivelestat also improved lung structure and elastin deposition in the hyperoxia-based BPD animal model in mice (98). In this study, it is also noted that administration of anti-elastin antibodies in the mouse hyperoxia model of BPD prevented inflammatory infiltration into the lungs. Thus, these investigators raised the exciting possibility that neutrophil elastase-generated elastin fragments acted as pro-inflammatory matrikines (143), suggesting a mechanism by which hyperoxia exposure provoked lung inflammation. These data also raise further questions, for example, while neutrophil elastase inhibition clearly improved alveolarization in two different animal models of BPD, the underlying mechanisms remain unclear. The organization of elastin fibers was improved in both models, and inflammation and TGF-β activation was blunted. However, it remains unclear whether the improved alveolarization was a direct or indirect consequence of elastase inhibition (144). For example, was the generation of elastin fragments sufficient to provoke lung inflammation, or did the elastase-mediated activation of TGF-β play a role in this process as well? Elastase inhibition in the background of TGF-β neutralization would go some distance to resolving these open questions.

One vexing controversy in the lung alveolarization field is: are elastin protein levels elevated or reduced in the aberrantly developing lungs in the hyperoxia-based animal models of BPD? In mechanically ventilated lambs and mice, multiple reports document increased *Eln* mRNA levels, which were consistent with increased elastin protein levels in the lung (23, 102). However, this was not the case with normobaric hyperoxia-based models in mice, where many reports also confirm that Eln mRNA levels were up-regulated by hyperoxia exposure, but there appeared to be a paucity of lung insoluble elastin, when (iso)desmosine was used as a surrogate for mature, insoluble elastin fibers (89, 96). However, these observations are complicated by other reports of *increased* elastin protein in the hyperoxia models, employing either slot–blots (98) or immunoblots (51, 93). This controversy must still be resolved. These discordant data might be attributable to the methodology employed, where protein extraction by sodium dodecyl sulfate (SDS)-polyacrylamide gel electrophoresis (PAGE) for the blot-based protocols may have a different capacity for the extraction of insoluble elastin compared with the whole-lung hydrolyzates used in the (iso)desmosine approaches. Irrespectively, neither approach address the quantification of elastin specifically in the developing septa, which represents a major limitation of all of the approaches currently employed.

The current state of the field seems to suggest less lung elastin and more lung collagen, at least in the hyperoxia models of BPD. Given that, collagen imparts rigidity and elastin imparts elasticity to the lung, a shift in the collagen:elastin ratio may impact alveologenesis. This shift in collagen:elastin ratio may be as much as threefold increased by hyperoxia exposure (89). This is likely to dramatically impact lung compliance, and given the importance of the physical forces generated by breathing motions in "pulling the alveoli into shape," a shift in the lung collagen:elastin ratio cannot be discounted as a possible contributing factor to lung alveolar development.

ADDITIONAL STRUCTURAL COMPONENTS OF THE ECM

Fibrillins

Fibrillins are elastin-binding glycoproteins (**Figure 2**) that make up the bulk of the microfibril component of elastic fibers, and act as a scaffold for elastic fiber deposition (28). Fibrillin-1 (Fbn1) and fibrillin-2 (Fbn2) are the main microfibril proteins (145). Fbn1 is clearly important for alveolarization and the structural homeostasis of the alveoli, since *Fbn1$^{-/-}$* mice exhibited an alveolarization defect (146), and fibrillin fibers were fragmented and disorganized in emphysema (147). In addition to imparting structural properties to elastic fibers, fibrillins may also help to mediate elastic fiber assembly, such as lysyl oxidase cross-linking of elastin fibers (28), which is thought to be highly relevant to lung development (27, 64, 72, 89, 148, 149). Similarly, Fbn1 played a role in anchoring LTBP to ECM components (58). Changes in fibrillin expression have been noted in animal models of BPD. In mechanically ventilated mice, the ratio of Fbn1:Fbn2 was increased, with elevated Fbn1 expression and reduced Fbn2 expression noted (23, 99). By contrast, in the mouse hyperoxia model of BPD, the expression of both *Fbn1* and *Fbn2* mRNA was elevated (51). With these ideas in mind, disturbances to fibrillin expression may impact lung development either by directly modulating the physical properties of elastic fibers or by altering TGF-β dynamics in the ECM. These ideas await experimental investigation.

Tenascin C

Tenascins are a five-member family of large ECM glycoproteins, with tenascin C (Tnc), which is expressed in myofibroblasts, and endothelial, smooth muscle, and type II cells (81, 83), being the most studied in lung development (84) (**Table 1**). Tnc was comparatively highly expressed during human and animal development, including in the lung, particularly during the pseudoglandular and canalicular stages (84), at sites of active branching. Tnc is important for alveolarization, since *Tnc$^{-/-}$* mice exhibited an alveolarization defect (150). Along these lines, administration of dexamethasone to developing mouse pups blunted alveolarization, which was accompanied by decreased Tnc expression (56), although the impact of dexamethasone on Tnc expression was not causally linked to the blunted alveolarization. In contrast to these findings, *TNC* expression was elevated in the lungs of patients with BPD (83), which is consistent with the ability of TGF-β to drive *Tnc* expression in primary mouse fibroblasts *in vitro* (95). Tnc clearly plays a role in normal lung alveolarization; however, a causal role for changes on Tnc expression in aberrant lung alveolarization has yet to be demonstrated.

Fibronectin

Fibronectin (Fn1) is a large (440 kDa) glycoprotein dimer, consisting of two almost identical subunits. Fn1 has been reported both as a soluble form in plasma and as an insoluble form associated with the ECM, where Fn1 binds collagen (**Figure 2**), as well as Tnc, and other ECM components (151). Fn1 is expressed in the lung (152), in interstitial fibroblasts, endothelial cells, and smooth muscle cells, but not in epithelial cells (**Table 1**). Fn1 expression was highest during lung development, and very low in adult lung tissue (152). $Fn1^{-/-}$ mice exhibited early embryonic lethality (153), and a role for *Fn1* in lung development has not been demonstrated but is assumed. Several studies have documented the increased expression of Fn1 in clinical BPD, including in plasma, in endotracheal aspirates, and in BAL fluid (60, 104, 154, 155), as well as in lung tissue (60). This is consistent with the ability of TGF-β to drive Fb1 expression in lung fibroblasts (152). To date, no causal role for Fb1 in normal or aberrant lung development has been demonstrated. However, one exciting observation has suggested that decreased miR-206 expression in both clinical and experimental BPD may underlie the increased levels of *FB1* noted in the lungs of BPD patients (60, 105), since *FB1* has been described to be a target of miR-206 (105). Furthermore, miR-206 levels were decreased, whereas *Fb1* levels were increased in lungs from hyperoxia-exposed mouse pups (105). Taken together, these data make a compelling argument for the miR-206/Fb1 axis in aberrant alveolarization associated with BPD, although this idea requires experimental demonstration.

Fibulins and Emilins

Fibulins and emilins promote proper elastin fiber formation, by mediating protein–protein interactions between ECM proteins, or between the ECM and ECM remodeling enzymes, such as lysyl oxidases (156). Fibulins are small calcium-dependent glycoproteins that bind elastin (**Figure 2**). Fibulin-5 (Fbln5; also called developmental arteries and neural crest EGF-like protein, DANCE) has been reported to play a role in lung alveolarization. $Fbln5^{-/-}$ mice exhibited short, fragmented, and thickened elastin fibers, as well as a pronounced arrest of alveolarization (29, 157). No studies have examined a role for fibulins in clinical BPD; however, studies in animal models of BPD consistently revealed increased expression of Fbln5 in mouse pups exposed to hyperoxia (51, 72). Since TGF-β can drive Fbln5 expression (158), increased Fbln5 production after hyperoxia exposure may have been due to the attendant increased TGF-β signaling seen in this model (95). Changes in fibulin expression also appear to be sensitive to mechanical ventilation, where Martin Post's group demonstrated that *Fbln5* expression was impacted by the duration and intensity of tidal volume ventilation, and breathing frequency, when rats were mechanically ventilated with room air (103). Conversely, Richard Bland's group did not detect any impact of mechanical ventilation on Fbln5 expression when mice were ventilated with room air; however, ventilation with 40% O_2 reduced Fbln5 levels in the lung, which was accompanied by blunted alveolarization. While the $Fbln5^{-/-}$ mouse studies have implied a role for Fbln5 in alveolarization, the impact of increased Fbln5 expression on secondary septation and the development of the alveoli await

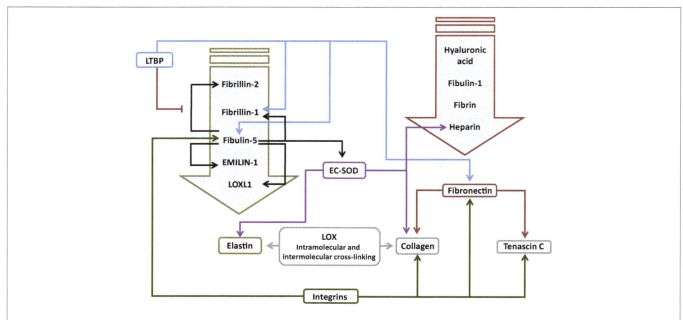

FIGURE 2 | Interactions between components of the extracellular matrix in the lung. The primary interacting molecules for elastin and fibronectin are collected together above the respective target molecules in the downward-pointing block arrows. Abbreviations: EC-SOD, extracellular superoxide dismutase; EMILIN-1, elastin microfibril interfacer 1; LOX, lysyl oxidase; LOXL1, lysyl oxidase-like 1; LTBP, latent transforming growth factor-β-binding protein.

demonstration. By way of speculation, Fbln5 promoted activation of MMP-2 and MMP-9 (159), which have also been associated with clinical and experimental BPD (see below). This, together with the possibility that Fbln5 over-expression might disturb elastic fiber formation, and might regulate the association of superoxide dismutase (SOD) (160) and lysyl oxidase-like 1 (LoxL1) (64) with the ECM, suggests avenues by which fibulin over-expression may influence lung development.

Like fibulins, emilins are a related group of elastic fiber-associated proteins (**Figure 2**), which impact elastogenesis, and have been reported to be expressed in the lung (161). Elastin microfibril interfacer 1 (Emilin-1) expression has not been studied in clinical BPD. However, Emilin1 expression has been reported to be dysregulated in animal models of BPD, including the hyperoxia exposure [*Emilin1* mRNA expression up-regulated; (23, 72)] and mechanical ventilation [Emilin1 protein expression down-regulated; (23)] in mice. *Emilin1*$^{-/-}$ knockout mice do exist (162), although no lung phenotype has been reported. However, the reported dramatic (2,000-fold) up-regulation of *Emilin1* expression in c-Jun N-terminal kinase (Jnk) knockout mice was reported to be accompanied by an alveolarization defect, perhaps implicating Emilin1 in the alveolarization process (163), although a dramatic up-regulation of *Fbln1*, *Fbln5*, and *Eln* expression was also noted in that study.

Latent TGF-β-Binding Proteins

The LTBP family consists of four extracellular MAGPs (164), which interact with, thereby modulate the activity of TGF-β. Ltbp1, Ltbp3, and Ltbp4 are reported to all associate with the small latent complex of TGF-β ligands and latency-associated propeptide (LAP), to generate the large latent complex (164). The LTBP family members are structurally related to fibrillins and were reported to interact with the ECM and play a role in ECM assembly. *Ltbp1*$^{-/-}$ mice exhibited perinatal lethality with heart defects, while a lung phenotype was not studied or reported (165). By contrast, both *Ltbp3*$^{-/-}$ and *Ltbp4*$^{-/-}$ mice exhibited an arrest of alveolarization (166) that was more pronounced in *Ltbp4*$^{-/-}$ mice (167). Ltbp4, which is known to bind Fbln5 (167), is believed to independently modulate elastogenesis and TGF-β activity, and thus, regulate lung development (168). The function of Ltbp2 remains elusive (164), but it has been suggested that Ltbp2 plays a TGF-β-independent role in elastogenesis (141), and Ltbp2 has been co-localized with fibronectin and Fbn1 in lung fibroblast cultures (58). Studies on Ltbp2 are complicated by the embryonic lethality reported in *Ltbp2*$^{-/-}$ mice (169). Interestingly, despite a clear role in alveolarization, no studies, to date, have examined the expression of LTBP family members in clinical or experimental BPD. These exciting studies await experimental investigation.

Polysaccharide Conjugates

Heparin, heparan sulfate, hyaluronic acid (hyaluronan), and chondroitin sulfate are polysaccharides or polysaccharide conjugates that have been reported to be mediators of lung alveolarization (170–172). Proteins carrying these conjugates, such as syndecan, which contains both heparan sulfate and chondroitin sulfate, exhibited molecular polymorphism – notably changes

in the length of the heparin sulfate chains – over the course of lung development (173), implicating a role for heparan sulfate proteoglycans in lung development.

Temporal and spatial changes in glycosaminoglycan synthesis by lung fibroblasts have also been reported during lung development (174). Notably, fibroblasts in close proximity to the epithelium secreted hyaluronan, while more distant fibroblasts produced heparan sulfate and chondroitin sulfate during the pseudoglandular stage of lung development. During later stages of lung development, these fibroblasts switched to producing more hyaluronan, which was coincident with the thinning of the alveolar walls during the canalicular and later developmental stages. These authors postulated that developmentally regulated glycosaminoglycan generation by lung fibroblasts facilitated lung epithelial–mesenchymal interactions, which guided aspects of lung development (174).

Heparin and heparan sulfate have been reported to be the predominant glycosaminoglycans in epithelial basement membranes of the alveolus, and granules associated with collagen fibers of the basement membrane contained proteoglycan aggregates, which included chondroitin or dermatan sulfate (175). Heparan sulfate has been localized in the basement membrane during the embryonic, canalicular, and later phases of lung development (176). Heparan sulfate has received particular attention as a growth factor-binding protein, particularly in the context of fibroblast growth factor (FGF)-10, where Wellington Cardoso's group has provided evidence that FGF-10 induction of local budding during early lung development is directed by developmentally regulated regional patterns of heparan sulfate sulfation (177). This idea has also been extended to cytokines, such as interleukin (IL)-1 in the developing chick lung (178), as well as members of the bone morphogenetic protein (BMP) family (179).

Several studies in transgenic mice have highlighted causal roles for enzymes of the heparan sulfate biosynthetic pathway in lung development. For example, deletion of *N*-deacetylase/*N*-sulfotransferase (heparan glucosaminyl) 1 (Ndst1) led to pulmonary hyperplasia and acute respiratory distress in mice, possibly due to decreased surfactant production as a result of type II cells to mature (180). Similarly, deletion of glucuronyl C5-epimerase (Glce) in mice caused embryonic lethality, and stunted embryonic lung development, which was accompanied by a total loss of L-iduronic acid in heparan sulfate conjugates (181). Specifically concerning late lung development, defects in the development of the airspaces have been noted in both heparan sulfate 6-O-sulfotransferase 1 (Hs6st1) (182) and sulfatase 2 (Sulf2) (183) knockout mice. Apart from mice lacking enzymes involved in the heparan sulfate biosynthetic pathway, mice lacking heparan sulfate proteoglycans also exhibit lung development phenotypes. For example, deletion of glypican-3, a member of a family of heparan sulfate proteoglycans linked to the cell surface through a glycosyl-phosphatidylinositol anchor, generated abnormal lung structures in mice (184). These studies validated the earlier suggestion that heparin and heparan sulfate are mediators of lung development, although most work has been confined to the earlier stages of lung development that precede alveolarization. The generation of antibodies that detect specific heparan sulfate epitopes has facilitated the identification of spatio-temporal changes in heparan sulfate structure during normal lung development, and aberrant lung development associated with congenital diaphragmatic hernia (CDH) (65, 185), which will facilitate further mechanistic work in this area. To date, exactly how these structural abnormalities to heparan sulfate proteoglycans results in disturbed alveolar structure remains to be clarified.

In addition to heparan sulfate proteoglycans, some work in embryonic lung explants has also revealed a role for chondroitin sulfate proteoglycans in early lung development (186). Furthermore, an interesting connection with inflammatory cells has been made, with the suggestion that CD44-positive macrophages, which take up hyaluronan, may regulate the steady-state levels of hyaluronan during lung development (187). Further work in this area should examine *how* defined alterations to proteoglycan structures direct proper development of the lung. The existence of transgenic mice and monoclonal antibodies that allow the specific detection of proteoglycan structures will facilitate these efforts. Additionally, no studies, to date, have examined changes in the expression of proteoglycan biosynthetic enzymes, or proteoglycan structures, in animal models of BPD.

ECM-INTERACTING MOLECULES

Integrins

Integrins are large heterodimeric transmembrane glycoproteins associated with various elements of the ECM. Integrin ligands include collagen I, Tnc, Fb1, laminins, TGF-β, and tissue transglutaminase (Tgm2), among many others. Each integrin dimer consists of a single α and β subunit. There are many integrin subunits, with 18 α and 8 β subunits having been identified in humans, to date (67). Expression of integrins is known to be dynamically regulated during lung development, where integrin-mediated cell–ECM interactions are known to play an important role (68, 188). Integrin expression has been noted during alveolarization, with the α2, α3, α6, and β1 subunits having been reported to be expressed in the bronchial and alveolar epithelium during the alveolar stage of lung development, as well as in adult lungs. By contrast, the α4 subunit was reported to be expressed in the respiratory epithelium only during lung development and has not been detected in adult lungs (68, 69, 188). The fibronectin receptor, integrin α8β1 (189) has been demonstrated to play a particularly noteworthy role in early and late lung development, where the Lawrence Prince's group demonstrated that *in utero* exposure of developing embryos to bacterial lipopolysaccharide (LPS) caused a reduction in expression of *Itga8*, which encodes the α8 integrin subunit, in mesenchymal cells (30). Thus, these authors examined lung structure in *Itga8$^{-/-}$* mice, which exhibited a pronounced disturbance to the developing lung structure, including lobar fusion and alveolar simplification. Additionally, elastin fibers in these mouse lungs were described to be "wavy and short." This led these authors to suggest that integrin–ECM interactions played a notable role in late lung development. This idea is supported by observations made in the mouse hyperoxia BPD model, where increased expression of *Itgav*, encoding the α$_v$ integrin subunit [which also binds fibronectin; (67)], was

noted (51), and was accompanied by impaired alveolarization and increased *Fbln5* expression and TGF-β activity, and aberrant elastin fiber deposition. These studies have opened up an exciting new avenue, that is, the role of integrin-mediated ECM interactions in the regulation of alveolarization.

Extracellular Superoxide Dismutase

Extracellular superoxide dismutase (EC-SOD or Sod3), is one of three forms of SOD, a group of antioxidant enzymes representing the major cellular defense against the superoxide anion $\left(O_2^-\right)$ (54, 190). EC-SOD is the only ECM-related antioxidant and has been reported to be the most abundant SOD in the lung (191). EC-SOD was reported to be expressed primarily in vessels, large airways, and alveolar septa. EC-SOD binds heparin (192) and heparan sulfate proteoglycans on the cell surface, and components of the ECM (54). EC-SOD binds collagen I (**Figure 2**) and is thought to protect against oxidative damage to collagen I (193). EC-SOD is also known to bind to tropoelastin, a process that is mediated by Fbln5 (160). EC-SOD is believed to play a role in protecting the ECM from oxidative damage, since reactive oxygen species (ROS) drive elastin degradation and increased collagen cross-linking (194, 195). Thus, EC-SOD might protect the developing and adult lung from oxidative damage (54), since EC-SOD was reported to be expressed throughout life (196), although EC-SOD protein expression and activity were blunted by hyperoxia exposure in adult mice (197). Along these lines, adult *Sod$^{-/-}$* mice exhibited increased sensitivity to hyperoxic damage, with reduced survival and more pronounced alveolar edema, compared to wild-type mice; thus, supporting a role for EC-SOD in protection against oxidative damage to the lung (198). In support of this idea, over-expression of EC-SOD in transgenic neonatal mice protected against the damaging effects of hyperoxia on lung alveolarization (196), and expression of EC-SOD in a mouse lung epithelial cell-line protected against oxidative damage-induced cell death (55). The protective effects of EC-SOD over-expression on lung epithelial cells has also been demonstrated *in vivo* in hyperoxia-exposed newborn mice (199). None of these studies addressed collagen or elastin fiber integrity.

A wide spectrum of other ECM-interacting proteins still remains to be studied in the context of lung alveolarization. These proteins include the MAGP family members (142), as well as the small leucine-rich proteoglycans, such as decorin and related molecules, which play key roles in driving collagen fiber formation (200, 201). These future studies will no doubt add to the list of ECM-associated proteins that impact normal and aberrant late lung development.

ECM REMODELING ENZYMES

Matrix Metalloproteinases and Their Inhibitors

Matrix metalloproteinases are a large family of endopeptidases responsible for ECM breakdown and remodeling, which are necessary processes for proper formation of the ECM (9, 202). Different MMPs preferentially degrade different components of the ECM, with MMP-1 and MMP-8 active against fibrillar collagens, and MMP-2 and MMP-9 preferentially active against basement membrane collagen (collagen IV), fibronectin, and elastin (77, 203–206). The proteolytic activity of MMPs can be regulated by MMP binding to cognate inhibitors, such as tissue inhibitor of metalloproteinases (TIMPs) (110, 207) (**Figure 3**). The expression of MMPs in the lung is known to be dynamically regulated over the course of lung development (**Figure 1**), with a progressive decrease in MMP-2 and MMP-14 [also called membrane-type-1 (MT1)-MMP] expression, but a progressive increase in MMP-9 expression between E10 and P21. These trends imply a role in lung alveolarization (9, 75, 78). Expression of MMP-2 and MMP-14 has been noted in airway and alveolar epithelial cells, endothelial cells, and fibroblasts (74–76), whereas MMP-9 was reported to be expressed in epithelial cells, fibroblasts, and inflammatory cells, including neutrophils and alveolar macrophages (61, 77, 79) (**Table 1**). MMP expression in the lung was driven by exposure of adult (77) and neonatal (93) rodents to hyperoxia. Similarly, elevated MMP expression has been noted in endotracheal aspirates or BAL fluid from preterm infants with BPD (109, 111–113). MMPs also played a role in alveolar destruction in experimental emphysema in mice (208). MMPs might impact alveolarization directly, through degradation of ECM components, or indirectly, through activation of growth factor pathways. For example, MMP-9 activated TGF-β signaling, which in turn stimulated lung fibroblasts to contract (61, 209). MMP-9 appeared to be able to influence lung alveolarization, since $Mmp9^{-/-}$ mice exhibited worsened lung development, in a mouse model where lung alveolarization was blocked by over-expression of IL-1β (210). In an alternative hyperoxia-based BPD model, $Mmp9^{-/-}$ mice were protected against the blunted alveolarization usually seen in the mouse hyperoxia BPD model (93). The reasons for these two discordant observations are currently unclear, however, may be related to the different models employed. Along the same lines, $Mmp14^{-/-}$ mice initially exhibited a 40% decrease in alveolar surface area compared to wild-type mice early during post-natal lung development (76), which was accompanied by thickened elastin fibers. By contrast, $Mmp2^{-/-}$ mice exhibited a "delayed" alveolarization, where an alveolarization defect was noted at P7, but alveolarization was normalized at P14 (76). It would be interesting to explore the impact of hyperoxia or mechanical ventilation of the $Mmp2^{-/-}$ and $Mmp14^{-/-}$ mice on alveolarization.

Several studies have addressed MMP expression in clinical BPD cases, where reduced MMP-2 levels were noted in endotracheal aspirates (109) and plasma (211), but increased MMP-8 levels were noted in endotracheal aspirates (111) and BAL fluid (112) from preterm infants with BPD. Increased MMP-9:TIMP-1 ratios have also been detected in BAL fluids from preterm infants that developed BPD (114) (**Figure 4**). Additionally, Ekekezie and coworkers (113) observed an increased MMP-9:TIMP-1 ratio in endotracheal aspirates from BPD patients, which correlated with poor patient outcome. These trends largely parallel observations made in animal models of BPD, where increased levels of MMP-2 and MMP-9 proteins were noted in hyperoxia-exposed mouse pups (93). Similarly, MMP-9 levels were modulated in the lungs of hyperoxia-exposed rats (78), and increased MMP-9 levels and an increased MMP-9:TIMP-1 ratio were noted in a premature baboon BPD model (107). Not all trends in MMP expression are consistent between investigations. For example, Hosford and co-workers reported the *decreased* expression of MMP-9 and *increased* expression of TIMP-1 in the rat hyperoxia model of BPD (110), which was also accompanied by blunted alveolarization. These discordant observations might be attributed to the extraordinary variation in the application of the BPD models: (i) newborn rats exposed to >90% O_2 for 9 days versus (ii) ventilated, premature baboons versus (iii) rats exposed to >95% O_2 between P4 and P14. Irrespectively, the general trend is toward increased MMP-9 activity in aberrantly developing lungs.

Lysyl Oxidases

Lysyl oxidases constitute a family of five members: the archetypical lysyl oxidase (Lox) and four lysyl oxidase-like enzymes (Loxl1–LoxL4) (212, 213). All lysyl oxidases catalyze the oxidative deamination of lysine and hydroxylysine residues, generating reactive semialdehydes, which then form intramolecular and intermolecular covalent cross-links in both elastin and collagen molecules (212, 213). Lysyl oxidases have been reported to play an essential role in normal lung development and have been implicated in the pathogenesis of several lung diseases, including pulmonary hypertension (73), lung adenocarcinoma (214), and BPD (72). Lysyl oxidases are known to play an important role in organogenesis, with $Lox^{-/-}$ mice exhibiting perinatal lethality, ostensibly due to a failure of the cardio-respiratory system (215, 216). Furthermore, Lox has been specifically implicated in the development of the respiratory system, where Lox has been reported to be required for the integrity of elastic and collagen fibers in multiple tissues (27). Interestingly, genetic ablation

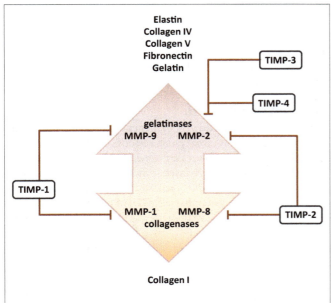

FIGURE 3 | Cognate inhibitors and target substrates of matrix metalloproteinases. The target substrates of the gelatinase and collagenase members of the matrix metalloproteinase (MMP) family are indicated, together with selected target MMP substrates. Abbreviation: TIMPs, tissue inhibitor of matrix metalloproteinases.

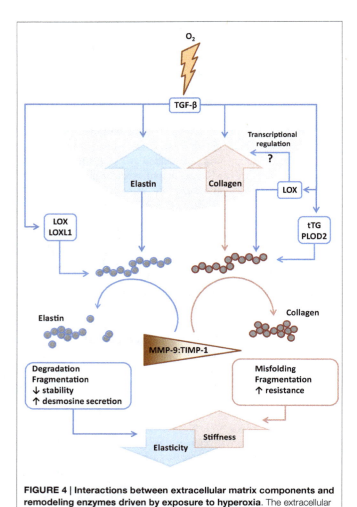

FIGURE 4 | **Interactions between extracellular matrix components and remodeling enzymes driven by exposure to hyperoxia**. The extracellular matrix remodeling processes that are described to be driven by exposure of the developing lung to hyperoxia that lead to increased stiffness and decreased elasticity of the developing lungs. Abbreviations: LOX, lysyl oxidase; LOXL1, lysyl oxidase-like 1; MMP, matrix metalloproteinase; TGF-β, transforming growth factor-β; TIMPs, tissue inhibitor of matrix metalloproteinases; tTG, tissue transglutaminase.

exclusively of Lox expression significantly reduced total lysyl oxidase activity, suggesting that Lox is the primary contributor out of the five family members, to lysyl oxidase-mediated effects. In $Lox^{-/-}$ mouse lungs, both desmosine and hydroxyproline levels were decreased relative to wild-type mice (216). While viable, $Loxl1^{-/-}$ mice exhibited connective tissue weakness, and developed pelvic organ prolapse and *cutis laxa* (64). Furthermore, $Loxl1^{-/-}$ mice exhibited alveolar simplification and reduced lung desmosine levels, implying a role in lung development, as well as perturbed elastin fiber structures throughout the organism (64).

Lysyl oxidase expression has been studied in animal models of BPD. Increased Lox and Loxl1 expression has been noted in the lungs of preterm ventilated lambs (24). Lox expression was also increased by mechanical ventilation in mouse pups (23), but lung Loxl1 levels were reduced in mechanically ventilated mice (23). Elevated lysyl oxidase activity (72, 89, 94), and elevated Lox and Loxl1 levels (72, 89) were detected in newborn mice exposed to

normobaric hyperoxia. This has led some investigators to propose that the ECM in affected lungs might be "over cross-linked," and thus excessively stabilized, which has been proposed to be a potential contributing factor in arrested alveologenesis associated with clinical and experimental BPD (72, 89). Consistent with elevated Lox expression and activity, exposure to hyperoxia also generated increased amounts of insoluble collagen and the dihydroxylysinonorleucine (DHLNL) collagen cross-link, as well as an increased DHLNL:hydroxylysinonorleucine (HLNL) ratio, and disordered elastin organization in the alveolar septa (89). To address a causal role for lysyl oxidases in blunted alveolarization in the hyperoxia BPD model, newborn mice were treated with the pan-lysyl oxidase inhibitor β-aminopropionitrile (BAPN), which did not improve lung alveolarization, but did improve elastin organization assessed by visual inspection (89). This might indicate that the partial normalization of elastin organization in developing septa alone (through normalization of lysyl oxidase activity) was not sufficient to normalize lung alveolarization in the mouse hyperoxia BPD model. Several questions regarding lysyl oxidases and alveolarization come to mind, among them: what role do the different lysyl oxidases play in lung development, and in which tissues? Lysyl oxidases are expressed in several different cell types (**Table 1**), and it may be that different lysyl oxidases have different contributions to lung alveolarization, acting in different cell types. The generation of conditional, inducible deletions of the various lysyl oxidase genes would help to address this question. Additionally, "non-matrix" roles for lysyl oxidases should also be considered, where lysyl oxidases have been reported to modulate gene regulation in the nucleus, for example, the expression of *COL3A1* (217). This has revealed nuclear functions – primarily of LoxL2 – which modulated epigenetic effects in the nucleus by deamination of trimethylated Lys[4] in histone H3, which was linked to transcriptional repression (218). Furthermore, LoxL2 regulated keratinocyte differentiation independent of lysyl oxidase catalytic activity (219). Similar studies have yet to be performed with other lysyl oxidases, but highlight possible roles for lysyl oxidases in lung alveolarization that are not related to ECM cross-linking.

Lysyl Hydroxylases

The ability of lysyl oxidases to generate covalent cross-links requires lysine or hydroxylysine residues in ECM substrates. These hydroxylysine residues are generated by another family of enzymes, the lysyl hydroxylases (officially named procollagen-lysine, 2-oxoglutarate 5-dioxygenases, or PLODs) (220), which consist of three family members: PLOD1–PLOD3. A role for lysyl hydroxylases in organ development was underscored by the early embryonic lethality of $Plod3^{-/-}$ mice (221), while $Plod1^{-/-}$ mice were viable, but exhibited vascular pathology and abnormal collagen fiber structure (222). This family of ECM-modifying enzymes is relatively poorly characterized. Some evidence does exist illustrating that lysyl hydroxylases play a role in aberrant late lung development, both in humans and in mice. A recent study by Witsch and colleagues (80) revealed that the lung expression of PLOD family member PLOD2 was up-regulated in premature infants with BPD. Furthermore, *Plod1*, *Plod2*, and *Plod3* expression was elevated in the lungs of mice in the hyperoxia BPD model

(80), and the elevated *Plod2* expression was mediated by TGF-β. These data indicate that the lysyl hydroxylases may play a role in normal and abnormal lung development, and this possibility awaits experimental attention.

Transglutaminases

The transglutaminases constitute an eight-member family of calcium-dependent enzymes, which cross-link collagens and fibronectin, among other proteins (223). Of the transglutaminases, largely transglutaminase 2 (Tgm2; also called tissue transglutaminase, tTG) has been studied in lung disease and was reported to be expressed in fibroblasts, as well as epithelial, endothelial, and smooth muscle cells (85, 224). In addition to cross-linking activity, Tgm2 is an integrin-binding adhesion co-receptor for fibronectin (225). Tgm2 has also been implicated in lung fibrosis (86, 226, 227), allergy (87), cystic fibrosis (228, 229), and pulmonary hypertension (230). Tgm2 has further been credited with a role in organogenesis (231), including lung development (232). In preterm infants with BPD, *TGM2* mRNA levels were elevated (85), which was also seen in the lungs of hyperoxia-exposed newborn mice with experimental BPD (85). In the case of hyperoxia-exposed newborn mice, increased *Tgm2* levels were driven by TGF-β, most likely in lung epithelial cells. This is particularly noteworthy because not only can TGF-β drive Tgm2 expression but Tgm2 can also activate TGF-β (233), suggesting a possible vicious circle of Tgm2 expression and TGF-β activation in aberrant lung alveolarization. These studies indicate that changes in transglutaminase expression are associated with normal and aberrant alveolarization; however, a causal role for transglutaminases in lung development has yet to be experimentally documented. The existing *Tmg2*$^{-/-}$ knockout mice would be an ideal starting point for these studies (234).

PERSPECTIVE

Given that, the ECM plays a pivotal role in lung development, it comes as no surprise that perturbations to ECM production and remodeling accompany defective secondary septation and aberrant alveolarization associated with BPD. Identification of the perturbations to ECM organization that play a causal role in aberrant alveolarization would assist in our understanding of the pathological processes that disturb late lung development. Equally important is the delineation of pathogenic pathways that drive these causal disturbances to ECM structure.

Roles for ECM structural proteins and ECM remodeling enzymes in lung alveolarization have been identified using gene knockout approaches. These studies have provided a very solid foundation for future work but are complicated by the pre- or peri-natal lethal phenotype of some knockout mice. This has been partially remedied by the parallel over-expression of human genes, or genes with altered promoter activity, in the background of a homozygous-null strain (such as the expression of the human *ELN* gene in *Eln*$^{-/-}$ mice, described above), which overcome the lethality of the homozygous-null mutants, and facilitated further studies on the gene products of interest. However, this has been more the exception than the norm. Additionally, it is widely recognized that the discrete expression of particular *genes*, in

particular, *cell types* at particular *stages* of lung development is the basis of the highly coordinated program of the generation of a very complex organ (1, 2). This makes the use of constitutive global knockout mouse strains problematic.

Rapidly evolving mouse transgenic technology makes an increasing number of conditional-ready gene-deletion strains available through the use of floxed alleles. In combination with inducible Cre-recombinase systems, these conditional strains become inducible, conditional strains, which facilitate gene deletion in developing mouse pups at particular time points during post-natal lung development, in restricted cell types. These approaches rely largely on the use of doxycycline-inducible rtTA (*tetO*)$_7$-Cre and tamoxifen-inducible Cre^{ERT2} systems. These inducible, conditional-ready mouse strains will prove invaluable in assessing how the temporal and tissue-specific expression of particular genes during lung development impacts lung development *per se* (235). Among the drawbacks of this approach are the limitations of some floxed allele strains, which would have to be created *de novo*, and also, the lack of – or technical difficulties with the use of – some driver lines. For example, no suitable driver line currently exists that can exclusively target lung fibroblasts, or that can discriminate between airway and vascular smooth muscle cells (235). Remaining with transgenic mice, most studies, to date, have evaluated the loss of a particular gene on lung development. However, particularly in the context of animal models of BPD, genes might be over-expressed or up-regulated, rather than down-regulated. As such, to be able to "phenocopy" a lung phenotype by over-expressing a gene of interest, *in the correct cell-type at the correct time*, would go a long way to validate candidate pathogenic mediators of arrested alveolarization. Along these lines, many knockout and pharmacological intervention studies have identified new "players" in normal lung alveolarization (such as LTBP and elastin and collagen cross-linking enzymes), but a contribution to pathological lung development in animal models of BPD has not been undertaken. These exciting studies may well reveal new pathogenic pathways that drive aberrant lung alveolarization.

While elastin has received a tremendous amount of attention as a regulator of lung development, the collagens remained largely neglected. Since many candidate pathogenic mediators (such as elastin cross-linking enzymes) also influence collagen structure and function, it would be interesting to explore roles for disturbed collagen organization during lung development. Along these lines, the ratio of elastin:collagen is also noteworthy. In the hyperoxia models of BPD, there is a reported shift toward an increased collagen:elastin ratio. This would impact lung rigidity and elasticity, and thus lung development, which is dependent on physical forces generated by, for example, breathing motions.

Animal models of BPD have proved very important for the identification of candidate pathogenic mediators of normal and aberrant late lung development. These studies are often not followed up with validation studies that pin-point a role (*if any*) for a particular candidate mediator that exhibited changes in gene or protein expression in a BPD model. These studies are important, since changes in the gene or protein expression of a particular molecule may be (i) epiphenomenal (i.e., that the molecule in question was a bystander without any role in the alveolarization process), (ii) causal (i.e., that molecule in question was a mediator of arrested alveolarization), or (iii) reparative (i.e., that molecule in question mediated a lung defense or repair program that was engaged during aberrant alveolarization, which aimed to restore proper alveolarization). It is very important to determine which of these three categories a "candidate" mediator of aberrant lung development falls into.

Interestingly, in many studies, once a candidate mediator of aberrant lung alveolarization was identified in an animal model of BPD, much effort was then expended on identifying how the candidate mediator impacted ECM structures during alveolarization. Rather, less energy is usually invested in understanding how the expression of the candidate mediator was altered by the injurious stimulus (for example, inflammation, hyperoxia, or mechanical ventilation). The identification of such proximal pathways would be important in a translational sense, where addressing the very proximal causes of arrested lung development might be therapeutically targeted, ultimately in affected patients. With this in mind, physical forces and oxidative stress might be good starting points to understand the activation of pathways that produce or remodel the ECM. Furthermore, ECM structures have recently

been credited with a role in driving pluripotent cell differentiation in acellular lung scaffolds (236). Thus, how the ECM may shape stem cell niches in the developing lung, and direct phenotypic transformation of the constituent cell types of the developing lung are further areas that will no doubt receive attention in the coming years.

With the rapidly expanding repertoire of genetic tools, and the development of state-of-the-art methodology to study both lung alveolar architecture and the biochemical nature of the ECM, we have never been better positioned to explore the complex interactions of the ECM during lung alveolarization. It is clear that there is much exciting work to be done!

ACKNOWLEDGMENTS

This study was supported by the Max Planck Society; von Behring-Röntgen Foundation grant 51-0031, Rhön Klinikum AG grant Fl_66; the Federal Ministry of Higher Education, Research and the Arts of the State of Hessen *LOEWE* Programme; the German Center for Lung Research; and the German Research Foundation through Excellence Cluster 147 "Cardio-Pulmonary System" (ECCPS) and Mo 1789/1.

REFERENCES

1. Herriges M, Morrisey EE. Lung development: orchestrating the generation and regeneration of a complex organ. *Development* (2014) 141(3):502–13. doi:10.1242/dev.098186
2. Morrisey EE, Cardoso WV, Lane RH, Rabinovitch M, Abman SH, Ai X, et al. Molecular determinants of lung development. *Ann Am Thorac Soc* (2013) 10(2):S12–6. doi:10.1513/AnnalsATS.201207-036OT
3. Morrisey EE, Hogan BL. Preparing for the first breath: genetic and cellular mechanisms in lung development. *Dev Cell* (2010) 18(1):8–23. doi:10.1016/j.devcel.2009.12.010
4. Rawlins EL. The building blocks of mammalian lung development. *Dev Dyn* (2011) 240(3):463–76. doi:10.1002/dvdy.22482
5. Minoo P, Li C. Cross-talk between transforming growth factor-beta and Wingless/int pathways in lung development and disease. *Int J Biochem Cell Biol* (2010) 42(6):809–12. doi:10.1016/j.biocel.2010.02.011
6. McCulley D, Wienhold M, Sun X. The pulmonary mesenchyme directs lung development. *Curr Opin Genet Dev* (2015) 32:98–105. doi:10.1016/j.gde.2015.01.011
7. Volckaert T, De Langhe SP. Wnt and FGF mediated epithelial-mesenchymal crosstalk during lung development. *Dev Dyn* (2015) 244(3):342–66. doi:10.1002/dvdy.24234
8. Mariani TJ, Reed JJ, Shapiro SD. Expression profiling of the developing mouse lung: insights into the establishment of the extracellular matrix. *Am J Respir Cell Mol Biol* (2002) 26(5):541–8. doi:10.1165/ajrcmb.26.5.2001-00080c
9. Greenlee KJ, Werb Z, Kheradmand F. Matrix metalloproteinases in lung: multiple, multifarious, and multifaceted. *Physiol Rev* (2007) 87(1):69–98. doi:10.1152/physrev.00022.2006
10. Northway WH Jr, Rosan RC, Porter DY. Pulmonary disease following respirator therapy of hyaline-membrane disease. Bronchopulmonary dysplasia. *N Engl J Med* (1967) 276(7):357–68. doi:10.1056/NEJM196702162760701
11. Jobe AH, Ikegami M. Mechanisms initiating lung injury in the preterm. *Early Hum Dev* (1998) 53(1):81–94. doi:10.1016/S0378-3782(98)00045-0
12. Northway WH Jr. Bronchopulmonary dysplasia: twenty-five years later. *Pediatrics* (1992) 89(5 Pt 1):969–73.
13. Madurga A, Mižíková I, Ruiz-Camp J, Morty RE. Recent advances in late lung development and the pathogenesis of bronchopulmonary dysplasia. *Am J Physiol Lung Cell Mol Physiol* (2013) 305(12):L893–905. doi:10.1152/ajplung.00267.2013

14. Jobe AH. The new bronchopulmonary dysplasia. *Curr Opin Pediatr* (2011) 23(2):167–72. doi:10.1097/MOP.0b013e3283423e6b
15. Baraldi E, Filippone M. Chronic lung disease after premature birth. *N Engl J Med* (2007) 357(19):1946–55. doi:10.1056/NEJMra067279
16. Wong PM, Lees AN, Louw J, Lee FY, French N, Gain K, et al. Emphysema in young adult survivors of moderate-to-severe bronchopulmonary dysplasia. *Eur Respir J* (2008) 32(2):321–8. doi:10.1183/09031936.00127107
17. Hilgendorff A, O'Reilly MA. Bronchopulmonary dysplasia early changes leading to long-term consequences. *Front Med* (2015) 2:2. doi:10.3389/fmed.2015.00002
18. Baker CD, Abman SH. Impaired pulmonary vascular development in bronchopulmonary dysplasia. *Neonatology* (2015) 107(4):344–51. doi:10.1159/000381129
19. Bruce MC, Wedig KE, Jentoft N, Martin RJ, Cheng PW, Boat TF, et al. Altered urinary excretion of elastin cross-links in premature infants who develop bronchopulmonary dysplasia. *Am Rev Respir Dis* (1985) 131(4):568–72.
20. Thibeault DW, Mabry SM, Ekekezie II, Truog WE. Lung elastic tissue maturation and perturbations during the evolution of chronic lung disease. *Pediatrics* (2000) 106(6):1452–9. doi:10.1542/peds.106.6.1452
21. Thibeault DW, Mabry SM, Ekekezie II, Zhang X, Truog WE. Collagen scaffolding during development and its deformation with chronic lung disease. *Pediatrics* (2003) 111(4 Pt 1):766–76. doi:10.1542/peds.111.4.766
22. McGowan SE. Extracellular matrix and the regulation of lung development and repair. *FASEB J* (1992) 6(11):2895–904.
23. Bland RD, Ertsey R, Mokres LM, Xu L, Jacobson BE, Jiang S, et al. Mechanical ventilation uncouples synthesis and assembly of elastin and increases apoptosis in lungs of newborn mice. Prelude to defective alveolar septation during lung development? *Am J Physiol Lung Cell Mol Physiol* (2008) 294(1):L3–14. doi:10.1152/ajplung.00362.2007
24. Bland RD, Xu L, Ertsey R, Rabinovitch M, Albertine KH, Wynn KA, et al. Dysregulation of pulmonary elastin synthesis and assembly in preterm lambs with chronic lung disease. *Am J Physiol Lung Cell Mol Physiol* (2007) 292(6):L1370–84. doi:10.1152/ajplung.00367.2006
25. Ozbek S, Balasubramanian PG, Chiquet-Ehrismann R, Tucker RP, Adams JC. The evolution of extracellular matrix. *Mol Biol Cell* (2010) 21(24):4300–5. doi:10.1091/mbc.E10-03-0251
26. Lang MR, Fiaux GW, Gillooly M, Stewart JA, Hulmes DJ, Lamb D. Collagen content of alveolar wall tissue in emphysematous and non-emphysematous lungs. *Thorax* (1994) 49(4):319–26. doi:10.1136/thx.49.4.319

27. Mäki JM, Sormunen R, Lippo S, Kaarteenaho-Wiik R, Soininen R, Myllyharju J. Lysyl oxidase is essential for normal development and function of the respiratory system and for the integrity of elastic and collagen fibers in various tissues. *Am J Pathol* (2005) **167**(4):927–36. doi:10.1016/s0002-9440(10)61183-2

28. Trask TM, Trask BC, Ritty TM, Abrams WR, Rosenbloom J, Mecham RP. Interaction of tropoelastin with the amino-terminal domains of fibrillin-1 and fibrillin-2 suggests a role for the fibrillins in elastic fiber assembly. *J Biol Chem* (2000) **275**(32):24400–6. doi:10.1074/jbc.M003665200

29. Nakamura T, Lozano PR, Ikeda Y, Iwanaga Y, Hinek A, Minamisawa S, et al. Fibulin-5/DANCE is essential for elastogenesis in vivo. *Nature* (2002) **415**(6868):171–5. doi:10.1038/415171a

30. Benjamin JT, Gaston DC, Halloran BA, Schnapp LM, Zent R, Prince LS. The role of integrin alpha8beta1 in fetal lung morphogenesis and injury. *Dev Biol* (2009) **335**(2):407–17. doi:10.1016/j.ydbio.2009.09.021

31. Adamson SL. Regulation of breathing at birth. *J Dev Physiol* (1991) **15**(1):45–52.

32. Bourbon J, Boucherat O, Chailley-Heu B, Delacourt C. Control mechanisms of lung alveolar development and their disorders in bronchopulmonary dysplasia. *Pediatr Res* (2005) **57**(5 Pt 2):38R–46R. doi:10.1203/01.PDR.0000159630.35883.BE

33. Wessells NK. Mammalian lung development: interactions in formation and morphogenesis of tracheal buds. *J Exp Zool* (1970) **175**(4):455–66. doi:10.1002/jez.1401750405

34. Bradley K, McConnell-Breul S, Crystal RG. Lung collagen heterogeneity. *Proc Natl Acad Sci U S A* (1974) **71**(7):2828–32. doi:10.1073/pnas.71.7.2828

35. Bradley KH, McConnell SD, Crystal RG. Lung collagen composition and synthesis. Characterization and changes with age. *J Biol Chem* (1974) **249**(8):2674–83.

36. Hance AJ, Bradley K, Crystal RG. Lung collagen heterogeneity. Synthesis of type I and type III collagen by rabbit and human lung cells in culture. *J Clin Invest* (1976) **57**(1):102–11. doi:10.1172/JCI108250

37. Arden MG, Spearman MA, Adamson IY. Degradation of type IV collagen during the development of fetal rat lung. *Am J Respir Cell Mol Biol* (1993) **9**(1):99–105. doi:10.1165/ajrcmb/9.1.99

38. Chen JM, Little CD. Cellular events associated with lung branching morphogenesis including the deposition of collagen type IV. *Dev Biol* (1987) **120**(2):311–21. doi:10.1016/0012-1606(87)90234-X

39. Powell JT, Whitney PL. Postnatal development of rat lung. Changes in lung lectin, elastin, acetylcholinesterase and other enzymes. *Biochem J* (1980) **188**(1):1–8. doi:10.1042/bj1880001

40. Shibahara SU, Davidson JM, Smith K, Crystal RG. Modulation of tropoelastin production and elastin messenger ribonucleic acid activity in developing sheep lung. *Biochemistry* (1981) **20**(23):6577–84. doi:10.1021/bi00526a009

41. Myers B, Dubick M, Last JA, Rucker RB. Elastin synthesis during perinatal lung development in the rat. *Biochim Biophys Acta* (1983) **761**(1):17–22. doi:10.1016/0304-4165(83)90357-4

42. Das RM. The effect of beta-aminopropionitrile on lung development in the rat. *Am J Pathol* (1980) **101**(3):711–22.

43. Margraf LR, Tomashefski JF Jr, Bruce MC, Dahms BB. Morphometric analysis of the lung in bronchopulmonary dysplasia. *Am Rev Respir Dis* (1991) **143**(2):391–400. doi:10.1164/ajrccm/143.2.391

44. Nakamura Y, Fukuda S, Hashimoto T. Pulmonary elastic fibers in normal human development and in pathological conditions. *Pediatr Pathol* (1990) **10**(5):689–706. doi:10.3109/15513819009064705

45. Wakafuji S. Pathological and histometrical studies on alveolar ducts and respiratory bronchioli. *Kobe J Med Sci* (1985) **31**(5):203–20.

46. Thibeault DW, Truog WE, Ekekezie II. Acinar arterial changes with chronic lung disease of prematurity in the surfactant era. *Pediatr Pulmonol* (2003) **36**(6):482–9. doi:10.1002/ppul.10349

47. Frantz C, Stewart KM, Weaver VM. The extracellular matrix at a glance. *J Cell Sci* (2010) **123**(Pt 24):4195–200. doi:10.1242/jcs.023820

48. Kaarteenaho-Wiik R, Paakko P, Herva R, Risteli J, Soini Y. Type I and III collagen protein precursors and mRNA in the developing human lung. *J Pathol* (2004) **203**(1):567–74. doi:10.1002/path.1547

49. Lohler J, Timpl R, Jaenisch R. Embryonic lethal mutation in mouse collagen I gene causes rupture of blood vessels and is associated with erythropoietic and mesenchymal cell death. *Cell* (1984) **38**(2):597–607. doi:10.1016/0092-8674(84)90514-2

50. Kratochwil K, Dziadek M, Lohler J, Harbers K, Jaenisch R. Normal epithelial branching morphogenesis in the absence of collagen I. *Dev Biol* (1986) **117**(2):596–606. doi:10.1016/0012-1606(86)90328-3

51. Han W, Guo C, Liu Q, Yu B, Liu Z, Yang J, et al. Aberrant elastin remodeling in the lungs of O(2)-exposed newborn mice; primarily results from perturbed interaction between integrins and elastin. *Cell Tissue Res* (2015) **359**(2):589–603. doi:10.1007/s00441-014-2035-1

52. Olsen KC, Sapinoro RE, Kottmann RM, Kulkarni AA, Iismaa SE, Johnson GV, et al. Transglutaminase 2 and its role in pulmonary fibrosis. *Am J Respir Crit Care Med* (2011) **184**(6):699–707. doi:10.1164/rccm.201101-0013OC

53. Nakamura T, Liu M, Mourgeon E, Slutsky A, Post M. Mechanical strain and dexamethasone selectively increase surfactant protein C and tropoelastin gene expression. *Am J Physiol Lung Cell Mol Physiol* (2000) **278**(5):L974–80.

54. Fattman CL, Schaefer LM, Oury TD. Extracellular superoxide dismutase in biology and medicine. *Free Radic Biol Med* (2003) **35**(3):236–56. doi:10.1016/S0891-5849(03)00275-2

55. Poonyagariyagorn HK, Metzger S, Dikeman D, Mercado AL, Malinina A, Calvi C, et al. Superoxide dismutase 3 dysregulation in a murine model of neonatal lung injury. *Am J Respir Cell Mol Biol* (2014) **51**(3):380–90. doi:10.1165/rcmb.2013-0043OC

56. Roth-Kleiner M, Berger TM, Gremlich S, Tschanz SA, Mund SI, Post M, et al. Neonatal steroids induce a down-regulation of tenascin-C and elastin and cause a deceleration of the first phase and an acceleration of the second phase of lung alveolarization. *Histochem Cell Biol* (2014) **141**(1):75–84. doi:10.1007/s00418-013-1132-7

57. Quondamatteo F, Reinhardt DP, Charbonneau NL, Pophal G, Sakai LY, Herken R. Fibrillin-1 and fibrillin-2 in human embryonic and early fetal development. *Matrix Biol* (2002) **21**(8):637–46. doi:10.1016/S0945-053X(02)00100-2

58. Vehvilainen P, Hyytiainen M, Keski-Oja J. Matrix association of latent TGF-beta binding protein-2 (LTBP-2) is dependent on fibrillin-1. *J Cell Physiol* (2009) **221**(3):586–93. doi:10.1002/jcp.21888

59. Lima BL, Santos EJ, Fernandes GR, Merkel C, Mello MR, Gomes JP, et al. A new mouse model for Marfan syndrome presents phenotypic variability associated with the genetic background and overall levels of Fbn1 expression. *PLoS One* (2010) **5**(11):e14136. doi:10.1371/journal.pone.0014136

60. Sinkin RA, Roberts M, LoMonaco MB, Sanders RJ, Metlay LA. Fibronectin expression in bronchopulmonary dysplasia. *Pediatr Dev Pathol* (1998) **1**(6):494–502. doi:10.1007/s100249900068

61. Kobayashi T, Kim H, Liu X, Sugiura H, Kohyama T, Fang Q, et al. Matrix metalloproteinase-9 activates TGF-beta and stimulates fibroblast contraction of collagen gels. *Am J Physiol Lung Cell Mol Physiol* (2014) **306**(11):L1006–15. doi:10.1152/ajplung.00015.2014

62. Rennard SI, Crystal RG. Fibronectin in human bronchopulmonary lavage fluid. Elevation in patients with interstitial lung disease. *J Clin Invest* (1982) **69**(1):113–22. doi:10.1172/JCI110421

63. Kuang PP, Goldstein RH, Liu Y, Rishikof DC, Jean JC, Joyce-Brady M. Coordinate expression of fibulin-5/DANCE and elastin during lung injury repair. *Am J Physiol Lung Cell Mol Physiol* (2003) **285**(5):L1147–52. doi:10.1152/ajplung.00098.2003

64. Liu X, Zhao Y, Gao J, Pawlyk B, Starcher B, Spencer JA, et al. Elastic fiber homeostasis requires lysyl oxidase-like 1 protein. *Nat Genet* (2004) **36**(2):178–82. doi:10.1038/ng1297

65. Thompson SM, Connell MG, van Kuppevelt TH, Xu R, Turnbull JE, Losty PD, et al. Structure and epitope distribution of heparan sulfate is disrupted in experimental lung hypoplasia: a glycobiological epigenetic cause for malformation? *BMC Dev Biol* (2011) **11**:38. doi:10.1186/1471-213X-11-38

66. Yue X, Li X, Nguyen HT, Chin DR, Sullivan DE, Lasky JA. Transforming growth factor-beta1 induces heparan sulfate 6-O-endosulfatase 1 expression in vitro and in vivo. *J Biol Chem* (2008) **283**(29):20397–407. doi:10.1074/jbc.M802850200

67. Sheppard D. Functions of pulmonary epithelial integrins: from development to disease. *Physiol Rev* (2003) **83**(3):673–86. doi:10.1152/physrev.00033.2002

68. Coraux C, Meneguzzi G, Rousselle P, Puchelle E, Gaillard D. Distribution of laminin 5, integrin receptors, and branching morphogenesis during human fetal lung development. *Dev Dyn* (2002) **225**(2):176–85. doi:10.1002/dvdy.10147

69. Caniggia I, Liu J, Han R, Wang J, Tanswell AK, Laurie G, et al. Identification of receptors binding fibronectin and laminin on fetal rat lung cells. *Am J Physiol* (1996) **270**(3 Pt 1):L459–68.

70. Wu JE, Santoro SA. Differential expression of integrin alpha subunits supports distinct roles during lung branching morphogenesis. *Dev Dyn* (1996) **206**(2):169–81. doi:10.1002/(SICI)1097-0177(199606)206:2<169::AID-AJA6>3.0.CO;2-G

71. Damjanovich L, Albelda SM, Mette SA, Buck CA. Distribution of integrin cell adhesion receptors in normal and malignant lung tissue. *Am J Respir Cell Mol Biol* (1992) **6**(2):197–206. doi:10.1165/ajrcmb/6.2.197

72. Kumarasamy A, Schmitt I, Nave AH, Reiss I, van der Horst I, Dony E, et al. Lysyl oxidase activity is dysregulated during impaired alveolarization of mouse and human lungs. *Am J Respir Crit Care Med* (2009) **180**(12):1239–52. doi:10.1164/rccm.200902-0215OC

73. Nave AH, Mizikova I, Niess G, Steenbock H, Reichenberger F, Talavera ML, et al. Lysyl oxidases play a causal role in vascular remodeling in clinical and experimental pulmonary arterial hypertension. *Arterioscler Thromb Vasc Biol* (2014) **34**(7):1446–58. doi:10.1161/ATVBAHA.114.303534

74. Fukuda Y, Ishizaki M, Okada Y, Seiki M, Yamanaka N. Matrix metalloproteinases and tissue inhibitor of metalloproteinase-2 in fetal rabbit lung. *Am J Physiol Lung Cell Mol Physiol* (2000) **279**(3):L555–61.

75. Boucherat O, Bourbon JR, Barlier-Mur AM, Chailley-Heu B, D'Ortho MP, Delacourt C. Differential expression of matrix metalloproteinases and inhibitors in developing rat lung mesenchymal and epithelial cells. *Pediatr Res* (2007) **62**(1):20–5. doi:10.1203/PDR.0b013e3180686cc5

76. Atkinson JJ, Holmbeck K, Yamada S, Birkedal-Hansen H, Parks WC, Senior RM. Membrane-type 1 matrix metalloproteinase is required for normal alveolar development. *Dev Dyn* (2005) **232**(4):1079–90. doi:10.1002/dvdy.20267

77. Pardo A, Barrios R, Maldonado V, Melendez J, Perez J, Ruiz V, et al. Gelatinases A and B are up-regulated in rat lungs by subacute hyperoxia: pathogenetic implications. *Am J Pathol* (1998) **153**(3):833–44. doi:10.1016/S0002-9440(10)65625-8

78. Buckley S, Warburton D. Dynamics of metalloproteinase-2 and -9, TGF-beta, and uPA activities during normoxic vs. hyperoxic alveolarization. *Am J Physiol Lung Cell Mol Physiol* (2002) **283**(4):L747–54. doi:10.1152/ajplung.00415.2001

79. Dik WA, van Kaam AH, Dekker T, Naber BA, Janssen DJ, Kroon AA, et al. Early increased levels of matrix metalloproteinase-9 in neonates recovering from respiratory distress syndrome. *Biol Neonate* (2006) **89**(1):6–14. doi:10.1159/000088193

80. Witsch TJ, Turowski P, Sakkas E, Niess G, Becker S, Herold S, et al. Deregulation of the lysyl hydroxylase matrix cross-linking system in experimental and clinical bronchopulmonary dysplasia. *Am J Physiol Lung Cell Mol Physiol* (2014) **306**(3):L246–59. doi:10.1152/ajplung.00109.2013

81. Paakko P, Kaarteenaho-Wiik R, Pollanen R, Soini Y. Tenascin mRNA expression at the foci of recent injury in usual interstitial pneumonia. *Am J Respir Crit Care Med* (2000) **161**(3 Pt 1):967–72. doi:10.1164/ajrccm.161.3.9809115

82. Estany S, Vicens-Zygmunt V, Llatjos R, Montes A, Penin R, Escobar I, et al. Lung fibrotic tenascin-C upregulation is associated with other extracellular matrix proteins and induced by TGFbeta1. *BMC Pulm Med* (2014) **14**:120. doi:10.1186/1471-2466-14-120

83. Kaarteenaho-Wiik R, Kinnula VL, Herva R, Soini Y, Pollanen R, Paakko P. Tenascin-C is highly expressed in respiratory distress syndrome and bronchopulmonary dysplasia. *J Histochem Cytochem* (2002) **50**(3):423–31. doi:10.1177/002215540205000313

84. Kaarteenaho-Wiik R, Kinnula V, Herva R, Paakko P, Pollanen R, Soini Y. Distribution and mRNA expression of tenascin-C in developing human lung. *Am J Respir Cell Mol Biol* (2001) **25**(3):341–6. doi:10.1165/ajrcmb.25.3.4460

85. Witsch TJ, Niess G, Sakkas E, Likhoshvay T, Becker S, Herold S, et al. Transglutaminase 2: a new player in bronchopulmonary dysplasia? *Eur Respir J* (2014) **44**(1):109–21. doi:10.1183/09031936.00075713

86. Oh K, Park HB, Byoun OJ, Shin DM, Jeong EM, Kim YW, et al. Epithelial transglutaminase 2 is needed for T cell interleukin-17 production and subsequent pulmonary inflammation and fibrosis in bleomycin-treated mice. *J Exp Med* (2011) **208**(8):1707–19. doi:10.1084/jem.20101457

87. Oh K, Seo MW, Lee GY, Byoun OJ, Kang HR, Cho SH, et al. Airway epithelial cells initiate the allergen response through transglutaminase 2 by inducing IL-33 expression and a subsequent Th2 response. *Respir Res* (2013) **14**:35. doi:10.1186/1465-9921-14-35

88. Kononov S, Brewer K, Sakai H, Cavalcante FS, Sabayanagam CR, Ingenito EP, et al. Roles of mechanical forces and collagen failure in the development of elastase-induced emphysema. *Am J Respir Crit Care Med* (2001) **164**(10 Pt 1):1920–6. doi:10.1164/ajrccm.164.10.2101083

89. Mižíková I, Ruiz-Camp J, Steenbock H, Madurga A, Vadász I, Herold S, et al. Collagen and elastin cross-linking is altered during aberrant late lung development associated with hyperoxia. *Am J Physiol Lung Cell Mol Physiol* (2015) **308**(11):L1145–58. doi:10.1152/ajplung.00039.2015

90. Shoemaker CT, Reiser KM, Goetzman BW, Last JA. Elevated ratios of type I/III collagen in the lungs of chronically ventilated neonates with respiratory distress. *Pediatr Res* (1984) **18**(11):1176–80. doi:10.1203/00006450-198411000-00025

91. Ohki Y, Kato M, Kimura H, Nako Y, Tokuyama K, Morikawa A. Elevated type IV collagen in bronchoalveolar lavage fluid from infants with bronchopulmonary dysplasia. *Biol Neonate* (2001) **79**(1):34–8. doi:10.1159/000047063

92. Moore AM, Buch S, Han RN, Freeman BA, Post M, Tanswell AK. Altered expression of type I collagen, TGF-beta 1, and related genes in rat lung exposed to 85% O2. *Am J Physiol* (1995) **268**(1 Pt 1):L78–84.

93. Chetty A, Cao GJ, Severgnini M, Simon A, Warburton R, Nielsen HC. Role of matrix metalloprotease-9 in hyperoxic injury in developing lung. *Am J Physiol Lung Cell Mol Physiol* (2008) **295**(4):L584–92. doi:10.1152/ajplung.00441.2007

94. Mammoto T, Jiang E, Jiang A, Mammoto A. Extracellular matrix structure and tissue stiffness control postnatal lung development through the lipoprotein receptor-related protein 5/Tie2 signaling system. *Am J Respir Cell Mol Biol* (2013) **49**(6):1009–18. doi:10.1165/rcmb.2013-0147OC

95. Alejandre-Alcázar MA, Kwapiszewska G, Reiss I, Amarie OV, Marsh LM, Sevilla-Perez J, et al. Hyperoxia modulates TGF-beta/BMP signaling in a mouse model of bronchopulmonary dysplasia. *Am J Physiol Lung Cell Mol Physiol* (2007) **292**(2):L537–49. doi:10.1152/ajplung.00050.2006

96. Hirakawa H, Pierce RA, Bingol-Karakoc G, Karaaslan C, Weng M, Shi GP, et al. Cathepsin S deficiency confers protection from neonatal hyperoxia-induced lung injury. *Am J Respir Crit Care Med* (2007) **176**(8):778–85. doi:10.1164/rccm.200704-519OC

97. Bozyk PD, Bentley JK, Popova AP, Anyanwu AC, Linn MD, Goldsmith AM, et al. Neonatal periostin knockout mice are protected from hyperoxia-induced alveolar simplification. *PLoS One* (2012) **7**(2):e31336. doi:10.1371/journal.pone.0031336

98. Masood A, Yi M, Belcastro R, Li J, Lopez L, Kantores C, et al. Neutrophil elastase-induced elastin degradation mediates macrophage influx and lung injury in 60% O2-exposed neonatal rats. *Am J Physiol Lung Cell Mol Physiol* (2015) **309**(1):L53–62. doi:10.1152/ajplung.00298.2014

99. Hilgendorff A, Parai K, Ertsey R, Navarro E, Jain N, Carandang F, et al. Lung matrix and vascular remodeling in mechanically ventilated elastin haploinsufficient newborn mice. *Am J Physiol Lung Cell Mol Physiol* (2015) **308**(5):L464–78. doi:10.1152/ajplung.00278.2014

100. Hilgendorff A, Parai K, Ertsey R, Jain N, Navarro EF, Peterson JL, et al. Inhibiting lung elastase activity enables lung growth in mechanically ventilated newborn mice. *Am J Respir Crit Care Med* (2011) **184**(5):537–46. doi:10.1164/rccm.201012-2010OC

101. Hilgendorff A, Parai K, Ertsey R, Juliana Rey-Parra G, Thebaud B, Tamosiuniene R. Neonatal mice genetically modified to express the elastase inhibitor elafin are protected against the adverse effects of mechanical ventilation on lung growth. *Am J Physiol Lung Cell Mol Physiol* (2012) **303**(3):L215–27. doi:10.1152/ajplung.00405.2011

102. Pierce RA, Albertine KH, Starcher BC, Bohnsack JF, Carlton DP, Bland RD. Chronic lung injury in preterm lambs: disordered pulmonary elastin deposition. *Am J Physiol* (1997) **272**(3 Pt 1):L452–60.

103. Kroon AA, Wang J, Post M. Alterations in expression of elastogenic and angiogenic genes by different conditions of mechanical ventilation in newborn rat lung. *Am J Physiol Lung Cell Mol Physiol* (2015) **308**(7):L639–49. doi:10.1152/ajplung.00293.2014

104. Watts CL, Fanaroff AA, Bruce MC. Elevation of fibronectin levels in lung secretions of infants with respiratory distress syndrome and development of bronchopulmonary dysplasia. *J Pediatr* (1992) **120**(4 Pt 1):614–20. doi:10.1016/S0022-3476(05)82492-8

105. Zhang X, Xu J, Wang J, Gortner L, Zhang S, Wei X, et al. Reduction of microRNA-206 contributes to the development of bronchopulmonary dysplasia through up-regulation of fibronectin 1. *PLoS One* (2013) **8**(9):e74750. doi:10.1371/journal.pone.0074750

106. Sinkin RA, LoMonaco MB, Finkelstein JN, Watkins RH, Cox C, Horowitz S. Increased fibronectin mRNA in alveolar macrophages following in vivo

hyperoxia. *Am J Respir Cell Mol Biol* (1992) **7**(5):548–55. doi:10.1165/ajrcmb/7.5.548

107. Tambunting F, Beharry KD, Hartleroad J, Waltzman J, Stavitsky Y, Modanlou HD. Increased lung matrix metalloproteinase-9 levels in extremely premature baboons with bronchopulmonary dysplasia. *Pediatr Pulmonol* (2005) **39**(1):5–14. doi:10.1002/ppul.20135

108. Hadchouel A, Decobert F, Franco-Montoya ML, Halphen I, Jarreau PH, Boucherat O, et al. Matrix metalloproteinase gene polymorphisms and bronchopulmonary dysplasia: identification of MMP16 as a new player in lung development. *PLoS One* (2008) **3**(9):e3188. doi:10.1371/journal.pone.0003188

109. Danan C, Jarreau PH, Franco ML, Dassieu G, Grillon C, Abd Alsamad I, et al. Gelatinase activities in the airways of premature infants and development of bronchopulmonary dysplasia. *Am J Physiol Lung Cell Mol Physiol* (2002) **283**(5):L1086–93. doi:10.1152/ajplung.00066.2002

110. Hosford GE, Fang X, Olson DM. Hyperoxia decreases matrix metalloproteinase-9 and increases tissue inhibitor of matrix metalloproteinase-1 protein in the newborn rat lung: association with arrested alveolarization. *Pediatr Res* (2004) **56**(1):26–34. doi:10.1203/01.PDR.0000130658.45564.1F

111. Cederqvist K, Sorsa T, Tervahartiala T, Maisi P, Reunanen K, Lassus P, et al. Matrix metalloproteinases-2, -8, and -9 and TIMP-2 in tracheal aspirates from preterm infants with respiratory distress. *Pediatrics* (2001) **108**(3):686–92. doi:10.1542/peds.108.3.686

112. Sweet DG, McMahon KJ, Curley AE, O'Connor CM, Halliday HL. Type I collagenases in bronchoalveolar lavage fluid from preterm babies at risk of developing chronic lung disease. *Arch Dis Child Fetal Neonatal Ed* (2001) **84**(3):F168–71. doi:10.1136/fn.84.3.F168

113. Ekekezie II, Thibeault DW, Simon SD, Norberg M, Merrill JD, Ballard RA, et al. Low levels of tissue inhibitors of metalloproteinases with a high matrix metalloproteinase-9/tissue inhibitor of metalloproteinase-1 ratio are present in tracheal aspirate fluids of infants who develop chronic lung disease. *Pediatrics* (2004) **113**(6):1709–14. doi:10.1542/peds.113.6.1709

114. Sweet DG, Curley AE, Chesshyre E, Pizzotti J, Wilbourn MS, Halliday HL, et al. The role of matrix metalloproteinases -9 and -2 in development of neonatal chronic lung disease. *Acta Paediatr* (2004) **93**(6):791–6. doi:10.1111/j.1651-2227.2004.tb03020.x

115. Kotecha S, Wangoo A, Silverman M, Shaw RJ. Increase in the concentration of transforming growth factor beta-1 in bronchoalveolar lavage fluid before development of chronic lung disease of prematurity. *J Pediatr* (1996) **128**(4):464–9. doi:10.1016/S0022-3476(96)70355-4

116. McAnulty RJ, Campa JS, Cambrey AD, Laurent GJ. The effect of transforming growth factor beta on rates of procollagen synthesis and degradation in vitro. *Biochim Biophys Acta* (1991) **1091**(2):231–5. doi:10.1016/0167-4889(91)90066-7

117. Nakanishi H, Sugiura T, Streisand JB, Lonning SM, Roberts JD Jr. TGF-beta-neutralizing antibodies improve pulmonary alveologenesis and vasculogenesis in the injured newborn lung. *Am J Physiol Lung Cell Mol Physiol* (2007) **293**(1):L151–61. doi:10.1152/ajplung.00389.2006

118. Vicencio AG, Lee CG, Cho SJ, Eickelberg O, Chuu Y, Haddad GG, et al. Conditional overexpression of bioactive transforming growth factor-beta1 in neonatal mouse lung: a new model for bronchopulmonary dysplasia? *Am J Respir Cell Mol Biol* (2004) **31**(6):650–6. doi:10.1165/rcmb.2004-0092OC

119. Tarantal AF, Chen H, Shi TT, Lu CH, Fang AB, Buckley S, et al. Overexpression of transforming growth factor-beta1 in fetal monkey lung results in prenatal pulmonary fibrosis. *Eur Respir J* (2010) **36**(4):907–14. doi:10.1183/09031936.00011810

120. Pierce RA, Mariani TJ, Senior RM. Elastin in lung development and disease. *Ciba Found Symp* (1995) **192**:199–212.

121. Burri PH, Weibel ER. Ultrastructure and morphometry of the developing lung. In: Hodson WA, editor. *Development of the Lung, Part 1: Structural Development.* New York, NY: Marcel Decker (1977). p. 215–68.

122. Emery JL. The post natal development of the human lung and its implications for lung pathology. *Respiration* (1970) **27**(Suppl):41–50. doi:10.1159/000192718

123. Noguchi A, Reddy R, Kursar JD, Parks WC, Mecham RP. Smooth muscle isoactin and elastin in fetal bovine lung. *Exp Lung Res* (1989) **15**(4):537–52. doi:10.3109/01902148909069617

124. Wendel DP, Taylor DG, Albertine KH, Keating MT, Li DY. Impaired distal airway development in mice lacking elastin. *Am J Respir Cell Mol Biol* (2000) **23**(3):320–6. doi:10.1165/ajrcmb.23.3.3906

125. Shifren A, Durmowicz AG, Knutsen RH, Hirano E, Mecham RP. Elastin protein levels are a vital modifier affecting normal lung development and susceptibility to emphysema. *Am J Physiol Lung Cell Mol Physiol* (2007) **292**(3):L778–87. doi:10.1152/ajplung.00352.2006

126. Bruce MC, Schuyler M, Martin RJ, Starcher BC, Tomashefski JF Jr, Wedig KE. Risk factors for the degradation of lung elastic fibers in the ventilated neonate. Implications for impaired lung development in bronchopulmonary dysplasia. *Am Rev Respir Dis* (1992) **146**(1):204–12. doi:10.1164/ajrccm/146.1.204

127. Mascaretti RS, Mataloun MM, Dolhnikoff M, Rebello CM. Lung morphometry, collagen and elastin content: changes after hyperoxic exposure in preterm rabbits. *Clinics (Sao Paulo)* (2009) **64**(11):1099–104. doi:10.1590/S1807-59322009001100010

128. Pierce RA, Joyce B, Officer S, Heintz C, Moore C, McCurnin D, et al. Retinoids increase lung elastin expression but fail to alter morphology or angiogenesis genes in premature ventilated baboons. *Pediatr Res* (2007) **61**(6):703–9. doi:10.1203/pdr.0b013e318053661d

129. Albertine KH, Jones GP, Starcher BC, Bohnsack JF, Davis PL, Cho SC, et al. Chronic lung injury in preterm lambs. Disordered respiratory tract development. *Am J Respir Crit Care Med* (1999) **159**(3):945–58. doi:10.1164/ajrccm.159.3.9804027

130. McGowan SE, McNamer R. Transforming growth factor-beta increases elastin production by neonatal rat lung fibroblasts. *Am J Respir Cell Mol Biol* (1990) **3**(4):369–76. doi:10.1165/ajrcmb/3.4.369

131. McGowan SE. Paracrine cellular and extracellular matrix interactions with mesenchymal progenitors during pulmonary alveolar septation. *Birth Defects Res A Clin Mol Teratol* (2014) **100**(3):227–39. doi:10.1002/bdra.23230

132. Noguchi A, Nelson T. IGF-I stimulates tropoelastin synthesis in neonatal rat pulmonary fibroblasts. *Pediatr Res* (1991) **30**(3):248–51. doi:10.1203/00006450-199109000-00009

133. Sproul EP, Argraves WS. A cytokine axis regulates elastin formation and degradation. *Matrix Biol* (2013) **32**(2):86–94. doi:10.1016/j.matbio.2012.11.004

134. McGowan SE, Jackson SK, Olson PJ, Parekh T, Gold LI. Exogenous and endogenous transforming growth factors-beta influence elastin gene expression in cultured lung fibroblasts. *Am J Respir Cell Mol Biol* (1997) **17**(1):25–35. doi:10.1165/ajrcmb.17.1.2686

135. Li J, Masood A, Yi M, Lau M, Belcastro R, Ivanovska J, et al. The IGF-I/IGF-R1 pathway regulates postnatal lung growth and is a nonspecific regulator of alveologenesis in the neonatal rat. *Am J Physiol Lung Cell Mol Physiol* (2013) **304**(9):L626–37. doi:10.1152/ajplung.00198.2012

136. Chetty A, Andersson S, Lassus P, Nielsen HC. Insulin-like growth factor-1 (IGF-1) and IGF-1 receptor (IGF-1R) expression in human lung in RDS and BPD. *Pediatr Pulmonol* (2004) **37**(2):128–36. doi:10.1002/ppul.10415

137. Popova AP, Bentley JK, Cui TX, Richardson MN, Linn MJ, Lei J, et al. Reduced platelet-derived growth factor receptor expression is a primary feature of human bronchopulmonary dysplasia. *Am J Physiol Lung Cell Mol Physiol* (2014) **307**(3):L231–9. doi:10.1152/ajplung.00342.2013

138. Dubick MA, Rucker RB, Cross CE, Last JA. Elastin metabolism in rodent lung. *Biochim Biophys Acta* (1981) **672**(3):303–6. doi:10.1016/0304-4165(81)90297-X

139. Zhang P, Huang A, Ferruzzi J, Mecham RP, Starcher BC, Tellides G, et al. Inhibition of microRNA-29 enhances elastin levels in cells haploinsufficient for elastin and in bioengineered vessels – brief report. *Arterioscler Thromb Vasc Biol* (2012) **32**(3):756–9. doi:10.1161/ATVBAHA.111.238113

140. Leimeister C, Steidl C, Schumacher N, Erhard S, Gessler M. Developmental expression and biochemical characterization of Emu family members. *Dev Biol* (2002) **249**(2):204–18. doi:10.1006/dbio.2002.0764

141. Hirai M, Horiguchi M, Ohbayashi T, Kita T, Chien KR, Nakamura T. Latent TGF-beta-binding protein 2 binds to DANCE/fibulin-5 and regulates elastic fiber assembly. *EMBO J* (2007) **26**(14):3283–95. doi:10.1038/sj.emboj.7601768

142. Mecham RP, Gibson MA. The microfibril-associated glycoproteins (MAGPs) and the microfibrillar niche. *Matrix Biol* (2015) **47**:13–33. doi:10.1016/j.matbio.2015.05.003

143. Burgess JK, Weckmann M. Matrikines and the lungs. *Pharmacol Ther* (2012) **134**(3):317–37. doi:10.1016/j.pharmthera.2012.02.002

144. Morty RE. Targeting elastase in bronchopulmonary dysplasia. *Am J Respir Crit Care Med* (2011) **184**(5):496–7. doi:10.1164/rccm.201105-0930ED

145. Kielty CM, Sherratt MJ, Shuttleworth CA. Elastic fibres. *J Cell Sci* (2002) **115**(Pt 14):2817–28.

146. Neptune ER, Frischmeyer PA, Arking DE, Myers L, Bunton TE, Gayraud B, et al. Dysregulation of TGF-beta activation contributes to pathogenesis in Marfan syndrome. *Nat Genet* (2003) **33**(3):407–11. doi:10.1038/ng1116

147. Robbesom AA, Koenders MM, Smits NC, Hafmans T, Versteeg EM, Bulten J, et al. Aberrant fibrillin-1 expression in early emphysematous human lung: a proposed predisposition for emphysema. *Mod Pathol* (2008) **21**(3):297–307. doi:10.1038/modpathol.3801004

148. Kida K, Thurlbeck WM. Lack of recovery of lung structure and function after the administration of beta-amino-propionitrile in the postnatal period. *Am Rev Respir Dis* (1980) **122**(3):467–75.

149. Kida K, Thurlbeck WM. The effects of beta-aminopropionitrile on the growing rat lung. *Am J Pathol* (1980) **101**(3):693–710.

150. Roth-Kleiner M, Hirsch E, Schittny JC. Fetal lungs of tenascin-C-deficient mice grow well, but branch poorly in organ culture. *Am J Respir Cell Mol Biol* (2004) **30**(3):360–6. doi:10.1165/rcmb.2002-0266OC

151. Mosher DF. Physiology of fibronectin. *Annu Rev Med* (1984) **35**:561–75. doi:10.1146/annurev.me.35.020184.003021

152. Dean DC. Expression of the fibronectin gene. *Am J Respir Cell Mol Biol* (1989) **1**(1):5–10. doi:10.1165/ajrcmb/1.1.5

153. George EL, Georges-Labouesse EN, Patel-King RS, Rayburn H, Hynes RO. Defects in mesoderm, neural tube and vascular development in mouse embryos lacking fibronectin. *Development* (1993) **119**(4):1079–91.

154. Gerdes JS, Yoder MC, Douglas SD, Paul M, Harris MC, Polin RA. Tracheal lavage and plasma fibronectin: relationship to respiratory distress syndrome and development of bronchopulmonary dysplasia. *J Pediatr* (1986) **108**(4):601–6. doi:10.1016/S0022-3476(86)80847-2

155. Dyke MP, Forsyth KD. Plasma fibronectin levels in extremely preterm infants in the first 8 weeks of life. *J Paediatr Child Health* (1994) **30**(1):36–9. doi:10.1111/j.1440-1754.1994.tb00563.x

156. Timpl R, Sasaki T, Kostka G, Chu ML. Fibulins: a versatile family of extracellular matrix proteins. *Nat Rev Mol Cell Biol* (2003) **4**(6):479–89. doi:10.1038/nrm1130

157. Yanagisawa H, Davis EC, Starcher BC, Ouchi T, Yanagisawa M, Richardson JA, et al. Fibulin-5 is an elastin-binding protein essential for elastic fibre development in vivo. *Nature* (2002) **415**(6868):168–71. doi:10.1038/415168a

158. Schiemann WP, Blobe GC, Kalume DE, Pandey A, Lodish HF. Context-specific effects of fibulin-5 (DANCE/EVEC) on cell proliferation, motility, and invasion. Fibulin-5 is induced by transforming growth factor-beta and affects protein kinase cascades. *J Biol Chem* (2002) **277**(30):27367–77. doi:10.1074/jbc.M200148200

159. Lee YH, Albig AR, Regner M, Schiemann BJ, Schiemann WP. Fibulin-5 initiates epithelial-mesenchymal transition (EMT) and enhances EMT induced by TGF-beta in mammary epithelial cells via a MMP-dependent mechanism. *Carcinogenesis* (2008) **29**(12):2243–51. doi:10.1093/carcin/bgn199

160. Nguyen AD, Itoh S, Jeney V, Yanagisawa H, Fujimoto M, Ushio-Fukai M, et al. Fibulin-5 is a novel binding protein for extracellular superoxide dismutase. *Circ Res* (2004) **95**(11):1067–74. doi:10.1161/01.RES.0000149568.85071.FB

161. Colombatti A, Doliana R, Bot S, Canton A, Mongiat M, Mungiguerra G, et al. The EMILIN protein family. *Matrix Biol* (2000) **19**(4):289–301. doi:10.1016/S0945-053X(00)00074-3

162. Zanetti M, Braghetta P, Sabatelli P, Mura I, Doliana R, Colombatti A, et al. EMILIN-1 deficiency induces elastogenesis and vascular cell defects. *Mol Cell Biol* (2004) **24**(2):638–50. doi:10.1128/MCB.24.2.638-650.2004

163. Liu S, Parameswaran H, Young SM, Varisco BM. JNK suppresses pulmonary fibroblast elastogenesis during alveolar development. *Respir Res* (2014) **15**:34. doi:10.1186/1465-9921-15-34

164. Robertson IB, Horiguchi M, Zilberberg L, Dabovic B, Hadjiolova K, Rifkin DB. Latent TGF-beta-binding proteins. *Matrix Biol* (2015) **47**:44–53. doi:10.1016/j.matbio.2015.05.005

165. Todorovic V, Frendewey D, Gutstein DE, Chen Y, Freyer L, Finnegan E, et al. Long form of latent TGF-beta binding protein 1 (Ltbp1L) is essential for cardiac outflow tract septation and remodeling. *Development* (2007) **134**(20):3723–32. doi:10.1242/dev.008599

166. Dabovic B, Chen Y, Choi J, Davis EC, Sakai LY, Todorovic V, et al. Control of lung development by latent TGF-beta binding proteins. *J Cell Physiol* (2011) **226**(6):1499–509. doi:10.1002/jcp.22479

167. Dabovic B, Robertson IB, Zilberberg L, Vassallo M, Davis EC, Rifkin DB. Function of latent TGFbeta binding protein 4 and fibulin 5 in elastogenesis and lung development. *J Cell Physiol* (2015) **230**(1):226–36. doi:10.1002/jcp.24704

168. Dabovic B, Chen Y, Choi J, Vassallo M, Dietz HC, Ramirez F, et al. Dual functions for LTBP in lung development: LTBP-4 independently modulates elastogenesis and TGF-beta activity. *J Cell Physiol* (2009) **219**(1):14–22. doi:10.1002/jcp.21643

169. Shipley JM, Mecham RP, Maus E, Bonadio J, Rosenbloom J, McCarthy RT, et al. Developmental expression of latent transforming growth factor beta binding protein 2 and its requirement early in mouse development. *Mol Cell Biol* (2000) **20**(13):4879–87. doi:10.1128/MCB.20.13.4879-4887.2000

170. Thompson SM, Jesudason EC, Turnbull JE, Fernig DG. Heparan sulfate in lung morphogenesis: the elephant in the room. *Birth Defects Res C Embryo Today* (2010) **90**(1):32–44. doi:10.1002/bdrc.20169

171. Smits NC, Shworak NW, Dekhuijzen PN, van Kuppevelt TH. Heparan sulfates in the lung: structure, diversity, and role in pulmonary emphysema. *Anat Rec (Hoboken)* (2010) **293**(6):955–67. doi:10.1002/ar.20895

172. Becchetti E, Evangelisti R, Stabellini G, Pagliarini A, del Borrello E, Calastrini C, et al. Developmental heterogeneity of mesenchymal glycosaminoglycans (GAG) distribution in chick embryo lung anlagen. *Am J Anat* (1988) **181**(1):33–42. doi:10.1002/aja.1001810105

173. Brauker JH, Trautman MS, Bernfield M. Syndecan, a cell surface proteoglycan, exhibits a molecular polymorphism during lung development. *Dev Biol* (1991) **147**(2):285–92. doi:10.1016/0012-1606(91)90286-C

174. Caniggia I, Tanswell K, Post M. Temporal and spatial differences in glycosaminoglycan synthesis by fetal lung fibroblasts. *Exp Cell Res* (1992) **202**(2):252–8. doi:10.1016/0014-4827(92)90072-G

175. Vaccaro CA, Brody JS. Ultrastructural localization and characterization of proteoglycans in the pulmonary alveolus. *Am Rev Respir Dis* (1979) **120**(4):901–10.

176. Jaskoll TF, Slavkin HC. Ultrastructural and immunofluorescence studies of basal-lamina alterations during mouse-lung morphogenesis. *Differentiation* (1984) **28**(1):36–48. doi:10.1111/j.1432-0436.1984.tb00264.x

177. Izvolsky KI, Shoykhet D, Yang Y, Yu Q, Nugent MA, Cardoso WV. Heparan sulfate-FGF10 interactions during lung morphogenesis. *Dev Biol* (2003) **258**(1):185–200. doi:10.1016/S0012-1606(03)00114-3

178. Calvitti M, Baroni T, Calastrini C, Lilli C, Caramelli E, Becchetti E, et al. Bronchial branching correlates with specific glycosidase activity, extracellular glycosaminoglycan accumulation, TGF beta(2), and IL-1 localization during chick embryo lung development. *J Histochem Cytochem* (2004) **52**(3):325–34. doi:10.1177/002215540405200303

179. Hu Z, Wang C, Xiao Y, Sheng N, Chen Y, Xu Y, et al. NDST1-dependent heparan sulfate regulates BMP signaling and internalization in lung development. *J Cell Sci* (2009) **122**(Pt 8):1145–54. doi:10.1242/jcs.034736

180. Fan G, Xiao L, Cheng L, Wang X, Sun B, Hu G. Targeted disruption of NDST-1 gene leads to pulmonary hypoplasia and neonatal respiratory distress in mice. *FEBS Lett* (2000) **467**(1):7–11. doi:10.1016/S0014-5793(00)01111-X

181. Li JP, Gong F, Hagner-McWhirter A, Forsberg E, Abrink M, Kisilevsky R, et al. Targeted disruption of a murine glucuronyl C5-epimerase gene results in heparan sulfate lacking L-iduronic acid and in neonatal lethality. *J Biol Chem* (2003) **278**(31):28363–6. doi:10.1074/jbc.C300219200

182. Habuchi H, Nagai N, Sugaya N, Atsumi F, Stevens RL, Kimata K. Mice deficient in heparan sulfate 6-O-sulfotransferase-1 exhibit defective heparan sulfate biosynthesis, abnormal placentation, and late embryonic lethality. *J Biol Chem* (2007) **282**(21):15578–88. doi:10.1074/jbc.M607434200

183. Lum DH, Tan J, Rosen SD, Werb Z. Gene trap disruption of the mouse heparan sulfate 6-O-endosulfatase gene, Sulf2. *Mol Cell Biol* (2007) **27**(2):678–88. doi:10.1128/MCB.01279-06

184. Cano-Gauci DF, Song HH, Yang H, McKerlie C, Choo B, Shi W, et al. Glypican-3-deficient mice exhibit developmental overgrowth and some of the abnormalities typical of Simpson-Golabi-Behmel syndrome. *J Cell Biol* (1999) **146**(1):255–64. doi:10.1083/jcb.146.999.255

185. Thompson SM, Connell MG, Fernig DG, Ten Dam GB, van Kuppevelt TH, Turnbull JE, et al. Novel 'phage display antibodies identify distinct heparan

185. sulfate domains in developing mammalian lung. *Pediatr Surg Int* (2007) 23(5):411–7. doi:10.1007/s00383-006-1864-8

186. Shannon JM, McCormick-Shannon K, Burhans MS, Shangguan X, Srivastava K, Hyatt BA. Chondroitin sulfate proteoglycans are required for lung growth and morphogenesis in vitro. *Am J Physiol Lung Cell Mol Physiol* (2003) 285(6):L1323–36. doi:10.1152/ajplung.00226.2003

187. Underhill CB, Nguyen HA, Shizari M, Culty M. CD44 positive macrophages take up hyaluronan during lung development. *Dev Biol* (1993) 155(2):324–36. doi:10.1006/dbio.1993.1032

188. Coraux C, Delplanque A, Hinnrasky J, Peault B, Puchelle E, Gaillard D. Distribution of integrins during human fetal lung development. *J Histochem Cytochem* (1998) 46(7):803–10. doi:10.1177/002215549804600703

189. Roman J. Fibronectin and fibronectin receptors in lung development. *Exp Lung Res* (1997) 23(2):147–59. doi:10.3109/01902149709074027

190. Fukai T, Folz RJ, Landmesser U, Harrison DG. Extracellular superoxide dismutase and cardiovascular disease. *Cardiovasc Res* (2002) 55(2):239–49. doi:10.1016/S0008-6363(02)00328-0

191. Oury TD, Chang LY, Marklund SL, Day BJ, Crapo JD. Immunocytochemical localization of extracellular superoxide dismutase in human lung. *Lab Invest* (1994) 70(6):889–98.

192. Oury TD, Crapo JD, Valnickova Z, Enghild JJ. Human extracellular superoxide dismutase is a tetramer composed of two disulphide-linked dimers: a simplified, high-yield purification of extracellular superoxide dismutase. *Biochem J* (1996) 317(Pt 1):51–7. doi:10.1042/bj3170051

193. Petersen SV, Oury TD, Ostergaard L, Valnickova Z, Wegrzyn J, Thogersen IB, et al. Extracellular superoxide dismutase (EC-SOD) binds to type i collagen and protects against oxidative fragmentation. *J Biol Chem* (2004) 279(14):13705–10. doi:10.1074/jbc.M310217200

194. Hayashi A, Ryu A, Suzuki T, Kawada A, Tajima S. In vitro degradation of tropoelastin by reactive oxygen species. *Arch Dermatol Res* (1998) 290(9):497–500. doi:10.1007/s004030050342

195. Ryu A, Naru E, Arakane K, Masunaga T, Shinmoto K, Nagano T, et al. Cross-linking of collagen by singlet oxygen generated with UV-A. *Chem Pharm Bull (Tokyo)* (1997) 45(8):1243–7. doi:10.1248/cpb.45.1243

196. Ahmed MN, Suliman HB, Folz RJ, Nozik-Grayck E, Golson ML, Mason SN, et al. Extracellular superoxide dismutase protects lung development in hyperoxia-exposed newborn mice. *Am J Respir Crit Care Med* (2003) 167(3):400–5. doi:10.1164/rccm.200202-108OC

197. Oury TD, Schaefer LM, Fattman CL, Choi A, Weck KE, Watkins SC. Depletion of pulmonary EC-SOD after exposure to hyperoxia. *Am J Physiol Lung Cell Mol Physiol* (2002) 283(4):L777–84. doi:10.1152/ajplung.00011.2002

198. Carlsson LM, Jonsson J, Edlund T, Marklund SL. Mice lacking extracellular superoxide dismutase are more sensitive to hyperoxia. *Proc Natl Acad Sci U S A* (1995) 92(14):6264–8. doi:10.1073/pnas.92.14.6264

199. Auten RL, O'Reilly MA, Oury TD, Nozik-Grayck E, Whorton MH. Transgenic extracellular superoxide dismutase protects postnatal alveolar epithelial proliferation and development during hyperoxia. *Am J Physiol Lung Cell Mol Physiol* (2006) 290(1):L32–40. doi:10.1152/ajplung.00133.2005

200. Chen S, Birk DE. The regulatory roles of small leucine-rich proteoglycans in extracellular matrix assembly. *FEBS J* (2013) 280(10):2120–37. doi:10.1111/febs.12136

201. Godoy-Guzmán C, San Martin S, Pereda J. Proteoglycan and collagen expression during human air conducting system development. *Eur J Histochem* (2012) 56(3):e29. doi:10.4081/ejh.2012.e29

202. Nagase H, Woessner JF Jr. Matrix metalloproteinases. *J Biol Chem* (1999) 274(31):21491–4. doi:10.1074/jbc.274.31.21491

203. Ohbayashi H. Matrix metalloproteinases in lung diseases. *Curr Protein Pept Sci* (2002) 3(4):409–21. doi:10.2174/1389203023380549

204. Collier IE, Wilhelm SM, Eisen AZ, Marmer BL, Grant GA, Seltzer JL, et al. H-ras oncogene-transformed human bronchial epithelial cells (TBE-1) secrete a single metalloprotease capable of degrading basement membrane collagen. *J Biol Chem* (1988) 263(14):6579–87.

205. Wilhelm SM, Collier IE, Marmer BL, Eisen AZ, Grant GA, Goldberg GI. SV40-transformed human lung fibroblasts secrete a 92-kDa type IV collagenase which is identical to that secreted by normal human macrophages. *J Biol Chem* (1989) 264(29):17213–21.

206. Senior RM, Griffin GL, Fliszar CJ, Shapiro SD, Goldberg GI, Welgus HG. Human 92- and 72-kilodalton type IV collagenases are elastases. *J Biol Chem* (1991) 266(12):7870–5.

207. Ruiz V, Ordonez RM, Berumen J, Ramirez R, Uhal B, Becerril C, et al. Unbalanced collagenases/TIMP-1 expression and epithelial apoptosis in experimental lung fibrosis. *Am J Physiol Lung Cell Mol Physiol* (2003) 285(5):L1026–36. doi:10.1152/ajplung.00183.2003

208. Hautamaki RD, Kobayashi DK, Senior RM, Shapiro SD. Requirement for macrophage elastase for cigarette smoke-induced emphysema in mice. *Science* (1997) 277(5334):2002–4. doi:10.1126/science.277.5334.2002

209. Yu Q, Stamenkovic I. Cell surface-localized matrix metalloproteinase-9 proteolytically activates TGF-beta and promotes tumor invasion and angiogenesis. *Genes Dev* (2000) 14(2):163–76.

210. Lukkarinen H, Hogmalm A, Lappalainen U, Bry K. Matrix metalloproteinase-9 deficiency worsens lung injury in a model of bronchopulmonary dysplasia. *Am J Respir Cell Mol Biol* (2009) 41(1):59–68. doi:10.1165/rcmb.2008-0179OC

211. Schulz CG, Sawicki G, Lemke RP, Roeten BM, Schulz R, Cheung PY. MMP-2 and MMP-9 and their tissue inhibitors in the plasma of preterm and term neonates. *Pediatr Res* (2004) 55(5):794–801. doi:10.1203/01.PDR.0000120683.68630.FB

212. Csiszar K. Lysyl oxidases: a novel multifunctional amine oxidase family. *Prog Nucleic Acid Res Mol Biol* (2001) 70:1–32. doi:10.1016/S0079-6603(01)70012-8

213. Kagan HM, Li W. Lysyl oxidase: properties, specificity, and biological roles inside and outside of the cell. *J Cell Biochem* (2003) 88(4):660–72. doi:10.1002/jcb.10413

214. Zhan P, Shen XK, Qian Q, Zhu JP, Zhang Y, Xie HY, et al. Down-regulation of lysyl oxidase-like 2 (LOXL2) is associated with disease progression in lung adenocarcinomas. *Med Oncol* (2012) 29(2):648–55. doi:10.1007/s12032-011-9959-z

215. Mäki JM, Rasanen J, Tikkanen H, Sormunen R, Makikallio K, Kivirikko KI, et al. Inactivation of the lysyl oxidase gene Lox leads to aortic aneurysms, cardiovascular dysfunction, and perinatal death in mice. *Circulation* (2002) 106(19):2503–9. doi:10.1161/01.CIR.0000038109.84500.1E

216. Hornstra IK, Birge S, Starcher B, Bailey AJ, Mecham RP, Shapiro SD. Lysyl oxidase is required for vascular and diaphragmatic development in mice. *J Biol Chem* (2003) 278(16):14387–93. doi:10.1074/jbc.M210144200

217. Giampuzzi M, Botti G, Di Duca M, Arata L, Ghiggeri G, Gusmano R, et al. Lysyl oxidase activates the transcription activity of human collagene III promoter. Possible involvement of Ku antigen. *J Biol Chem* (2000) 275(46):36341–9. doi:10.1074/jbc.M003362200

218. Herranz N, Dave N, Millanes-Romero A, Morey L, Diaz VM, Lorenz-Fonfria V, et al. Lysyl oxidase-like 2 deaminates lysine 4 in histone H3. *Mol Cell* (2012) 46(3):369–76. doi:10.1016/j.molcel.2012.03.002

219. Lugassy J, Zaffryar-Eilot S, Soueid S, Mordoviz A, Smith V, Kessler O, et al. The enzymatic activity of lysyl oxidas-like-2 (LOXL2) is not required for LOXL2-induced inhibition of keratinocyte differentiation. *J Biol Chem* (2012) 287(5):3541–9. doi:10.1074/jbc.M111.261016

220. Myllyla R, Wang C, Heikkinen J, Juffer A, Lampela O, Risteli M, et al. Expanding the lysyl hydroxylase toolbox: new insights into the localization and activities of lysyl hydroxylase 3 (LH3). *J Cell Physiol* (2007) 212(2):323–9. doi:10.1002/jcp.21036

221. Rautavuoma K, Takaluoma K, Sormunen R, Myllyharju J, Kivirikko KI, Soininen R. Premature aggregation of type IV collagen and early lethality in lysyl hydroxylase 3 null mice. *Proc Natl Acad Sci U S A* (2004) 101(39):14120–5. doi:10.1073/pnas.0404966101

222. Takaluoma K, Hyry M, Lantto J, Sormunen R, Bank RA, Kivirikko KI, et al. Tissue-specific changes in the hydroxylysine content and cross-links of collagens and alterations in fibril morphology in lysyl hydroxylase 1 knock-out mice. *J Biol Chem* (2007) 282(9):6588–96. doi:10.1074/jbc.M608830200

223. Beninati S, Bergamini CM, Piacentini M. An overview of the first 50 years of transglutaminase research. *Amino Acids* (2009) 36(4):591–8. doi:10.1007/s00726-008-0211-x

224. Iismaa SE, Mearns BM, Lorand L, Graham RM. Transglutaminases and disease: lessons from genetically engineered mouse models and inherited disorders. *Physiol Rev* (2009) 89(3):991–1023. doi:10.1152/physrev.00044.2008

225. Akimov SS, Krylov D, Fleischman LF, Belkin AM. Tissue transglutaminase is an integrin-binding adhesion coreceptor for fibronectin. *J Cell Biol* (2000) 148(4):825–38. doi:10.1083/jcb.148.4.825

226. Olsen KC, Epa AP, Kulkarni AA, Kottmann RM, McCarthy CE, Johnson GV, et al. Inhibition of transglutaminase 2, a novel target for pulmonary fibrosis, by two small electrophilic molecules. *Am J Respir Cell Mol Biol* (2014) **50**(4):737–47. doi:10.1165/rcmb.2013-0092OC

227. Griffin M, Smith LL, Wynne J. Changes in transglutaminase activity in an experimental model of pulmonary fibrosis induced by paraquat. *Br J Exp Pathol* (1979) **60**(6):653–61.

228. Luciani A, Villella VR, Esposito S, Brunetti-Pierri N, Medina DL, Settembre C, et al. Cystic fibrosis: a disorder with defective autophagy. *Autophagy* (2011) **7**(1):104–6. doi:10.4161/auto.7.1.13987

229. Maiuri L, Luciani A, Giardino I, Raia V, Villella VR, D'Apolito M, et al. Tissue transglutaminase activation modulates inflammation in cystic fibrosis via PPARgamma down-regulation. *J Immunol* (2008) **180**(11):7697–705. doi:10.4049/jimmunol.180.11.7697

230. Penumatsa KC, Fanburg BL. Transglutaminase 2-mediated serotonylation in pulmonary hypertension. *Am J Physiol Lung Cell Mol Physiol* (2014) **306**(4):L309–15. doi:10.1152/ajplung.00321.2013

231. Piacentini M, Rodolfo C, Farrace MG, Autuori F. "Tissue" transglutaminase in animal development. *Int J Dev Biol* (2000) **44**(6):655–62. doi:10.1007/bfb0102308

232. Schittny JC, Paulsson M, Vallan C, Burri PH, Kedei N, Aeschlimann D. Protein cross-linking mediated by tissue transglutaminase correlates with the maturation of extracellular matrices during lung development. *Am J Respir Cell Mol Biol* (1997) **17**(3):334–43. doi:10.1165/ajrcmb.17.3.2737

233. Kojima S, Nara K, Rifkin DB. Requirement for transglutaminase in the activation of latent transforming growth factor-beta in bovine endothelial cells. *J Cell Biol* (1993) **121**(2):439–48. doi:10.1083/jcb.121.2.439

234. Nanda N, Iismaa SE, Owens WA, Husain A, Mackay F, Graham RM. Targeted inactivation of Gh/tissue transglutaminase II. *J Biol Chem* (2001) **276**(23):20673–8. doi:10.1074/jbc.M010846200

235. Rawlins EL, Perl AK. The a"MAZE"ing world of lung-specific transgenic mice. *Am J Respir Cell Mol Biol* (2012) **46**(3):269–82. doi:10.1165/rcmb.2011-0372PS

236. Shojaie S, Ermini L, Ackerley C, Wang J, Chin S, Yeganeh B, et al. Acellular lung scaffolds direct differentiation of endoderm to functional airway epithelial cells: requirement of matrix-bound HS proteoglycans. *Stem Cell Reports* (2015) **4**(3):419–30. doi:10.1016/j.stemcr.2015.01.004

11

The Correlation Between Bronchopulmonary Dysplasia and Platelet Metabolism in Preterm Infants

Longli Yan, Zhuxiao Ren[†], Jianlan Wang[†], Xin Xia, Liling Yang, Jiayu Miao, Fang Xu, Weiwei Gao and Jie Yang*

Department of Neonatology, Guangdong Women and Children Hospital, Guangzhou Medical University, Guangzhou, China

*Correspondence:
Jie Yang
jieyang0830@126.com

[†] These authors have contributed equally to this work

Background: Platelets play an important role in the formation of pulmonary blood vessels, and thrombocytopenia is common in patients with pulmonary diseases. However, a few studies have reported on the role of platelets in bronchopulmonary dysplasia.

Objective: The objective of the study was to explore the relationship between platelet metabolism and bronchopulmonary dysplasia in premature infants.

Methods: A prospective case-control study was performed in a cohort of premature infants (born with a gestational age < 32 weeks and a birth weight $< 1,500$ g) from June 1, 2017 to June 1, 2018. Subjects were stratified into two groups according to the diagnostic of bronchopulmonary dysplasia: with bronchopulmonary dysplasia (BPD group) and without bronchopulmonary dysplasia (control group). Platelet count, circulating megakaryocyte count (MK), platelet-activating markers (CD62P and CD63), and thrombopoietin (TPO) were recorded and compared in two groups 28 days after birth; then serial thrombopoietin levels and concomitant platelet counts were measured in infants with BPD.

Results: A total of 252 premature infants were included in this study. Forty-eight premature infants developed BPD, 48 premature infants without BPD in the control group who were matched against the study infants for gestational age, birth weight, and admission diagnosis at the age of postnatal day 28. Compared with the controls, infants with BPD had significantly lower peripheral platelet count [BPD vs. controls: 180.3 (24.2) $\times 10^9$/L vs. 345.6 (28.5) $\times 10^9$/L, $p = 0.001$]. Circulating MK count in the BPD group was significantly more abundant than that in the control group [BPD vs. controls: 30.7 (4.5)/ml vs. 13.3 (2.6)/ml, $p = 0.025$]. The level of CD62p, CD63, and TPO in BPD group was significantly higher than the control group [29.7 (3.1%) vs. 14.5 (2.5%), 15.4 (2.0%) vs. 5.8 (1.7%), 301.4 (25.9) pg/ml vs. 120.4 (14.2) pg/ml, all $p < 0.05$]. Furthermore, the concentration of TPO was negatively correlated with platelet count in BPD group with thrombocytopenia.

Conclusions: Our findings suggest that platelet metabolism is involved in the development of BPD in preterm infants. The possible mechanism might be through increased platelet activation and promoted TPO production by feedback.

Keywords: bronchopulmonary dysplasia, platelet, TPO, megakaryocyte, CD62P, CD63

INTRODUCTION

Bronchopulmonary dysplasia (BPD) is one of the common complications in neonatal intensive care units (NICU) and is considered to be the main cause of death in preterm infants (1). In recent years, with advances in perinatal and neonatal care of preterm infants such as antenatal steroid usage, surfactant therapy, and ventilation strategies, the survival rate of premature infants also increases, resulting in an increasing incidence of BPD. BPD severely influences premature infants by increasing their risk of respiratory infection, asthma, and chronic obstructive pulmonary distress in their later life (2–4).

Currently, alveolar and microvascular arrest is considered as the pathological feature of clinical bronchopulmonary dysplasia (5), the development of alveolar microvascular can promote the formation of alveoli structure; therefore, the role of pulmonary vascular development, especially in pulmonary microvascular development in BPD is getting more and more attention.

The platelet has been recognized as a multifunctional cell, besides hemostasis and thrombosis. The platelet plays an essential role in the formation and development of pulmonary blood vessels, as demonstrated by numerous studies (6, 7). Some clinical retrospective studies (8, 9) found that mean platelet volume might predict the occurrence of BPD, and also, a study (10) has shown that higher platelet count is an independent factor of the development of moderate–severe BPD, and the research (11) found that a higher platelet transfusion threshold can increase the risk of BPD in premature infants. So, we speculate that platelets are involved in the occurrence of BPD, and a few studies have been reported in this regard.

In the present study, we evaluated this hypothesis by comparing peripheral platelet count, circulating MK count, platelet-activating markers, (CD62P and CD63) 28 days after birth in two groups, and the relationship between TPO expression and platelet count in infants with BPD.

MATERIALS AND METHODS
Study Design and Population

This is a prospective study performed at the Neonatal Intensive Care Unit (NICU), Guangdong Women and Children Hospital from June 1, 2017 to June 1, 2018. This study was approved by the ethics committee of Guangdong Women and Children Hospital. Preterm infants cared for in our center were enrolled if they satisfied the following recruitment criteria: (1) gestation <32 weeks, (2) birth weight <1.5 kg, (3) requiring mechanical ventilation for the treatment of respiratory distress syndrome for at least 3 days during the first weeks of life, (4) ventilator and/or oxygen dependent at the time of

enrollment, and (5) presence of clinical and radiologic signs of BPD.

Prospectively determined exclusion criteria included the following conditions: (1) congenital abnormalities; (2) infection (bacterial infection confirmed by positive blood culture or viral infection confirmed by serological test or viral culture); (3) evidence of complications of perinatal asphyxia including an Apgar score <3 at 1 or 5 min after birth, evidence of hypoxic–ischemic encephalopathy, acute tubular necrosis, or transient myocardial ischemia; and (4) identifiable hematologic disease.

The infants who were matched against the study infant for gestational age, birth weight, and admission diagnosis were recruited as control group at their age of postnatal day 28.

Definition of Clinical Variables

The diagnosis of BPD in preterm birth was assessed using the consensus definition of the National Institute of Child Health and Human Development (NICHD). Briefly, BPD was defined as the need for supplemental oxygen for more than 28 days and the severity was assessed according to the oxygen concentration required at 36 weeks PMA or discharge (12). Neonatal thrombocytopenia was defined arbitrarily as a platelet count of <150,000 mm^3. Neonatal respiratory distress syndrome (NRDS) was defined according to Gomella's Neonatology (13).

Data Collection

The following data were retrieved from the electronic medical record, including maternal disease, gestation, birth weight, gender, Apgar score, NRDS, ventilation mode, blood testing (hemoglobin, white cell count, platelet count, blood gas) using the samples collected within 1 h after birth from the peripheral arterial of the infants.

Measurements
Blood Sampling

In enrolled premature infants at their age of postnatal day 28, during blood sampling for routine laboratory investigation, 1 ml of blood was drawn from the peripheral arterial and placed into an EDTA tube. After mixing gently, 40 μl of whole blood was used as an aliquot for the detection of CD62P and CD63 expressions by flow cytometry. After centrifugation at $400 \times g$, plasma was separated from the blood and preserved at −80°C for TPO level detection. The cell pellet was resuspended in phosphate-buffered saline (PBS) for circulating MK isolation. All samples were processed within 1 h of collection.

Platelet Counts and Circulating Megakaryocyte Counts

Blood platelets were quantified by a Japanese Sysmex KX221 automatic blood cell analyzer. Circulating MK count was

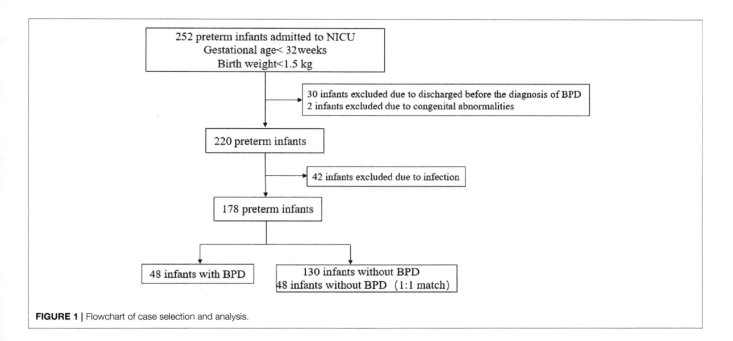

FIGURE 1 | Flowchart of case selection and analysis.

estimated as previously described (14). Briefly, samples were passed through a syringe filter holder (Millipore, Ireland) containing a polycarbonate membrane with an aperture of 5 μm at 37°C and then washed with 2 ml of saline. After the removal of the membrane, it was dried quickly and slightly with a heater and was left overnight at room temperature.

CD62P and CD63 Expressions

CD62P and CD63 were estimated by flow cytometry (FACSCalibur, Becton-Dickinson, San Jose, CA, USA) with the procedure details as previously described (14). In short, 40 μl of whole blood was taken at room temperature and stained with the monoclonal antibody at a saturated concentration for 30 min in dark. FITC-conjugated CD61 is regarded as a platelet-specific monoclonal antibody, and anti-cd62p and anti-cd63 combined with PE in dichroism analysis were used as platelet activation markers. After incubation, 1 ml of PBS containing 1% paraformaldehyde was added to each tube. The samples were fixed at 4°C for 24 h for flow cytometry detection. CD62P and CD63 were detected in 20,000 platelets. All antibodies were purchased from Abcam.

Plasma Thrombopoietin Concentration

TPO levels were measured using a commercially available ELISA (R&D Systems Quantikine Human TPO ELISA kit, Minneapolis, MN, USA), with a lower limit of detection of 15 pg/ml.

Statistical Analysis

Statistical analyses between the two groups were performed using two-tailed Student's t-test. One-way analysis of variance was performed to compare the relationship between TPO concentration and platelet count at each time point in BPD group. A value of $p < 0.05$ was considered statistically significant.

All values were expressed as mean (SEM) unless otherwise stated. All statistical analyses were done using SPSS 20.0.

RESULTS

Demography Characteristics

A total of 252 eligible premature infants were admitted to our NICU during the study period, after applying exclusion criteria, 178 premature infants were included, in which 48 premature infants diagnosed with BPD, 134 premature infants without BPD, and 48 premature infants in the control group were matched 1:1 according to gestational age, birth weight, and admission diagnosis at their age of postnatal day 28 (**Figure 1**).

The demographic characteristics of the study infants are shown in **Table 1**.

We studied 48 infants in the BPD group (female: 27; male: 21) and 48 infants in the control group (female: 24; male: 24). The infants in the BPD group and control group were similar in their demographic characteristics including gestational age and birth weight. However, the infants with BPD had been exposed to a significantly higher FiO_2 and had a significantly longer ventilation duration (**Table 1**). Among the infants with BPD, 30 infants had a peripheral platelet count $<150 \times 10^9$/L, while none of the infants in the control group had a platelet count $<150 \times 10^9$/L. Infants in both groups received similar conventional treatment according to the unit protocol.

Thirty thrombocytopenic infants in the BPD group were studied serially at postnatal age of day 28, day 35, and day 42, respectively. The platelet count in all these infants returned to normal by the age of day 42.

Peripheral Platelet Count

Peripheral platelet count in the BPD group was significantly lower than that in the control group [BPD vs. controls: 180.3

TABLE 1 | Demographic characteristics of infants with BPD.

Variable	BPD (n = 48)	Control (n = 48)	p-Value
Gestation (weeks)	28.5 (0.5)	29.7 (0.43)	0.17
Birth weight (g)	1,040 (60)	1,220 (60)	0.14
Gender			
Female	27	24	0.23
Male	21	14	0.25
Maternal disease			
PIH	20	16	0.32
IUGR	4	2	0.25
PROM	6	4	0.30
Oligohydramnios	3	1	0.22
Twin–twin transfusion	1	1	0.5
APH	3	4	0.36
Nil	4	2	0.42
Apgar score			
At 1 min	7	7	0.55
At 5 min	8	9	0.45
Admission diagnosis			
Prematurity	48	48	
RDS	48	44	
Hemoglobin (g/ml)	11.0 (0.3)	10.4 (0.4)	0.18
White cell count (x10^5/L)	10.5 (0.3)	11.8 (1.5)	0.55
Platelet count (x10^9/L)	170.1 (15.4)	343.1 (23.4)	<0.001
Ventilation duration (days)			
IPPV	20 (0.8)	9 (0.4)	<0.001
CPAP	29 (1.7)	15 (0.7)	<0.001
HFOV	12 (1.3)	7 (0.4)	0.08
Blood gas			
PH	7.37 (0.04)	7.39 (0.03)	0.25
PaO$_2$	6.31 (0.4)	5.7 (0.4)	0.34
PaCO$_2$	5.0 (0.4)	5.1 (0.3)	0.83
FiO$_2$	0.27 (0.03)	0.21 (0.3)	<0.001

PIH, pregnancy-induced hypertension; IUGR, intra-uterine growth retardation; PROM, prolonged rupture of membrane; SLE, systemic lupus erythematosus; IPPV, intermittent positive pressure ventilation; CPAP, continuous positive airway pressure; HFOV, high-frequency oscillatory ventilation; BPD, bronchopulmonary dysplasia.

(24.2) × 10^9/L vs. 345.6 (28.5) × 10^9/L, $p = 0.001$], as shown in **Figure 2**.

Circulating Megakaryocyte Count
Circulating MK count in the BPD group was significantly more abundant than that in the control group [BPD vs. controls: 30.7 (4.5)/ml vs. 13.3 (2.6)/ml, $p = 0.025$], as shown in **Figure 3**.

CD62P and CD63 Expressions on Platelets
When compared with the controls, premature infants with BPD had significantly greater expressions of CD62P [BPD vs. controls: 29.70 (3.1%) platelets vs. 14.5 (2.5%) platelets, $p = 0.023$] and CD63 [BPD vs. controls: 15.4 (2.0%) platelets vs. 5.8 (1.7%) platelets, $p = 0.015$)], as shown in **Figures 4–6**.

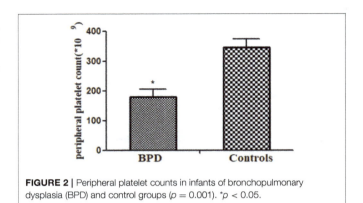

FIGURE 2 | Peripheral platelet counts in infants of bronchopulmonary dysplasia (BPD) and control groups ($p = 0.001$). *$p < 0.05$.

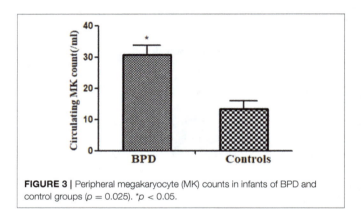

FIGURE 3 | Peripheral megakaryocyte (MK) counts in infants of BPD and control groups ($p = 0.025$). *$p < 0.05$.

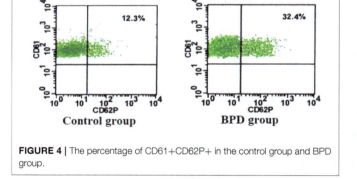

FIGURE 4 | The percentage of CD61+CD62P+ in the control group and BPD group.

Plasma Thrombopoietin Concentration
Circulating MK count in the BPD group was significantly higher than that in the control group [BPD vs. controls: 301.4 (25.9) pg/ml vs. 120.4 (14.2) pg/ml, $p = 0.032$], as shown in **Figure 7**.

Plasma Thrombopoietin Response to Thrombocytopenia in Infants With Bronchopulmonary Dysplasia
TPO levels showed an inverse relationship with peripheral platelet count, peaking near the nadir and decreasing as platelet count increased, as shown in **Figure 8**.

DISCUSSION

In this prospective study, we studied the relevant indicators of platelet metabolism in premature infants with BPD and analyzed its relationship with the occurrence of BPD. Our finding in this study was consistent with our observation in the rat model (15).

In previous studies (16, 17), we have known that CD62p and CD63 are sensitive indicators of platelet activation, and we found that CD62p and CD63 were increased in premature infants who developed BPD compared with those who did not, and the platelet count in the BPD group was significantly lower than in the non-BPD group. Our observation suggested that in infants with BPD, platelet consumption was at least partly responsible for the low peripheral platelet count. The new type of BPD is characterized by alveolar and microvascular dysplasia (5), and endothelial cell injury will impair lung vascular and alveolar growth. Previous workers have reported that pulmonary endothelium was the earliest cell damaged by oxygen free radicals (18), which was followed by an influx of inflammatory cells, such as neutrophils. Once endothelial damage occurs, the activated platelets cause inflammation by the migration of central granulocytes, which play a key role in the arrested lung development (19). In addition, the intercellular adhesion molecule-1, one of the markers in estimating neutrophil attachment to endothelial cells, was elevated in infants with BPD (20). Furthermore, the vascular endothelial growth factor, one of the markers in evaluating the growth and repair of vascular endothelial cell, was lower in infants with BPD than those without BPD (21). In addition, activated polymorphonuclear leukocytes can cause lung tissue injury by the release of toxic oxygen radicals, all of which can further damage the endothelium and increase platelet

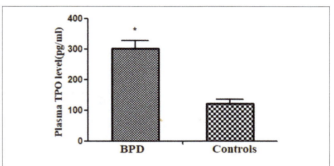

FIGURE 7 | Plasma thrombopoietin (TPO) level in infants of BPD and control groups ($p = 0.032$). *$p < 0.05$.

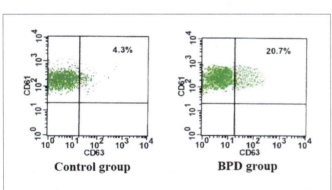

FIGURE 5 | The percentage of CD61 + CD63 in the control group and BPD group.

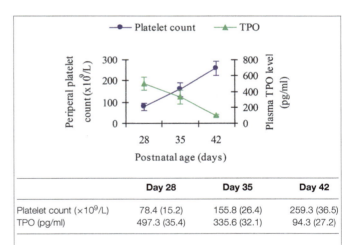

FIGURE 8 | Response of plasma TPO to thrombocytopenia in infants with BPD.

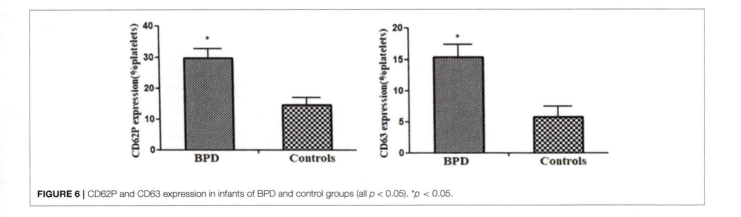

FIGURE 6 | CD62P and CD63 expression in infants of BPD and control groups (all $p < 0.05$). *$p < 0.05$.

activation (22). These observations, together with ours, indicated that pulmonary endothelial damage in infants with BPD may lead to platelet activation and, most likely, increased platelet consumption, resulting in the reduction of peripheral platelet count. Therefore, inhibition of platelet activation may improve the occurrence of BPD.

Our previous study (15) confirmed that the lung is an important site for MK fragmentation and platelet release by comparing the MK and platelet counts between the pre-pulmonary and post-pulmonary blood in rats. Using state-of-the-art intravital microscopy, Lefracais et al. (23) observed the dynamic release of platelets by intravascular megakaryocytes in the lung microcirculation of mice, and intravascular lung megakaryocytes account for about 50% of total platelet production. In this study, as the central arterial and venous catheters were rarely simultaneously available in infants at their postnatal 28 days, we were not able to estimate the platelet and MK count at the pre-pulmonary and post-pulmonary circulation. Thus, we cannot confirm the effect of lung damage in BPD on platelet production. However, it is possible that in infants with BPD, there were lots of pulmonary capillary beds or the damaged endothelium was unable to retain MK for platelet release. On the other hand, mechanical ventilation may damage the pulmonary blood–gas barrier, which causes leakage of fluid, protein, and blood cells into tissue and air spaces. This leakage may result in leakage of MK cells into the alveoli and impairment of MK fragmentation into platelets due to functional impairment of the filtration and sequestration functions of pulmonary capillaries. In this experiment, we found that circulating MK count in the preterm with BPD was higher than that without BPD. The circulating MK, reflecting the MK progenitor in bone marrow, suggests that thrombocytopenia may initiate a feedback mechanism to stimulate the generation of bone marrow megakaryocytes, to increase the number of megakaryocytes in circulation.

Thrombocytopenia is the common complication of newborns in NICU. To our knowledge, TPO is a major regulator of platelet production. So far, there are no reports on plasma TPO level in infants with BPD or its relationship with platelet count. Therefore, in our study, serial TPO and platelet count measurements were obtained in some subjects. Platelet count in infants with BPD showed significantly increased plasma TPO level when compared with the infants in the control group. Our finding that TPO showed a decrease at the time of resolution of thrombocytopenia has also been observed in both adults and children (24, 25). The mechanism might be that plasma TPO concentration is dependent on circulating platelet mass (26). Elevated platelet levels lead to increased binding of cytokines to platelet receptors, which increases the activity of antiplatelet antibodies and reduces plasma concentration. Conversely, lower platelet levels lead to decreased absorption and catabolic metabolism, which leads to higher plasma TPO concentrations. This theory supports our findings.

In conclusion, platelets may play an important role in the formation and development of pulmonary microvascularization in premature infants with BPD. The mechanism may be related to platelet activation and TPO regulation. However, the specific mechanism of TPO-regulating platelets in infants with BPD needs to be further studied, which provides a new idea for the study of BPD.

AUTHOR CONTRIBUTIONS

LYan and ZR conceived and coordinated the study, and wrote the paper. LYan, JW, XX, and LYang performed the experiments. FX and WG collected and analyzed the data. JM collected the references. JY edited the manuscript and provided guidance. All authors reviewed the results and approved the final version of the manuscript.

REFERENCES

1. Stoll BJ, Hansen NI, Bell EF, Walsh MC, Carlo WA, Shankaran S, et al. Trends in care practices, morbidity, and mortality of extremely preterm neonates, 1993-2012. *JAMA*. (2015) 314:1039–51. doi: 10.1001/jama.2015.10244
2. Postma DS, Bush A, van den Berge M. Risk factors and early origins of chronic obstructive pulmonary disease. *Lancet*. (2015) 385:899–909. doi: 10.1016/S0140-6736(14)60446-3
3. Moschino L, Carraro S, Baraldi E. Early-life origin and prevention of chronic obstructive pulmonary diseases. *Pediatr Allergy Immunol*. (2020) 31:16–8. doi: 10.1111/pai.13157
4. Islam JY, Keller RL, Aschner JL, Hartert TV, Moore PE. Understanding the short- and long-term respiratory outcomes of prematurity and bronchopulmonary dysplasia. *Am J Respir Crit Care Med*. (2015) 192:134–56. doi: 10.1164/rccm.201412-2142PP
5. Thébaud B, Goss KN, Laughon M, Whitsett JA, Abman SH, Steinhorn RH, et al. Bronchopulmonary dysplasia. *Nat Rev Dis Primers*. (2019) 5:78–131. doi: 10.1038/s41572-019-0127-7
6. Jiménez J, Richter J, Nagatomo T, Salaets T, Quarck R, Wagennar A, et al. Progressive vascular functional and structural damage in a bronchopulmonary dysplasia model in preterm rabbits exposed to hyperoxia. *Int J Mol Sci*. (2016) 17:e1776. doi: 10.3390/ijms17101776
7. Kroll MH, Afshar-Kharghan V. Platelets in pulmonary vascular physiology and pathology. *Plum Circ*. (2012) 2:291–308. doi: 10.4103/2045-8932.101398
8. Bolouki MK, Zarkesh M, Kamali A, Dalili S, Heidarzadeh A, Rad AH. The association of mean platelet volume with intra ventricular hemorrhage and broncho pulmonary dysplasia in preterm infants. *J Pediat Hematol Onc*. (2015) 15:227–32.
9. Dani C, Poggi C, Barp J, Berti E, Fontanelli G. Mean platelet volume and risk of bronchopulmonary dysplasia and intraventricular hemorrhage in extremely preterm infants. *Am J Perinatol*. (2011) 28:551–7. doi: 10.1055/s-0031-1274503
10. Chen X, Li H, Qiu X, Yang CZ, Walther FJ. Neonatal hematological parameters and the risk of moderate-severe bronchopulmonary dysplasia in extremely premature infants. *BMC Pediatr*. (2019) 19:138–44. doi: 10.1186/s12887-019-1515-6
11. Curley A, Stanworth SJ, Willoughby K, Fustolo-Gunnink SF, Venkatesh V, Hudson C, et al. Randomized trial of platelet-transfusion thresholds in neonates. *N Engl J Med*. (2019) 3:242–51. doi: 10.1056/NEJMoa1807320
12. Ehrenkranz RA, Walsh MC, Vohr BR, Jobe AH, Wright LL, Fanaroff AA. et al. *Validation of the National Institutes of Health consensus definition of bronchopulmonary dysplasia[J]Pediatrics*. (2005) 116:1353–60. doi: 10.1542/peds.2005-0249
13. Gomella T, Cummingham M, Fabien E. *Neonatology*. 6th ed. New York, NY: Lange (2009).
14. Yang J, Zhang HC, Niu JM, Mu XP, Zhang XL, Ying Liu Y, et al. Impact of preeclampsia on megakaryocytopoesis and platelet homeostasis of preterm infants. *Platelets*. (2016) 27:123–7. doi: 10.3109/09537104.2015.1048213

15. Yang J, Yang M, Xu F, Li K, Lee SKM, Ng PC, et al. Effects of oxygen-induced lung damage on megakaryocytopoiesis and platelet homeostasis in a rat model. *Pediatr Res.* (2003) 54:344–52. doi: 10.1203/01.PDR.0000079186.86219.29

16. Ergelen M, Uyarel H. Plateletcrit: a novel prognostic marker for acute coronary syndrome. *Int J Cardiol.* (2014) 177:161. doi: 10.1016/j.ijcard.2014.09.054

17. Taylor ML, Misso NL, Stewart GA, Thompson PJ. differential expression of platelet activation markers CD62P and CD63 following stimulation with PAF, arachidonic acid and collagen. *Platelets.* (2009) 6:394–401. doi: 10.3109/09537109509078478

18. Mittal M, Siddiqui MR, Tran K, Reddy SP, Malik AB. Reactive oxygen species in inflammation and tissue injury. *Antioxid Redox Signal.* (2014) 20:1126–67. doi: 10.1089/ars.2012.5149

19. Bui CB, Pang MA, Sehgal A, Theda C, Lao JC, Berger PJ, et al. Pulmonary hypertension associated with bronchopulmonary dysplasia in preterm infants. *J Reprod Immunol.* (2017) 124:21–9. doi: 10.1016/j.jri.2017.09.013

20. Wang XH, Jia HL, Deng L, Huang WM. Astragalus polysaccharides mediated preventive effects on bronchopulmonary dysplasia in rats. *Pediatr Res.* (2014) 76:347–54. doi: 10.1038/pr.2014.107

21. Baker CD, Abman SH. Impaired pulmonary vascular development in bronchopulmonary dysplasia. *Neonatology.* (2015) 107:344–51. doi: 10.1159/000381129

22. Middleton EA, Rondina MT, Schwertz H, Zimmerman GA. Amicus or adversary revisited: platelets in acute lung injury and acute respiratory distress syndrome. *Am J Respir Cell Mol Biol.* (2018) 59:18–35. doi: 10.1165/rcmb.2017-0420TR

23. Lefrancais E, Ortiz-Munoz G, Caudrillier A, Mallavia B, Liu FC, Sayah DM, et al. The lung is a site of platelet biogenesis and a reservoir for haematopoietic progenitors. *Nature.* (2017) 544:105–9. doi: 10.1038/nature21706

24. Temel T, Cansu DU, Temel HE, Ozakyol AH. Serum thrombopoietin levels and its relationship with thrombocytopenia in patients with cirrhosis. *Hepat Mon.* (2014) 14:e18556–9. doi: 10.5812/hepatmon.18556

25. Del Vecchio GC, Giordano P, Tesse R, Piacente L, Altomare M. De Mattia, D. Clinical significance of serum cytokine levels and thrombopoietic markers in childhood idiopathic thrombocytopenic purpura. *Blood Transfus.* (2012) 10:194–9. doi: 10.2450/2011.0055-11

26. de Graaf CA, Kauppi M, Baldwin T, Hyland CD, Metcalf D, Willson TA, et al. Regulation of hematopoietic stem cells by their mature progeny. *Proc Natl Acad Sci U S A.* (2010) 107:21689–94. doi: 10.1073/pnas.1016166108

12

A Breath of Fresh Air on the Mesenchyme: Impact of Impaired Mesenchymal Development on the Pathogenesis of Bronchopulmonary Dysplasia

Cho-Ming Chao[1,2,3], Elie El Agha[2,3], Caterina Tiozzo[4], Parviz Minoo[5] and Saverio Bellusci[2,3,6,7]*

[1] Department of General Pediatrics and Neonatology, University Children's Hospital Giessen, Giessen, Germany, [2] Department of Internal Medicine II, Universities of Giessen and Marburg Lung Center, Giessen, Germany, [3] Member of the German Center for Lung Research (DZL), Giessen, Germany, [4] Division of Neonatology, Department of Pediatrics, Columbia University, New York, NY, USA, [5] Division of Newborn Medicine, Department of Pediatrics, Children's Hospital Los Angeles, University of Southern California, Los Angeles, CA, USA, [6] Saban Research Institute, Childrens Hospital Los Angeles, University of Southern California, Los Angeles, CA, USA, [7] Kazan Federal University, Kazan, Russia

*Correspondence:
*Saverio Bellusci,
Department of Internal Medicine II,
Universities of Giessen and Marburg
Lung Center (UGMLC), Klinikstraße
36, Giessen, Hessen 35392, Germany
saverio.bellusci@innere.med.uni-
giessen.de*

The early mouse embryonic lung, with its robust and apparently reproducible branching pattern, has always fascinated developmental biologists. They have extensively used this embryonic organ to decipher the role of mammalian orthologs of *Drosophila* genes in controlling the process of branching morphogenesis. During the early pseudoglandular stage, the embryonic lung is formed mostly of tubes that keep on branching. As the branching takes place, progenitor cells located in niches are also amplified and progressively differentiate along the proximo-distal and dorso-ventral axes of the lung. Such elaborate processes require coordinated interactions between signaling molecules arising from and acting on four functional domains: the epithelium, the endothelium, the mesenchyme, and the mesothelium. These interactions, quite well characterized in a relatively simple lung tubular structure remain elusive in the successive developmental and postnatal phases of lung development. In particular, a better understanding of the process underlying the formation of secondary septa, key structural units characteristic of the alveologenesis phase, is still missing. This structure is critical for the formation of a mature lung as it allows the subdivision of saccules in the early neonatal lung into alveoli, thereby considerably expanding the respiratory surface. Interruption of alveologenesis in preterm neonates underlies the pathogenesis of chronic neonatal lung disease known as bronchopulmonary dysplasia. *De novo* formation of secondary septae appears also to be the limiting factor for lung regeneration in human patients with emphysema. In this review, we will therefore focus on what is known in terms of interactions between the different lung compartments and discuss the current understanding of mesenchymal cell lineage formation in the lung, focusing on secondary septae formation.

Keywords: lung development, alveologenesis, bronchopulmonary dysplasia, epithelial–mesenchymal interaction, endothelial–mesenchymal interaction, secondary septae formation

Bronchopulmonary Dysplasia is Characterized by Impaired Alveologenesis

Bronchopulmonary dysplasia (BPD) is a chronic lung disease of prematurely born infants and remains a leading cause of morbidity and mortality. Currently, there is no curative therapy available. Based on the severity-based definition of BPD (inclusion of infants with mild BPD) 68% of premature infants born with a gestational age (GA) $\leq$28 weeks develop BPD (1–3). The risk of developing BPD correlates inversely with the GA and birth weight (BW) (4). Since premature infants (24–28 weeks of gestation) are born with a lung, which is in the canalicular or saccular stages of development, the lung structure (characterized by thickened airspace walls and surfactant deficiency) is therefore not adequate to provide sufficient ventilation and gas exchange. Thus, mechanical ventilation and high-oxygen concentration are often necessary at birth. Barotrauma induced by mechanical ventilation as well as oxygen toxicity and inflammation are major contributing factors responsible for the pulmonary damages in the morphological and functional immature lung. In addition, some studies have suggested a strong genetic component in BPD (5). For example, using genome-wide association study, it has been shown that polymorphisms (SNPs) in *MMP16* and *SPOCK2* might be associated with BPD (6). Due to remarkable advances in the management and therapy (e.g., gentle ventilation, restricted oxygen supplementation, antenatal steroids, and exogenous surfactant use) survival rate for premature infants has increased over the last decades. These advances in treatment have changed the histological characteristics of what is now called the old BPD since it was first described by Northway in 1967. The "old" BPD was mostly an airway disease characterized by interstitial fibrosis and squamous metaplasia of airways. The prominent histological findings in the lungs of "new" BPD are simplification of alveolar formation (fewer and larger alveoli) and dysmorphic pulmonary microvasculature (7, 8). Pulmonary hypertension is also a common complication in infants with BPD, resulting in high mortality (9). According to these findings, the "new" BPD is considered as a consequence of the premature lung interrupted in its development by postnatal lung injury leading to the growth arrest of the lung in the canalicular/saccular phase of normal lung development. BPD, as a chronic lung disease, leads to long-term morbidity (e.g., pulmonary infection, neurodevelopmental impairment) affecting quality of life during childhood and in some severely affected patients even into adulthood. Treatment for BPD represents a considerable health care burden (10–12).

The mechanisms responsible for alveolar simplification in BPD remain understudied and poorly understood. However, autopsy samples from premature infants from pre- and post-surfactant era, who died from BPD consistently showed abnormalities in the mesenchyme (interstitial fibrosis and dysmorphic microvasculature). In the new BPD, there is clear evidence for decreased number of secondary septae, a derivative of the lung mesoderm. Furthermore, animal models mimicking the premature lung and the risk factors for BPD provide more evidence that indeed the mesenchyme plays a pivotal role in late lung development/alveologenesis and therefore in BPD. This review will summarize the current understanding of the impaired mesenchymal compartment of the BPD lungs, with a focus on mesenchymal–endothelial and mesenchymal–epithelial crosstalk known to contribute to disease pathogenesis.

Normal Lung Development in Human and Mouse

In human and mouse, the lung arises from two germ layers: the gut endoderm gives rise to the lung epithelium and the splanchnic mesoderm is the origin of the lung mesenchyme. The human lung consists of three lobes on the right and two lobes on the left side; in mice four lobes form on the right (cranial, medial, caudal, and accessory lobe) and one on the left. Compared to the 12 airway generations observed in mice, human lungs comprise 23 airway generations.

In humans, lung development arises from the laryngo-tracheal groove and starts at week 4 of gestation as an outgrowth from the ventral wall of the caudal primitive foregut. During the further growth of the lung, the prospective trachea separates from the foregut by the formation of the so-called tracheo-esophageal septum. At the most distal part of the tracheal tube, two buds that will form the right and left primary bronchial buds appear. These primary buds are further ramified to form three secondary bronchial buds on the right and two secondary bronchial buds on the left side. These buds are the origin of the five lobes in the mature lung (13).

In mice, at embryonic day 8 (E8), signaling molecules and growth factors (e.g., Fgf1, Fgf2) emanate from the cardiac mesoderm and specify the prospective lung field in the primitive foregut endoderm, which is positive for the transcription factor *Nkx2.1* (or *Ttf1*). These pre-lung epithelial progenitor cells represent the earliest and most likely the most pluripotent epithelial cells for the lung. At E9.5, the ventral foregut endoderm evaginates and elongates caudally dividing into two buds that form the prospective trachea and the first generation of bronchi (main bronchi). The process of lung development (human and mouse) has been divided into four distinct histological phases: pseudoglandular, canalicular, saccular, and alveolar (**Figure 1**).

During the pseudoglandular stage (human: week 4–17; mouse: E9.5–E16.5), the process of branching morphogenesis generates the basic tree-like structure of the lung including the conducting airways and the numerous terminal bronchioles surrounded by thick mesenchyme. Concurrently, epithelial cell progenitors undergo differentiation to give rise to basal, neuroendocrine, ciliated, and secretory cells. The mesodermal lung compartment serves as progenitors for the smooth muscle, lymphatic, endothelial, nerve, and chondrocytic cells.

In the subsequent canalicular stage (human: week 17–26; mouse: E16.5–E17.5), the lung undergoes further subdivision of the respiratory bronchioles accompanied by thinning of the surrounding mesenchyme and the massive formation of capillaries. For the first time during development, a primitive respiratory epithelium competent of gas exchange is formed by differentiation of distal lung epithelial progenitors. Recently, it has been shown that type I and type II alveolar epithelial cells (AEC I and II) emerge from a common alveolar bipotential progenitor (14). In mice, interstitial fibroblasts containing cytoplasmic lipid droplets (so called lipofibroblast, LIF) emerge in

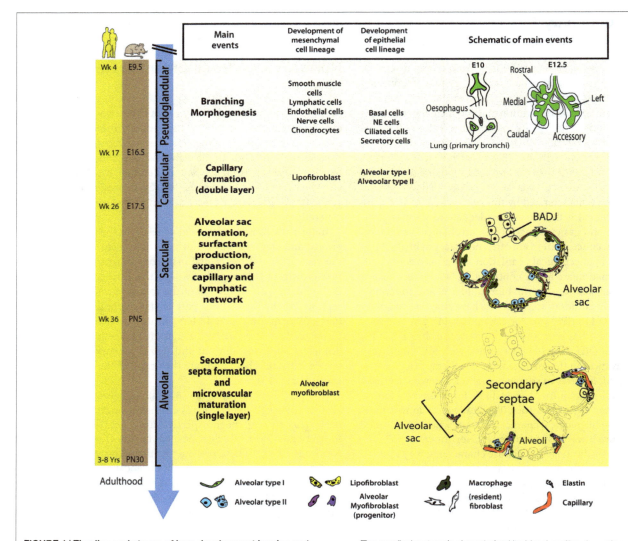

FIGURE 1 | Timeline and stages of lung development in mice and humans. Lung development starts with the specification of the lung domain in the foregut endoderm followed by the formation of primary lung buds. These buds will later give rise to the respiratory tree via the process of branching morphogenesis. The latter is a characteristic of the pseudoglandular stage of lung development. Most epithelial and mesenchymal cell types start to form during the pseudoglandular stage. The canalicular stage is characterized by blood capillary formation and the appearance of AECI/II. During the saccular stage, primitive alveoli (sac-like structures) start to form and this is accompanied by surfactant production and the expansion of capillary and lymphatic networks. The alveolar stage of lung developments starts *in utero* in humans whereas in mice, it starts postnatally. Wk, week; E, embryonic; PN, postnatal; NE, neuroendocrine.

the mesenchyme. Additionally, this is the earliest time point of pregnancy (23–24 weeks of gestation) where a preterm infant can be born with a chance to survive. Those who died from BPD showed pathologic characteristics of the lung (interstitial fibrosis and dysmorphic microvasculature) similar to the morphology of the immature lung at this developmental stage thus reinforcing the concept that BPD results from interruption of normal lung development by deleterious environmental events. The introduction of antenatal steroids treatment and exogenous surfactant supplementation drastically increased survival of premature infants born at this stage (15).

The saccular stage of lung development occurs approximately between 26 and 36 weeks of gestation (mouse: E17.5–PN5). This stage is characterized by the formation of alveolar sacs, surfactant production, and thinning of the mesenchyme to facilitate gas exchange. Kresch demonstrated that the thinning of the mesenchyme results from apoptosis of mesenchymal cells (16). Furthermore, the capillary and lymphatic networks also expand in the saccular stage of lung development.

The last stage of lung development is termed alveolar stage (human: ~36 weeks to 8 years; mouse: PN5–PN30). During this stage, the alveolar surface area increases massively at the expense of the mesenchyme through subdividing the alveolar sacs (also called primitive alveoli) into mature alveoli by a process termed alveolarization (or alveologenesis) (**Figure 2**). This process starts with the deposition of elastin in primary septae (wall of alveolar sacs) and subsequently secondary septae emerge at the place of elastin and elongate toward the alveolar sac airspace to subdivide

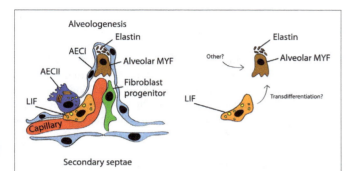

FIGURE 2 | Schematic representation of the secondary septum during alveologenesis. Most of the alveolar surface is occupied by AECI (gas exchange) whereas a minor surface is occupied by AECII (surfactant production). The alveolar wall consists of the blood capillary, LIF, resident fibroblast progenitor, alveolar MYF, and ECM (mostly elastin). It has been proposed that alveolar MYF can originate from LIF (right panel) but this concept needs further validation.

it into the smallest respiratory units of the lung – the mature alveoli. Importantly, concomitant with this process, primary septae, still containing a double layer of capillaries, become thinner and a single capillary network emerges allowing more efficient gas exchange (microvascular maturation). The bulk of alveolarization takes place during the first 6 months after birth in humans (mouse: PN5–PN15) (17). The alveolar myofibroblast (MYF), localized in the mesenchyme at the tip of the emerging secondary septae, is the cell responsible for secondary septae formation. A more detailed description of this mesenchymal cell lineage will be provided in the following sections.

In summary, the lung is a complex ramified organ that develops through continuous and elaborate interaction among the epithelium, mesenchyme, mesothelium, and endothelium. During this process, an intricate signaling network controls the amplification, proliferation, migration, and differentiation of diverse progenitor cells to populate these different compartments. Importantly, most of the epithelial and mesenchymal cell types in the lung are formed during the late pseudoglandular stage (E13.5–E16.6). This means that any deleterious factors present prenatally (such as inflammations due to chorioamnionitis) or postnatally (such as barotrauma injury and subsequent inflammation due to oxygen or mechanical ventilation), interfering with normal lung development at that time, could lead to impaired pulmonary function postnatally. Since preterm infants who die from BPD commonly display abnormal mesenchyme, a better understanding of aberrant signaling pathways in the lung mesenchyme of BPD lungs is important for improving the existing, and may facilitate the development of new preventive and curative therapies. In the next section, the current knowledge, mostly obtained from animal models of BPD, about abnormalities occurring in the lung mesenchyme will be reviewed.

The Embryonic Lung Mesenchyme

During the pseudoglandular stage of lung development (~E13.5), the distal lung bud is composed of three morphologically distinguishable layers: the mesothelium (outer layer), the mesenchyme (middle layer), and the epithelium (inner layer). The mesenchyme can be further divided into two domains, the submesothelial mesenchyme (SMM) and the subepithelial mesenchyme (SEM). Whereas mesenchymal cells constituting the SEM display high density and circumferential orientation, those of the SMM display low density and organization. Lineage-tracing experiments have identified markers for some mesenchymal progenitors such as Wnt2/Gli1/Isl1 (originating from the heart and invading the lung), Ret, Pdgfrα, Vegfr2, Prox1, and Fgf10 (18–20). Progenitors in these two compartments give rise to various cell types such as airway smooth muscle cells (ASMCs), vascular smooth muscle cells (VSMCs), resident mesenchymal stem cells (MSCs), LIFs, endothelial cells, chondrocytes, nerve cells, alveolar MYFs, lymphatic cells, and others. Mesenchymal progenitor cells are believed to play important roles not only in development but also in homeostasis and regeneration after injury.

Epithelial–Mesenchymal Crosstalk in Normal Lung Development and BPD

During development, the lung is formed through an elaborated epithelial–mesenchymal crosstalk that drives lung specification, budding, and branching. Signaling molecules like fibroblast growth factors (Fgf), Wnt (wingless and int), Sonic hedgehog (Shh), and bone morphogenetic proteins (Bmp) are key ligands initiating the pulmonary cell fate and specifying the early lung domain at the ventral foregut endoderm (21). So far, the most convincing evidence for epithelial–mesenchymal interactions during lung development came from recombination studies where distal lung mesenchyme, grafted on the tracheal epithelium led to ectopic budding accompanied by expression of surfactant protein C as a distal epithelial marker (22–24).

The mammalian Fgf family consists of 22 members subdivided in 7 subfamilies, based on phylogenetic as well as gene loci analyses (25). Fgfs acts in a paracrine, endocrine, or intracrine fashion and have diverse biological activities during embryonic organogenesis. These growth factors act via seven main receptors (Fgfrs 1b, 1c, 2b, 2c, 3b, 3c, and 4), exhibiting different ligand-binding specificity. The Fgf receptors are encoded by four *Fgfr* genes (*Fgfr1*–*Fgfr4*), which undergo alternative splicing to produce the different isoforms. Each receptor comprises an extracellular ligand-binding domain with three immunoglobulin-like loops (D I, D II, D III), a transmembrane domain and an intracellular tyrosine kinase domain. Human diseases involving gain or loss of function mutations have been described. For example, loss of function of *FGF3* causes deafness, heterozygous loss of function of *FGF10* results in lacrimo-auriculo-dento-digital syndrome (LADD syndrome), *FGF10* haploinsufficiency is also associated with chronic obstructive pulmonary disease and *FGF23* gain of function leads to autosomal dominant hypophosphataemic rickets (26–29). During early (E12.5) embryonic mouse lung development, Fgf9 and Fgf10 have been shown to play an important role in branching morphogenesis and the associated differentiation of the epithelium and mesenchyme. Fgf9 is expressed in the mesothelium and the epithelium and acts through Fgfr2c- and Fgfr1c-expressing cells in the mesenchyme to maintain Fgf10 expression as well as mesenchymal progenitors proliferative and undifferentiated (30). It also can signal directly to the epithelium to promote epithelial branching by induction of *Dkk1* expression and inhibition of Wnt signaling (31). Fgf10 is a diffusible key molecule orchestrating branching morphogenesis during early lung development in mice (32, 33) but the exact mechanism of action remains unknown. During the early pseudoglandular stage, Fgf10 is secreted by cells located adjacent to the mesothelium in the distal mesenchyme and signals in a paracrine manner mainly through fibroblast growth factor receptor 2-IIIb (Fgfr2b) expressed on epithelial cells. Fgf10 has a high affinity for heparan sulfate and is therefore unlikely to diffuse over a long distance. Instead, Fgf10 promotes outgrowth of the distal epithelium via a chemotactic mechanism. Several studies using transgenic mouse lines that display abnormal Fgf10/Fgfr2 signaling confirmed the importance of this pathway (**Table 1**). *Fgf10* and *Fgfr2b* knockout pups display similar phenotypes. The mutant pups die shortly after birth due to lung agenesis and multiple organ agenesis/defects (salivary gland, limb, inner ear, teeth, skin, pancreas, kidney, thyroid, pituitary gland, mammary gland) (34–38).

In order to identify epithelial-specific gene expressions mediated by recombinant human FGF10 during bud morphogenesis, Lu and colleagues (39) used mesenchyme-free epithelium in culture. By using microarray analysis, they identified a panel of transcriptional *Fgf10* targets, which are associated with cell rearrangement, migration, inflammatory processes, lipid metabolism, cell cycle, and tumor invasion. Interestingly, the authors did not observe a remarkable induction of genes responsible for proliferation. Moreover, Fgf10 is proposed to control the angle of the mitotic spindle in distal epithelial cells during development. Thus, Tang et al. argued that Fgf10 signals via a Ras-regulated Erk1/2

signaling pathway to shape the lung tube (40). Fgf10 is also critical for the amplification of distal epithelial cell progenitors and for the formation of multiple mesenchymal lineages during lung development. Hypomorphic $Fgf10^{lacZ/-}$ pups expressing ~20% $Fgf10$ compared to wild type (WT) died within 24–48 h after birth due to lung defects, which included decreased branching, thickened primary septae, and vascular abnormalities with intrapulmonary hemorrhages. At the cellular level, *Fgf10* deficiency led to decrease in Nkx2.1 and Sftpb-expressing cells, suggesting that adequate *Fgf10* expression level is critical for the amplification of epithelial progenitors. Apart from the epithelium, constitutive decrease in *Fgf10* expression also affects mesenchymal cell lineages as *Pecam* and α*Sma*-positive cells are also diminished (41). Interestingly, recent experiments conducted in our lab to investigate the impact of *Fgf10* levels on lung function demonstrate that even a 50% decrease in *Fgf10* expression (*Fgf10* heterozygous pups) leads to changes in the expression of genes relevant for lung development such as *Epcam*, *Sftpc*, *Fgfr2b*, *Tgf-*β, and *Collagen*. Additionally, *Fgf10* heterozygous neonatal mice survive and do not display any obvious phenotypic differences compared to WT mice. However, when exposed to hyperoxia between PN0 and PN8 to trigger lung injury and mimic some of the clinical manifestations of BPD (impaired alveologenesis and inflammation), *Fgf10*-deficient pups display drastically increased mortality compared to WT controls. Further analysis indicates that under physiological conditions, *Fgf10*-deficient mice already show structural abnormalities during embryonic lung development supporting that *Fgf10*-deficient pups carry congenital defects. These findings suggest that *Fgf10*-deficient lung epithelium is more susceptible to oxygen toxicity and does not undergo normal repair after injury

TABLE 1 | Overview of proteins that are known to be involved in alveologenesis.

Protein name	Origin	Localization/ targets	Function in alveologenesis	Alterations in BPD	Alterations in animal model of BPD	Effect of genetic modulation in the animal model
Elastin	Alveolar myofibroblast	Tip of growing secondary septae	Secondary septae formation (tips)	Increased and disorganized in saccular walls (66, 67)	Decreased in hyperoxia (133)	KO: inhibited alveolarization (87)
Pdgfa	Epithelial cells, macrophages	Pdgfrα-expressing cells (ASMC, alv. MYF, LIF)	Chemotactic attractant for fibroblasts (134)	Not known	Delayed in hyperoxia (135)	KO: inhibited alveolarization (93, 94)
Fgf10	Mesenchymal cells located in SMM	Distal epithelial cells expressing Fgfr2b	Under investigation	Decreased (75)	Decreased in LPS-model (76)	KO: lung agenesis
						Partial deficiency: delayed/disturbed lung branching (41)
Tgf-β/ Tgf-β1	Epithelial cells	Epithelial and mesenchymal cells	Modulation of cell survival, differentiation and ECM (Elastin) deposition (136, 137)	Increased in tracheal aspirate (138)	Increased in hyperoxia (139, 140)	Overexpression: inhibition of branching morphogenesis and alveolarization (141) Inhibition: attenuated hyperoxia-induced hypoalveolarization (140)
Vegf	Epithelial (during embryonic development also in mesenchymal cells)	Endothelial cells (Vegfr1/2)	Stimulation of endothelial cells for angio-/vasculogenesis (essential for alveolarization)	Decreased (8, 127)	Decreased in hyperoxia (125); (126)	Inhibition: hypoalveolarization (142, 143)

(Chao and Bellusci, in preparation). Additionally, recent studies suggest that Fgf10 may control basal cell density in the tracheal epithelium (42–45). This is not surprising as it has already been previously shown, by our group and others, that Fgf10 is part of the stem cell niche in the lung (20, 46, 47).

Wnt (Wnt2, Wnt2b) ligands are expressed in the mesenchyme and are important for lung domain specification of the foregut endoderm from E9.0 to E10.5. Wnt signaling is also essential for the proximo-distal patterning of the epithelium during embryonic lung development. Genetic deletion of *Wnt2/2b* or β-*catenin* leads to lung agenesis due to loss of *Nkx2.1* (48, 49). *Wnt2* null mice display lung hypoplasia and abnormal development of ASMCs (50). Furthermore, Mucenski and colleagues demonstrated, by using *Spc-rtTA;tet(O)Cre* double transgenic mice, that loss of function of β-*catenin* in the distal lung epithelium leads to the inhibition of distal airway formation (51). The authors showed an opposite phenotype by inducing gain of function of β-*catenin* signaling (52). The absence of *Wnt7b* results in a phenotype similar to *Wnt2* null mice (53) but a combination of *Wnt7b* and *Wnt2* loss of function leads to a more severe phenotype with decreased branching and abnormal distal endoderm patterning (54). The constitutive deletion of *Wnt5a* – a non-canonical Wnt ligand expressed in the mesenchyme and the epithelium – leads to increased proliferation of the mesenchyme and the distal epithelium as well as disrupted lung maturation (55). β-*catenin* inactivation in the mesenchyme (*Dermo1-Cre* line) leads to abnormal mesenchyme development with disrupted amplification of ASMC progenitors and defects in angioblast differentiation (56). Kumar and colleagues demonstrated by using a clonal cell labeling approach that ASMC progenitors are located exclusively at the tip mesenchyme and that mesenchymal Wnt signaling is able to prime the stalk mesenchyme to form an ASMC progenitor pool at the tip (57).

Bmp4 is dynamically expressed in the endoderm and in the mesenchyme during early embryonic lung development (E11.5). It is also expressed at the distal epithelial buds and has been shown to be an inhibitor of Fgf10-induced chemotaxis in the epithelium. Bmp4 controls intraepithelial crosstalk to form ASMCs. It has been shown that *Fgf10* is able to upregulate *Bmp4* mRNA expression. *In vitro* experiments demonstrated that exogenous recombinant human BMP4 inhibits Fgf10-induced bud outgrowth, providing evidence that Bmp4 is acting downstream of Fgf10 to inhibit its signaling cascade (58–61).

Other Fgf10 inhibitors are Sonic hedgehog (Shh) and Sprouty homolog 2 (Spry2), both expressed in the epithelium of the outgrowing buds. Shh is a secreted growth factor that acts through its mesenchymal receptor Patched (Ptc) to induce mesenchymal cell proliferation and differentiation. In E11.5 lung explants, exogenous recombinant SHH is able to induce expression of mesenchymal markers (*Noggin, Acta2, Myosin*) (19, 62). Spry2 is an intracellular inhibitor of receptor tyrosine kinase signaling (63, 64); (32). Using *in vitro* approaches, it has been shown that *Spry2* reduction leads to increased epithelial branching and vice versa.

Apart from its important role in development, the mesenchyme is crucial in disease pathogenesis. Indeed, it has been reproducibly shown that the lung mesenchyme in preterm infants dying from BPD includes interstitial fibrosis and thickening with increased total collagen content (65–67). Similar findings were obtained

in diverse animal models (rat, mice, baboon) recapitulating the conditions of preterm infants after birth (mechanical ventilation, oxygen supplementation, exogenous surfactant) leading to a human BPD-like phenotype (68–72). These pathological changes in the lung mesenchyme in BPD strengthen the concept that alveolarization depends on an intact and normally developed mesenchyme. Several studies using animal models of BPD to identify molecules located in the altered lung mesenchyme contributed to our understanding of disease pathogenesis. Some of them will be reviewed in the following section.

One of the major causes of BPD is believed to be inflammation. Inflammation is caused prenatally by chorioamnionitis and postnatally by mechanical stretch (ventilation), oxygen toxicity, as well as infection. Emerging evidence gained from *in vitro* and *in vivo* studies support this hypothesis (73–77). For example, it has been shown that lipopolysaccharides (LPS from *Escherichia coli*) inhibit branching morphogenesis *in vitro* (73). Blackwell et al. published similar results using activated resident macrophages to inhibit epithelial branching. The proposed mechanism is that LPS activates nuclear factor kappa beta (NF-kappa B), which is then accompanied by increased expression of *interleukin-1beta* (IL-1β) and *tumor necrosis factor-a* (TNF-a) in resident macrophages (74). This branching inhibitory effect caused by macrophage-mediated inflammation has been confirmed by a macrophage-depletion study in the lung. Benjamin et al. explained this inhibitory effect by linking Fgf10 signaling with inflammatory signals. Using *in vitro* experiments, they demonstrated that NF-kappa B, IL-1β, and TNF-a are capable of reducing *Fgf10* expression in LPS-treated primary mesenchymal cells. The mechanism involved activation of toll-like receptors 2 and 4 (TLR2/4). The authors showed that FGF10-positive cells were decreased in lung samples of premature infants who died from BPD (75).

Tgf-β1 has been demonstrated to induce epithelial–mesenchymal transition (EMT) of AEC to MYF-like cells leading to extracellular matrix (ECM) deposition and thereby contributing to fibrosis and destruction of alveolar structure (78–80) (see also **Table 1**). Endogenous nitric oxide is proposed to attenuate EMT in AECs in an *in vitro* approach using primary culture of AEC II (81).

As previously mentioned, the alveologenesis phase leads to a dramatic increase in alveolar surface, which is essential for gas exchange. The current consensus is that this process is interrupted by exogenous deleterious factors leading to simplification of alveoli in BPD. Many studies confirmed that the alveolar MYF, located in the mesenchyme, is the unique cell type responsible for secondary septae formation. During alveologenesis, the alveolar myofibroblast is characterized by expression of alpha-smooth-muscle-actin (αSMA or Acta2) compared to other mesenchymal fibroblast population. By deposition of elastin and collagen, the alveolar myofibroblast initiates the process of secondary septation (82, 83). Both elastin and alveolar myofibroblast have been shown to be critical for secondary septae formation (83, 84). Expression of tropoelastin starts in the pseudoglandular stage of lung development and reaches the highest level during the alveolar stage (85, 86). The strongest evidence so far showing the importance of elastin for secondary septae formation came from the *Elastin*-knock-out mice that reveal a complete failure of alveologenesis leading to an emphysematous-like phenotype (87, 88) (**Table 1**). Interestingly, both hyperoxia and mechanical ventilation lead to increased expression of Elastin (89–91). Fgfr3 and Fgfr4 have been shown to direct alveologenesis in the murine lung by controlling elastogenesis (92). By using mice homozygous for *Pdgfa*-null allele, Boström and colleagues demonstrated failed alveolar formation due to loss of alveolar myofibroblasts and consequent loss of Elastin fibers (93, 94). Likewise, blocking antibody against Pdgfrα in newborn mice (PN1–PN7) led to aberrant Elastin fiber deposition and impaired alveolar septation, resulting in long-term failure in alveologenesis that lasted into adulthood. Pdgfa is expressed in the epithelium and targets its receptor (Pdgfrα) on mesenchymal cells such as alveolar myofibroblast and LIF (**Table 1**). Given the many mesenchymal targets of Pdgfa, it is not clear whether the impact of Pdgfa or Pdgfrα deletion on myofibroblast formation is via a direct effect of Pdgfa on alveolar myofibroblasts (and or alveolar myofibroblast progenitors) or indirectly via Pdgfa action on other targets (ASMCs and LIF). Gain and loss of function for Pdgfa/Pdgfrα signaling using cell autonomous-based approaches in specific lineages should be carried out in the future to sort out these issues.

Interestingly, increased levels of *Fgf* signaling in the mesenchyme also leads to arrested development of terminal airways accompanied by reduced Elastin deposition (95). The authors achieved this condition by taking advantage of $Fgfr2c^{+/\Delta}$ mice that develop an autocrine Fgf10–Fgfr2b signaling loop in the mesenchyme due to a splicing switch, resulting in the ectopic expression of *Fgfr2b* instead of *Fgfr2c*. The proposed mechanism of action is that mesenchymal *Fgf* signaling suppresses the differentiation of alveolar myofibroblast progenitors. Furthermore, the blockade of Fgfr2b ligands in the lung from E14.5 to E18.5 by overexpression of a soluble dominant negative receptor of *Fgfr2b* (*Sftpc-rtTA/+;tetOsolFgfr2b/+*) blocking all Fgfr2b ligands also leads to arrest in secondary septae formation and alveolar simplification (96) suggesting that Fgfr2b ligands, during this time period, are also important for the formation of alveolar myofibroblasts. Subsequent treatment with retinoic acid (RA, biologically active derivative of vitamin A) induced re-alveolarization and was accompanied by increased *Pdgfra*-positive cells and decreased αSma/Acta2-positive cells. Concurrent induction of the dominant negative *Fgfr2b* in these experimental conditions is able to prevent the RA-mediated alveolar regeneration. These data suggest that re-alveolarization is dependent on Fgfr2b ligands. Furthermore, the authors proposed a conceptual model that alveolar myofibroblasts (αSma/Acta2-positive) arise from *Pdgfra*-positive LIF. Specific lineage-tracing studies targeting subsets of lung fibroblasts (e.g., *Adrp* for LIF) are needed to validate this model. Chen and colleagues also demonstrated that Fgfr2b ligands are necessary for alveolar myofibroblast formation during compensatory lung growth after pneumonectomy (97). However, the blockade of Fgfr2b ligands by soluble Fgfr2b (decoy receptor) postnatally during alveolarization does not impair alveologenesis in mice. Recently, it has been shown that reduced *Pdgfra* expression is a primary feature of human BPD. The authors showed decreased mRNA and protein expression of *PDGFR-α* and *PDGFR-β* in MSCs isolated from tracheal aspirates of premature neonates with BPD. Similarly, lungs of infants dying from BPD display less PDGFRα-positive cells in the alveolar septae. These findings were confirmed using a BPD mouse model exposed to hyperoxia (75% oxygen) for 14 days (98).

The LIF remains a poorly characterized lipid-containing interstitial cell located in the mesenchyme in close proximity to AEC II. LIFs, which accumulate lipid vacuoles (83, 99), are abundant in the early postnatal lung and regress significantly in number after alveolar septation. The presence of LIF in rodent lungs has been demonstrated extensively. However, whether LIF reside in adult human lung remains controversial (100, 101). Because of their close localization to AEC II, LIF have been proposed to interact with AEC II. Indeed, it has been shown convincingly that LIF are involved in the trafficking of lipids to the AEC II for surfactant production (102, 103). Apart from triglycerides, LIF also secrete leptin and retinoic acid, both important for surfactant production and alveolar septation (104, 105). On the other hand, AECII secrete parathyroid hormone-related protein (Pthrp) to signal through Pthrp receptor expressed on LIF to induce expression of adipose differentiation-related protein (*Adrp*) via peroxisome proliferator-activated receptor gamma (Pparg) pathway (**Figure 3**). The current consensus is that this signaling pathway is essential for the maintenance of the LIF phenotype as well as for regulation of surfactant production (104, 106–108). By performing co-culture experiments it has been proposed recently that LIF constitute a niche for AECII cells postnatally. Co-culture of LIF with AECII cells allows the formation of alveolospheres (109).

The contribution of LIF to lung regeneration and structural maintenance in later phases of life is currently unknown. Several lung injury models including cigarette-smoke exposure induce the transdifferentiation of LIF to αSma/Acta2$^+$ MYF *in vitro*. These αSma/Acta2$^+$ MYF are highly proliferative and express high levels of collagen (110). For this reason, it has been proposed that LIF are progenitors for alveolar MYF (**Figure 2**). However, an alternative and more plausible possibility is that LIF give rise to the activated MYF. Activated MYF, unlike the alveolar MYF, is involved in pathological situations and is responsible for fibrosis. Supporting this possibility, we have recently shown that during alveologenesis, *Fgf10*-positive cells give rise to LIF

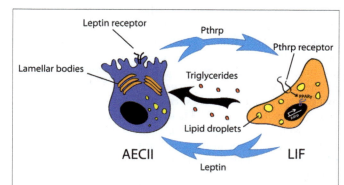

FIGURE 3 | Interaction between type II alveolar epithelial cells (AEC II) and lipofibroblasts (LIF) for surfactant production. The Pthrp (parathyroid hormone-related protein)/Pparg (peroxisome proliferator-activated receptor gamma) axis is important for LIF formation and maintenance. LIF secrete triglycerides and leptin that are essential for surfactant production.

rather than alveolar MYF and during adult life, a subpopulation of *Fgf10*-expressing cells represents a pool of resident MSCs (Cd45$^-$ Cd31$^-$ Sca-1$^+$) (20). In addition, the LIF-to-"activated MYF" transdifferentiation would translate indeed into loss of pulmonary integrity by smoke *in vivo*. Such transdifferentiation can be prevented and reversed *in vitro* using Pparg agonists such as rosiglitazone (111). However, it remains unclear whether such transdifferentiation occurs *in vivo*. Of note, exposure of premature neonates to hyperoxia induces arrest of alveolar septation and thickened primary septae due to MYF hyperplasia and excessive ECM production. Therefore, LIFs are unlikely progenitors for alveolar MYF. In the future, these results will have to be confirmed by lineage-tracing experiments in the context of injury using more specific knock-in lines to target the LIF and determine their fate.

Endothelial–Mesenchymal Crosstalk in Normal Lung Development and BPD

In parallel to branching morphogenesis during early embryonic lung development the lung vasculature begins to form in the mesenchyme at around E10.0 (112). This process involves angiogenesis and vasculogenesis. Angiogenesis occurs when pre-existing endothelial cells sprout to form capillaries. In comparison, vasculogenesis is characterized by migration and differentiation of endothelial progenitor cells (or hemangioblasts) in the distal mesenchyme to form new blood vessels. DeMello and colleagues investigated the early fetal development of lung vasculature by employing light and transmission electron microscopy as well as vascular casts and scanning electron microscopy. They demonstrated three features of the lung vasculature occurring between E9.0 and E20.0 in mice: (1) angiogenesis occurs in the proximal (central) lung vasculature, (2) peripheral lung vessels are established by vasculogenesis, and (3) at E13.0/E14.0 the central and peripheral parts of lung vasculature begin to connect to each other via a lytic process (113, 114). Finally, the main event of microvascular maturation takes place during the alveolar stage of lung development where the transition from a double capillary network to a single capillary system within alveolar walls occurs.

Although BPD has long been regarded as an epithelial disease due to its emphysematous aspect, much emphasis has now been placed also on the role of the lung vasculature in this disease. The temporal–spatial proximity of lung vasculature development and branching morphogenesis suggests a close interaction between these two important structures via endothelial–epithelial tissue crosstalk. The better understanding of this crosstalk in development and disease condition might be highly relevant for future therapies. Vascular endothelial growth factor receptor 2 (Vegfr2 or Flk-1) is an early marker for endothelial progenitors located in the SEM (115, 116). However, it is not yet clear whether these progenitors arise from the mesothelium or the mesenchyme (117, 118). Progenitors for VSMCs are believed to arise from Fgf10$^+$ cells (20), Wnt2$^+$, Gli1$^+$ and Isl1$^+$ cells (coming from the second heart field) (18), Pdgfrb$^+$ cells (119), and mesothelial cells (117, 118).

During murine embryonic development, Vegfr2-positive cells receive the Vegfa signal from epithelial and mesenchymal cells until E14.5, after which *Vegfa* expression becomes restricted to the epithelium (120) (**Table 1**). Furthermore, it has been shown that Shh and Fgf9, secreted by the epithelium, are able to induce expression of *Vegfa* in the mesenchyme (121). Reciprocally, mesenchymally secreted Fgf10 leads to the upregulation of Vegf in the distal epithelium (122). In our previous work, we showed that treatment of embryonic lung explants with recombinant Vegfa not only upregulates *Vegfr2* in the mesenchyme but also induces branching of the epithelium (123). However, it is unclear whether the effect of Vegfa on epithelial branching is direct or indirect. This endothelial–epithelial tissue crosstalk has been extensively examined by using *in vitro* recombination studies (co-culture of epithelium and mesenchyme respectively and mesenchyme alone) as well as in *in vivo* lung agenesis model (β-*catenin* knockout) (112). Using an *in vivo* inducible decoy receptor of Vegfr1 (solubleVegfr1), Lazarus and colleagues demonstrated that Spry2 is upregulated in the epithelium upon inhibition of Vegfr1-mediated signaling, suggesting an inhibition of Fgf signaling (as mentioned before Spry2 is an inhibitor of Fgf10), which is essential for branching morphogenesis (124). Another link in the endothelial–epithelial crosstalk came from the *Pecam1*-deficient mice that display a failure in endothelial cell formation accompanied by simplified alveolarization (125).

During a pathological process, Vegfa has been found downregulated in preterm infants with BPD (8, 126, 127). Furthermore, Thebaud and colleagues demonstrated that *Vegf* and *Vegfr2* are decreased in the hyperoxia model of BPD in newborn rats and that adenoviral administration of VEGF improved alveolar architecture and promoted capillary formation (128, 129). Although the trophic and angiogenic potential of VEGF on the lung vasculature is known, the aforementioned study, and the studies from other groups, suggest that vascular growth serves as a driving force for alveolar growth and maturation, leading to improvement of lung structure, and promoting secondary septae formation. A recent report revealed the association of a *VEGF* polymorphism with BPD in Japanese preterm newborns (130).

Newborn mice that are hypomorphic for *Fgf10* also display reduced expression of *Vegfa* and *Pecam*. These mice suffer from an oversimplified lung with an abnormally developed lung vasculature (41). Interestingly, *Fgf10* expression is reduced in lungs from BPD patients (75). Whether the effect of mesenchyme-derived growth factors (such as Fgf10) on the lung endothelium is direct needs to be demonstrated. Another animal injury model demonstrating the importance of endothelial–epithelial interactions is the pneumonectomy model in mice. An inducible endothelium-specific deletion of *Vegfr2* and *Fgfr1* leads to reduction of Mmp14 secretion. Mmp14 is critical for expansion of epithelial progenitor cells during compensatory lung growth by unmasking Egfr ecto-domains. This was confirmed convincingly by rescue-experiments where EGF/MMP14 administration resulted in restored alveologenesis (131).

Conclusion

Although advances in pharmacotherapy and medical technology (e.g., gentle ventilation) have improved the management of premature infants, BPD remains the most common incurable chronic lung disease of infancy with considerable mortality and long-term morbidity. An unintended consequence of these advances has been the survival rate of premature infants born before the 24th week of gestation who represent the highest risk group for pathogenesis of BPD. This means that the number of infants born with an immature lung (in the canalicular stage of lung development) is increased, leading to an increase in the incidence of BPD. Thus, it is urgent to find a treatment for BPD. The treatment of BPD has been confounded by its multifactorial causes. Therefore, only a comprehensive and individualized therapy adjusted to the profile of risk factors of each prematurely born infant will likely be able to provide a meaningful and effective strategy. The early identification of infants predisposed to BPD is essential. Several studies have been conducted to detect biomarkers in premature infants indicating their level of risk for BPD (132). Yet, the results remain inconclusive due to the low numbers of infants considered for the study. Importantly, more effort should be made in establishing preventive therapy. For example, more research should be conducted to understand the pathogenesis of preterm labor, a common cause of preterm delivery, which is one of the main risk factor associated with BPD. In addition, the current knowledge about the mechanisms of alveolarization must be expanded. Due to lack of human lung samples, the establishment of animal models precisely resembling the disease condition of BPD in humans will be helpful. Single cell transcriptomic studies should be carried out on alveolar myofibroblasts in physiological and pathological conditions to unravel the aberrant gene expression patterns and/or gene mutations responsible for impaired secondary septae formation. Furthermore, the use of the pneumonectomy mouse model and cell specific lineage-tracing approaches to understand the process of *de novo* alveolarization should contribute significantly to our understanding of lung regeneration. Last, but not least, the knowledge about progenitor/stem cells located in niches of the postnatal lung will be a valuable source of information that would be useful in triggering lung regeneration subsequent to injury.

Acknowledgments

We thank all the members of the Bellusci lab for their input. We apologize to those colleagues whose references have been omitted from this discussion; due to space restrictions and our focus, we were unable to include all articles on this interesting and diverse subject matter. PM acknowledges the support from the Hastings foundation. PM and SB acknowledge the NHLBI support (HL107307). SB was also supported by grants from the DFG (BE4443/4-1 and BE4443/6-1), LOEWE and UKGM as well as the program of competitive growth of Kazan Federal University.

References

1. Northway WH Jr, Rosan RC, Porter DY. Pulmonary disease following respirator therapy of hyaline-membrane disease. Bronchopulmonary dysplasia. *N Engl J Med* (1967) **276**:357–68. doi:10.1056/NEJM196702162760701
2. Stoll BJ, Hansen NI, Bell EF, Shankaran S, Laptook AR, Walsh MC, et al. Neonatal outcomes of extremely preterm infants from the NICHD Neonatal Research Network. *Pediatrics* (2010) **126**:443–56. doi:10.1542/peds.2009-2959
3. Baraldi E, Filippone M. Chronic lung disease after premature birth. *N Engl J Med* (2007) **357**:1946–55. doi:10.1056/NEJMra067279
4. Bhandari A, Bhandari V. Pitfalls, problems, and progress in bronchopulmonary dysplasia. *Pediatrics* (2009) **123**:1562–73. doi:10.1542/peds.2008-1962
5. Shaw GM, O'Brodovich HM. Progress in understanding the genetics of bronchopulmonary dysplasia. *Semin Perinatol* (2013) **37**:85–93. doi:10.1053/j.semperi.2013.01.004
6. Hadchouel A, Durrmeyer X, Bouzigon E, Incitti R, Huusko J, Jarreau PH, et al. Identification of SPOCK2 as a susceptibility gene for bronchopulmonary dysplasia. *Am J Respir Crit Care Med* (2011) **184**:1164–70. doi:10.1164/rccm.201103-0548OC
7. Jobe AJ. The new BPD: an arrest of lung development. *Pediatr Res* (1999) **46**:641–3. doi:10.1203/00006450-199912000-00007
8. Bhatt AJ, Pryhuber GS, Huyck H, Watkins RH, Metlay LA, Maniscalco WM. Disrupted pulmonary vasculature and decreased vascular endothelial growth factor, Flt-1, and TIE-2 in human infants dying with bronchopulmonary dysplasia. *Am J Respir Crit Care Med* (2001) **164**:1971–80. doi:10.1164/ajrccm.164.10.2101140
9. Rossor T, Greenough A. Advances in paediatric pulmonary vascular disease associated with bronchopulmonary dysplasia. *Expert Rev Respir Med* (2015) **9**:35–43. doi:10.1586/17476348.2015.986470
10. Furman L, Baley J, Borawski-Clark E, Aucott S, Hack M. Hospitalization as a measure of morbidity among very low birth weight infants with chronic lung disease. *J Pediatr* (1996) **128**:447–52. doi:10.1016/S0022-3476(96)70353-0
11. Schmidt B, Asztalos EV, Roberts RS, Robertson CM, Sauve RS, Whitfield MF. Impact of bronchopulmonary dysplasia, brain injury, and severe retinopathy on the outcome of extremely low-birth-weight infants at 18 months: results from the trial of indomethacin prophylaxis in preterms. *JAMA* (2003) **289**:1124–9. doi:10.1001/jama.289.9.1124
12. El Mazloum D, Moschino L, Bozzetto S, Baraldi E. Chronic lung disease of prematurity: long-term respiratory outcome. *Neonatology* (2014) **105**:352–6. doi:10.1159/000360651
13. Moore KL, Persaud TVN. *The Developing Human: Clinically Oriented Embryology.* Philadelphia, PA: W.B. Saunders Co (2002).
14. Treutlein B, Brownfield DG, Wu AR, Neff NF, Mantalas GL, Espinoza FH, et al. Reconstructing lineage hierarchies of the distal lung epithelium using single-cell RNA-seq. *Nature* (2014) **509**:371–5. doi:10.1038/nature13173
15. Roberts D, Dalziel S. Antenatal corticosteroids for accelerating fetal lung maturation for women at risk of preterm birth. *Cochrane Database Syst Rev* (2006) **3**:CD004454. doi:10.1002/14651858.CD004454.pub2
16. Kresch MJ, Christian C, Wu F, Hussain N. Ontogeny of apoptosis during lung development. *Pediatr Res* (1998) **43**:426–31. doi:10.1203/00006450-199803000-00020
17. Schittny JC, Mund SI, Stampanoni M. Evidence and structural mechanism for late lung alveolarization. *Am J Physiol Lung Cell Mol Physiol* (2008) **294**:L246–54. doi:10.1152/ajplung.00296.2007
18. Peng T, Tian Y, Boogerd CJ, Lu MM, Kadzik RS, Stewart KM, et al. Coordination of heart and lung co-development by a multipotent cardiopulmonary progenitor. *Nature* (2013) **500**:589–92. doi:10.1038/nature12358
19. El Agha E, Bellusci S. Walking along the fibroblast growth factor 10 route: a Key pathway to understand the control and regulation of epithelial and mesenchymal cell-lineage formation during lung development and repair after injury. *Scientifica (Cairo)* (2014) **2014**:538379. doi:10.1155/2014/538379
20. El Agha E, Herold S, Al Alam D, Quantius J, Mackenzie B, Carraro G, et al. Fgf10-positive cells represent a progenitor cell population during lung development and postnatally. *Development* (2014) **141**:296–306. doi:10.1242/dev.099747
21. Hines EA, Sun X. Tissue crosstalk in lung development. *J Cell Biochem* (2014) **115**:1469–77. doi:10.1002/jcb.24811
22. Shannon JM. Induction of alveolar type II cell differentiation in fetal tracheal epithelium by grafted distal lung mesenchyme. *Dev Biol* (1994) **166**:600–14. doi:10.1006/dbio.1994.1340
23. Shannon JM, Nielsen LD, Gebb SA, Randell SH. Mesenchyme specifies epithelial differentiation in reciprocal recombinants of embryonic lung and trachea. *Dev Dyn* (1998) **212**:482–94. doi:10.1002/(SICI)1097-0177(199808)212:4<482::AID-AJA2>3.0.CO;2-D
24. Hyatt BA, Shangguan X, Shannon JM. FGF-10 induces SP-C and Bmp4 and regulates proximal-distal patterning in embryonic tracheal epithelium.

Am J Physiol Lung Cell Mol Physiol (2004) **287**:L1116–26. doi:10.1152/ajplung.00033.2004

25. Itoh N, Ornitz DM. Fibroblast growth factors: from molecular evolution to roles in development, metabolism and disease. *J Biochem* (2011) **149**:121–30. doi:10.1093/jb/mvq121

26. Tekin M, Hismi BO, Fitoz S, Ozdag H, Cengiz FB, Sirmaci A, et al. Homozygous mutations in fibroblast growth factor 3 are associated with a new form of syndromic deafness characterized by inner ear agenesis, microtia, and microdontia. *Am J Hum Genet* (2007) **80**:338–44. doi:10.1086/510920

27. Milunsky JM, Zhao G, Maher TA, Colby R, Everman DB. LADD syndrome is caused by FGF10 mutations. *Clin Genet* (2006) **69**:349–54. doi:10.1111/j.1399-0004.2006.00597.x

28. Klar J, Blomstrand P, Brunmark C, Badhai J, Hakansson HF, Brange CS, et al. Fibroblast growth factor 10 haploinsufficiency causes chronic obstructive pulmonary disease. *J Med Genet* (2011) **48**:705–9. doi:10.1136/jmedgenet-2011-100166

29. White KE, Carn G, Lorenz-Depiereux B, Benet-Pages A, Strom TM, Econs MJ. Autosomal-dominant hypophosphatemic rickets (ADHR) mutations stabilize FGF-23. *Kidney Int* (2001) **60**:2079–86. doi:10.1046/j.1523-1755.2001.00064.x

30. del Moral PM, De Langhe SP, Sala FG, Veltmaat JM, Tefft D, Wang K, et al. Differential role of FGF9 on epithelium and mesenchyme in mouse embryonic lung. *Dev Biol* (2006) **293**:77–89. doi:10.1016/j.ydbio.2006.01.020

31. Ornitz DM, Yin Y. Signaling networks regulating development of the lower respiratory tract. *Cold Spring Harb Perspect Biol* (2012) **4**:a008318. doi:10.1101/cshperspect.a008318

32. Bellusci S, Furuta Y, Rush MG, Henderson R, Winnier G, Hogan BL. Involvement of Sonic hedgehog (Shh) in mouse embryonic lung growth and morphogenesis. *Development* (1997) **124**:53–63.

33. Bellusci S, Grindley J, Emoto H, Itoh N, Hogan BL. Fibroblast growth factor 10 (FGF10) and branching morphogenesis in the embryonic mouse lung. *Development* (1997) **124**:4867–78.

34. Peters K, Werner S, Liao X, Wert S, Whitsett J, Williams L. Targeted expression of a dominant negative FGF receptor blocks branching morphogenesis and epithelial differentiation of the mouse lung. *EMBO J* (1994) **13**:3296–301.

35. Arman E, Haffner-Krausz R, Gorivodsky M, Lonai P. Fgfr2 is required for limb outgrowth and lung-branching morphogenesis. *Proc Natl Acad Sci U S A* (1999) **96**:11895–9. doi:10.1073/pnas.96.21.11895

36. Sekine K, Ohuchi H, Fujiwara M, Yamasaki M, Yoshizawa T, Sato T, et al. Fgf10 is essential for limb and lung formation. *Nat Genet* (1999) **21**:138–41. doi:10.1038/5096

37. De Moerlooze L, Spencer-Dene B, Revest JM, Hajihosseini M, Rosewell I, Dickson C. An important role for the IIIb isoform of fibroblast growth factor receptor 2 (FGFR2) in mesenchymal-epithelial signalling during mouse organogenesis. *Development* (2000) **127**:483–92.

38. Mailleux AA, Spencer-Dene B, Dillon C, Ndiaye D, Savona-Baron C, Itoh N, et al. Role of FGF10/FGFR2b signaling during mammary gland development in the mouse embryo. *Development* (2002) **129**:53–60.

39. Lu J, Izvolsky KI, Qian J, Cardoso WV. Identification of FGF10 targets in the embryonic lung epithelium during bud morphogenesis. *J Biol Chem* (2005) **280**:4834–41. doi:10.1074/jbc.M410714200

40. Tang W, Wei Y, Le K, Li Z, Bao Y, Gao J, et al. Mitogen-activated protein kinases ERK 1/2- and p38-GATA4 pathways mediate the Ang II-induced activation of FGF2 gene in neonatal rat cardiomyocytes. *Biochem Pharmacol* (2011) **81**:518–25. doi:10.1016/j.bcp.2010.11.012

41. Ramasamy SK, Mailleux AA, Gupte VV, Mata F, Sala FG, Veltmaat JM, et al. Fgf10 dosage is critical for the amplification of epithelial cell progenitors and for the formation of multiple mesenchymal lineages during lung development. *Dev Biol* (2007) **307**:237–47. doi:10.1016/j.ydbio.2007.04.033

42. Hines EA, Jones MK, Verheyden JM, Harvey JF, Sun X. Establishment of smooth muscle and cartilage juxtaposition in the developing mouse upper airways. *Proc Natl Acad Sci U S A* (2013) **110**:19444–9. doi:10.1073/pnas.1313223110

43. Turcatel G, Rubin N, Menke DB, Martin G, Shi W, Warburton D. Lung mesenchymal expression of Sox9 plays a critical role in tracheal development. *BMC Biol* (2013) **11**:117. doi:10.1186/1741-7007-11-117

44. Sala FG, Del Moral PM, Tiozzo C, Alam DA, Warburton D, Grikscheit T, et al. FGF10 controls the patterning of the tracheal cartilage rings via Shh. *Development* (2011) **138**:273–82. doi:10.1242/dev.051680

45. Volckaert T, Campbell A, Dill E, Li C, Minoo P, De Langhe S. Localized Fgf10 expression is not required for lung branching morphogenesis but prevents differentiation of epithelial progenitors. *Development* (2013) **140**:3731–42. doi:10.1242/dev.096560

46. Volckaert T, Dill E, Campbell A, Tiozzo C, Majka S, Bellusci S, et al. Parabronchial smooth muscle constitutes an airway epithelial stem cell niche in the mouse lung after injury. *J Clin Invest* (2011) **121**:4409–19. doi:10.1172/JCI58097

47. McQualter JL, Yuen K, Williams B, Bertoncello I. Evidence of an epithelial stem/progenitor cell hierarchy in the adult mouse lung. *Proc Natl Acad Sci U S A* (2010) **107**:1414–9. doi:10.1073/pnas.0909207107

48. Goss AM, Tian Y, Tsukiyama T, Cohen ED, Zhou D, Lu MM, et al. Wnt2/2b and beta-catenin signaling are necessary and sufficient to specify lung progenitors in the foregut. *Dev Cell* (2009) **17**:290–8. doi:10.1016/j.devcel.2009.06.005

49. Harris-Johnson KS, Domyan ET, Vezina CM, Sun X. Beta-catenin promotes respiratory progenitor identity in mouse foregut. *Proc Natl Acad Sci U S A* (2009) **106**:16287–92. doi:10.1073/pnas.0902274106

50. Goss AM, Tian Y, Cheng L, Yang J, Zhou D, Cohen ED, et al. Wnt2 signaling is necessary and sufficient to activate the airway smooth muscle program in the lung by regulating myocardin/Mrtf-B and Fgf10 expression. *Dev Biol* (2011) **356**:541–52. doi:10.1016/j.ydbio.2011.06.011

51. Mucenski ML, Wert SE, Nation JM, Loudy DE, Huelsken J, Birchmeier W, et al. Beta-catenin is required for specification of proximal/distal cell fate during lung morphogenesis. *J Biol Chem* (2003) **278**:40231–8. doi:10.1074/jbc.M305892200

52. Mucenski ML, Nation JM, Thitoff AR, Besnard V, Xu Y, Wert SE, et al. Beta-catenin regulates differentiation of respiratory epithelial cells in vivo. *Am J Physiol Lung Cell Mol Physiol* (2005) **289**:L971–9. doi:10.1152/ajplung.00172.2005

53. Shu W, Jiang YQ, Lu MM, Morrisey EE. Wnt7b regulates mesenchymal proliferation and vascular development in the lung. *Development* (2002) **129**:4831–42.

54. Miller MF, Cohen ED, Baggs JE, Lu MM, Hogenesch JB, Morrisey EE. Wnt ligands signal in a cooperative manner to promote foregut organogenesis. *Proc Natl Acad Sci U S A* (2012) **109**:15348–53. doi:10.1073/pnas.1201583109

55. Li C, Xiao J, Hormi K, Borok Z, Minoo P. Wnt5a participates in distal lung morphogenesis. *Dev Biol* (2002) **248**:68–81. doi:10.1006/dbio.2002.0729

56. De Langhe SP, Carraro G, Tefft D, Li C, Xu X, Chai Y, et al. Formation and differentiation of multiple mesenchymal lineages during lung development is regulated by beta-catenin signaling. *PLoS One* (2008) **3**:e1516. doi:10.1371/journal.pone.0001516

57. Kumar ME, Bogard PE, Espinoza FH, Menke DB, Kingsley DM, Krasnow MA. Mesenchymal cells. Defining a mesenchymal progenitor niche at single-cell resolution. *Science* (2014) **346**:1258810. doi:10.1126/science.1258810

58. Weaver M, Dunn NR, Hogan BL. Bmp4 and Fgf10 play opposing roles during lung bud morphogenesis. *Development* (2000) **127**:2695–704.

59. Mailleux AA, Kelly R, Veltmaat JM, De Langhe SP, Zaffran S, Thiery JP, et al. Fgf10 expression identifies parabronchial smooth muscle cell progenitors and is required for their entry into the smooth muscle cell lineage. *Development* (2005) **132**:2157–66. doi:10.1242/dev.01795

60. Weaver M, Yingling JM, Dunn NR, Bellusci S, Hogan BL. Bmp signaling regulates proximal-distal differentiation of endoderm in mouse lung development. *Development* (1999) **126**:4005–15.

61. Weaver M, Batts L, Hogan BL. Tissue interactions pattern the mesenchyme of the embryonic mouse lung. *Dev Biol* (2003) **258**:169–84. doi:10.1016/S0012-1606(03)00117-9

62. Minowada G, Jarvis LA, Chi CL, Neubuser A, Sun X, Hacohen N, et al. Vertebrate Sprouty genes are induced by FGF signaling and can cause chondrodysplasia when overexpressed. *Development* (1999) **126**:4465–75.

63. Mailleux AA, Tefft D, Ndiaye D, Itoh N, Thiery JP, Warburton D, et al. Evidence that SPROUTY2 functions as an inhibitor of mouse embryonic lung growth and morphogenesis. *Mech Dev* (2001) **102**:81–94. doi:10.1016/S0925-4773(01)00286-6

64. Tefft D, Lee M, Smith S, Crowe DL, Bellusci S, Warburton D. mSprouty2 inhibits FGF10-activated MAP kinase by differentially binding to upstream target proteins. *Am J Physiol Lung Cell Mol Physiol* (2002) **283**:L700–6. doi:10.1152/ajplung.00372.2001

65. Husain AN, Siddiqui NH, Stocker JT. Pathology of arrested acinar development in postsurfactant bronchopulmonary dysplasia. *Hum Pathol* (1998) **29**:710–7. doi:10.1016/S0046-8177(98)90280-5

66. Thibeault DW, Mabry SM, Ekekezie II, Truog WE. Lung elastic tissue maturation and perturbations during the evolution of chronic lung disease. *Pediatrics* (2000) **106**:1452–9. doi:10.1542/peds.106.6.1452

67. Thibeault DW, Mabry SM, Ekekezie II, Zhang X, Truog WE. Collagen scaffolding during development and its deformation with chronic lung disease. *Pediatrics* (2003) **111**:766–76. doi:10.1542/peds.111.4.766

68. Warner BB, Stuart LA, Papes RA, Wispe JR. Functional and pathological effects of prolonged hyperoxia in neonatal mice. *Am J Physiol* (1998) **275**:L110–7.

69. Dauger S, Ferkdadji L, Saumon G, Vardon G, Peuchmaur M, Gaultier C, et al. Neonatal exposure to 65% oxygen durably impairs lung architecture and breathing pattern in adult mice. *Chest* (2003) **123**:530–8. doi:10.1378/chest.123.2.530

70. Auten RL, Mason SN, Auten KM, Brahmajothi M. Hyperoxia impairs postnatal alveolar epithelial development via NADPH oxidase in newborn mice. *Am J Physiol Lung Cell Mol Physiol* (2009) **297**:L134–42. doi:10.1152/ajplung.00112.2009

71. Velten M, Heyob KM, Rogers LK, Welty SE. Deficits in lung alveolarization and function after systemic maternal inflammation and neonatal hyperoxia exposure. *J Appl Physiol (1985)* (2010) **108**:1347–56. doi:10.1152/japplphysiol.01392.2009

72. Coalson JJ, Winter VT, Siler-Khodr T, Yoder BA. Neonatal chronic lung disease in extremely immature baboons. *Am J Respir Crit Care Med* (1999) **160**:1333–46. doi:10.1164/ajrccm.160.4.9810071

73. Prince LS, Dieperink HI, Okoh VO, Fierro-Perez GA, Lallone RL. Toll-like receptor signaling inhibits structural development of the distal fetal mouse lung. *Dev Dyn* (2005) **233**:553–61. doi:10.1002/dvdy.20362

74. Blackwell TS, Hipps AN, Yamamoto Y, Han W, Barham WJ, Ostrowski MC, et al. NF-kappaB signaling in fetal lung macrophages disrupts airway morphogenesis. *J Immunol* (2011) **187**:2740–7. doi:10.4049/jimmunol.1101495

75. Benjamin JT, Smith RJ, Halloran BA, Day TJ, Kelly DR, Prince LS. FGF-10 is decreased in bronchopulmonary dysplasia and suppressed by toll-like receptor activation. *Am J Physiol Lung Cell Mol Physiol* (2007) **292**:L550–8. doi:10.1152/ajplung.00329.2006

76. Benjamin JT, Carver BJ, Plosa EJ, Yamamoto Y, Miller JD, Liu JH, et al. NF-kappaB activation limits airway branching through inhibition of Sp1-mediated fibroblast growth factor-10 expression. *J Immunol* (2010) **185**:4896–903. doi:10.4049/jimmunol.1001857

77. Carver BJ, Plosa EJ, Stinnett AM, Blackwell TS, Prince LS. Interactions between NF-kappaB and SP3 connect inflammatory signaling with reduced FGF-10 expression. *J Biol Chem* (2013) **288**:15318–25. doi:10.1074/jbc.M112.447318

78. Kim KK, Kugler MC, Wolters PJ, Robillard L, Galvez MG, Brumwell AN, et al. Alveolar epithelial cell mesenchymal transition develops in vivo during pulmonary fibrosis and is regulated by the extracellular matrix. *Proc Natl Acad Sci U S A* (2006) **103**:13180–5. doi:10.1073/pnas.0605669103

79. Willis BC, Liebler JM, Luby-Phelps K, Nicholson AG, Crandall ED, Du Bois RM, et al. Induction of epithelial-mesenchymal transition in alveolar epithelial cells by transforming growth factor-beta1: potential role in idiopathic pulmonary fibrosis. *Am J Pathol* (2005) **166**:1321–32. doi:10.1016/S0002-9440(10)62351-6

80. Phan SH. The myofibroblast in pulmonary fibrosis. *Chest* (2002) **122**:286S–9S. doi:10.1378/chest.122.6_suppl.286S

81. Vyas-Read S, Shaul PW, Yuhanna IS, Willis BC. Nitric oxide attenuates epithelial-mesenchymal transition in alveolar epithelial cells. *Am J Physiol Lung Cell Mol Physiol* (2007) **293**:L212–21. doi:10.1152/ajplung.00475.2006

82. Noguchi A, Reddy R, Kursar JD, Parks WC, Mecham RP. Smooth muscle isoactin and elastin in fetal bovine lung. *Exp Lung Res* (1989) **15**:537–52. doi:10.3109/01902148909069617

83. Vaccaro C, Brody JS. Ultrastructure of developing alveoli. I. The role of the interstitial fibroblast. *Anat Rec* (1978) **192**:467–79. doi:10.1002/ar.1091920402

84. Dickie R, Wang YT, Butler JP, Schulz H, Tsuda A. Distribution and quantity of contractile tissue in postnatal development of rat alveolar interstitium. *Anat Rec (Hoboken)* (2008) **291**:83–93. doi:10.1002/ar.20622

85. Mariani TJ, Sandefur S, Pierce RA. Elastin in lung development. *Exp Lung Res* (1997) **23**:131–45. doi:10.3109/01902149709074026

86. Willet KE, McMenamin P, Pinkerton KE, Ikegami M, Jobe AH, Gurrin L, et al. Lung morphometry and collagen and elastin content: changes during normal development and after prenatal hormone exposure in sheep. *Pediatr Res* (1999) **45**:615–25. doi:10.1203/00006450-199905010-00002

87. Wendel DP, Taylor DG, Albertine KH, Keating MT, Li DY. Impaired distal airway development in mice lacking elastin. *Am J Respir Cell Mol Biol* (2000) **23**:320–6. doi:10.1165/ajrcmb.23.3.3906

88. Shifren A, Durmowicz AG, Knutsen RH, Hirano E, Mecham RP. Elastin protein levels are a vital modifier affecting normal lung development and susceptibility to emphysema. *Am J Physiol Lung Cell Mol Physiol* (2007) **292**:L778–87. doi:10.1152/ajplung.00352.2006

89. Bruce MC, Bruce EN, Janiga K, Chetty A. Hyperoxic exposure of developing rat lung decreases tropoelastin mRNA levels that rebound postexposure. *Am J Physiol* (1993) **265**:L293–300.

90. Albertine KH, Jones GP, Starcher BC, Bohnsack JF, Davis PL, Cho SC, et al. Chronic lung injury in preterm lambs. Disordered respiratory tract development. *Am J Respir Crit Care Med* (1999) **159**:945–58. doi:10.1164/ajrccm.159.3.9804027

91. Nakamura T, Liu M, Mourgeon E, Slutsky A, Post M. Mechanical strain and dexamethasone selectively increase surfactant protein C and tropoelastin gene expression. *Am J Physiol Lung Cell Mol Physiol* (2000) **278**:L974–80.

92. Weinstein M, Xu X, Ohyama K, Deng CX. FGFR-3 and FGFR-4 function cooperatively to direct alveogenesis in the murine lung. *Development* (1998) **125**:3615–23.

93. Bostrom H, Willetts K, Pekny M, Leveen P, Lindahl P, Hedstrand H, et al. PDGF-A signaling is a critical event in lung alveolar myofibroblast development and alveogenesis. *Cell* (1996) **85**:863–73. doi:10.1016/S0092-8674(00)81270-2

94. Lindahl P, Karlsson L, Hellstrom M, Gebre-Medhin S, Willetts K, Heath JK, et al. Alveogenesis failure in PDGF-A-deficient mice is coupled to lack of distal spreading of alveolar smooth muscle cell progenitors during lung development. *Development* (1997) **124**:3943–53.

95. De Langhe SP, Carraro G, Warburton D, Hajihosseini MK, Bellusci S. Levels of mesenchymal FGFR2 signaling modulate smooth muscle progenitor cell commitment in the lung. *Dev Biol* (2006) **299**:52–62. doi:10.1016/j.ydbio.2006.07.001

96. Perl AK, Gale E. FGF signaling is required for myofibroblast differentiation during alveolar regeneration. *Am J Physiol Lung Cell Mol Physiol* (2009) **297**:L299–308. doi:10.1152/ajplung.00008.2009

97. Chen L, Acciani T, Le Cras T, Lutzko C, Perl AK. Dynamic regulation of platelet-derived growth factor receptor alpha expression in alveolar fibroblasts during realveolarization. *Am J Respir Cell Mol Biol* (2012) **47**:517–27. doi:10.1165/rcmb.2012-0030OC

98. Popova AP, Bentley JK, Cui TX, Richardson MN, Linn MJ, Lei J, et al. Reduced platelet-derived growth factor receptor expression is a primary feature of human bronchopulmonary dysplasia. *Am J Physiol Lung Cell Mol Physiol* (2014) **307**:L231–9. doi:10.1152/ajplung.00342.2013

99. O'Hare KH, Sheridan MN. Electron microscopic observations on the morphogenesis of the albino rat lung, with special reference to pulmonary epithelial cells. *Am J Anat* (1970) **127**:181–205. doi:10.1002/aja.1001270205

100. Rehan VK, Sugano S, Wang Y, Santos J, Romero S, Dasgupta C, et al. Evidence for the presence of lipofibroblasts in human lung. *Exp Lung Res* (2006) **32**:379–93. doi:10.1080/01902140600880257

101. Tahedl D, Wirkes A, Tschanz SA, Ochs M, Muhlfeld C. How common is the lipid body-containing interstitial cell in the mammalian lung? *Am J Physiol Lung Cell Mol Physiol* (2014) **307**:L386–94. doi:10.1152/ajplung.00131.2014

102. Torday J, Hua J, Slavin R. Metabolism and fate of neutral lipids of fetal lung fibroblast origin. *Biochim Biophys Acta* (1995) **1254**:198–206. doi:10.1016/0005-2760(94)00184-Z

103. Tordet C, Marin L, Dameron F. Pulmonary di-and-triacylglycerols during the perinatal development of the rat. *Experientia* (1981) **37**:333–4. doi:10.1007/BF01959845

104. Torday JS, Rehan VK. Stretch-stimulated surfactant synthesis is coordinated by the paracrine actions of PTHrP and leptin. *Am J Physiol Lung Cell Mol Physiol* (2002) **283**:L130–5. doi:10.1152/ajplung.00380.2001

105. Simon DM, Mariani TJ. Role of PPARs and retinoid X receptors in the regulation of lung maturation and development. *PPAR Res* (2007) **2007**:91240. doi:10.1155/2007/91240

106. Schultz CJ, Torres E, Londos C, Torday JS. Role of adipocyte differentiation-related protein in surfactant phospholipid synthesis by type II cells. *Am J Physiol Lung Cell Mol Physiol* (2002) 283:L288–96. doi:10.1152/ajplung.00204.2001

107. Rubin LP, Kovacs CS, De Paepe ME, Tsai SW, Torday JS, Kronenberg HM. Arrested pulmonary alveolar cytodifferentiation and defective surfactant synthesis in mice missing the gene for parathyroid hormone-related protein. *Dev Dyn* (2004) 230:278–89. doi:10.1002/dvdy.20058

108. Rehan VK, Torday JS. PPARgamma signaling mediates the evolution, development, homeostasis, and repair of the lung. *PPAR Res* (2012) 2012:289867. doi:10.1155/2012/289867

109. Barkauskas CE, Cronce MJ, Rackley CR, Bowie EJ, Keene DR, Stripp BR, et al. Type 2 alveolar cells are stem cells in adult lung. *J Clin Invest* (2013) 123:3025–36. doi:10.1172/JCI68782

110. Rehan VK, Wang Y, Sugano S, Romero S, Chen X, Santos J, et al. Mechanism of nicotine-induced pulmonary fibroblast transdifferentiation. *Am J Physiol Lung Cell Mol Physiol* (2005) 289:L667–76. doi:10.1152/ajplung.00358.2004

111. Milam JE, Keshamouni VG, Phan SH, Hu B, Gangireddy SR, Hogaboam CM, et al. PPAR-gamma agonists inhibit profibrotic phenotypes in human lung fibroblasts and bleomycin-induced pulmonary fibrosis. *Am J Physiol Lung Cell Mol Physiol* (2008) 294:L891–901. doi:10.1152/ajplung.00333.2007

112. Gebb SA, Shannon JM. Tissue interactions mediate early events in pulmonary vasculogenesis. *Dev Dyn* (2000) 217:159–69. doi:10.1002/(SICI)1097-0177(200002)217:2<159::AID-DVDY3>3.3.CO;2-0

113. deMello DE, Sawyer D, Galvin N, Reid LM. Early fetal development of lung vasculature. *Am J Respir Cell Mol Biol* (1997) 16:568–81. doi:10.1165/ajrcmb.16.5.9160839

114. Schachtner SK, Wang Y, Scott Baldwin H. Qualitative and quantitative analysis of embryonic pulmonary vessel formation. *Am J Respir Cell Mol Biol* (2000) 22:157–65. doi:10.1165/ajrcmb.22.2.3766

115. Kappel A, Ronicke V, Damert A, Flamme I, Risau W, Breier G. Identification of vascular endothelial growth factor (VEGF) receptor-2 (Flk-1) promoter/enhancer sequences sufficient for angioblast and endothelial cell-specific transcription in transgenic mice. *Blood* (1999) 93:4284–92.

116. Yamaguchi TP, Dumont DJ, Conlon RA, Breitman ML, Rossant J. flk-1, an flt-related receptor tyrosine kinase is an early marker for endothelial cell precursors. *Development* (1993) 118:489–98.

117. Que J, Wilm B, Hasegawa H, Wang F, Bader D, Hogan BL. Mesothelium contributes to vascular smooth muscle and mesenchyme during lung development. *Proc Natl Acad Sci U S A* (2008) 105:16626–30. doi:10.1073/pnas.0808649105

118. Dixit R, Ai X, Fine A. Derivation of lung mesenchymal lineages from the fetal mesothelium requires hedgehog signaling for mesothelial cell entry. *Development* (2013) 140:4398–406. doi:10.1242/dev.098079

119. Greif DM, Kumar M, Lighthouse JK, Hum J, An A, Ding L, et al. Radial construction of an arterial wall. *Dev Cell* (2012) 23:482–93. doi:10.1016/j.devcel.2012.07.009

120. Bhatt AJ, Amin SB, Chess PR, Watkins RH, Maniscalco WM. Expression of vascular endothelial growth factor and Flk-1 in developing and glucocorticoid-treated mouse lung. *Pediatr Res* (2000) 47:606–13. doi:10.1203/00006450-200005000-00009

121. White AC, Lavine KJ, Ornitz DM. FGF9 and SHH regulate mesenchymal Vegfa expression and development of the pulmonary capillary network. *Development* (2007) 134:3743–52. doi:10.1242/dev.004879

122. Scott CL, Walker DJ, Cwiklinski E, Tait C, Tee AR, Land SC. Control of HIF-1{alpha} and vascular signaling in fetal lung involves cross talk between mTORC1 and the FGF-10/FGFR2b/Spry2 airway branching periodicity clock. *Am J Physiol Lung Cell Mol Physiol* (2010) 299:L455–71. doi:10.1152/ajplung.00348.2009

123. Del Moral PM, Sala FG, Tefft D, Shi W, Keshet E, Bellusci S, et al. VEGF-A signaling through Flk-1 is a critical facilitator of early embryonic lung epithelial to endothelial crosstalk and branching morphogenesis. *Dev Biol* (2006) 290:177–88. doi:10.1016/j.ydbio.2005.11.022

124. Lazarus A, Del-Moral PM, Ilovich O, Mishani E, Warburton D, Keshet E. A perfusion-independent role of blood vessels in determining branching stereotypy of lung airways. *Development* (2011) 138:2359–68. doi:10.1242/dev.060723

125. DeLisser HM, Helmke BP, Cao G, Egan PM, Taichman D, Fehrenbach M, et al. Loss of PECAM-1 function impairs alveolarization. *J Biol Chem* (2006) 281:8724–31. doi:10.1074/jbc.M511798200

126. Lassus P, Ristimaki A, Ylikorkala O, Viinikka L, Andersson S. Vascular endothelial growth factor in human preterm lung. *Am J Respir Crit Care Med* (1999) 159:1429–33. doi:10.1164/ajrccm.159.5.9806073

127. Lassus P, Turanlahti M, Heikkila P, Andersson LC, Nupponen I, Sarnesto A, et al. Pulmonary vascular endothelial growth factor and Flt-1 in fetuses, in acute and chronic lung disease, and in persistent pulmonary hypertension of the newborn. *Am J Respir Crit Care Med* (2001) 164:1981–7. doi:10.1164/ajrccm.164.10.2012036

128. Thebaud B, Ladha F, Michelakis ED, Sawicka M, Thurston G, Eaton F, et al. Vascular endothelial growth factor gene therapy increases survival, promotes lung angiogenesis, and prevents alveolar damage in hyperoxia-induced lung injury: evidence that angiogenesis participates in alveolarization. *Circulation* (2005) 112:2477–86. doi:10.1161/CIRCULATIONAHA.105.541524

129. Kunig AM, Balasubramaniam V, Markham NE, Morgan D, Montgomery G, Grover TR, et al. Recombinant human VEGF treatment enhances alveolarization after hyperoxic lung injury in neonatal rats. *Am J Physiol Lung Cell Mol Physiol* (2005) 289:L529–35. doi:10.1152/ajplung.00336.2004

130. Fujioka K, Shibata A, Yokota T, Koda T, Nagasaka M, Yagi M, et al. Association of a vascular endothelial growth factor polymorphism with the development of bronchopulmonary dysplasia in Japanese premature newborns. *Sci Rep* (2014) 4:4459. doi:10.1038/srep04459

131. Ding BS, Nolan DJ, Guo P, Babazadeh AO, Cao Z, Rosenwaks Z, et al. Endothelial-derived angiocrine signals induce and sustain regenerative lung alveolarization. *Cell* (2011) 147:539–53. doi:10.1016/j.cell.2011.10.003

132. Bhandari A, Bhandari V. Biomarkers in bronchopulmonary dysplasia. *Paediatr Respir Rev* (2013) 14:173–9. doi:10.1016/j.prrv.2013.02.008

133. Bruce MC, Pawlowski R, Tomashefski JF Jr. Changes in lung elastic fiber structure and concentration associated with hyperoxic exposure in the developing rat lung. *Am Rev Respir Dis* (1989) 140:1067–74. doi:10.1164/ajrccm/140.4.1067

134. Prodhan P, Kinane TB. Developmental paradigms in terminal lung development. *Bioessays* (2002) 24:1052–9. doi:10.1002/bies.10177

135. Buch S, Han RN, Cabacungan J, Wang J, Yuan S, Belcastro R, et al. Changes in expression of platelet-derived growth factor and its receptors in the lungs of newborn rats exposed to air or 60% O(2). *Pediatr Res* (2000) 48:423–33. doi:10.1203/00006450-200010000-00003

136. McGowan SE, McNamer R. Transforming growth factor-beta increases elastin production by neonatal rat lung fibroblasts. *Am J Respir Cell Mol Biol* (1990) 3:369–76. doi:10.1165/ajrcmb/3.4.369

137. McGowan SE, Jackson SK, Olson PJ, Parekh T, Gold LI. Exogenous and endogenous transforming growth factors-beta influence elastin gene expression in cultured lung fibroblasts. *Am J Respir Cell Mol Biol* (1997) 17:25–35. doi:10.1165/ajrcmb.17.1.2686

138. Kotecha S, Wangoo A, Silverman M, Shaw RJ. Increase in the concentration of transforming growth factor beta-1 in bronchoalveolar lavage fluid before development of chronic lung disease of prematurity. *J Pediatr* (1996) 128:464–9. doi:10.1016/S0022-3476(96)70355-4

139. Alejandre-Alcazar MA, Kwapiszewska G, Reiss I, Amarie OV, Marsh LM, Sevilla-Perez J, et al. Hyperoxia modulates TGF-beta/BMP signaling in a mouse model of bronchopulmonary dysplasia. *Am J Physiol Lung Cell Mol Physiol* (2007) 292:L537–49. doi:10.1152/ajplung.00050.2006

140. Nakanishi H, Sugiura T, Streisand JB, Lonning SM, Roberts JD Jr. TGF-beta-neutralizing antibodies improve pulmonary alveologenesis and vasculogenesis in the injured newborn lung. *Am J Physiol Lung Cell Mol Physiol* (2007) 293:L151–61. doi:10.1152/ajplung.00389.2006

141. Gauldie J, Galt T, Bonniaud P, Robbins C, Kelly M, Warburton D. Transfer of the active form of transforming growth factor-beta 1 gene to newborn rat lung induces changes consistent with bronchopulmonary dysplasia. *Am J Pathol* (2003) 163:2575–84. doi:10.1016/S0002-9440(10)63612-7

142. Le Cras TD, Markham NE, Tuder RM, Voelkel NF, Abman SH. Treatment of newborn rats with a VEGF receptor inhibitor causes pulmonary hypertension and abnormal lung structure. *Am J Physiol Lung Cell Mol Physiol* (2002) 283:L555–62. doi:10.1152/ajplung.00408.2001

143. McGrath-Morrow SA, Cho C, Zhen L, Hicklin DJ, Tuder RM. Vascular endothelial growth factor receptor 2 blockade disrupts postnatal lung development. *Am J Respir Cell Mol Biol* (2005) 32:420–7. doi:10.1165/rcmb.2004-0287OC

13

Early Life Microbial Exposure and Immunity Training Effects on Asthma Development and Progression

Andressa Daronco Cereta[1], Vinícius Rosa Oliveira[2,3], Ivan Peres Costa[4],
Letícia Lopes Guimarães[1], João Pedro Ribeiro Afonso[5], Adriano Luís Fonseca[5],
Alan Robson Trigueiro de Sousa[5], Guilherme Augusto Moreira Silva[5],
Diego A. C. P. G. Mello[5], Luis Vicente Franco de Oliveira[5] and Renata Kelly da Palma[1,2,6]*

[1] School of Veterinary Medicine and Animal Sciences, University of São Paulo, São Paulo, Brazil, [2] Department of Physical Therapy, EUSES University School, University of Barcelona-University of Girona (UB-UdG), Barcelona, Spain, [3] Research Group on Methodology, Methods, Models and Outcomes of Health and Social Sciences (M3O), University of VIC-Central University of Catalonia, Vic, Spain, [4] Master's and Doctoral Programs in Rehabilitation Sciences, Nove de Julho University, São Paulo, Brazil, [5] Human Movement and Rehabilitation, Post Graduation Program Medical School, University Center of Anápolis-UniEVANGELICA, Anápolis, Brazil, [6] Institute for Bioengineering of Catalonia, Barcelona, Spain

*Correspondence:
Renata Kelly da Palma
rekellyp@hotmail.com

Asthma is the most common inflammatory disease affecting the lungs, which can be caused by intrauterine or postnatal insults depending on the exposure to environmental factors. During early life, the exposure to different risk factors can influence the microbiome leading to undesired changes to the immune system. The modulations of the immunity, caused by dysbiosis during development, can increase the susceptibility to allergic diseases. On the other hand, immune training approaches during pregnancy can prevent allergic inflammatory diseases of the airways. In this review, we focus on evidence of risk factors in early life that can alter the development of lung immunity associated with dysbiosis, that leads to asthma and affect childhood and adult life. Furthermore, we discuss new ideas for potential prevention strategies that can be applied during pregnancy and postnatal period.

Keywords: asthma, lung microbiome, dysbiosis, early life immunity, prevention strategies

INTRODUCTION

Asthma is the most common heterogeneous inflammatory lung disease appearing generally in childhood. Adults are also affected, and more than 339 million people of all ages are living with asthma worldwide. Over 80% of asthma-related deaths occur in low-and lower-middle income countries (1). The pathophysiology of asthma is complex including phenotypes (visible properties) and Endotypes (mechanisms). Regarding phenotypes, the most common are allergic, in early onset, mild, or moderate-to-severe remodeled asthma or non-allergic with late-onset eosinophilic asthma or non-eosinophilic asthma (2). In addition, several factors such environmental, genetic polymorphisms, epigenetic regulations, aberrant immune maturation during pregnancy, and other factors in early life can contribute to the development of asthma. Regarding these factors we can find respiratory infections (mainly the viral ones), the exposure to airborne environment agents (tobacco smoke, pollutants), and most recently comes to light the important role in microbiome imbalance (3).

In this sense, there is not a unique cause or major determinant risk factor that contributes to the development of asthma. Apparently, the combination of several factors in early life and inflammatory response due to it in a period of rapid growth and development of the lung causes structural and immune impairments that leading to asthma (4). Therefore, the key for developing prevention and strategies treatment in asthma is trying to understand the early-life exposures. In this review, we focus on evidence of risk factors in early life that can alter the development of lung immunity associated with dysbiosis, that leads to asthma and affect childhood and adult life.

EVENTS IN EARLY LIFE AND DYSBIOSIS IN ASTHMA

As above mentioned, asthma is developed due to several risk factors and can be linked with prenatal or early life events, causing it to appear specially in childhood. During early life, asthma can be associated with factors (**Figure 1**) such as delivery by cesarean section, antibiotics usage during the neonatal period, maternal low fiber diet, formula feeding, pollution and the variety of microbes due to environmental exposure (5). Therefore, perturbations on microbial composition (dysbiosis) can consequently alter immune development in mucosal tissues and lead to an increased susceptibility to asthma. Alterations in the microbiome in asthma are due to an association between changes in diversity and composition of lung microbiota along with modifications of functional genes (6). Besides that of the lung, nasal and bronchial microbiomes, asthmatic children also have alterations in the gut microbiome (7). Instances of crosstalk between gut and lung, called the "gut-lung" axis, have been demonstrated. For example, several studies have demonstrated that gut microbiome modulate Tregs in immune function by producing local and systemic mediators which impact on asthma development mediated by gut-lung axis (5, 8, 9).

In the recent years there were many advances in gene sequencing technology, expanding the knowledge on lung and gut microbiome, and on the significant role of the interactions between these two niches in the development and incidence of chronic airway disease. The airways are composed by a resident microbiota that develops after birth and interacts with different body sites, such as the gut, and its composition changes in health and disease (10).

Previous studies have suggested a strong correlation between mode of delivery and asthma incidence (11, 12). At the time of birth, maternal bacterial population is transferred to the baby. Stokholm et al. (13) demonstrated that vaginal delivery was associated with neonatal colonization of the intestinal tract by *Escherichia coli* at age 1 week while colonization by *Citrobacter freundii*, *Clostridium species*, *Enterobacter cloacae*, *Enterococcus faecalis*, *Klebsiella oxytoca*, *Klebsiella pneumoniae*, and *Staphylococcus aureus* were associated with cesarean section. However, at age 1 year this gut microbial perturbations were not apparent. Therefore, the same group conducted a cohort prospectively study with 700 children to investigate a risk of developing asthma in the first 6 years of life (14). Children who retained a cesarean gut microbial

profile at age 1 year were more susceptible to developing asthma by age 6. On the other hand, Boker et al. (15) demonstrated no association between the mode of delivery and asthma incidence. However, this study has some limitations regarding sample size and information about exposition of the neonatal to maternal microflora due to premature rupture of membranes. Therefore, further research should be addressed to answer the questions regarding mode of delivery and asthma incidence.

In addition to mode of delivery, the antibiotics usage during the pregnancy seems alter both the maternal and neonatal microbiomes which may lead to subsequent allergy diseases in childhood (16, 17). Moreover, evidence suggesting that maternal antibiotic usage before and after pregnancy can increase the childhood asthma's risk (18). Furthermore, it should be noted that child exposed to antibiotics in the first days of life can reduced abundance and diversity of *Bifidobacterium* species (18) and increase the abundancy of *Enterobacteriaceae* species (19), which may induce the development of asthma. Therefore, it is important to raise the question about the contributions of antibiotics and infection on microbiome disturbance during and after pregnancy, further studies regarding this topic should be address.

The microbiota colonization of the child may be promoted by maternal gut microbiota *in utero*, after delivery and finally through breastfeeding. Maternal nutrition seems to play an important role on gut microbiota composition alterations in the child. Mother who intake a high-fat diet alters the child microbiome during pregnancy and lactation. The high-fat diet induces increase in *Enterococcus* and decreases *Bacteroides* in the third trimester of pregnancy, aside from decrease *Bacteroides* at delivery (20). Moreover, obese breastfeeding mothers has showed *Bacteroides* decreases in breast milk (21) which can induce a risk of asthma development in the early life (22).

On the other hand, human milk from mother who intake adequate nutrition, induces a general health benefits for the child and the World Health Organization recommends breastfeeding for at least 6 months after birth. Le Doare et al. (23) suggested that human milk can provide nutrition for the microbiome and prevent pathogenic bacterial adhesion. However, in nowadays some mothers has been replaced the breastfeeding and/or supplemented with cow's milk formula. In this sense, several studies have been demonstrated that the food sensitization in the early life may be associated with an increased risk of asthma (24) which can be mediated by an inflammatory immune response driven by Th2 cells. Liang et al. (25) demonstrated that neonatal fed by breast milk had an increase in *Bifidobacterium* and *Lactobacillus* and less viruses in stool samples in compared to those fed with cow's milk, which suggest that breastfeeding can be a potential protection against asthma. A Randomized Clinical Trial with a total of 312 newborns in 6 years follow-up, demonstrated that the cow's formula milk should be avoiding in the first 3 days of life especially in neonatal with higher levels of total Immunoglobulin-E (IgE) that can presents food sensitization

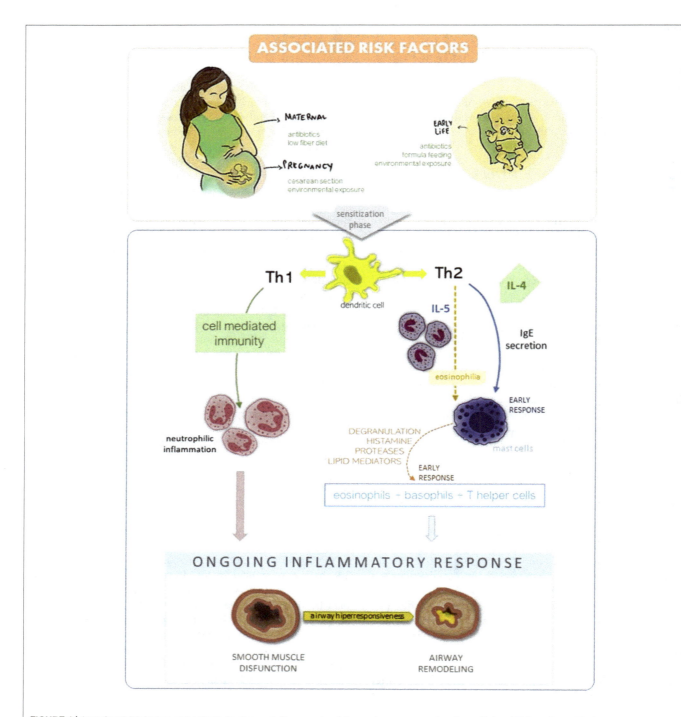

FIGURE 1 | Associated risk factors and asthma development. There are two inflammatory responses in asthma: Th1 and Th2 mediated. Th2 is the most common and leads to an early response by IgE production, presence of eosinophilia and mast cell recruitment. Late response in Th2 mediated asthma recruits' eosinophils, basophils and T helper cells to the mucosa leads to inflammatory response. Th1 mediate cell immunity in asthma, with neutrophilic inflammation affecting the epithelial layer. Both Th1 and Th2 cause airway hyper responsiveness, smooth muscle disfunction and airway remodeling.

in the early life (26). On the "Prevention strategies and immune training" section, we can observer that as earlier we introduce the allergic food the child can development a protective allergic effect.

Apart from food, the pollution and smoking exposure can be a risk for allergic sensitization and enhancement the probability of allergic asthma. Zheng et al. (27) collected fecal samples from 21 children in clean and smog days. Air pollution alters the intestinal microbiome in asthmatic children, increasing *Bacteroidetes* and decreasing *Firmicutes*, these changes can be associated with asthma development. Besides air pollution, tobacco smoke exposure *in utero* and after birth may be associated with a risk of respiratory symptoms in childhood (28).

Children of mothers who smoked during their entire pregnancy present with a higher abundance of *Enterobacteriaceae* (29) at birth and increased abundance of *Bacteroides* and *Staphylococcus* at 6 months of age (30).

Therefore, we can suggest that the gut microbiota presents an important role in asthma development, probably due to the transfer of metabolites and immunomodulatory signals to the lung by gut-lung axis. Although are evidence regarding this connection, the appropriate pathway is not well-elucidated. Previous study demonstrated that gut dysbiosis can increase the allergic lung inflammation through both dendritic cells and T cells (31). Further studies should be address in this field. However, knowing the factor risks which induce a gut dysbiosis and may developed asthma, we can trace potential prevention strategies that can be applied during pregnancy and postnatal period.

PREVENTION STRATEGIES AND IMMUNE TRAINING

Pinning down strategies for asthma prevention in pregnancy and childhood has attracted great interest lately. The identification of potentially modifiable environmental and host risk factors for asthma development appears to be the cornerstone for the paradigm shift from disease treatment toward primary asthma prevention (32). Childhood asthma risk can be dampened by an appropriate maternal asthma control. The latter includes components such as monthly monitoring of lung function, patient education on inhaler technique, avoidance of environmental triggers (e.g., cigarette smoking, pollen, air pollution), and pharmacological treatment of comorbid conditions (e.g., depression, rhinitis, gastroesophageal reflux) (33).

The capacity of immune training the fetus by maternal environment provides possibilities for prevention of asthma after birth. Management of microbial dysbiosis could be a potential target for this training. Maternal diet and nutritional supplementation can shape immune *in utero* regarding to the airway's response later in life. Evidence suggests that a mother who intake high-fiber diet during pregnancy, leads to changes in the microbiota, enhancing T-regulatory cell numbers and function (34). Moreover, recent randomized clinical trials showed positive results on asthma prevention in offspring derived from adequate levels of vitamin D, antioxidants and fish oil intake during pregnancy (35–38).

In the postnatal period, prevention measures include the control of severe neonatal respiratory infections (e.g., respiratory syncytial virus and human rhinovirus), incentive for breastfeeding and enhancing other microbial exposure through the "farm effect," as endorsed by the hygiene hypothesis (39,

40). Beyond that, after the LEAP study (41), the old-fashioned avoidance allergenic foods strategy from the diets of infants began to be replaced by the tolerance strategy toward early exposure to allergens. This remarkable study demonstrated that early exposure to allergen can increase the levels of allergic-specific IgG and IgG4 which may induce an absence allergic reaction. Afterward, Pitt et al. (42) demonstrated a reduced risk of allergic sensitization following exposure through breast-feeding. In this sense, as early allergic foods are introduced its possible to training the immune system against allergic sensitization and it can be a strategy for asthma prevention.

Furthermore, supplementation with probiotic and vitamin could be a good strategy for immune training. Administration of probiotic—*Lactobacillus rhamnosus*- on postnatal period, showed a reduced risk of childhood asthma (43) probably because the probiotics can modulate the levels of short chain fatty acid and alters the microbiome composition. On the other side, the role of vitamin D on asthma management relies on its effects on immune cell function (44), corticosteroid responsiveness mediated by pathways involving IL-10 (45), IL-17 (46), oxidative stress (47), and airway remodeling (48). Results from observational studies are still mixed and limited, with more studies showing a beneficial effect for supplementation with vitamin D (49).

Prevention strategies involved in the translation of the environmental exposures elucidated in epidemiological studies mainly focus on asthma protective environmental microbial exposures associated with rural lifestyle activities. This led to some preclinical studies with bacterial lysates (ongoing clinical trial NCT02148796) and metabolites, dietary derivatives and helminthic compounds in order to prevent the disease development (50).

Moreover, The Finnish Allergy prevention program (51) describe practical advices regarding early life exposure: (i) Support breastfeeding, with solid foods from 4–6 months, (ii) do not avoid exposure to environmental allergens (foods, pets), (iii) do not smoke, (iv) probiotic bacteria in fermented food or other preparations and (v) Antibiotics should be taken only if is really necessary. All this simple practical approach can shape the immune system during early life and prevent asthma.

CONCLUSIONS

The changes in microbiome composition due to diseases is called *dysbiosis*. Understanding its roles and the immune responses due to this imbalance in asthma are promising both to comprehend the disease pathophysiology and to elaborate preventive strategies. Dietary interventions are considered safe and promising to boost the immune system and attenuate asthma symptomatology in children. Nevertheless, tackling asthma prevention is challenging because of the existing knowledge gap on the immune pathways that predispose some infants to develop asthma and not others.

It seems that the beneficial effects resulting from prevention approaches are due to the combination of them, instead of just one strategy. However, further research is needed on observational studies and clinical trials on the effects of using different combined strategies vs. a sole intervention for asthma prevention.

AUTHOR CONTRIBUTIONS

LG, JA, AF, AS, GS, DM, and LO conceived the design and concepts. RP, AC, VO, and IC wrote the manuscript. All authors contributed to the editing and revision of the manuscript and approved the submission.

REFERENCES

1. World Health Organization. *Chronic Respiratory Disease: Asthma.* (2020). Available online at: http:// www.who.int/news-room/q-a-detail/chronic-respiratory-diseases-asthma (accessed December 05, 2020).
2. Kaur R, Chupp G. Phenotypes and endotypes of adult asthma: moving toward precision medicine. *J Allergy Clin Immunol.* (2019) 144:1–12. doi: 10.1016/j.jaci.2019.05.031
3. Mims JW. Asthma: definitions and pathophysiology. *Int Forum Allergy Rhinol.* (2015) 5(Suppl. 1):S2–6. doi: 10.1002/alr.21609
4. Decrue F, Gorlanova O, Usemann J, Frey U. Lung functional development and asthma trajectories. *Semin Immunopathol.* (2020) 42:17–27. doi: 10.1007/s00281-020-00784-2
5. Gollwitzer ES, Marsland BJ. Impact of early-life exposures on immune maturation and susceptibility to disease. *Trends Immunol.* (2015) 36:684–96. doi: 10.1016/j.it.2015.09.009
6. Huang C, Yu Y, Du W, Liu Y, Dai R, Tang W, et al. Fungal and bacterial microbiome dysbiosis and imbalance of trans-kingdom network in asthma. *Clin Transl Allergy.* (2020) 10:42. doi: 10.1186/s13601-020-00345-8
7. Stokholm J, Blaser MJ, Thorsen J, Rasmussen MA, Waage J, Vinding RK, et al. Maturation of the gut microbiome and risk of asthma in childhood. *Nat Commun.* (2018) 9:141. doi: 10.1038/s41467-017-02573-2
8. Trompette A, Gollwitzer ES, Yadava K, Sichelstiel AK, Sprenger N, Ngom-Bru C, et al. Gut microbiota metabolism of dietary fiber influences allergic airway disease and hematopoiesis. *Nat Med.* (2014) 20:159–66. doi: 10.1038/nm.3444
9. Frati F, Salvatori C, Incorvaia C, Bellucci A, Di Cara G, Marcucci F, et al. The role of the microbiome in asthma: the gut$^-$lung axis. *Int J Mol Sci.* (2018) 20:123. doi: 10.3390/ijms20010123
10. Santacroce L, Charitos IA, Ballini A, Inchingolo F, Luperto P, De Nitto E, et al. The human respiratory system and its microbiome at a glimpse. *Biology.* (2020) 9:318. doi: 10.3390/biology9100318
11. Black M, Bhattacharya S, Philip S, Norman JE, McLernon DJ. Planned cesarean delivery at term and adverse outcomes in childhood health. *JAMA.* (2015) 314:2271–9. doi: 10.1001/jama.2015.16176
12. van Berkel AC, den Dekker HT, Jaddoe VW, Reiss IK, Gaillard R, Hofman A, et al. Mode of delivery and childhood fractional exhaled nitric oxide, interrupter resistance and asthma: the Generation R study. *Pediatr Allergy Immunol.* (2015) 26:330–6. doi: 10.1111/pai.12385
13. Stokholm J, Thorsen J, Chawes BL, Schjørring S, Krogfelt KA, Bønnelykke K, et al. Cesarean section changes neonatal gut colonization. *J Allergy Clin Immunol.* (2016) 138:881–9.e2. doi: 10.1016/j.jaci.2016.01.028
14. Stokholm J, Thorsen J, Blaser MJ, Rasmussen MA, Hjelmsø M, Shah S, et al. Delivery mode and gut microbial changes correlate with an increased risk of childhood asthma. *Sci Transl Med.* (2020) 12:eaax9929. doi: 10.1126/scitranslmed.aax9929
15. Boker F, Alzahrani A, Alsaeed A, Alzhrani M, Albar R. Cesarean section and development of childhood bronchial asthma: is there a risk? *J Med Sci.* (2019) 7:347–51. doi: 10.3889/oamjms.2019.085
16. Meropol SB, Edwards A. Development of the infant intestinal microbiome: a bird's eye view of a complex process. *Birth Defects Res.* (2015) 105:228–39. doi: 10.1002/bdrc.21114
17. Baron R, Taye M, der Vaart IB, Ujčič-Voortman J, Szajewska H, Seidell JC, et al. The relationship of prenatal antibiotic exposure and infant antibiotic administration with childhood allergies: a systematic review. *BMC Pediatr.* (2020) 20:312. doi: 10.1186/s12887-020-02042-8
18. Uzan-Yulzari A, Turta O, Belogolovski A, Ziv O, Kunz C, Perschbacher S, et al. Neonatal antibiotic exposure impairs child growth during the first six years

of life by perturbing intestinal microbial colonization. *Nat Commun.* (2021) 12:443. doi: 10.1038/s41467-020-20495-4
19. Greenwood C, Morrow AL, Lagomarcino AJ, Altaye M, Taft DH, Yu, et al. Early empiric antibiotic use in preterm infants is associated with lower bacterial diversity and higher relative abundance of Enterobacter. *J Pediatr.* (2014) 165:23–9. doi: 10.1016/j.jpeds.2014.01.010
20. Chu DM, Antony KM, Ma J, Prince AL, Showalter L, Moller M, et al. The early infant gut microbiome varies in association with a maternal high-fat diet. *Genome Med.* (2016) 8:77. doi: 10.1186/s13073-016-0330-z
21. Williams JE, Carrothers JM, Lackey KA, Beatty NF, York MA, Brooker SL, et al. Human milk microbial community structure is relatively stable and related to variations in macronutrient and micronutrient intakes in healthy lactating women. *J Nutr.* (2017) 147:1739–48. doi: 10.3945/jn.117.248864
22. Mesa MD, Loureiro B, Iglesia I, Fernandez Gonzalez S, Llurba Olivé E, García Algar O, et al. The evolving microbiome from pregnancy to early infancy: a comprehensive review. *Nutrients.* (2020) 12:133. doi: 10.3390/nu12010133
23. Le Doare K, Holder B, Bassett A, Pannaraj PS. Mother's milk: a purposeful contribution to the development of the infant microbiota and immunity. *Front Immunol.* (2018) 9:361. doi: 10.3389/fimmu.2018.00361
24. Alduraywish SA, Lodge CJ, Campbell B, Allen KJ, Erbas B, Lowe AJ, et al. The march from early life food sensitization to allergic disease: a systematic review and meta-analyses of birth cohort studies. *Allergy.* (2016) 71:77–89. doi: 10.1111/all.12784
25. Liang G, Zhao C, Zhang H, Mattei L, Sherrill-Mix S, Bittinger K, et al. The stepwise assembly of the neonatal virome is modulated by breastfeeding. *Nature.* (2020) 581:470–4. doi: 10.1038/s41586-020-2192-1
26. Tachimoto H, Imanari E, Mezawa H, Okuyama M, Urashima T, Hirano D, et al. Effect of avoiding cow's milk formula at birth on prevention of asthma or recurrent wheeze among young children: extended follow-up from the ABC randomized clinical trial. *JAMA Netw Open.* (2020) 3:e2018534. doi: 10.1001/jamanetworkopen.2020.18534
27. Zheng P, Zhang B, Zhang K, Lv X, Wang Q, Bai X. The impact of air pollution on intestinal microbiome of asthmatic children: a panel study. *BioMed Res Int.* (2020) 2020:5753427. doi: 10.1155/2020/5753427
28. Vardavas CI, Hohmann C, Patelarou E, Martinez D, Henderson AJ, Granell R, et al. The independent role of prenatal and postnatal exposure to active and passive smoking on the development of early wheeze in children. *Eur Respir J.* (2016) 48:115–24. doi: 10.1183/13993003.01016-2015
29. Gosalbes MJ, Llop S, Vallès Y, Moya A, Ballester F, Francino MP. Meconium microbiota types dominated by lactic acid or enteric bacteria are differentially associated with maternal eczema and respiratory problems in infants. *Clin Exp Allergy.* (2013) 43:198–211. doi: 10.1111/cea.12063
30. Levin AM, Sitarik AR, Havstad SL, Fujimura KE, Wegienka G, Cassidy-Bushrow AE, et al. Joint effects of pregnancy, sociocultural, and environmental factors on early life gut microbiome structure and diversity. *Sci Rep.* (2016) 6:31775. doi: 10.1038/srep31775
31. Cait A, Hughes MR, Antignano F, Cait J, Dimitriu PA, Maas KR, et al. Microbiome-driven allergic lung inflammation is ameliorated by short-chain fatty acids. *Mucosal Immunol.* (2018) 11:785–95. doi: 10.1038/mi.2017.75
32. Polk BI, Bacharier LB. Potential strategies and targets for the prevention of pediatric asthma. *Immunol Allergy Clin North Am.* (2019) 39:151–62. doi: 10.1016/j.iac.2018.12.010
33. Bonham CA, Patterson KC, Strek ME. Asthma outcomes and management during pregnancy. *Chest.* (2018) 153:515–27. doi: 10.1016/j.chest.2017.08.029
34. Thorburn AN, McKenzie CI, Shen S, Stanley D, Macia L, Mason LJ, et al. Evidence that asthma is a developmental origin disease influenced by maternal diet and bacterial metabolites. *Nat Commun.* (2015) 6:7320. doi: 10.1038/ncomms8320

35. Bisgaard H, Stokholm J, Chawes BL, Vissing NH, Bjarnadóttir E, Schoos AM, et al. Fish oil-derived fatty acids in pregnancy and wheeze and asthma in offspring. *N Eng J Med.* (2016) 375:2530–9. doi: 10.1056/NEJMoa1503734

36. Hansen S, Strøm M, Maslova E, Dahl R, Hoffmann HJ, Rytter D, et al. Fish oil supplementation during pregnancy and allergic respiratory disease in the adult offspring. *J Allergy Clin Immunol.* (2017) 139:104–11.e4. doi: 10.1016/j.jaci.2016.02.042

37. Litonjua AA, Carey VJ, Laranjo N, Harshfield BJ, McElrath TF, O'Connor GT, et al. Effect of prenatal supplementation with vitamin D on asthma or recurrent wheezing in offspring by age 3 years: the VDAART randomized clinical trial. *JAMA.* (2016) 315:362–70. doi: 10.1001/jama.2015.18589

38. Wolsk HM, Harshfield BJ, Laranjo N, Carey VJ, O'Connor G, Sandel M, et al. Vitamin D supplementation in pregnancy, prenatal 25(OH)D levels, race, and subsequent asthma or recurrent wheeze in offspring: secondary analyses from the Vitamin D antenatal asthma reduction trial. *J Allergy Clin Immunol.* (2017) 140:1423–9.e5. doi: 10.1016/j.jaci.2017.01.013

39. Chung KF. Airway microbial dysbiosis in asthmatic patients: a target for prevention and treatment? *J Allergy Clin Immunol.* (2017) 139:1071–81. doi: 10.1016/j.jaci.2017.02.004

40. Gur M, Hakim F, Bentur L. Better understanding of childhood asthma, towards primary prevention - are we there yet? *Consideration of pertinent literature. F1000Res.* (2017) 6:2152. doi: 10.12688/f1000research.11601.1

41. Du Toit G, Roberts G, Sayre PH, Bahnson HT, Radulovic S, Santos AF, et al. Randomized trial of peanut consumption in infants at risk for peanut allergy. *N Eng J Med.* (2015) 372:803–13. doi: 10.1056/NEJMoa1414850

42. Pitt TJ, Becker AB, Chan-Yeung M, Chan ES, Watson W, Chooniedass R, et al. Reduced risk of peanut sensitization following exposure through breast-feeding and early peanut introduction. *J Allergy Clin Immunol.* (2018) 141:620–25.e1. doi: 10.1016/j.jaci.2017.06.024

43. Du X, Wang L, Wu S, Yuan L, Tang S, Xiang Y, et al. Efficacy of probiotic supplementary therapy for asthma, allergic rhinitis, and wheeze: a meta-analysis of randomized controlled trials. *Allergy Asthma Proc.* (2019) 40:250–60. doi: 10.2500/aap.2019.40.4227

44. Pfeffer PE, Hawrylowicz CM. Vitamin D in asthma: mechanisms of action and considerations for clinical trials. *Chest.* (2018) 153:1229–39. doi: 10.1016/j.chest.2017.09.005

45. Xystrakis E, Kusumakar S, Boswell S, Peek E, Urry Z, Richards DF, et al. Reversing the defective induction of IL-10-secreting regulatory T cells in glucocorticoid-resistant asthma patients. *J Clin Invest.* (2006) 116:146–55. doi: 10.1172/JCI21759

46. Chambers ES, Nanzer AM, Pfeffer PE, Richards DF, Timms PM, Martineau AR, et al. Distinct endotypes of steroid-resistant asthma characterized by IL-17A(high) and IFN-γ(high) immunophenotypes: potential benefits of calcitriol. *J Allergy Clin Immunol.* (2015) 136:628–37.e4. doi: 10.1016/j.jaci.2015.01.026

47. Lan N, Luo G, Yang X, Cheng Y, Zhang Y, Wang X, et al. 25-Hydroxyvitamin D3-deficiency enhances oxidative stress and corticosteroid resistance in severe asthma exacerbation. *PLoS ONE.* (2014) 9:e111599. doi: 10.1371/journal.pone.0111599

48. Gupta A, Sjoukes A, Richards D, Banya W, Hawrylowicz C, Bush A, et al. Relationship between serum vitamin D, disease severity, and airway remodeling in children with asthma. *Am J Respir Crit Care Med.* (2011) 184:1342–9. doi: 10.1164/rccm.201107-1239OC

49. Litonjua AA. Vitamin D and childhood asthma: causation and contribution to disease activity. *Curr Opin Allergy Clin Immunol.* (2019) 19:126–31. doi: 10.1097/ACI.0000000000000509

50. von Mutius E, Smits HH. Primary prevention of asthma: from risk and protective factors to targeted strategies for prevention. *Lancet.* (2020) 396:854–66. doi: 10.1016/S0140-6736(20)31861-4

51. Haahtela T, Valovirta E, Bousquet J, Mäkelä M, Allergy Programme Steering Group. The Finnish Allergy Programme 2008-2018 works. *Eur Respir J.* (2017) 49:1700470. doi: 10.1183/13993003.00470-2017

14

Understanding the Impact of Infection, Inflammation and their Persistence in the Pathogenesis of Bronchopulmonary Dysplasia

Jherna Balany and Vineet Bhandari*

Section of Neonatology, Department of Pediatrics, St. Christopher's Hospital for Children, Drexel University College of Medicine, Philadelphia, PA, USA

*Correspondence:
Vineet Bhandari
vineet.bhandari@drexelmed.edu

The concerted interaction of genetic and environmental factors acts on the preterm human immature lung with inflammation being the common denominator leading to the multifactorial origin of the most common chronic lung disease in infants – bronchopulmonary dysplasia (BPD). Adverse perinatal exposure to infection/inflammation with added insults like invasive mecha nical ventilation, exposure to hyperoxia, and sepsis causes persistent immune dysregulation. In this review article, we have attempted to analyze and consolidate current knowledge about the role played by persistent prenatal and postnatal inflammation in the pathogenesis of BPD. While some parameters of the early inflammatory response (neutrophils, cytokines, etc.) may not be detectable after days to weeks of exposure to noxious stimuli, they have already initiated the signaling pathways of the inflammatory process/immune cascade and have affected permanent defects structurally and functionally in the BPD lungs. Hence, translational research aimed at prevention/amelioration of BPD needs to focus on dampening the inflammatory response at an early stage to prevent the cascade of events leading to lung injury with impaired healing resulting in the pathologic pulmonary phenotype of alveolar simplification and dysregulated vascularization characteristic of BPD.

Keywords: premature newborn, chronic lung disease, cytokines, sepsis, hyperoxia, mechanical ventilation

INTRODUCTION

Bronchopulmonary dysplasia (BPD) is the most common chronic respiratory disease affecting infants wherein the developmental program of the lung is altered secondary to preterm birth of the baby (1). Lung development progresses in five distinct stages: embryonic, pseudoglandular, canalicular, saccular, and alveolar (2, 3). Human preterm babies who develop BPD are born in the late canalicular or early saccular stage of lung development. The late canalicular stage is characterized by development of the primitive alveoli and the alveolar capillary barrier, and the differentiation of type I and type II pneumocytes. The early saccular stage is marked by initiation of surfactant production, pulmonary vascularization, and enlargement of terminal airways (2–5). Unique to lung development is the fact that unlike other organs, the lungs complete their development after birth (up to 8 years of age) (6). Alveolar sacs are formed by secondary septation of alveolar ducts. With preterm birth, this programed development is disrupted, and in the setting of inflammation [whether it is due to infection, mechanical ventilation (MV), or hyperoxia] causes impaired alveolarization leading to BPD. We need to remember that while in sheep, baboons, and humans, the saccular stage occurs *in utero*; in rodent models, it begins at embryonic day 18 and continues through postnatal (PN) day 5 (4, 5).

In spite of many advances in neonatal medicine in the past few decades, like the introduction of better MV strategies and the use of surfactant and antenatal steroids, the incidence of BPD has not declined (7). The incidence of BPD in the United States is about 10,000–15,000 new cases each year out of which the majority of those affected have a birth weight <1250 g (8). Pulmonary and neurodevelopmental sequelae of this devastating disease extend even into adulthood (9).

Genetic (10) and environmental factors (pre- and/or postnatal sepsis, invasive MV, and hyperoxia) (1) act on the preterm human immature lung with inflammation being the common denominator in all these interactions leading to the multifactorial origins of this disease. As shown in **Figure 1**, it is postulated that adverse perinatal exposure/infection with added insults like invasive MV, exposure to hyperoxia, and sepsis causes persistent immune dysregulation. This on top of genetic susceptibility and prematurity leads to persistent inflammation leading to lung remodeling and evolution of BPD.

In this review article, we have attempted to analyze and consolidate current knowledge about the role played by persistent prenatal and postnatal inflammation in the pathogenesis of BPD. We searched PubMed for articles limited to English language with the keywords: "Bronchopulmonary dysplasia or BPD," "inflammation," "chorioamnionitis," "mechanical ventilation," "hyperoxia," "postnatal sepsis," either individually or in combination.

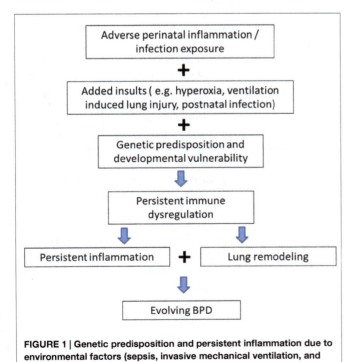

FIGURE 1 | Genetic predisposition and persistent inflammation due to environmental factors (sepsis, invasive mechanical ventilation, and hyperoxia) acting on the foundation of immature lung underlie the pathogenesis of BPD.

We focused on articles published over the last 10 years and used the most relevant ones for this review.

MEDIATORS OF INFLAMMATION IN BPD

Bronchopulmonary dysplasia has been linked to the development of an inflammatory response that can occur in absence of clinical infection. Systemic fetal inflammatory response (11) and neonatal leukemoid reactions (12) have been implicated as a risk factor for BPD. Pulmonary inflammation in BPD is characterized by the presence of inflammatory cells like neutrophils and monocytes, pro-inflammatory cytokines, and other mediators, including soluble adhesion molecules.

The innate immunity and adaptive immunity reinforce each other and act in unison. Cells of the innate immune system secrete cytokines, which can prime lymphocytes thereby modulating adaptive immunity (13). Exposure to a specific antigen causes these primed lymphocytes to have a more rapid and intense immune response (14, 15). Naïve T cells express CD62L (L-selectin) (16). Upon activation, the T cells shed their surface CD62L molecules. In infants with BPD, the expression of the CD62L is decreased on these CD4+ T-cells thereby suggesting T cell activation. CD54 (intercellular adhesion molecule-1 or ICAM-1) is an adhesion molecule that mediates a co-stimulatory signal in T cell activation. CD54 expression is increased upon cell activation (17).

The premature lung is exposed to ongoing oxidative and cellular damage. Damaged lung tissue releases chemotactic factors and inflammatory cytokines, such as interleukin (IL)-1, IL-8 (CXCL-8), and tumor necrosis factor alpha (TNF-α). This leads to an influx of neutrophils and other inflammatory cells with increased release/production of additional pro-inflammatory cytokines (**Table 1**). Multiple studies have shown that IL-1β, IL-6, and IL-8 are elevated very early in the respiratory course of the human preterm population that ultimately develop BPD, and in tracheal aspirates of those with BPD. In contrast, decreased levels of IL-10 in serum and tracheal aspirates have been shown in studies of those infants who developed BPD. In addition to ILs, a large variety of other biomarkers have been detected and associated with the development of BPD in tracheal aspirates, as well as blood and urine samples of premature infants (9, 18). The ones that have been implicated in the animal models include inflammatory cytokines, matrix proteins, growth factors, and vascular factors (9, 18–33). Their role is illustrated in **Table 1**.

We will now describe the major environmental factors that contribute to inflammation, and its persistence, in the pathogenesis of BPD. These include prenatal influences (chorioamnionitis) and postnatal influences, namely early- and late- onset sepsis, invasive MV, and hyperoxia.

PRENATAL FACTORS CAUSING INFLAMMATION – CHORIOAMNIONITIS

As the name suggests, chorioamnionitis is inflammation of the chorion and amnion membranes of the placenta (34).

TABLE 1 | Selected mediators of inflammation, their role, and corresponding expression in BPD.

Mediators of inflammation	Role	Expression in BPD
Inflammatory cytokines		
Interleukins: anti-inflammatory		
IL-10	Suppresses inflammatory response by inhibiting NF-κB	↓/↔
IL-4, IL-13	Suppresses inflammation by inhibiting pro-inflammatory cytokine production	↔
Interleukins: pro-inflammatory		
IL-1, IL-6	Acute phase inflammatory response	↑
IL-8 (CXCL-8)	Main chemoattractant for neutrophils	↑
CC chemokines		
Monocyte chemoattractant protein (MCP)-1, 1α, 1β, 2, 3	Recruit inflammatory cells to area of injury	↑
Macrophage migration inhibitory factor (MIF)	Upstream regulator of innate immune response	↓
Tumor necrosis factor alpha (TNF-α)	Enhances expression of other pro-inflammatory cytokines	↑
Transforming growth factor-beta 1 (TGF-β1)	Pro-inflammatory	↑
Matrix proteins		
Matrix metalloproteinase-8	Disordered pulmonary remodeling after inflammation	↑
Matrix metalloproteinase-9	Pro-inflammatory, interferon-gamma (IFN-γ) signaling	↑
Growth factors		
Endothelin-1	Pro-inflammatory	↑
Vascular endothelial growth factor	Pro-inflammatory	↑/↓
Connective tissue growth factor (CTGF)	Pro-inflammatory	↑
Bombesin-like peptide (BLP)	Increases mast cells in the lung	↑
Breast regression protein-39 (human analog is YKL-40)	Anti-inflammatory	↓
Pulmonary hepatocyte growth factor (HGF)	Alveolar septation, repair	↓
Keratinocyte growth factor (KGF)	Regulates proliferation of alveolar epithelial cells	↓
Miscellaneous		
Interferon-inducible protein 9 (IP-9 – also known as CXCL11)	Pro-inflammatory, IFN-γ signaling	↑
Cyclooxygenase-2 (Cox-2)	Pro-inflammatory, IFN-γ signaling	↑
CCAAT/enhancer-binding protein (C/EBP)	Pro-inflammatory, IFN-γ signaling	↑
Endoglin	Pro-inflammatory	↑
Periostin	Pro-inflammatory	↑
Clara cell secretory protein	Modulates acute pulmonary inflammation	↓
Parathyroid hormone-related protein (PTHrP)	Alveolar growth	↓
Angiopoietin-2	Pro-inflammatory	↑
Lactoferrin	Anti-inflammatory	↓

↑ – increase; ↔ – no change; ↓ – decrease.

Although commonly seen in clinical practice, chorioamnionitis is a complex syndrome associated with pregnancy leading to preterm deliveries (34). Chorioamnionitis has been classified as either histological or clinical. With histological chorioamnionitis, there is infiltration of polymorphonuclear leukocytes and other inflammatory cells like macrophages and T cells as seen microscopically (35–37). Clinical chorioamnionitis is evidenced by fever >37.5°C, uterine tenderness, foul smelling vaginal discharge, abdominal pain, maternal tachycardia with a heart rate >100 bpm, fetal tachycardia HR >160 bpm, and white blood cell (WBC) count >15,000/mm³ (38, 39).

It has been shown in *in vitro* studies that bacterial products like phospholipase A2, peptidoglycan polysaccharide, proteolytic enzymes, and endotoxins can initiate an inflammatory response. Inoculation of the amniotic cavity with *E. coli* lipopolysaccharide (LPS) or live *Ureaplasma* organisms has been shown to induce structural and functional fetal lung maturation (40–43). Antenatal lung inflammation impacts a variety of signaling pathway regulators like toll-like receptors 2 and 4 (TLR2 and TLR4), growth factors like TGF-β and CTGF, and mesenchymal structural proteins like bone morphogenetic protein-4 leading to vascular remodeling and alveolar simplification, which could be considered akin to a mild BPD phenotype (40–43). However, repetitive LPS exposure and/or chronic chorioamnionitis leads to immune tolerance and a dampened inflammatory response, which in turn allows the lungs to develop close to normal in experimental BPD animals (40–42).

Adverse perinatal outcomes are seen with intra-amniotic inflammation irrespective of the presence of intra-amniotic infection. Colonization *per se*, without inflammation is not associated with adverse outcomes (44). The severity of the adverse outcomes is directly related to the severity of the intra-amniotic inflammation (44). Maternal antibiotic use has been associated with decreased BPD (45).

To summarize, in experimental animals, antenatal inflammation causes lung maturation and some degrees of lung injury, which is modified by the not fully developed innate immune response, exposure to antenatal steroids, and noxious postnatal factors. Not surprisingly, given the variability in definition and impact of various confounding factors, the issue of antenatal inflammation causing BPD in human infants is controversial (42, 46–49). Chorioamnionitis increases the incidence of preterm birth, and if accompanied by lung inflammation could result in surfactant dysfunction allowing for prolonged exposure to supplemental oxygen and invasive MV (11, 48). This "multiple hit" of events could explain the propensity to BPD in such infants (48), though this has not been consistently shown (50). In addition, persistence and non-resolution of lung inflammation lead to BPD by inhibiting secondary septation, alveolarization and normal vascular development, and the compromised ability of the lungs to heal.

POSTNATAL FACTORS CAUSING INFLAMMATION – SEPSIS

Preterm infants are more susceptible to infections since their immune defenses are not fully developed, have vulnerable skin barrier, and require multiple invasive procedures (51). Postnatal infection/inflammation could either be localized to the lung or could be systemic in origin. Chorioamnionitis increases the risk of early-onset neonatal sepsis, which sets off an inflammatory cascade (48). Also, it has been shown that late-onset sepsis induces a pro-inflammatory and pro-fibrotic response in the preterm lung predisposing it to BPD (51).

Local (intra-tracheal) exposure to LPS (bacterial endotoxin) or dsRNA (a marker of viral replication) in the neonatal rat led to acute cellular and cytokine inflammatory responses, which were associated with histologic features of impaired alveolar development (52, 53).

Neonatal mice injected with intraperitoneal LPS demonstrated reduced lung inflammation and apoptosis after 24 h as compared to adults, and this was associated with activation of the transcription factor, nuclear factor kappa B (NF-κB) (54). Inhibition of NF-κB resulted in increased cell death and alveolar simplification and disruption of angiogenesis via vascular growth factor (VEGF)-R2 (55). It has also been shown that using a targeted deletion of NF-κB signaling (using a lung epithelium-specific deletion of IKKβ – which is a known activating kinase upstream of NF-κB) in a mouse model results in alveolar hypoplasia with decreased VEGF expression (56). In addition, there was increased expression of CXCL-1, as well as its receptor CXCR2. Pretreatment with CXCR2-neutralizing antibody was able to reverse the effects in the developing lung (53). In summary, exposure to either bacterial or viral agents in the rodent model led to features of inflammation, with pulmonary histology suggestive of BPD.

Inflammatory response secondary to viral infections in early post natal stages could be worth considering in the evolution of BPD. Increased neutrophil accumulation, increased expression of CXCL-1 and its receptor CXCR2, and decreased lung alveolarization have been seen with intra-tracheal delivery of viral pro-inflammatory dsRNA in 10-day-old mouse model (53).

POSTNATAL FACTORS CAUSING INFLAMMATION – INVASIVE MECHANICAL VENTILATION

Mechanical ventilation is a risk factor for the development of BPD in premature infants. Lung injury from MV results due to volutrauma, barotrauma, or atelectrauma (57).

When lungs are exposed to high tidal volumes, over distension leads to production of pro-inflammatory cytokines like IL-6, IL-8, and TNFα and reduced expression of anti-inflammatory cytokines like IL-10 (58). Even ventilation at low tidal volumes is deleterious because of the stretch injury it can induce by overdistending partially collapsed lungs. Sustained lung inflation (SLI) has been shown to increase levels of pro-inflammatory cytokines and BPD-like changes in the lungs of preterm lambs (59). There is great need to find non-invasive ventilation strategies for preterm neonates because even "gentle" invasive MV for a shorter duration can induce an inflammatory response (60).

In neonatal rats (7- to 14-day-old – in the alveolar phase of lung development), high tidal volume ventilation increased IL-6 mRNA and upregulated the TGF-β signaling molecule, CTGF

mRNA, and protein expression compared to controls (61). In an 8-day-old rat ventilation model, high tidal volumes increased the neutrophilic and inflammatory cytokine mRNA and/or protein expression (IL-1β, IL-6, CXCL-1 and 2) response (62). In a 7-day-old rat model, exposure to MV for 24 h in room air led to cell cycle arrest (63), suggesting a harbinger to alveolar simplification, the pathologic hallmark of BPD.

In an invasive MV model in 2-week-old mice (well into the alveolar phase of lung development) for 1 h, IL-6 lung levels were increased in the high tidal volume ventilation group (64). Studies conducted in 2- to 6-day-old mice (late saccular to early alveolar phase of lung development) ventilated for 8–24 h with room air or 40% O_2 revealed dysregulated elastin (ELN) assembly, a threefold to fivefold increase in cell death, TGF-β activation, and a decrease in VEGF-R2 expression (65, 66). Inhibiting lung elastase activity by using recombinant human elafin or genetically modified mice that expressed elafin in the vascular endothelium was protective of the lung injury (67, 68).

Early studies using a chronically ventilated (3–4 weeks) preterm lamb model of BPD showed evidence of non-uniform inflation patterns and impaired alveolar formation with an abnormal abundance of elastin (69). Inflammation was evident by the presence of inflammatory cells, namely alveolar macrophages, neutrophils, and mononuclear cells and edema (69). In this model, there was also reduced lung expression of growth factors that regulate alveolarization and differential alteration of matrix proteins that regulate ELN assembly (70). A non-invasive (nasal) ventilation approach preserved alveolar architecture (71) and had a positive effect on parathyroid hormone-related protein-peroxisome proliferator-activated receptor-gamma (PTHrP-PPARγ)-driven alveolar homeostatic epithelial–mesenchymal signaling in the preterm lamb model (72).

It has been seen in preterm fetal sheep that there is increased expression of early response gene-1 (Egr-1) as well as pro- and anti-inflammatory cytokines and dynamic changes in heat shock protein 70 (HSP70) (57). This stretch injury also increases expression of granulocyte/macrophage colony-stimulating factor mRNA leading to maturation of lung monocytes to alveolar macrophages (57). Induction of surfactant proteins A, B, and C mRNA is also increased (57). More recently, even short-term stretch injury (15 min) secondary to invasive MV in preterm fetal sheep led to increased levels of pro-inflammatory cytokines, IL-1β, IL-6, monocyte chemoattractant protein (MCP)-1, and MCP-2 mRNA by 1 h (57). This was accompanied by increased presence of inflammatory cells in the bronchoalveolar lavage fluid (BALF) with initial increases in neutrophils and monocytes by 1 h and a transition to macrophages by 24 h (57).

The preterm ventilated baboon model of BPD (delivered at 125 days – at 68% of gestation) showed evidence of alveolar hypoplasia and dysmorphic vasculature, akin to that seen in human BPD (73). Importantly, there were significant elevations of TNF-α, IL-6, IL-8 levels, but not of IL-1β and IL-10, in tracheal aspirate fluids at various times during the period of ventilator support, supporting a role for inflammation (73). In addition, increased matrix metalloproteinase-9 (MMP-9) levels were associated with lung inflammation and edema seen in this invasive ventilation model (74). Alteration of VEGF was also noted in the lungs of various baboon models (75, 76). Bombesin is a 14-amino acid peptide, initially detected in amphibian skin, but immunoreactive studies have shown the presence of bombesin-like peptide (BLP) in multiple organ systems in mammals (77). In the lung, BLP have been shown to be released by pulmonary neuroendocrine cells (77). BLP blockade improved alveolar septation and angiogenesis in the preterm baboon models (78, 79).

In the 125-day baboon model, treatment with early nasal continuous positive airway pressure (NCPAP) for 28 days led to a pulmonary phenotype similar to 156 days gestational control lungs, suggesting that this non-invasive approach could minimize lung injury (80). In the same model, delayed extubation (till 5 days) versus early extubation to NCPAP at 24 h led to significantly increased BALF IL-6, IL-8, MCP-1, macrophage inflammatory protein-1 alpha (MIP-1α), and growth-regulated oncogene-alpha (GRO-α) in the delayed NCPAP group (81).

Some epidemiological studies showed that replacing invasive MV with NCPAP was associated with BPD reduction (82). No reduction in the incidence of BPD or mortality in the NCPAP group was seen in the COIN study that randomized infants born at 25–28 weeks to receive either NCPAP or intubation with MV in the delivery room (83). The INSURE (IN: intubation, SUR: surfactant, E: extubation) technique has been shown to reduce the need for MV and incidence of BPD (84). Non-invasive ventilation strategies like nasal intermittent-positive pressure ventilation (NIPPV) not only reduce the need for intubation within the first 48–72 h of life, but also have been associated with decreased mortality and/or BPD and hence is a feasible option for the newborn (85–87), though additional studies are required (88). The optimal mode of non-invasive ventilation (for example: type of NCPAP, maximum level of NCPAP, synchronized or non-synchronized method of nasal ventilation), selection of the best nasal interface (short-prongs or mask), and choice of ventilator need to be determined, and this information would be helpful in management of the disease.

To summarize, while the lamb/sheep/baboon ventilation models are in the saccular stage (akin to the human premature babies who are at most risk for BPD at birth), the rat/mouse ventilation models are in the alveolar phase of lung development. However, it is quite obvious that mechanical stretch injury generates an inflammatory response (mostly neutrophils, IL-1β, IL-6, CXCL-1/-2, TGF-β signaling), along with alterations in matrix proteins (ELN, MMP-9) and VEGF. In addition, there is increased cell death and cell cycle arrest. Thus, it appears that an initial inflammatory cascade triggers the signaling of additional molecular mediators that lead to dysregulated vascularization and impaired alveolarization. Interestingly, non-invasive (nasal) ventilation approaches were protective of these responses. Thus, prolonged invasive MV sets off a persistent cascade of inflammatory response that in the setting of hyperoxia takes the "multiple hit" pathway of leading to BPD.

POSTNATAL FACTORS CAUSING INFLAMMATION – HYPEROXIA

Many studies have documented the injurious effects of perinatal supplemental oxygen on lung development. Target levels of O_2 in

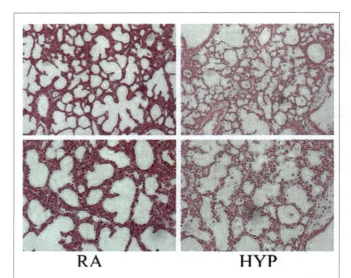

FIGURE 2 | Photomicrographs (×10, upper panel; ×20 lower panel; hematoxylin and eosin stain) of neonatal lung injury noted in newborn mice at postnatal day 2, after 100% O_2 exposure since birth. Note the alveolar exudates and presence of inflammatory cells in the hyperoxia-exposed lungs compared with litter-mate controls in room air. RA, room air; HYP, hyperoxia [with permission from Semin Fetal Neonatal Med (2010) 15(4):223–9].

extremely low birth weight (ELBW) have been studied extensively. The morphologic changes of human BPD resemble hyperoxic lung injury in newborn animals (73). Prolonged exposure to hyperoxia in the neonatal mouse for 14 days or longer results in a phenotype of "old" BPD (89, 90). Exposure to hyperoxia in the critical saccular stage of lung development replicates human BPD, with effects that are dose-dependent on the fraction of inspired oxygen (FiO_2) concentration; the effects last lifelong with increased susceptibility to respiratory tract infections (91–95). Acute lung injury caused by hyperoxia (**Figure 2**) occurs secondary to an inflammatory response, which causes destruction of the alveolar–capillary barrier, vascular leak, influx of inflammatory mediators, pulmonary edema, and ultimately cell death (96). With continued exposure to hyperoxia this inflammatory response and pulmonary edema improve initially but chronic pulmonary inflammation ensues in the following weeks (97). At the cellular level, alveolar or interstitial macrophages express early response cytokines when exposed to hyperoxia, which in turn attract inflammatory cells to the lungs (19).

It has been shown that there exists a dose-dependent effect of hyperoxia on severity of BPD in the murine model. Mice exposed to varying concentrations of oxygen ranging from 40 to 100% at PN days 1–4 had more severe disease at higher concentrations of oxygen (92). An oxygen dose-dependent inflammatory response to influenza-A viral infection in adult mice that had been exposed to hyperoxia as neonates has been reported (95). Furthermore, this response was dependent upon the cumulative exposure to oxygen (98).

The specific role of individual inflammatory molecular mediators in the pathogenesis of BPD has been particularly well illustrated by utilizing lung-targeted overexpressing transgenic models, in room air, resulting in pulmonary phenotypes reminiscent of human BPD. These include IL-1β (99, 100) and IFN-γ (25, 91). In the case of IL-1β transgenic mice, absence of the beta6 integrin subunit was protective of the BPD phenotype (101). Interestingly, inhibition of cyclooxygenase-2 (Cox-2) ameliorated the BPD phenotype in the hyperoxia-induced as well as the IFN-γ lung overexpressing transgenic mouse model in room air. A recent paper has reported that increased Cox-2 activity may contribute to proinflammatory responses in hyperoxia-exposed developing mouse lungs (102).

There is increased expression of IL-1α mRNA in neonatal mice exposed to hyperoxia (89). Lung mRNA for IL-1β also increases in neonatal mice exposed to hyperoxia (103). Transgenic IL-1β overexpression in lung epithelium resulted in BPD phenotype in neonatal mice (100). In hyperoxia-exposed newborn rabbits, the pattern of IL-1β rise and fall matches the rise and fall of histologic inflammation (104). However, in the immature baboon model of BPD, no such pattern between IL-1β levels and inflammation was seen in the tracheal aspirates (73). CINC-1 in premature rat lungs (105) and newborn rabbits (104) exposed to hyperoxia was upregulated. Also, IL-8 levels in tracheal aspirates of the premature baboon model of BPD have been shown to be increased (73).

The lungs of hyperoxia-exposed neonatal mice had no change in IL-10 mRNA expression (103). Also tracheal aspirates of baboon model of BPD show no difference in IL-10 levels (73). IL-1β, IL-6, and IL-8 are pro-inflammatory cytokines and are elevated very early in the course of BPD.

Typically viewed as pro-inflammatory, these cytokines have been shown to be elevated very early in the respiratory course of the human preterm population that ultimately develops BPD (20). Studies have found that serum and tracheal aspirate IL-10 levels were decreased in those infants who developed BPD (20).

A variety of potential therapeutic agents have been used in hyperoxia-exposed mice models that have been shown to decrease inflammation and/or attenuate other parameters of lung injury/BPD phenotype. These include rosiglitazone (106, 107), hepatocyte growth factor (HGF) (108), B-naphthoflavone (109), arginyl-glutamine as well as docosahexaenoic acid (110), and a combination of vitamin A and retinoic acid (111). Treatment with human amnion epithelial cells attenuated some parameters of hyperoxia-induced inflammatory lung injury (mRNA expression of IL-1α, IL-6, TGF-β, platelet-derived growth factor-beta or PDGF-β, mean linear intercept, and septal crest density), but not other aspects, for example, alveolar airspace volume, collagen content, or leukocyte infiltration in neonatal mice (112).

To summarize, while variable initiation and duration of exposure to hyperoxia animal models have been reported as models of human BPD, exposure to hyperoxia for a relatively short (PN1–4) duration in mice, which is at the critical saccular stage of lung development, can result in an inflammatory response sufficient to create the BPD pulmonary phenotype. This can be recapitulated using transgenic mice models of the inflammatory mediators, but kept in room air. Importantly, exposure to 0.4, 0.6, >0.8 FiO$_2$ can mimic mild, moderate, and severe BPD, respectively. A vast array of therapeutic agents has been reported to be effective in improving alveolar and/or vascular architecture of the hyperoxia-exposed neonatal lung in lambs, rats, and mice.

While hyperoxia exposure is a good starting point for testing the efficacy of potential therapeutic agents, it is important to be able to delineate the responsible molecule/signaling pathway in developmentally appropriate room air models and confirm the results in preventing/ameliorating the BPD phenotype. This would avoid the confounding variable of hyperoxia-induced alterations in multiple other molecular mediators, allowing delineation of targeted molecules in specific signaling pathways for maximal potential therapeutic relevance. Among the inflammatory mediators of hyperoxia-induced lung injury that can mimic the BPD phenotype in room air, the well-defined ones are IL-1β, TGF-β1, CTGF, IFN-γ, and MIF. It would be important to attempt to translate some of the newer targets in specific signaling pathways that have been recently reported, for example, inhibition of Cox-2 (91, 102) as a potential therapeutic option for prevention/amelioration of BPD.

PERSISTENT INFLAMMATION IN BPD

It is important to highlight the fact that for BPD to occur, it requires the known environmental factors to be exposed to the immature lung for a sustained duration, resulting in persistent inflammation. For the chorioamnionitis rodent models, the exposure to LPS is over a few days in the late canalicular/early saccular stage of lung development. For the relative short duration of exposure to invasive MV and hyperoxia in rodent models, 1 postnatal day in the saccular stage of lung development is equivalent to 3–4 weeks in a human preterm infant. Obviously, the larger animal models (sheep/lamb/baboon) also need few days to weeks of injury to develop the pulmonary phenotype of BPD. While some parameters of the early inflammatory response (neutrophils, cytokines such as IL-1, TNFα) may not be detectable after days to weeks of exposure to noxious stimuli, they have already initiated the signaling pathways of the inflammatory process/immune cascade and have affected permanent defects structurally and functionally in the BPD lungs. This is borne out by the facts that the pathologic appearance of large simplified alveoli is permanent following just the first 4 PN days of hyperoxia exposure in mice models (93). Furthermore, these mice have increased mortality when exposed to viral infectious challenge as adults (98, 113). In concordance, preterm neonates with BPD have anatomical and functional pulmonary deficits well into childhood and as adults (114–116). There is some clinical evidence that early interruption of the initial inflammatory response could result in amelioration and potential reversal of these effects (117).

SUMMARY AND CONCLUSION

It is important to remember that while *in vitro* studies are helpful in figuring out the mechanistic significance of a signaling pathway, these are usually conducted with cell lines or freshly isolated single cells of a particular phenotype. Thus, the results of such studies may not accurately reflect the *in vivo* situation of interaction with the multiple cell types found in the lung. In addition, while the significantly different responses between adult and neonatal lungs to the postnatal factors discussed here – invasive ventilation (118–121), local/systemic sepsis (52, 54, 122–124), and hyperoxia (19, 125–127) – are well established, it is also important to be cognizant of the stages of lung development when comparing animal data for relevance to humans. This is best exemplified by studies that highlight the differential responses in the various stages of lung development (mostly, saccular vs. alveolar) in animal models (99). Furthermore, the degree and duration of exposure to the noxious stimulus (hyperoxia, for example) in the animal models needs to be appropriate in order to attempt to extrapolate the data to humans. For example, a prolonged exposure to hyperoxia from birth to 2 weeks in the mouse, i.e., almost to the end of alveolarization is akin to exposing a preterm neonate to the same to at least up to 2 years of age.

To conclude, it is the preterm lung in the late canalicular/saccular phase of development that is most predisposed to BPD, when exposed to the pre- and postnatal factors. Inflammation and then its persistence in the preterm lung – whether initiated by prenatal factors like chorioamnionitis or whether propagated postnatally with the use of high FiO_2 and invasive MV or sepsis – culminates in BPD. Hence, translational research needs to be aimed at decreasing chorioamnionitis and finding better strategies for early non-invasive MV and optimum use of oxygen for the immature preterm lung for dampening the inflammatory response.

AUTHOR CONTRIBUTIONS

JB wrote the initial draft. VB did substantial re-organization and editing of the manuscript. Both authors have approved the final version of the manuscript as submitted.

REFERENCES

1. Bhandari V. Postnatal inflammation in the pathogenesis of bronchopulmonary dysplasia. *Birth Defects Res A Clin Mol Teratol* (2014) **100**(3):189–201. doi:10.1002/bdra.23220
2. Kotecha S. Lung growth: implications for the newborn infant. *Arch Dis Child Fetal Neonatal Ed* (2000) **82**(1):F69–74. doi:10.1136/fn.82.1.F69
3. Maeda Y, Dave V, Whitsett JA. Transcriptional control of lung morphogenesis. *Physiol Rev* (2007) **87**(1):219–44. doi:10.1152/physrev.00028.2006
4. Joshi S, Kotecha S. Lung growth and development. *Early Hum Dev* (2007) **83**(12):789–94. doi:10.1016/j.earlhumdev.2007.09.007
5. Kramer EL, Deutsch GH, Sartor MA, Hardie WD, Ikegami M, Korfhagen TR, et al. Perinatal increases in TGF-{alpha} disrupt the saccular phase of lung morphogenesis and cause remodeling: microarray analysis. *Am J Physiol Lung Cell Mol Physiol* (2007) **293**(2):L314–27. doi:10.1152/ajplung.00354.2006
6. Berger J, Bhandari V. Animal models of bronchopulmonary dysplasia. The term mouse models. *Am J Physiol Lung Cell Mol Physiol* (2014) **307**(12):L936–47. doi:10.1152/ajplung.00159.2014
7. Smith VC, Zupancic JA, McCormick MC, Croen LA, Greene J, Escobar GJ, et al. Trends in severe bronchopulmonary dysplasia rates between 1994 and 2002. *J Pediatr* (2005) **146**(4):469–73. doi:10.1016/j.jpeds.2004.12.023
8. Bhandari A, Bhandari V. "New" bronchopulmonary dysplasia: a clinical review. *Clin Pulm Med* (2011) **18**(3):137–43. doi:10.1097/CPM.0b013e318218a071
9. Bhandari A, Bhandari V. Pitfalls, problems, and progress in bronchopulmonary dysplasia. *Pediatrics* (2009) **123**(6):1562–73. doi:10.1542/peds.2008-1962
10. Bhandari V, Gruen JR. The genetics of bronchopulmonary dysplasia. *Semin Perinatol* (2006) **30**(4):185–91. doi:10.1053/j.semperi.2006.05.005
11. Hofer N, Kothari R, Morris N, Muller W, Resch B. The fetal inflammatory response syndrome is a risk factor for morbidity in preterm neonates. *Am J Obstet Gynecol* (2013) **209**(6):e1–11. doi:10.1016/j.ajog.2013.08.030
12. Zanardo V, Savio V, Giacomin C, Rinaldi A, Marzari F, Chiarelli S. Relationship between neonatal leukemoid reaction and bronchopulmonary dysplasia in low-birth-weight infants: a cross-sectional study. *Am J Perinatol* (2002) **19**(7):379–86. doi:10.1055/s-2002-35612
13. Hoebe K, Janssen E, Beutler B. The interface between innate and adaptive immunity. *Nat Immunol* (2004) **5**(10):971–4. doi:10.1038/ni1004-971
14. Vivier E, Malissen B. Innate and adaptive immunity: specificities and signaling hierarchies revisited. *Nat Immunol* (2005) **6**(1):17–21. doi:10.1038/ni1153
15. Lanzavecchia A, Sallusto F. From synapses to immunological memory: the role of sustained T cell stimulation. *Curr Opin Immunol* (2000) **12**(1):92–8. doi:10.1016/S0952-7915(99)00056-4

16. Hannet I, Erkeller-Yuksel F, Lydyard P, Deneys V, DeBruyere M. Developmental and maturational changes in human blood lymphocyte subpopulations. *Immunol Today* (1992) **13**(6):215–218. doi:10.1016/0167-5699(92)90157-3
17. Springer TA. Adhesion receptors of the immune system. *Nature* (1990) **346**(6283):425–34. doi:10.1038/346425a0
18. Bhandari A, Bhandari V. Biomarkers in bronchopulmonary dysplasia. *Paediatr Respir Rev* (2013) **14**(3):173–9. doi:10.1016/j.prrv.2013.02.008
19. Bhandari V, Elias JA. Cytokines in tolerance to hyperoxia-induced injury in the developing and adult lung. *Free Radic Biol Med* (2006) **41**(1):4–18. doi:10.1016/j.freeradbiomed.2006.01.027
20. Thompson A, Bhandari V. Pulmonary biomarkers of bronchopulmonary dysplasia. *Biomark Insights* (2008) **3**:361–73.
21. Alapati D, Rong M, Chen S, Hehre D, Rodriguez MM, Lipson KE, et al. Connective tissue growth factor antibody therapy attenuates hyperoxia-induced lung injury in neonatal rats. *Am J Respir Cell Mol Biol* (2011) **45**(6):1169–77. doi:10.1165/rcmb.2011-0023OC
22. Bozyk PD, Bentley JK, Popova AP, Anyanwu AC, Linn MD, Goldsmith AM, et al. Neonatal periostin knockout mice are protected from hyperoxia-induced alveolar simplification. *PLoS One* (2012) **7**(2):e31336. doi:10.1371/journal.pone.0031336
23. De Paepe ME, Patel C, Tsai A, Gundavarapu S, Mao Q. Endoglin (CD105) up-regulation in pulmonary microvasculature of ventilated preterm infants. *Am J Respir Crit Care Med* (2008) **178**(2):180–7. doi:10.1164/rccm.200608-1240OC
24. Choo-Wing R, Syed MA, Harijith A, Bowen B, Pryhuber G, Janér C, et al. Hyperoxia and interferon-γ–induced injury in developing lungs occur via cyclooxygenase-2 and the endoplasmic reticulum stress–dependent pathway. *Am J Respir Cell Mol Biol* (2013) **48**(6):749–57. doi:10.1165/rcmb.2012-0381OC
25. Harijith A, Choo-Wing R, Cataltepe S, Yasumatsu R, Aghai ZH, Janer J, et al. A role for matrix metalloproteinase 9 in IFNgamma-mediated injury in developing lungs: relevance to bronchopulmonary dysplasia. *Am J Respir Cell Mol Biol* (2011) **44**(5):621–30. doi:10.1165/rcmb.2010-0058OC
26. Bhatt AJ, Pryhuber GS, Huyck H, Watkins RH, Metlay LA, Maniscalco WM. Disrupted pulmonary vasculature and decreased vascular endothelial growth factor, Flt-1, and TIE-2 in human infants dying with bronchopulmonary dysplasia. *Am J Respir Crit Care Med* (2001) **164**(10 Pt 1):1971–80. doi:10.1164/ajrccm.164.10.2101140
27. Lassus P, Turanlahti M, Heikkila P, Andersson LC, Nupponen I, Sarnesto A, et al. Pulmonary vascular endothelial growth factor and Flt-1 in fetuses, in acute and chronic lung disease, and in persistent pulmonary hypertension of the newborn. *Am J Respir Crit Care Med* (2001) **164**(10 Pt 1):1981–7. doi:10.1164/ajrccm.164.10.2012036

28. Meller S, Bhandari V. VEGF levels in humans and animal models with RDS and BPD: temporal relationships. *Exp Lung Res* (2012) 38(4):192–203. doi:10.3109/01902148.2012.663454

29. Subramaniam M, Sugiyama K, Coy DH, Kong Y, Miller YE, Weller PF, et al. Bombesin-like peptides and mast cell responses: relevance to bronchopulmonary dysplasia? *Am J Respir Crit Care Med* (2003) 168(5):601–11. doi:10.1164/rccm.200212-1434OC

30. Bhattacharya S, Go D, Krenitsky DL, Huyck HL, Solleti SK, Lunger VA, et al. Genome-wide transcriptional profiling reveals connective tissue mast cell accumulation in bronchopulmonary dysplasia. *Am J Respir Crit Care Med* (2012) 186(4):349–58. doi:10.1164/rccm.201203-0406OC

31. Sohn MH, Kang MJ, Matsuura H, Bhandari V, Chen NY, Lee CG, et al. The chitinase-like proteins breast regression protein-39 and YKL-40 regulate hyperoxia-induced acute lung injury. *Am J Respir Crit Care Med* (2010) 182(7):918–28. doi:10.1164/rccm.200912-1793OC

32. Bhandari V, Choo-Wing R, Lee CG, Zhu Z, Nedrelow JH, Chupp GL, et al. Hyperoxia causes angiopoietin 2-mediated acute lung injury and necrotic cell death. *Nat Med* (2006) 12(11):1286–93. doi:10.1038/nm1494

33. Aghai ZH, Faqiri S, Saslow JG, Nakhla T, Farhath S, Kumar A, et al. Angiopoietin 2 concentrations in infants developing bronchopulmonary dysplasia: attenuation by dexamethasone. *J Perinatol* (2008) 28(2):149–55. doi:10.1038/sj.jp.7211886

34. Menon R, Taylor RN, Fortunato SJ. Chorioamnionitis – a complex pathophysiologic syndrome. *Placenta* (2010) 31(2):113–20. doi:10.1016/j.placenta.2009.11.012

35. Pankuch GA, Appelbaum PC, Lorenz RP, Botti JJ, Schachter J, Naeye RL. Placental microbiology and histology and the pathogenesis of chorioamnionitis. *Obstet Gynecol* (1984) 64(6):802–6.

36. Duff P, Sanders R, Gibbs RS. The course of labor in term patients with chorioamnionitis. *Am J Obstet Gynecol* (1983) 147(4):391–5.

37. Redline RW, Heller D, Keating S, Kingdom J. Placental diagnostic criteria and clinical correlation – a workshop report. *Placenta* (2005) 26(Suppl A):S114–7. doi:10.1016/j.placenta.2005.02.009

38. Miyazaki K, Furuhashi M, Matsuo K, Minami K, Yoshida K, Kuno N, et al. Impact of subclinical chorioamnionitis on maternal and neonatal outcomes. *Acta Obstet Gynecol Scand* (2007) 86(2):191–7. doi:10.1080/00016340601022793

39. Gibbs RS, Blanco JD, St Clair PJ, Castaneda YS. Quantitative bacteriology of amniotic fluid from women with clinical intraamniotic infection at term. *J Infect Dis* (1982) 145(1):1–8. doi:10.1093/infdis/145.1.1

40. Viscardi RM. Perinatal inflammation and lung injury. *Semin Fetal Neonatal Med* (2012) 17(1):30–5. doi:10.1016/j.siny.2011.08.002

41. Kramer BW, Kallapur S, Newnham J, Jobe AH. Prenatal inflammation and lung development. *Semin Fetal Neonatal Med* (2009) 14(1):2–7. doi:10.1016/j.siny.2008.08.011

42. Kunzmann S, Collins JJ, Kuypers E, Kramer BW. Thrown off balance: the effect of antenatal inflammation on the developing lung and immune system. *Am J Obstet Gynecol* (2013) 208(6):429–37. doi:10.1016/j.ajog.2013.01.008

43. Kallapur SG, Kramer BW, Jobe AH. Ureaplasma and BPD. *Semin Perinatol* (2013) 37(2):94–101. doi:10.1053/j.semperi.2013.01.005

44. Combs CA, Gravett M, Garite TJ, Hickok DE, Lapidus J, Porreco R, et al. Amniotic fluid infection, inflammation, and colonization in preterm labor with intact membranes. *Am J Obstet Gynecol* (2014) 210(2):e1–15. doi:10.1016/j.ajog.2013.11.032

45. Eriksson L, Haglund B, Odlind V, Altman M, Kieler H. Prenatal inflammatory risk factors for development of bronchopulmonary dysplasia. *Pediatr Pulmonol* (2014) 49(7):665–72. doi:10.1002/ppul.22881

46. Been JV, Zimmermann LJ. Histological chorioamnionitis and respiratory outcome in preterm infants. *Arch Dis Child Fetal Neonatal Ed* (2009) 94(3):F218–25. doi:10.1136/adc.2008.150458

47. Thomas W, Speer CP. Chorioamnionitis: important risk factor or innocent bystander for neonatal outcome? *Neonatology* (2011) 99(3):177–87. doi:10.1159/000320170

48. Thomas W, Speer CP. Chorioamnionitis is essential in the evolution of bronchopulmonary dysplasia – the case in favour. *Paediatr Respir Rev* (2014) 15(1):49–52. doi:10.1016/j.prrv.2013.09.004

49. Plakkal N, Soraisham AS, Trevenen C, Freiheit EA, Sauve R. Histological chorioamnionitis and bronchopulmonary dysplasia: a retrospective cohort study. *J Perinatol* (2013) 33(6):441–5. doi:10.1038/jp.2012.154

50. Nasef N, Shabaan AE, Schurr P, Iaboni D, Choudhury J, Church P, et al. Effect of clinical and histological chorioamnionitis on the outcome of preterm infants. *Am J Perinatol* (2013) 30(1):59–68. doi:10.1055/s-0032-1321501

51. Shah J, Jefferies AL, Yoon EW, Lee SK, Shah PS, Canadian Neonatal Network. Risk factors and outcomes of late-onset bacterial sepsis in preterm neonates born at <32 weeks' gestation. *Am J Perinatol* (2015) 32(7):675–82. doi:10.1055/s-0034-1393936

52. Franco ML, Waszak P, Banalec G, Levame M, Lafuma C, Harf A, et al. LPS-induced lung injury in neonatal rats: changes in gelatinase activities and consequences on lung growth. *Am J Physiol Lung Cell Mol Physiol* (2002) 282(3):L491–500. doi:10.1152/ajplung.00140.2001

53. Londhe VA, Belperio JA, Keane MP, Burdick MD, Xue YY, Strieter RM. CXCR2/CXCR2 ligand biological axis impairs alveologenesis during dsRNA-induced lung inflammation in mice. *Pediatr Res* (2005) 58(5):919–26. doi:10.1203/01.PDR.0000181377.78061.3E

54. Alvira CM, Abate A, Yang G, Dennery PA, Rabinovitch M. Nuclear factor-kappaB activation in neonatal mouse lung protects against lipopolysaccharide-induced inflammation. *Am J Respir Crit Care Med* (2007) 175(8):805–15. doi:10.1164/rccm.200608-1162OC

55. Iosef C, Alastalo TP, Hou Y, Chen C, Adams ES, Lyu SC, et al. Inhibiting NF-kappaB in the developing lung disrupts angiogenesis and alveolarization. *Am J Physiol Lung Cell Mol Physiol* (2012) 302(10):L1023–36. doi:10.1152/ajplung.00230.2011

56. Londhe VA, Maisonet TM, Lopez B, Jeng JM, Xiao J, Li C, et al. Conditional deletion of epithelial IKKbeta impairs alveolar formation through apoptosis and decreased VEGF expression during early mouse lung morphogenesis. *Respir Res* (2011) 12:134. doi:10.1186/1465-9921-12-134

57. Hillman NH, Polglase GR, Pillow JJ, Saito M, Kallapur SG, Jobe AH. Inflammation and lung maturation from stretch injury in preterm fetal sheep. *Am J Physiol Lung Cell Mol Physiol* (2011) 300(2):L232–41. doi:10.1152/ajplung.00294.2010

58. Carvalho CG, Silveira RC, Procianoy RS. Ventilator-induced lung injury in preterm infants. *Rev Bras Ter Intensiva* (2013) 25(4):319–26. doi:10.5935/0103-507X.20130054

59. Hillman NH, Kemp MW, Noble PB, Kallapur SG, Jobe AH. Sustained inflation at birth did not protect preterm fetal sheep from lung injury. *Am J Physiol Lung Cell Mol Physiol* (2013) 305(6):L446–53. doi:10.1152/ajplung.00162.2013

60. Allison BJ, Crossley KJ, Flecknoe SJ, Davis PG, Morley CJ, Harding R, et al. Ventilation of the very immature lung in utero induces injury and BPD-like changes in lung structure in fetal sheep. *Pediatr Res* (2008) 64(4):387–92. doi:10.1203/PDR.0b013e318181e05e

61. Wu S, Capasso L, Lessa A, Peng J, Kasisomayajula K, Rodriguez M, et al. High tidal volume ventilation activates Smad2 and upregulates expression of connective tissue growth factor in newborn rat lung. *Pediatr Res* (2008) 63(3):245–50. doi:10.1203/PDR.0b013e318163a8cc

62. Kroon AA, Wang J, Huang Z, Cao L, Kuliszewski M, Post M. Inflammatory response to oxygen and endotoxin in newborn rat lung ventilated with low tidal volume. *Pediatr Res* (2010) 68(1):63–9. doi:10.1203/00006450-201011001-00120

63. Kroon AA, Wang J, Kavanagh BP, Huang Z, Kuliszewski M, van Goudoever JB, et al. Prolonged mechanical ventilation induces cell cycle arrest in newborn rat lung. *PLoS One* (2011) 6(2):e16910. doi:10.1371/journal.pone.0016910

64. Cannizzaro V, Zosky GR, Hantos Z, Turner DJ, Sly PD. High tidal volume ventilation in infant mice. *Respir Physiol Neurobiol* (2008) 162(1):93–9. doi:10.1016/j.resp.2008.04.010

65. Bland RD, Ertsey R, Mokres LM, Xu L, Jacobson BE, Jiang S, et al. Mechanical ventilation uncouples synthesis and assembly of elastin and increases apoptosis in lungs of newborn mice. Prelude to defective alveolar septation during lung development? *Am J Physiol Lung Cell Mol Physiol* (2008) 294(1):L3–14. doi:10.1152/ajplung.00362.2007

66. Mokres LM, Parai K, Hilgendorff A, Ertsey R, Alvira CM, Rabinovitch M, et al. Prolonged mechanical ventilation with air induces apoptosis and causes failure of alveolar septation and angiogenesis in lungs of newborn mice. *Am J Physiol Lung Cell Mol Physiol* (2010) 298(1):L23–35. doi:10.1152/ajplung.00251.2009

67. Hilgendorff A, Parai K, Ertsey R, Jain N, Navarro EF, Peterson JL, et al. Inhibiting lung elastase activity enables lung growth in mechanically

67. ventilated newborn mice. *Am J Respir Crit Care Med* (2011) **184**(5):537–46. doi:10.1164/rccm.201012-2010OC

68. Hilgendorff A, Parai K, Ertsey R, Juliana Rey-Parra G, Thebaud B, Tamosiuniene R, et al. Neonatal mice genetically modified to express the elastase inhibitor elafin are protected against the adverse effects of mechanical ventilation on lung growth. *Am J Physiol Lung Cell Mol Physiol* (2012) **303**(3):L215–27. doi:10.1152/ajplung.00405.2011

69. Albertine KH, Jones GP, Starcher BC, Bohnsack JF, Davis PL, Cho SC, et al. Chronic lung injury in preterm lambs. Disordered respiratory tract development. *Am J Respir Crit Care Med* (1999) **159**(3):945–58. doi:10.1164/ajrccm.159.3.9804027

70. Bland RD, Xu L, Ertsey R, Rabinovitch M, Albertine KH, Wynn KA, et al. Dysregulation of pulmonary elastin synthesis and assembly in preterm lambs with chronic lung disease. *Am J Physiol Lung Cell Mol Physiol* (2007) **292**(6):L1370–84. doi:10.1152/ajplung.00367.2006

71. Reyburn B, Li M, Metcalfe DB, Kroll NJ, Alvord J, Wint A, et al. Nasal ventilation alters mesenchymal cell turnover and improves alveolarization in preterm lambs. *Am J Respir Crit Care Med* (2008) **178**(4):407–18. doi:10.1164/rccm.200802-359OC

72. Rehan VK, Fong J, Lee R, Sakurai R, Wang ZM, Dahl MJ, et al. Mechanism of reduced lung injury by high-frequency nasal ventilation in a preterm lamb model of neonatal chronic lung disease. *Pediatr Res* (2011) **70**(5):462–6. doi:10.1038/pr.2011.687

73. Coalson JJ, Winter VT, Siler-Khodr T, Yoder BA. Neonatal chronic lung disease in extremely immature baboons. *Am J Respir Crit Care Med* (1999) **160**(4):1333–46. doi:10.1164/ajrccm.160.4.9810071

74. Tambunting F, Beharry KD, Hartleroad J, Waltzman J, Stavitsky Y, Modanlou HD. Increased lung matrix metalloproteinase-9 levels in extremely premature baboons with bronchopulmonary dysplasia. *Pediatr Pulmonol* (2005) **39**(1):5–14. doi:10.1002/ppul.20135

75. Maniscalco WM, Watkins RH, Pryhuber GS, Bhatt A, Shea C, Huyck H. Angiogenic factors and alveolar vasculature: development and alterations by injury in very premature baboons. *Am J Physiol Lung Cell Mol Physiol* (2002) **282**(4):L811–23. doi:10.1152/ajplung.00325.2001

76. Tambunting F, Beharry KD, Waltzman J, Modanlou HD. Impaired lung vascular endothelial growth factor in extremely premature baboons developing bronchopulmonary dysplasia/chronic lung disease. *J Investig Med* (2005) **53**(5):253–62. doi:10.2310/6650.2005.53508

77. Ganter MT, Pittet JF. Bombesin-like peptides: modulators of inflammation in acute lung injury? *Am J Respir Crit Care Med* (2006) **173**(1):1–2. doi:10.1164/rccm.2510002

78. Sunday ME, Yoder BA, Cuttitta F, Haley KJ, Emanuel RL. Bombesin-like peptide mediates lung injury in a baboon model of bronchopulmonary dysplasia. *J Clin Invest* (1998) **102**(3):584–94. doi:10.1172/JCI2329

79. Subramaniam M, Bausch C, Twomey A, Andreeva S, Yoder BA, Chang L, et al. Bombesin-like peptides modulate alveolarization and angiogenesis in bronchopulmonary dysplasia. *Am J Respir Crit Care Med* (2007) **176**(9):902–12. doi:10.1164/rccm.200611-1734OC

80. Thomson MA, Yoder BA, Winter VT, Martin H, Catland D, Siler-Khodr TM, et al. Treatment of immature baboons for 28 days with early nasal continuous positive airway pressure. *Am J Respir Crit Care Med* (2004) **169**(9):1054–62. doi:10.1164/rccm.200309-1276OC

81. Thomson MA, Yoder BA, Winter VT, Giavedoni L, Chang LY, Coalson JJ. Delayed extubation to nasal continuous positive airway pressure in the immature baboon model of bronchopulmonary dysplasia: lung clinical and pathological findings. *Pediatrics* (2006) **118**(5):2038–50. doi:10.1542/peds.2006-0622

82. Aly H, Milner JD, Patel K, El-Mohandes AA. Does the experience with the use of nasal continuous positive airway pressure improve over time in extremely low birth weight infants? *Pediatrics* (2004) **114**(3):697–702. doi:10.1542/peds.2003-0572-L

83. Morley CJ, Davis PG, Doyle LW, Brion LP, Hascoet JM, Carlin JB. Nasal CPAP or intubation at birth for very preterm infants. *N Engl J Med* (2008) **358**(7):700–8. doi:10.1056/NEJMoa072788

84. Stevens TP, Harrington EW, Blennow M, Soll RF. Early surfactant administration with brief ventilation vs. selective surfactant and continued mechanical ventilation for preterm infants with or at risk for respiratory distress syndrome. *Cochrane Database Syst Rev* (2007) **4**:CD003063.

85. Bhandari V. The potential of non-invasive ventilation to decrease BPD. *Semin Perinatol* (2013) **37**(2):108–14. doi:10.1053/j.semperi.2013.01.007

86. Mehta P, Berger J, Bucholz E, Bhandari V. Factors affecting nasal intermittent positive pressure ventilation failure and impact on bronchopulmonary dysplasia in neonates. *J Perinatol* (2014) **34**(10):754–60. doi:10.1038/jp.2014.100

87. Jasani B, Nanavati R, Kabra N, Rajdeo S, Bhandari V. Comparison of non-synchronized nasal intermittent positive pressure ventilation versus nasal continuous positive airway pressure as post-extubation respiratory support in preterm infants with respiratory distress syndrome: a randomized controlled trial. *J Matern Fetal Neonatal Med* (2015) **10**:1–6. doi:10.3109/14767058.2015.1059809

88. Kirpalani H, Millar D, Lemyre B, Yoder BA, Chiu A, Roberts RS. A trial comparing noninvasive ventilation strategies in preterm infants. *N Engl J Med* (2013) **369**(7):611–20. doi:10.1056/NEJMoa1214533

89. Warner BB, Stuart LA, Papes RA, Wispe JR. Functional and pathological effects of prolonged hyperoxia in neonatal mice. *Am J Physiol* (1998) **275**(1 Pt 1):L110–7.

90. Zhang X, Wang H, Shi Y, Peng W, Zhang S, Zhang W, et al. Role of bone marrow-derived mesenchymal stem cells in the prevention of hyperoxia-induced lung injury in newborn mice. *Cell Biol Int* (2012) **36**(6):589–94. doi:10.1042/CBI20110447

91. Choo-Wing R, Syed MA, Harijith A, Bowen B, Pryhuber G, Janer C, et al. Hyperoxia and interferon-gamma-induced injury in developing lungs occur via cyclooxygenase-2 and the endoplasmic reticulum stress-dependent pathway. *Am J Respir Cell Mol Biol* (2013) **48**(6):749–57. doi:10.1165/rcmb.2012-0381OC

92. Yee M, Chess PR, McGrath-Morrow SA, Wang Z, Gelein R, Zhou R, et al. Neonatal oxygen adversely affects lung function in adult mice without altering surfactant composition or activity. *Am J Physiol Lung Cell Mol Physiol* (2009) **297**(4):L641–9. doi:10.1152/ajplung.00023.2009

93. O'Reilly MA, Marr SH, Yee M, McGrath-Morrow SA, Lawrence BP. Neonatal hyperoxia enhances the inflammatory response in adult mice infected with influenza A virus. *Am J Respir Crit Care Med* (2008) **177**(10):1103–10. doi:10.1164/rccm.200712-1839OC

94. Li Z, Choo-Wing R, Sun H, Sureshbabu A, Sakurai R, Rehan VK, et al. A potential role of the JNK pathway in hyperoxia-induced cell death, myofibroblast transdifferentiation and TGF-beta1-mediated injury in the developing murine lung. *BMC Cell Biol* (2011) **12**:54. doi:10.1186/1471-2121-12-54

95. Buczynski BW, Yee M, Paige Lawrence B, O'Reilly MA. Lung development and the host response to influenza A virus are altered by different doses of neonatal oxygen in mice. *Am J Physiol Lung Cell Mol Physiol* (2012) **302**(10):L1078–87. doi:10.1152/ajplung.00026.2012

96. Thickett DR, Armstrong L, Christie SJ, Millar AB. Vascular endothelial growth factor may contribute to increased vascular permeability in acute respiratory distress syndrome. *Am J Respir Crit Care Med* (2001) **164**(9):1601–5. doi:10.1164/ajrccm.164.9.2011071

97. Ben-Ari J, Makhoul IR, Dorio RJ, Buckley S, Warburton D, Walker SM. Cytokine response during hyperoxia: sequential production of pulmonary tumor necrosis factor and interleukin-6 in neonatal rats. *Isr Med Assoc J* (2000) **2**(5):365–9.

98. Maduekwe ET, Buczynski BW, Yee M, Rangasamy T, Stevens TP, Lawrence BP, et al. Cumulative neonatal oxygen exposure predicts response of adult mice infected with influenza A virus. *Pediatr Pulmonol* (2014) **50**(3):222–30. doi:10.1002/ppul.23063

99. Backstrom E, Hogmalm A, Lappalainen U, Bry K. Developmental stage is a major determinant of lung injury in a murine model of bronchopulmonary dysplasia. *Pediatr Res* (2011) **69**(4):312–8. doi:10.1203/PDR.0b013e31820bcb2a

100. Bry K, Whitsett JA, Lappalainen U. IL-1beta disrupts postnatal lung morphogenesis in the mouse. *Am J Respir Cell Mol Biol* (2007) **36**(1):32–42. doi:10.1165/rcmb.2006-0116OC

101. Hogmalm A, Sheppard D, Lappalainen U, Bry K. beta6 Integrin subunit deficiency alleviates lung injury in a mouse model of bronchopulmonary dysplasia. *Am J Respir Cell Mol Biol* (2010) **43**(1):88–98. doi:10.1165/rcmb.2008-0480OC

102. Britt RD Jr, Velten M, Tipple TE, Nelin LD, Rogers LK. Cyclooxygenase-2 in newborn hyperoxic lung injury. *Free Radic Biol Med* (2013) **61**:502–11. doi:10.1016/j.freeradbiomed.2013.04.012

103. Johnston CJ, Wright TW, Reed CK, Finkelstein JN. Comparison of adult and newborn pulmonary cytokine mRNA expression after hyperoxia. *Exp Lung Res* (1997) 23(6):537–52. doi:10.3109/01902149709039242

104. D'Angio CT, LoMonaco MB, Chaudhry SA, Paxhia A, Ryan RM. Discordant pulmonary proinflammatory cytokine expression during acute hyperoxia in the newborn rabbit. *Exp Lung Res* (1999) 25(5):443–65. doi:10.1080/019021499270187

105. Wagenaar GT, ter Horst SA, van Gastelen MA, Leijser LM, Mauad T, van der Velden PA, et al. Gene expression profile and histopathology of experimental bronchopulmonary dysplasia induced by prolonged oxidative stress. *Free Radic Biol Med* (2004) 36(6):782–801. doi:10.1016/j.freeradbiomed.2003.12.007

106. Dasgupta C, Sakurai R, Wang Y, Guo P, Ambalavanan N, Torday JS, et al. Hyperoxia-induced neonatal rat lung injury involves activation of TGF-{beta} and Wnt signaling and is protected by rosiglitazone. *Am J Physiol Lung Cell Mol Physiol* (2009) 296(6):L1031–41. doi:10.1152/ajplung.90392.2008

107. Takeda K, Okamoto M, de Langhe S, Dill E, Armstrong M, Reisdorf N, et al. Peroxisome proliferator-activated receptor-g agonist treatment increases septation and angiogenesis and decreases airway hyperresponsiveness in a model of experimental neonatal chronic lung disease. *Anat Rec (Hoboken)* (2009) 292(7):1045–61. doi:10.1002/ar.20921

108. Ohki Y, Mayuzumi H, Tokuyama K, Yoshizawa Y, Arakawa H, Mochizuki H, et al. Hepatocyte growth factor treatment improves alveolarization in a newborn murine model of bronchopulmonary dysplasia. *Neonatology* (2009) 95(4):332–8. doi:10.1159/000187651

109. Couroucli XI, Liang YH, Jiang W, Wang L, Barrios R, Yang P, et al. Prenatal administration of the cytochrome P4501A inducer, Beta-naphthoflavone (BNF), attenuates hyperoxic lung injury in newborn mice: implications for bronchopulmonary dysplasia (BPD) in premature infants. *Toxicol Appl Pharmacol* (2011) 256(2):83–94. doi:10.1016/j.taap.2011.06.018

110. Ma L, Li N, Liu X, Shaw L, Li Calzi S, Grant MB, et al. Arginyl-glutamine dipeptide or docosahexaenoic acid attenuate hyperoxia-induced lung injury in neonatal mice. *Nutrition* (2012) 28(11–12):1186–91. doi:10.1016/j.nut.2012.04.001

111. James ML, Ross AC, Nicola T, Steele C, Ambalavanan N. VARA attenuates hyperoxia-induced impaired alveolar development and lung function in newborn mice. *Am J Physiol Lung Cell Mol Physiol* (2013) 304(11):L803–12. doi:10.1152/ajplung.00257.2012

112. Vosdoganes P, Lim R, Koulaeva E, Chan ST, Acharya R, Moss TJ, et al. Human amnion epithelial cells modulate hyperoxia-induced neonatal lung injury in mice. *Cytotherapy* (2013) 15(8):1021–9. doi:10.1016/j.jcyt.2013.03.004

113. Reilly EC, Martin KC, Jin GB, Yee M, O'Reilly MA, Lawrence BP. Neonatal hyperoxia leads to persistent alterations in NK responses to influenza A virus infection. *Am J Physiol Lung Cell Mol Physiol* (2015) 308(1):L76–85. doi:10.1152/ajplung.00233.2014

114. Bhandari A, McGrath-Morrow S. Long-term pulmonary outcomes of patients with bronchopulmonary dysplasia. *Semin Perinatol* (2013) 37(2):132–7. doi:10.1053/j.semperi.2013.01.010

115. Islam JY, Keller RL, Aschner JL, Hartert TV, Moore PE. Understanding the short- and long-term respiratory outcomes of prematurity and broncho-pulmonary dysplasia. *Am J Respir Crit Care Med* (2015) 192(2):134–56. doi:10.1164/rccm.201412-2142PP

116. Saarenpaa HK, Tikanmaki M, Sipola-Leppanen M, Hovi P, Wehkalampi K, Siltanen M, et al. Lung function in very low birth weight adults. *Pediatrics* (2015) 136(4):642–50. doi:10.1542/peds.2014-2651

117. Berger J, Mehta P, Bucholz E, Dziura J, Bhandari V. Impact of early extubation and reintubation on the incidence of bronchopulmonary dysplasia in neonates. *Am J Perinatol* (2014) 31(12):1063–72. doi:10.1055/s-0034-1371702

118. Naik AS, Kallapur SG, Bachurski CJ, Jobe AH, Michna J, Kramer BW, et al. Effects of ventilation with different positive end-expiratory pressures on cytokine expression in the preterm lamb lung. *Am J Respir Crit Care Med* (2001) 164(3):494–8. doi:10.1164/ajrccm.164.3.2010127

119. Ikegami M, Moss TJ, Kallapur SG, Mulrooney N, Kramer BW, Nitsos I, et al. Minimal lung and systemic responses to TNF-alpha in preterm sheep. *Am J Physiol Lung Cell Mol Physiol* (2003) 285(1):L121–9. doi:10.1152/ajplung.00393.2002

120. Copland IB, Martinez F, Kavanagh BP, Engelberts D, McKerlie C, Belik J, et al. High tidal volume ventilation causes different inflammatory responses in newborn versus adult lung. *Am J Respir Crit Care Med* (2004) 169(6):739–48. doi:10.1164/rccm.200310-1417OC

121. Kornecki A, Tsuchida S, Ondiveeran HK, Engelberts D, Frndova H, Tanswell AK, et al. Lung development and susceptibility to ventilator-induced lung injury. *Am J Respir Crit Care Med* (2005) 171(7):743–52. doi:10.1164/rccm.200408-1053OC

122. Lee PT, Holt PG, McWilliam AS. Role of alveolar macrophages in innate immunity in neonates: evidence for selective lipopolysaccharide binding protein production by rat neonatal alveolar macrophages. *Am J Respir Cell Mol Biol* (2000) 23(5):652–61. doi:10.1165/ajrcmb.23.5.4016

123. Lee PT, Holt PG, McWilliam AS. Ontogeny of rat pulmonary alveolar mac-rophage function: evidence for a selective deficiency in il-10 and nitric oxide production by newborn alveolar macrophages. *Cytokine* (2001) 15(1):53–7. doi:10.1006/cyto.2001.0894

124. Martin TR, Ruzinski JT, Wilson CB, Skerrett SJ. Effects of endotoxin in the lungs of neonatal rats: age-dependent impairment of the inflammatory response. *J Infect Dis* (1995) 171(1):134–44. doi:10.1093/infdis/171.1.134

125. Choo-Wing R, Nedrelow JH, Homer RJ, Elias JA, Bhandari V. Developmental differences in the responses of IL-6 and IL-13 transgenic mice exposed to hyperoxia. *Am J Physiol Lung Cell Mol Physiol* (2007) 293(1):L142–50. doi:10.1152/ajplung.00434.2006

126. Bhandari V, Choo-Wing R, Lee CG, Yusuf K, Nedrelow JH, Ambalavanan N, et al. Developmental regulation of NO-mediated VEGF-induced effects in the lung. *Am J Respir Cell Mol Biol* (2008) 39(4):420–30. doi:10.1165/rcmb.2007-0024OC

127. Bhandari V. Developmental differences in the role of interleukins in hyperoxic lung injury in animal models. *Front Biosci* (2002) 7:d1624–33. doi:10.2741/bhan

Etiologies of Hospitalized Acute Bronchiolitis in Children 2 Years of Age and Younger: A 3 Years' Study during a *Pertussis* Epidemic

Sainan Chen[1†], Yuqing Wang[1*], Anrong Li[1], Wujun Jiang[1†], Qiuyan Xu[2], Min Wu[1], Zhengrong Chen[1], Chuangli Hao[1], Xunjun Shao[1] and Jun Xu[1]

[1] *Department of Respiratory Medicine, Children's Hospital of Soochow University, Suzhou, China,* [2] *Department of Pediatrics, Affiliated Suzhou Science and Technology Town Hospital of Nanjing Medical University, Suzhou, China*

*Correspondence:
Yuqing Wang
wang_yu_qing@126.com

† These authors have contributed equally to this work

Objective: In recent years, the incidence of *Bordetella pertussis* infection in infants and young children has been increasing. Multiple studies have suggested that *B. pertussis* may be one of the pathogens of bronchiolitis in infants and young children. However, the prevalence and clinic characteristic of *B. pertussis* in bronchiolitis is controversial. This prospective descriptive study evaluated the prevalence and clinical manifestations of infants and young children hospitalized for bronchiolitis with *B. pertussis*.

Methods: Children hospitalized with bronchiolitis were eligible for a prospective study for 36 months from January 1, 2017, to December 31, 2019. Besides *B. pertussis*, 10 common respiratory viruses and *Mycoplasma pneumoniae* (MP) were confirmed by laboratory tests. Medical records of patients were reviewed for demographic, clinical characteristics, and laboratory examination.

Results: A total of 1,092 patients with bronchiolitis were admitted. *B. pertussis* was detected in 78/1,092 (7.1%) patients. Of the 78 patients with *B. pertussis* bronchiolitis, coinfections occurred in 45 (57.7%) patients, most frequently with human rhinovirus (28/78, 35.9%), followed by MP (9/78, 11.4%), and human bocavirus (6/78, 7.7%). The peak incidence of *B. pertussis* infection was in May. A high leukocyte count could help distinguish *B. pertussis*–associated acute bronchiolitis from other acute bronchiolitis etiologies. After excluding coinfections, children with *B. pertussis*–only bronchiolitis exhibited a milder clinical presentation than those with RSV-only infection; also, children with MP-only and other pathogen infections revealed similar severity. The morbidity of *B. pertussis* was common (31/78, 39.7%) in infants with bronchiolitis under 3 months.

Conclusion: In summary, *B. pertussis* is one of the pathogens in children with bronchiolitis, and coinfection of *B. pertussis* with other viruses is common in bronchiolitis. *B. pertussis* should be considered when patients hospitalized with bronchiolitis present a longer course and have an elevated leukocyte count. Patients with *B. pertussis*–associated bronchiolitis present a milder clinical presentation.

Keywords: *Bordetella pertussis*, bronchiolitis, coinfection, immunization, disease progression, high leukocyte count

INTRODUCTION

Pertussis, caused by the bacterium *Bordetella pertussis*, is a highly contagious respiratory disease and one of the leading causes of death from infectious diseases in children. *B. pertussis*, a Gram-negative bacterium that was first described by Bordet and Gengou in 1906 (1), has recently reemerged as a major public health threat. The World Health Organization reported 141,074 confirmed pertussis cases worldwide in 2018 (2). Approximately 160,700 deaths were reported worldwide in 2014 from pertussis in children <5 years of age (3).

Bronchiolitis is the most common acute respiratory disease in infants and young children, and one of the most common causes of hospital admission (4, 5). A total of 40–80% of infection is caused by respiratory syncytial virus (RSV), followed by human rhinovirus (HRV), adenovirus (ADV), parainfluenza virus, human bocavirus (hBoV), and human metapneumovirus (hMPV) (6, 7).

In recent years, several studies suggested that *B. pertussis* is a possible pathogen causing bronchiolitis in infants and young children hospitalized for lower respiratory tract infections (8–10). However, studies reporting the prevalence and clinical characteristics of *B. pertussis* bronchiolitis are rare. This study aimed to assess the epidemiological features and clinical characteristics of *B. pertussis* infection and evaluate its impact on infants and young children hospitalized with acute bronchiolitis.

MATERIALS AND METHODS

Patients and Definitions

This prospective descriptive study was conducted on children presenting with acute bronchiolitis who were admitted to the Department of Respiratory Medicine in the Children's Hospital of Soochow University between January 1, 2017, and December 31, 2019. Acute bronchiolitis was characterized by age ≤ 2, cough, tachypnea, retraction, and expiratory wheezes, often accompanied by rales (11). *B. pertussis* was confirmed by polymerase chain reaction (PCR) assays (12). Patients requiring oxygen supply were considered with severe conditions. The exclusion criteria were as follows: (1) patients with incomplete clinical data; (2) patients with bronchopulmonary dysplasia, heredity metabolic diseases, neurological disorders, congenital heart disease, and immunodeficiency; and (3) patients with evidence suggesting that wheezing was caused by tuberculosis and non-infectious factors such as bronchial foreign bodies.

The study was approved by the ethics committees of Children's Hospital Soochow University (Approval No. 2016026). Informed consent was obtained from the parents of all children enrolled in this study.

Determination of Vaccination Status

Vaccination history was obtained by querying the "Suzhou Children's Vaccination Inquiry and Evaluation Platform." A diphtheria, tetanus, and acellular pertussis combination vaccine was administered as a primary series at 3, 4, and 5 months, followed by a booster dose at 24 months in China. The

TABLE 1 | Gene primer sequence and product length detected by real-time PCR.

Gene name	Primer sequence products	Length
IS481	5′GATTCAATAGGTTGTATGCATGGTT3′	145
	5′TGGACCATTTCGAGTCGACG3′	
PtxA-pr	5′CCAACGCGCATGCGTGCAGATTCGTC3′	191
	5′CCCTCTGCGTTTGATGGTGCCTATTTTA3′	

vaccination status was regarded as ever-vaccinated if one to three doses were received.

Data Collection

Data regarding demographic, clinical, and laboratory characteristics were documented. Demographic and clinical characteristics included age, gender, length of hospital stay, and requirement of supplemental oxygen. Laboratory specimens were obtained including blood and nasopharyngeal aspirates (NPAs). NPAs were obtained during the first 24 h of hospitalization, using a sterile plastic catheter briefly inserted into the lower pharynx *via* the nasal cavity. The blood samples were taken immediately after hospitalization. The laboratory data of leukocyte count, percentages of lymphocytes and neutrophils, and detection of common viruses were collected.

PCR Detection of *B. pertussis*

B. pertussis DNA was detected in NPAs by real-time PCR assays. The primer sequence was synthesized by Shanghai Sangon Biotech Company. The pertussis PtxA-pr and IS481 gene sequences were used as specific primers (**Table 1**). The RT-PCR assay result was considered negative if the cycle threshold (CT) was ≥ 40. Specimens that tested positive by PCR for both insertion sequence IS481 (CT < 40) and ptxS1 (CT < 40) were considered positive for *B. pertussis*. If a specimen was PtxA-pr target negative with an IS481 assay CT <35, it was also considered positive for *B. pertussis*.

Respiratory Pathogens

Direct immunofluorescence was used to detect RSV; ADV; influenza virus A (IV-A) and B (IV-B); and parainfluenza virus 1 (PIV I), 2 (PIV II), and 3 (PIV III) using a D³ Ultra Respiratory Virus Screening and LD Kit (Diagnostic Hybrids, Athens, OH, USA). A positive result was defined as over five inclusion bodies analyzed under a fluorescence microscope. *Mycoplasma pneumoniae* (MP), HRV, HMPV, and HBoV were detected by a PCR (nucleic acid amplification fluorescent reagent kit, Ann Gene Co., Guangdong, China) according to the manufacturer's instructions.

Statistical Analyses

Statistical analyses were conducted using SPSS 26.0 (IBM, SPSS, Chicago, IL, USA).

Data were shown as mean $\pm$ standard deviation and median and interquartile range. Quantitative variables among the three age groups were compared using one-way analysis of variance or the Kruskal–Wallis test when appropriate. Frequency

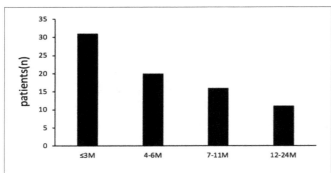

FIGURE 1 | Distribution of B. pertussis infection in infants and young children stratified by age.

distribution was compared by the chi-square test. A p value <0.05 was considered as a significant difference.

RESULTS
Demographic Characteristics
Of the total 1,092 patients admitted for bronchiolitis, one or more respiratory pathogens including virus and MP were detected in 1,057 of 1,092 patients (a positive rate of 96.8%) and B. pertussis was identified in 78 patients (7.1%, based on positive results by PCR). Of the 78 cases of bronchiolitis with B. pertussis infection, 47 (60.3%) were male and 31 (39.7%) were female. The male-to-female ratio was 1.52:1. The median age was 6.45 ± 4.94 months. The age distribution of patients is shown in **Figure 1**; 31 (39.7%) patients were aged ≤3 months, 20 (25.6%) patients were aged 4–6 months, 16 (20.5%) patients were aged 7–11 months, and 11 (14.1%) patients were aged ≥12 months.

Seasonality of B. pertussis Infection
The monthly distribution of B. pertussis infection is shown in **Figures 2A,B**. Bronchiolitis could occur throughout the year, and the peak incidence was in winter. The most common pathogen of bronchiolitis was RSV (534/1092, 48.9%), and the peak incidence was in December. MP was detected in 159/1,092 (14.6%) children with bronchiolitis, and the peak incidence was in September. Differing from the above two pathogens, the peak incidence of B. pertussis infection was in May, with a total of 10 (19.2%, 10/52) patients reported, and no patients were infected in October and December.

Coinfection Status
Overall, one or more respiratory pathogens including virus and MP were detected in 1,057 of 1,092 patients. The most commonly detected pathogens in patients with bronchiolitis were as follows: RSV (48.9%), HRV (25.9%), HMPV (13.0%), MP (14.6%), HBoV (12.1%), B. pertussis (7.1%), PIV III (7.0%), ADV (1.1%), and PIV I (1.1%).

Of the 78 B. pertussis-infected patients, B. pertussis was the sole pathogen detected in 33 (42.3%) patients. The remaining 45 patients (57.7%) were coinfected with other respiratory pathogens, most frequently with HRV ($n = 28$, 35.9%), followed by MP ($n = 9$, 11.4%), HBoV ($n = 6$, 7.7%), PIV III ($n = 4$, 5.1%), RSV ($n = 3$, 3.9%), IV-A ($n = 3$, 3.9%), and HMPV ($n = 2$, 2.6%) (**Figure 3**).

Clinical Features of B. pertussis–Only Infection Compared With Infections With Other Pathogens
In the present study, 33 patients with B. pertussis–only infection, 438 patients with RSV-only infection, 87 patients with MP-only infection, and 534 patients infected with other pathogens were analyzed. In unadjusted comparisons, children with B. pertussis–only infection were similar to children with RSV-only infection in age, but the number of children with age ≤ 3 months who were only infected with pertussis was less than that of children with RSV-only infection (**Table 2**). Children with B. pertussis–only infection were significantly more likely to have vomiting (36.4%), cyanosis (12.1%), leukocyte count >15 × 10^9 (57.6%), longer duration of symptoms before admission (media day, 14.0), and longer hospital stay (media day, 9.0) compared with those with RSV-only infection (17.8%, 2.7%, 7.5%, media 5.0, and 8.0 days, respectively; $p < 0.05$ for all comparisons). Patients with B. pertussis–only infection requiring supplement oxygen were fewer than patients with RSV-only infection (6.1 vs. 34.9%; $p < 0.05$).

In unadjusted comparisons, among 120 patients with B. pertussis and MP infections excluding co-detection with other pathogen types, children with B. pertussis–only infection were younger than children with MP-only infection (median 3.9 vs. 5.8 months, respectively) (**Table 2**). Children with B. pertussis–only infection were significantly more likely to have dyspnea (6.1%), rhinorrhea (15%), vomiting (15%), cyanosis (4%), and leukocyte count >15 × 10^9/L (57.6%) compared with those with MP-only infection (0.0, 24.1, 10.3, 0.0, and 6.9%, respectively; $p < 0.05$ for all comparisons). Children with B. pertussis–only infection had a higher number of leukocyte and higher percentage of lymphocyte compared with children with MP-only infection. Children with B. pertussis–only infection had a longer duration of hospital stay (median 9.0 days) than those with MP-only infection (median 8.0 days); however, no significant difference was observed in the duration of symptoms before admission.

B. pertussis Infection and Results of Laboratory Examination in Different Age Groups
B. pertussis–positive patients were divided into three age groups to assess the difference among different age groups (**Table 3**). A total of 31 patients aged ≤3 months, 36 patients aged 4–11 months, and 11 patients aged ≥12 months were analyzed. Patients aged ≤3 months had a longer duration of hospital stay than others ($p < 0.05$). The common clinic characteristics among the 78 confirmed patients were paroxysmal cough 92.3% (72/78), whoops 15.5% (12/78), post-tussive vomiting 38.5% (30/78), and cyanosis 12.8% (10/78). Patients with cyanosis aged ≤3 months were more compared with older ones ($p < 0.05$); the others exhibited no difference among three age groups ($p > 0.05$). Patients aged ≤3 months requiring supplemental oxygen were more compared

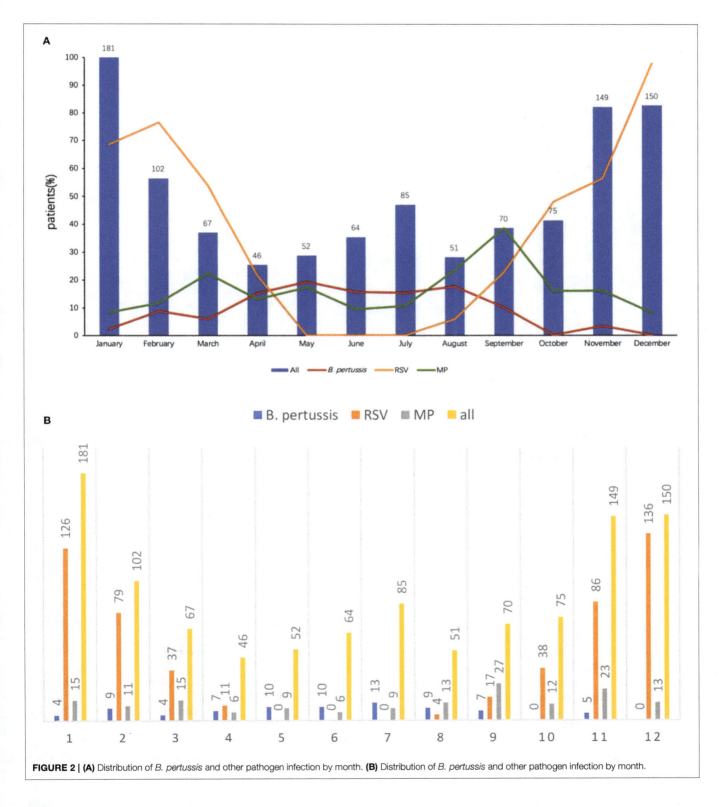

FIGURE 2 | (A) Distribution of B. pertussis and other pathogen infection by month. (B) Distribution of B. pertussis and other pathogen infection by month.

with older ones ($p < 0.05$). The gender ratio exhibited no significant difference among the three groups ($p < 0.05$). Coinfection among the three age groups was also compared, which showed no difference ($p > 0.05$). Although, patients aged ≥12 months had a higher number of leukocytes, and higher percentages of neutrophils and lymphocytes, no

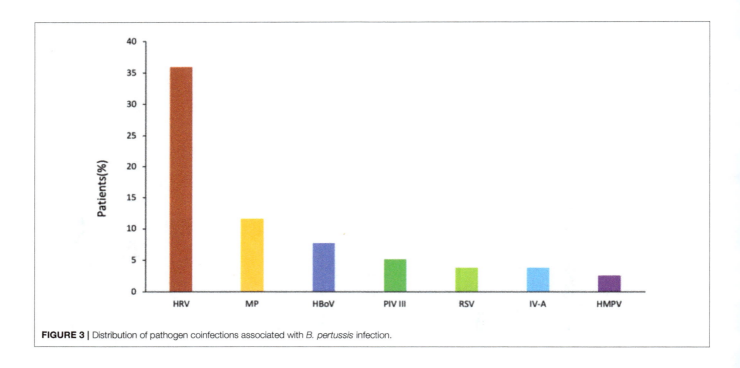

FIGURE 3 | Distribution of pathogen coinfections associated with *B. pertussis* infection.

significant difference was observed among the three groups ($p > 0.05$).

Clinical Features of *B. pertussis*–Only Infection Compared With Coinfection

Patients with *B. pertussis*-only infection were younger and had a high incidence of paroxysmal cough compared with patients with coinfection ($p < 0.05$). However, patients with coinfection had an increased demand for oxygen and showed more crackles in lungs ($p < 0.05$) (**Table 4**).

DISCUSSION

In recent years, an increasing incidence of pertussis has been reported in infants and young children (13). Several studies suggested that *B. pertussis* is a possible pathogen causing bronchiolitis in infants (8–10). Several investigators demonstrated that *B. pertussis* is a common pathogen of bronchiolitis (14, 15). A study conducted in Turkey identified 44 (25.6%) of the 172 infants with *B. pertussis* hospitalized for acute bronchiolitis (15). Another study showed *B. pertussis* involvement in 12 of 142 (8.5%) infants hospitalized for bronchiolitis in Finland (9). Yet other studies identified that *B. pertussis* was an uncommon pathogen in bronchiolitis (16). Pedro A. Piedra and his colleges found only four of 2,027 children admitted to the hospital as *B. pertussis* positive using PCR in the USA (10). Similarly, Walsh et al. found *B. Pertussis* infection in three of 488 patients (0.6%) in the emergency department (17). The present study found that 7.1% of infants and young children hospitalized with acute bronchiolitis had a positive *B. pertussis* test, which demonstrated that *B. pertussis* was a common pathogen in bronchiolitis. The variation in the prevalence of *B. pertussis* in children hospitalized with bronchiolitis among the studies might be due to the difference in climates, recruit criteria, and vaccination. According to the finding of this study, the peak incidence of *B. pertussis* infection was from May to July, with a total of 33 (50.15%) patients, which has not been reported before.

Studies reported that *B. pertussis* coinfection with other respiratory viruses was common in children hospitalized for bronchiolitis; the incidence rate was 36–67% (9, 14, 15, 18). However, the present study reported that 45 (57.7%) patients with *B. pertussis* were coinfected with other respiratory viruses, which was in agreement with previous studies. Some studies (6, 15, 19) suggested that coinfection with RSV was the most common in young children hospitalized for bronchiolitis with *B. pertussis* infection. However, in the present study, the most common coinfection respiratory viruses in children with *B. pertussis* hospitalized for bronchiolitis were HRV (35.9%), followed by MP (11.4%), and HBoV (7.7%); these differences in coinfection might be due to the heterogeneity of social demography and differences in study methods and periods.

Symptom duration before admission and hospital stay were more common in *B. pertussis*-only infection than in RSV-only infection ($p < 0.05$). It indicated that patients with *B. pertussis*-associated bronchiolitis often presented a longer course, which was consistent with the clinical symptoms of *B. pertussis* infection (20) and could help distinguish *B. pertussis*-associated acute bronchiolitis from other acute bronchiolitis etiologies. The present study compared *B. pertussis*-only infection with RSV-only infection in children with bronchiolitis. Children with *B. pertussis*-only infection requiring supplement oxygen

Etiologies of Hospitalized Acute Bronchiolitis in Children 2 Years of Age and Younger: A 3 Years' Study...

TABLE 2 | Select characteristics of hospitalized children with *B. pertussis*-only infection compared with RSV-only, MP-only, and other pathogens infection (*n* = 1,092).

	B. pertussis–only infection (*n* = 33)	RSV-only infection (*n* = 438)	*MP*-only infection (*n* = 87)	Other pathogens infection (*n* = 534)	*p*-value
Gender (male/female)	21/12	321/117	54/33	374/160	0.148
Median age, months	3.9 (2.5, 5.0)	2.8 (2.0, 4.9)	5.8 (3.0, 13.0)**	6.8 (3.7, 12.0)*	**<0.001**
Age group					
≤3 months	17 (51.5%)	300 (68.5%)**	30 (34.5%)	152 (28.5%)*	**<0.001**
4–6 months	10 (30.3%)	78 (17.8%)	18 (20.7%)	124 (23.2%)	0.107
7–11 months	4 (12.1%)	39 (8.9%)	12 (13.8%)	120 (22.5%)	**<0.001**
12–24 months	2 (6.1%)	21 (4.8%)	27 (31.0%)*	138 (25.8%)	**<0.001**
Duration of symptoms before admission (days)	14.0 (7.0, 15.0)	5.0 (4.0, 8.0)**	9.0 (5.0, 17.0)	10.0 (5.0, 15.0)	**0.001**
Duration of symptoms before admission group					
<7d *n* (%)	3 (9.1%)	285 (65.1%)*	30 (34.5%)*	200 (37.5%)*	**<0.001**
7–14d *n* (%)	12 (36.4%)	72 (16.4%)*	30 (34.5%)**	139 (26.0%)	**<0.001**
≥14d *n* (%)	17 (51.5%)	81 (18.5%)*	27 (31.0%)	195 (36.5%)	**<0.001**
Clinic presentation					
Cough	33 (100.0%)	430 (98.2%)	84 (96.6%)	529 (99.1%)	0.236
Dyspnea	2 (6.1%)	18 (4.1%)	0 (0.0%)**	54 (10.1%)	**<0.001**
Rhinorrhea	15 (45.5%)	195 (44.5%)	21 (24.1%)**	218 (40.8%)	**0.005**
Vomiting	12 (36.4%)	78 (17.8%)**	9 (10.3%)*	117 (21.9%)	**0.005**
Cyanosis *n* (%)	4 (12.1%)	12 (2.7%)*	0 (0.0%)*	36 (6.7%)	**<0.001**
O_2 requirement [*n* (%)]	2 (6.1%)	153 (34.9%)*	12 (13.8%)	100 (18.7%)	**<0.001**
Crackles *n* (%)	14 (42.4%)	291 (66.4%)*	54 (62.1%)	292 (54.7%)	**<0.001**
Laboratory findings					
Leukocyte count (× 109/L)	16.8 ± 6.7	9.0 ± 4.0*	9.5 ± 3.7*	11.3 ± 5.9*	**<0.001**
Leukocyte count >15 × 10^9	19 (57.6%)	33 (7.5%)*	6 (6.9%)*	106 (19.9%)*	**<0.001**
Lymphocyte count (%)	42.5 ± 28.6	60.8 ± 13.4*	48.2 ± 18.4	53.3 ± 24.4	**0.006**
Neutrophil count (%)	21.4 ± 21.7	32.9 ± 44.1	44.4 ± 18.6**	40.0 ± 21.0	**<0.001**
Hospital stay (day)	9.0 (7.0, 12.0)	8.0 (7.0, 9.3)**	8.0 (7.0, 9.0)**	8.0 (7.0, 10.0)	**0.011**

B. pertussis–only infection: detection of B. pertussis without coinfection with any other virus or MP; RSV-only: detection of RSV without coinfection with any other virus or B. pertussis; MP-only: detection of RSV without coinfection with any other virus or B. pertussis; other pathogens: pathogens excluding B. pertussis–only, RSV-only, and MP-only infection. Data are expressed as % of positive cases, mean (quartile), unless otherwise stated. p < 0.05 considered statistically significant, listed in bold text, and represents p values for comparisons across all groups. Asterisks indicate statistical significance (p < 0.05) in bivariate comparison (B. pertussis–only vs. RSV-only, MP-only, and other pathogens infection. **p < 0.008, *p < 0.05).

were fewer than children with RSV-only infection, indicating that the former had a milder clinical presentation compared with the latter. This study also compared *B. pertussis*–only infection with MP-only infection and infections with other pathogens in children and revealed similar severity among these pathogens. This is a novel report explaining such associations. Several other studies (9, 14, 15, 18, 20–22) assessed the influence of *B. pertussis* on acute bronchiolitis, but they could not exclude the possibility of other respiratory pathogens contributing to the illness. In the present study, the leukocyte count was higher in patients with *B. pertussis*–only bronchiolitis infection than that in patients with RSV-only infection, MP-only infection, and infections with other pathogens ($p < 0.008$ for all comparisons), which could also help distinguish *B. pertussis*–associated acute bronchiolitis from other acute bronchiolitis etiologies. One study showed that the leukocyte count $> 60 \times 10^9$/L was associated with death in children with *B. pertussis* infection (23). Another study

demonstrated that the leukocyte count $> 100 \times 10^9$/L was an independent risk factor of death in children with pertussis (24). However, no patent died of *B. pertussis* infection in the present study, which might be because the vast majority of infants and young children with mild-to-moderate bronchiolitis were considered, and severe bronchiolitis in the PICU setting was ignored.

Pertussis is a vaccine-preventable respiratory disease. *B. pertussis* could affect all individuals, but the highest morbidity and mortality rates were among newborns and unvaccinated or incompletely vaccinated young infants (21, 25, 26). In the present study, the morbidity of *B. pertussis* was common (31/78, 39.7%) in infants with bronchiolitis who had been unvaccinated (infants ≤3 months). The unvaccinated infants were associated with a longer hospital stay and more likely to require supplemental oxygen. Studies suggested that early identification and treatment of *B. pertussis* could shorten the duration of paroxysmal cough (27, 28),

TABLE 3 | Clinical characteristics and results of laboratory examination among the different age groups with *B. pertussis* infection.

	≤3 months (n = 31)	4-11 months (n = 36)	≥12 months (n = 11)	p-value
Clinical characteristics				
Hospital stay (day)	12.5 ± 6.69	9.91 ± 3.41	9 ± 1.56	0.049
Requirement for supplemental oxygen n (%)	10 (32.3%)	2 (5.6%)	1 (9.1%)	0.011
Paroxysmal cough n (%)	30 (96.8%)	33 (91.7%)	9 (81.8%)	0.237
Whoops n (%)	3 (9.7%)	9 (25.0%)	0 (0.0%)	0.076
Post-tussive vomiting n (%)	13 (41.9%)	12 (33.3%)	5 (45.5%)	0.694
Cyanosis n (%)	8 (25.8%)	2 (5.6%)	0 (0.0%)	0.030
Low oxygen saturation n (%)[a]	3 (9.7%)	2 (5.6%)	1 (9.1%)	0.728
Crackles n (%)	18 (58.1%)	27 (75.0%)	4 (36.5%)	0.051
Laboratory results				
Leukocyte count (× 10^9/L)	15.83 ± 6.58	17.72 ± 8.39	14.25 ± 5.52	0.356
Lymphocyte (%)	38.57 ± 28.89	51.42 ± 26.63	35.77 ± 25.29	0.102
Neutrophil (%)	22.31 ± 22.73	20.15 ± 14.76	24.70 ± 18.31	0.723

TABLE 4 | Comparison between *B. pertussis*–only infection and coinfection.

	B. pertussis–only infection (n = 33)	*B. pertussis* and virus coinfection (n = 45)	p-value
Gender (male) n (%)	21 (63.6%)	25 (55.6%)	0.473
Age ≤3 months n (%)	17 (51.5%)	12 (26.7%)	0.025
Vaccination	22 (66.7%)	27 (60.0%)	0.547
Oxygen n (%)	2 (6.1%)	11 (24.4%)	0.031
Paroxysmal cough n (%)	33 (100%)	39 (86.7%)	0.036
Whoops n (%)	6 (18.2%)	6 (13.3%)	0.558
Post-tussive vomiting n (%)	12 (36.4%)	18 (40%)	0.744
Cyanosis n (%)	4 (12.1%)	6 (13.3%)	0.874
Low oxygen saturation n (%)[a]	2 (6.1%)	4 (8.9%)	0.643
Crackles n (%)	14 (42.4%)	35 (77.8%)	0.001

B. pertussis–only infection: detection of B. pertussis without coinfection with any other virus or MP.
[a]*Low oxygen saturation is less than 92%.*

and antibiotics against pertussis could limit the severity of disease if started in the catarrhal phase (27, 29). In addition, several systematic reviews confirmed the safety and effectiveness of maternal pertussis vaccination during pregnancy (30–32). Therefore, it is important to early recognize and initiate treatment.

This study had potential limitations. It enrolled only inpatients hospitalized with *B. pertussis* infection, but more patients with *B. pertussis* infection were treated in the outpatient department. Therefore, patients with more severe symptoms might have been overrepresented, and the prevalence of *B. pertussis* in children with bronchiolitis-associated hospitalization might be affected.

In summary, *B. pertussis* is one of the pathogens in children with bronchiolitis, and coinfection of *B. pertussis* with other viruses is common in bronchiolitis. *B. pertussis* should be considered when patients hospitalized with bronchiolitis present a longer course and have an elevated leukocyte count. Patients with *B. pertussis*–associated bronchiolitis present a milder clinical presentation.

AUTHOR CONTRIBUTIONS

WJ and SC wrote the main manuscript text. CH and YW designed the study and revised the manuscript. ZC and MW carried out the initial analyses. XS and JX performed the microbiological detection. AL and QX performed the data collection. All authors read and approved the final manuscript.

REFERENCES

1. Bordet J, Gengou O. Le microbe de la coqueluche. *Ann. l'Institut Pasteur.* (1906) 20:731–741.
2. World Health Organization. *Immunization Vaccines and Biologicals: Pertussis* 2018 (2019). Available online at: https://www.who.int/immunization/monitoring_surveillance/burden/vpd/surveillance_type/passive/pertussis/en/.

3. Yeung K, Duclos P, Nelson E, Hutubessy R, Hutubessy RCW. An update of the global burden of pertussis in children younger than 5 years: a modelling study. *Lancet Infect Dis.* (2017) 17:974–80. doi: 10.1016/S1473-3099(17)30390-0
4. Carroll KN, Gebretsadik T, Griffin MR, Wu P, Dupont WD, Mitchel EF, et al. Increasing burden and risk factors for bronchiolitis-related medical visits in infants enrolled in a state health care insurance plan. *Pediatrics.* (2008) 122:58–64. doi: 10.1542/peds.2007-2087

5. Hasegawa K, Tsugawa Y, Brown D, Mansbach JM, Camargo CA. Trends in bronchiolitis hospitalizations in the United States, 2000-2009. *Pediatrics.* (2013) 132:28–36. doi: 10.1542/peds.2012-3877

6. Robledo-Aceves M, Moreno-Peregrina M, Velarde-Rivera F, Ascencio-Esparza E, Preciado-Figueroa FM, Caniza MA, et al. Risk factors for severe bronchiolitis caused by respiratory virus infections among Mexican children in an emergency department. *Medicine.* (2018) 97:e0057. doi: 10.1097/MD.0000000000010057

7. Cui D, Feng L, Chen Y, Lai S, Zhang Z, Yu F, et al. Clinical and epidemiologic characteristics of hospitalized patients with laboratory-confirmed respiratory syncytial virus infection in eastern China between 2009 and 2013: a retrospective study. *PLoS ONE.* (2016) 11:e0165437. doi: 10.1371/journal.pone.0165437

8. Heininger U, Burckhardt MA. Bordetella pertussis and concomitant viral respiratory tract infections are rare in children with cough illness. *Pediatr Infect Dis J.* (2011) 30:640–4. doi: 10.1097/INF.0b013e3182152d28

9. Nuolivirta K, Koponen P, He Q, Halkosalo A, Korppi M, Vesikari T, et al. Bordetella pertussis infection is common in nonvaccinated infants admitted for bronchiolitis. *Pediatr Infect Dis J.* (2010) 29:1013–5. doi: 10.1097/INF.0b013e3181f537c6

10. Piedra PA, Mansbach JM, Jewell AM, Thakar SD, Camargo CA. Bordetella pertussis is an uncommon pathogen in children hospitalized with bronchiolitis during the winter season. *Pediatr Infect Dis J.* (2015) 34:566–70. doi: 10.1097/INF.0000000000000596

11. Ralston SL, Lieberthal AS, Meissner HC, Alverson BK, Baley JE, Gadomski AM, et al. Clinical practice guideline: the diagnosis, management, and prevention of bronchiolitis. *Pediatrics.* (2014) 134:e1474–502. doi: 10.1542/peds.2014-2742

12. Cherry JD, Tan T, von König Carl-Heinz W, Forsyth KD, Usa T, David G, et al. Clinical definitions of pertussis: summary of a global pertussis initiative roundtable meeting, February 2011. *Clin Infect Dis.* (2012) 54:1756–64. doi: 10.1093/cid/cis302

13. Wood N, Mcintyre P. Pertussis: review of epidemiology, diagnosis, management and prevention. *Paediatr Respir Rev.* (2008) 9:201–11; quiz 211–2. doi: 10.1016/j.prrv.2008.05.010

14. Raya BA, Bamberger E, Kassis I, Kugelman A, Srugo I, Miron, et al. Bordetella pertussis infection attenuates clinical course of acute bronchiolitis. *Pediatr Infect Dis J.* (2013) 32:619–21. doi: 10.1097/INF.0b013e3182877973

15. Gökçe S, Kurugöl Z, Söhret Aydemir S, Çiçek C, Aslan A, Koturoglu G. Bordetella pertussis infection in hospitalized infants with acute bronchiolitis. *Indian J Pediatr.* (2018) 85:189–93. doi: 10.1007/s12098-017-2480-4

16. Efendiyeva E, Kara TT, Erat T, Yahi A, Ifti E. The incidence and clinical effects of Bordetella pertussis in children hospitalized with acute bronchiolitis. *Turk J Pediatr.* (2020) 62:726–33. doi: 10.24953/turkjped.2020.05.003

17. Walsh P, Overmeyer C, Kimmel L, Feola M, Adelson ME. Prevalence of Bordetella pertussis and Bordetella parapertussis in Samples Submitted for RSV screening. *West J Emerg Med.* (2008) 9:135–40.

18. Greenberg D, Bamberger E, Ben-Shimol S, Gershtein R, Srugo, I. Pertussis is under diagnosed in infants hospitalized with lower respiratory tract infection in the pediatric intensive care unit. *Med Sci Monit.* (2007) 13:CR475–480.

19. Sun H, Ji Y, Ji W, Hao C, Yan Y, Chen Z. Impact of RSV coinfection on human bocavirus in children with acute respiratory infections. *J Trop Pediatr.* (2019) 65:342–51. doi: 10.1093/tropej/fmy057

20. Melvin JA, Scheller EV, Miller JF, Cotter PA. Bordetella pertussis pathogenesis: current and future challenges. *Nat Rev Microbiol.* (2014) 12:274–88. doi: 10.1038/nrmicro3235

21. Somerville RL, Grant CC, Grimwood K, Murdoch D, Graham D, Jackson P, et al. Infants hospitalised with pertussis: estimating the true disease burden. *J Paediatr Child Health.* (2007) 43:617–22. doi: 10.1111/j.1440-1754.2007.01154.x

22. Jiang W, Wu M, Chen S, Li A, Xu J, Wang Y, et al. Share virus coinfection is a predictor of radiologically confirmed pneumonia in children with bordetella pertussis infection. *Infect Dis Ther.* (2020) 10:335–46. doi: 10.1007/s40121-020-00376-5

23. Paddock C, Sanden G, Cherry J, Langston C, Tatti K, Wu KH, et al. Pathology and pathogenesis of fatal bordetella pertussis infection in infants. *Clin Infect Dis.* (2008) 47:328–38. doi: 10.1086/589753

24. Pierce C, Klein N, Peters M. Is leukocytosis a predictor of mortality in severe pertussis infection? *Intens Care Med.* (2014) 26:1512–4. doi: 10.1007/s001340000587

25. Tanaka M, Vitek CR, Brain Pascual F, Bisgard KM, Tate JE, Murphy TV. Trends in pertussis among infants in the United States, 1980-1999. *JAMA.* (2003) 290:2968–75. doi: 10.1001/jama.290.22.2968

26. Masseria C, Martin CK, Krishnarajah G, Becker LK, Buikema A, Tan TQ, et al. Incidence and burden of pertussis among infants less than 1 year of age. *Pediatr Infect Dis J.* (2017) 36:e54–61. doi: 10.1097/INF.0000000000001440

27. Carlsson R, Segebaden KV, Bergstrom J, Kling A, Nilsson, L. Surveillance of infant pertussis in Sweden 1998-2012: severity of disease in relation to the national vaccination programme. *Euro Surveill.* (2015) 20:21032. doi: 10.2807/1560-7917.ES2015.20.6.21032

28. Tiwari TS BA, Clark TA. First pertussis vaccine dose and prevention of infant mortality. *Pediatrics.* (2015) 135:990–9. doi: 10.1542/peds.2014-2291

29. Bergquist SO, Brenander S, Dahnsjö H, Sundelöf B. Erythromycin in the treatment of pertussis- a study of bacteriologic and clinical effects. *Pediatr Infect Dis J.* (1987) 6:458–61. doi: 10.1097/00006454-198705000-00009

30. Switzer C, D'Heilly C, Macina D. Immunological and clinical benefits of maternal immunization against pertussis: a systematic review. *Infect Dis Ther.* (2019) 8:499–541. doi: 10.1007/s40121-019-00264-7

31. Heilly CD, Switzer C, Macina D. Safety of maternal immunization against pertussis: a systematic review. *Infect Dis Ther.* (2019) 8:543–68. doi: 10.1007/s40121-019-00265-6

32. Ashish A, Sanjeev S, Kolhapure S, Kandeil W, Pai R, Singhal T. Neonatal pertussis, an under-recognized health burden and rationale for maternal immunization: a systematic review of south and South-East Asian Countries. *Infect Dis Ther.* (2019) 8:139–53. doi: 10.1007/s40121-019-0245-2

16

Affect of Early Life Oxygen Exposure on Proper Lung Development and Response to Respiratory Viral Infections

William Domm [1,2]*, Ravi S. Misra[1] and Michael A. O'Reilly [1,2]

[1] Department of Pediatrics, School of Medicine and Dentistry, The University of Rochester, Rochester, NY, USA, [2] Department of Environmental Medicine, School of Medicine and Dentistry, The University of Rochester, Rochester, NY, USA

*Correspondence:
William Domm,
Department of Pediatrics, School of
Medicine and Dentistry, The
University of Rochester, 601
Elmwood Avenue, Box 850,
Rochester, NY 14642, USA
william_domm@urmc.rochester.edu

Children born preterm often exhibit reduced lung function and increased severity of response to respiratory viruses, suggesting that premature birth has compromised proper development of the respiratory epithelium and innate immune defenses. Increasing evidence suggests that premature birth promotes aberrant lung development likely due to the neonatal oxygen transition occurring before pulmonary development has matured. Given that preterm infants are born at a point of time where their immune system is also still developing, early life oxygen exposure may also be disrupting proper development of innate immunity. Here, we review current literature in hopes of stimulating research that enhances understanding of how the oxygen environment at birth influences lung development and host defense. This knowledge may help identify those children at risk for disease and ideally culminate in the development of novel therapies that improve their health.

Keywords: hyperoxia, influenza A virus, innate immunity, lung development, prematurity

Introduction

Growing evidence suggest gene–environment interactions during critical stages of development profoundly influence health later in life. This concept of "developmental origins of health and disease," also called DOHaD, originated with a study by Dr. David Barker who showed that low birth weight correlated with increased risk of coronary heart disease in adults (1). DOHaD has now been linked to a wide variety of diseases in children and adults. Preterm birth, infection, tobacco smoke, and exposure to many inhaled pollutants can permanently impact lung development and immune function (2–4). Similarly, exposure to exogenous chemicals, malnutrition, and low birth weight correlates with poorer immune function (5–8). Even socioeconomic status and child abuse have been shown to influence a healthy lifestyle later in life (9). In 1983, the comedy movie *Trading Places* starring Dan Aykroyd and Eddie Murphy "tested" whether nature or nurture were responsible for distinguishing social hierarchy between two individuals. Although the question was never resolved in the movie, we are now beginning to appreciate 30 years later that gene–environment interactions influence children's health, in part, through metabolic and epigenetic reprograming of cells required for organ growth, regeneration, and immunity.

The human lung is designed to efficiently exchange oxidant gases between the environment and blood, and exclude or defend against inhaled pollutants that otherwise disrupts this process. When considering gene–environment interactions that influence lung function, the transition to air at birth must surely be one of the most profound environmental changes that one will ever experience. In this singular moment, the delivery of oxygen and nutrients via the placenta is transferred, respectively, to the lung and gut. Both organs must therefore be developmentally mature and functional by this time. Proper development of the lung involves a complex set of transcription factors, morphogens, growth factors, and matrix molecules be expressed during precise developmental windows (10–13). Expression profiling studies have defined a pattern of gene expression wherein developmental genes are expressed first and genes involved in oxygen transport, protection against reactive oxygen species, and host defense are expressed near birth (14, 15). This "time-to-birth" program ensures that the lung is ready to breathe air and defend against environmental toxins at birth.

The interaction of genes with the oxygen environment at birth is disrupted when infants are born too soon. Many preterm infants develop bronchopulmonary dysplasia, a chronic form of lung disease characterized by alveolar simplification and restrictive airways (16). Mechanisms that promote BPD include genetics and maternal, fetal, or postnatal environments (17). It has been difficult to define which is most important for initiating or promoting disease, perhaps because BPD is clinically defined by the amount of oxygen used at a specific gestational age (18, 19). Fortunately, most preterm infants born >24 weeks gestation are surviving, albeit at the risk of developing a variety of lung and non-lung diseases later in life. Children born preterm often display reduced lung function, increased re-hospitalization following a respiratory viral infection, and incidence of non-atopic asthma (20, 21). They may also show neurodevelopmental delay and have greater risk for high blood pressure and heart disease as adults (22, 23). The annual cost of treating children in the United States who were born prematurely in 2005 was $26.2 billion dollars, of which 10% was just for treating infants with BPD (http://www.nhlbi.nih.gov/new/press/06-07-26.htm). Hence, there is an urgent need to understand how premature birth is a developmental antecedent of poorer health later in life.

The pathogenesis of BPD and the health sequela of survivors is a complex and poorly understood process, perhaps because it is a multi-organ disease originating from abnormal gene–environment interactions. Recognizing that there is a genetic program designed to create the lung and afford it anti-oxidant and innate immune defenses by birth, it seems rather obvious that preterm birth will disrupt the timing of when specific genetic programs need to be completed or in place to properly allow the lung to transition to an oxygen-rich environment. Therefore, identifying genetic variants that predispose to preterm birth may also identify variants that correlate with BPD. A screen of single-nucleotide polymorphisms identified two genes (CRHR1 and CYP2E1) acting in the fetus and four genes (ENPP1, IGFBP3, DHCR7, and TRAF2) in the mother that predisposes to preterm birth (24). But, interestingly none of these genes have been detected in other studies seeking to find variants that predispose preterm infants to BPD (25, 26). In fact, the few weak candidates detected in one study were not detected in another, suggesting that BPD is not entirely a genetic disorder. On the other hand, widespread methylation was detected in the blood of extremely preterm infants, suggesting that there were changes in blood cell development,

composition, and perhaps immune function (27). Since these changes in methylation resolved by 18 years of age, they may not be responsible for the long-term health effects reported in people born preterm. Therefore, genetic susceptibility to BPD is more likely to represent genetic variants that modify how cells respond to an environmental stress, such as infection or the transition to air too soon.

Environmental stresses known to promote BPD include prenatal and postnatal infections, and oxygen or ventilator-induced damage to the lung. In both cases, inflammation and oxidative stress or damage to the developing lung seems to be a primary driver of BPD. Preterm infants are deficient in anti-oxidant enzymes and are therefore susceptible to oxidative stress, whether initiated by inflammation or supplemental oxygen therapies in the preterm infant (28, 29). Lungs of preterm infants are often underdeveloped and cannot adequately exchange oxygen and carbon dioxide. Supplemental oxygen supported by ventilation is often used to improve blood oxygen levels and prevent hypoxemia. However, it is now clear that high levels of oxygen can disrupt development of the lung and is a risk factor for neurodevelopmental delay, retinopathy, and probably other diseases attributed to preterm birth (30). Oxygen-induced damage can also elicit an inflammatory response, subsequently compounding the oxidative stress to the lung. Consistent with oxygen playing a role in the pathogenesis of BPD and the long-term respiratory complications associated with preterm birth, anti-oxidant therapies have proven partially effective in alleviating lung disease in humans and in animals exposed to high oxygen (31–34). Because the pathogenesis of neonatal oxygen exposure in humans and in animal models has been recently reviewed (19, 35–40), the following discusses oxygen-induced changes in lung development in relationship to how it also perturbs host response to respiratory viral infections.

Proper Lung Development

The pulmonary system, in highly simplistic form, can be described as the co-branching of air conducting and blood circulating systems that, due to simultaneous and congruent branching, efficiently interact for proper gas-exchange and subsequent systemic circulation of oxygen. In humans, gas-exchange is accomplished by diffusion through squamous epithelial cells in the alveolar saccules of the mature lung. Branching morphogenesis of the airways that concludes with formation of the alveolus leads to an impressive pulmonary surface area of around 70 square meters with a thickness of 0.1 um capable of supporting an oxygen consumption of 250–5500 ml/min (41, 42). This developmental program progresses through five successive stages. The mammalian lung undergoes five stages of maturation that begin with the embryonic stage, followed by the pseudoglandular, canalicular, saccular, and ending with the alveolar stage (**Figure 1**). The timing of these stages during fetal and postnatal periods varies between species, including between humans and mice. This is important when attempting to model human diseases in experimental animals. For example, many preterm infants born today are in the saccular phase of lung development, which pathologically corresponds to e17.5 to postnatal day 4 in mice. Hence, the mouse

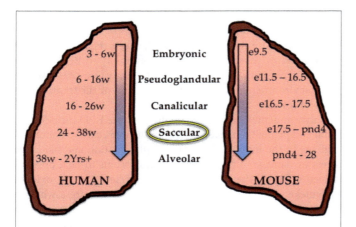

FIGURE 1 | **Stages of lung development in the human and mouse.** During development, the human (mouse) lung undergoes five successive stages of development; The Embryonic stage 3–6 weeks (e9.5–11.5), the Pseudoglandular stage 6–16 weeks (e11.5–16.5), the Canalicular stage 12–26 weeks (e16.5–17.5), the Saccular stage 24–38 weeks (e17.5–PND4), and the Alveolar stage 38 weeks–2+ years (PND4–28). Preterm children who survive are often born between 24 and 38 weeks of age and are in the saccular stage of development (circled) corresponding to the saccular stage in the mouse from e17.5–PND4.

is an appropriate experimental model for studying how too much oxygen can perturb saccular development in preterm humans. Additional details on factors controlling lung development have been reviewed elsewhere (10, 12, 41, 43).

Successive developmental stages are defined by changes in lung morphology. In the embryonic stage, the pulmonary branching pattern originates and two distinct lobes are formed. The pseudoglandular stage marks the appearance of numerous terminal buds projecting away from the initial two lung lobes and recent work has defined the patterns as domain branching, planar, and orthogonal bifurcation budding (44). During the canalicular stage, epithelial tubules form with large terminal buds while the mesenchyme separates into dense subsets between future alveolar septa. Specialized epithelial cell types and alveolar sacs emerge during the saccular stage of development. Squamous type I epithelial cells form the lining of the alveolar sacs with cuboidal type II epithelial cells interspersed. Thinning of the mesenchyme along with an increase in extracellular matrix allows for expansion of these alveolar sacs culminating in the alveolar stage where dense connective tissue, containing cartilage and smooth muscle, surrounds the airways. The timing of developmental completion, leading to the formation of alveolar sacs, varies between species. In mice and rats, alveolar development concludes mainly postnatally characterized by lung expansion and alveoli subdividing into smaller gas-exchanging units (45). Importantly, this morphogenic process has been accompanied by blood vessel morphogenesis that concludes with capillary networks residing in close proximity to the alveolar epithelium.

It is often written that the normal adult mammalian lung contains approximately 40 different cell types, yet the origin of this statement seems to have disappeared in the historical literature. However, it should not be surprising to find that this is a gross underestimation when one considers how expression of cell surface receptors has markedly increased the diversity of leukocytes present in the lung (46). The emerging use of microfluidic single-cell RNA sequencing is also uncovering an equally rich diversity among non-hematopoietic cell populations (47, 48). Pulse-chase labeling with H-thymidine, cell-restricted fluorescent reporter genes, and cell-specific ablation with toxins has identified region-specific niches containing stem cells required for proper lung development and repair (49). Unique specific stem cell niches may therefore have evolved to facilitate repair of specific areas of the lung damaged by region-specific toxins. Since perinatal exposures influence saccular and alveolar phases of development, the following briefly focuses on progenitor cells controlling distal airway and alveolar development and regeneration.

The region where the airway meets the alveolus has been termed the bronchoalveolar duct junction (BADJ) (50). The distal airway epithelium contains Clara (now called Club) cells defined by their cuboidal appearance and expression of secretoglobin family 1A, member 1 (Scgb1a1), also called Clara Cell Secretory Protein (CCSP) or uteroglobin. During recovery from naphthalene depletion, a population of Club cells proliferates from neuroendocrine bodies and from the BADJ (51, 52). These bronchoalveolar stem cells (BASC) express airway Scgb1a1, alveolar Type II surfactant protein (SP)-C, the stem cell markers Sca-1, and CD34, but not CD45 (53). These BASCs are able to self-renew and maintain expression of both airway Scgb1a1 and alveolar SP-C expression when cultured on irradiated mouse embryonic fibroblasts. However, their importance in defining airway and alveolar epithelial cell development and repair remains unclear because they proliferate less frequently than Type II cells in a post-pneumonectomy model of lung regeneration (54).

A label-retaining population of airway cells expressing Scgb1a1 and the stem cell markers Oct-4, Sca-1, and SSEA-1 has also been identified in BADJ (55). These cells can be maintained *ex vivo* for several weeks, but have the capacity to express SP-C and T1α when cultured on Type I collagen. Fate-mapping studies using Scgb1a1-driven reverse transcriptional transactivator (rtTA) gene or Cre fused to an estrogen responsive binding site (CreER) gene to durably label Scgb1a1+ cells with LacZ or fluorescent proteins has provided new insight into the ability of airway Scgb1a1+ progenitors to repopulate alveolar cells. Depending upon the model and the timing of activation, airway Scgb1a1+ progenitors contribute to ~10–50% of adult type II cells during normal postnatal lung development (56–60). These cells also contribute to alveolar repair when adult mice are infected with Influenza A Virus (IAV) or injured with bleomycin, both of which damage alveolar type II cells (59). Interestingly, they do not participate in repair when mice are exposed to hyperoxia or naphthalene (58). Since hyperoxia injures alveolar type I cells, and naphthalene injures airway Club cells, these two studies suggest Scgb1a1+ cells may serve as precursors for themselves and type II cells.

Analogous to studies using naphthalene to ablate airway Clara cells, exposure of adult mice, rats, or monkeys to oxidant gases (hyperoxia, ozone, or nitrogen dioxide) kills alveolar type I epithelial cells (61–63). Pulse-chase labeling studies with H-thymidine indicate type II epithelial cells proliferate and differentiate into type I cells following injury (64–66). Emerging evidence suggests that subpopulations of type II cells exist and T1α, a protein expressed by Type I cells, has been shown to co-localize with the Type II cell-specific lectin Maclura pomifera (67). Tri-transgenic mice containing the rat airway CCSP promoter driving rtTA, the otet-Cre gene, and the LacZ/EGFP (Z/EG) reporter identified a lineage of epithelial cells that defines airway Club and a small population of alveolar Type II cells (68). Recently, single-cell RNA sequencing revealed the existence of four distinct populations of type II cells (48). Alveolar type I cells have historically be thought to be the most terminally differentiated cell of the lung whose sole function was to facilitate gas-exchange and maintain barrier function (64–66). However, a study showing that type I cells isolated from rats can proliferate *ex vivo*, express the stem cell protein Oct-4, and can be induced to express SP-C and Scgb1a1 has challenged this conclusion (69).

Pulmonary Response to Influenza A Infection

As the lung evolved to efficiently exchange oxygen and carbon dioxide, so did an innate immune system comprised of specialized epithelial resident cells and circulating immune cells that function to recognize and clear a variety of inhaled pathogens and toxicants. Failure to detoxify the airspace can result in significant disease and even death. These defenses are most likely designed to respond to inhaled pathogens, like respiratory viruses, which were present in the environment before vertebrates migrated onto land. We therefore will discuss the current understanding of the pulmonary interactions with respiratory infections, primarily focusing on IAV, in an attempt to build a greater understanding of the poor response experienced by children born prematurely.

Viral respiratory infections have been found to afflict preterm infants at a higher rate than full term controls. Respiratory Syncytial Virus (RSV), human Rhinovirus (RV), and Bocavirus infection of children less than 14 years of age hospitalized over a 7-year study period were described (70). The authors found that children who were preterm exhibited a higher rate of infection with human metapneumovirus and parainfluenza virus as compared to controls (70). Additionally, a recent study describes extremely and moderately preterm infants facing a 3.6 times increased risk of being hospitalized due to respiratory infection, likely from RSV or RV, in the first year of life (71). Preterm infants hospitalized due to RSV were found more likely to wheeze in the first six years of life and experience decreased quality of life versus those infants who were not hospitalized due to RSV infection (72). RV infection of preterm infants also increases the risk of developing wheeze and requiring respiratory medicines in the first year of life, and can be the source of serious lower respiratory tract infections (73–76). A recent NHLBI workshop report recommends identifying prophylactic approaches to prevent RSV and RV infections to help lessen the burden of asthma development in childhood (77), however determining when the use of such prophylaxis is complicated (78). Thus, infants born preterm face serious consequences in response to respiratory viral infections.

In human pediatric populations, RSV is more common in infancy (first two years of life) while IAV is generally more common in school age children (79, 80). Gaining a better understanding of how early life oxygen exposure affects responses to respiratory viral infections necessitates the use of animal models. While different species have shown utilization in RSV modeling, each has advantages and disadvantages (81, 82). Human RSV does not efficiently replicate and leads to non-significant disease and mortality in mouse models, making it difficult to model how it is perturbed in preterm children (82). This is in contrast to IAV mouse models that have proven robust viral replication and disease that closely model human disease. Here, neonatal oxygen exposures that have been shown to promote BPD-like lung disease in mice have also been shown to alter the response to IAV infection (35). Understanding how the oxygen environment at birth disrupts the host response to IAV may provide insight into how it influences the response to RSV and other respiratory viruses.

IAV annually causes global seasonal epidemics but also novel IAV occasionally arise leading to global pandemics. The most notorious of which was the pandemic of 1918 and the most recent the 2009 swine-flu pandemic (83). Significant insight into IAV–host interactions has historically occurred through *in vitro* investigations. A much greater understanding of this virus–host interaction, prior to, during, and following significant pathological outcomes *in vivo*, has been hampered due to a lack of traceable reporter expressing IAV that retain full virulence as well as other technical problems. Recently, IAV–host interactions and *in vivo* dynamics following infection have been investigated utilizing reporter expressing recombinant IAV (84, 85).

The first step in IAV infection involves the recognition of sialic-acid (SA) moieties on the surface of susceptible cells by the viral hemagglutinin (HA) protein. Human IAV primarily infect via α2-6 SA residues and avian IAV by α2-3 linked residues. In healthy humans, α2-6 SA has been primarily found on the epithelial (ciliated and non-ciliated) and goblet cells of the upper respiratory tract in humans (86). Avian like α2-3 SA has primarily been found on non-ciliated bronchiolar and alveolar type II cells in the lower respiratory tract (86, 87). Viral attachment and histochemical studies have revealed human IAV primarily interacting with the upper respiratory tract through ciliated epithelial cells, goblet cells, as well as to type I alveolar epithelial cells, to varying extents (86–89). Contrasting with human IAV, avian IAV has been shown to primarily attach to alveolar epithelial type II cells, alveolar macrophages, and bronchiolar non-ciliated epithelial cells (89, 90). Sialic-acid receptor expression is a good correlate of IAV binding based upon histochemical studies. Although human IAV is of primary concern for understanding infection of the population discussed in this review, understanding avian IAV infection is imperative in the face of novel viruses entering the human population.

Both human and avian IAV can infect human airway epithelial cultures with human IAV preferentially target non-ciliated airway cells whereas avian IAV infect ciliated populations (91, 92). Alveolar type II cells have also been demonstrated as a site of IAV infection and replication although their importance to human disease is currently unclear. Human alveolar type II cells were infected by IAV in a primary cell culture system (93). Alveolar type II cells are imperative for the maintenance of the alveoli by producing and secreting surfactant as well as being a renewable source for themselves and type I alveolar cells. Although poorly understood, the affect of IAV infection of type II cells has been shown to affect their phenotype and subsequent innate immune responses (93). Taken together, IAV tropism as it relates to human disease requires further investigation. Differences based on the strain of IAV used and type of assay utilized must be clarified for a greater understanding of human disease.

The source of cells responsible for pulmonary regeneration following viral injury is currently an active area of research. Bronchiolar epithelial cells expressing p63 were found to rapidly expand and disseminate to areas of lung injury following IAV infection and repair (94). This cell population was also found to have the ability to form "pods" in both bronchiolar as well as alveolar regions following injury caused by IAV. Keratin 5 expression (Krt5) was also shown to map to these regions and, importantly, was only detected following IAV infection, during reparative processes (94). These p63/Krt5 + cell populations therefore may act as distal airway stem cells and serve as the source for alveoli cell regeneration following injury and recently these p63/Krt5 + cells were found to recapitulate alveoli following epithelial injury by IAV (95). This unique population also has the ability to form alveoli-like structures when delivered to IAV-infected lungs minimizing virus-induced pathology (95).

Oxygen Perturbation of Proper Lung Development and Innate Immunity

As discussed previously, the transition to an oxygen environment at birth may be one of the most profound environmental changes one will ever experience and can lead to disease when it occurs inappropriately. Lungs of infants born preterm are often in the saccular phase of development. Alveolar regions at this time have yet to develop into true gas-exchanging structures, which is why many preterm infants develop respiratory distress. Furthermore, the capillary network surrounding the alveolus, which shuttles oxygen to the circulation, has yet to effectively complement the alveolus (96). Despite the life-saving efficacy of supplemental oxygen treatment during this critical time, growing evidence suggests that this treatment contributes to bronchopulmonary dysplasia (BPD), a chronic lung disease that is characterized by alveolar simplification and restrictive airways (16, 30). Oxygen-dependent changes in genes specifying lung structure and cell phenotype are likely to impact cells and molecules involved in innate immunity required for a proper host response to respiratory viral infection (**Figure 2**). This includes alveolar epithelial type II cells, goblet cells, eosinophils, macrophages, dendritic cells, T cells, B cells, and innate lymphoid cells, in addition to soluble mediators produced by these cells, including SPs, cytokines, chemokines, and mucus proteins mediate innate immunity (97–100). In other words, early life oxygen exposure or other oxidative stresses may drive the development of long-term lung disease by disrupting a delicate balance of cell communication between genes controlling lung development and innate immunity.

One hallmark of supplemental oxygen treatment at birth is the development of a highly simplified alveolar epithelium. Although incompletely understood, this may develop due to oxidative stress

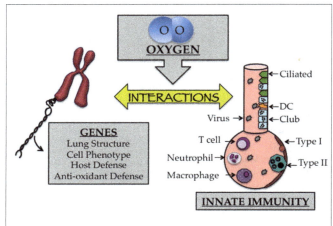

FIGURE 2 | The early life oxygen environment affects changes in genetic as well as innate immune mechanisms. Cartoon depicting the affect early life oxygen environment imparts on genes that specify lung structure and function with cells involved in innate immunity.

or an aberrant immune response that suppresses angiogenic factors (101). In mice, alveolar epithelial type II cells expand rapidly following neonatal hyperoxia compared to room air control littermates (102, 103). Following recovery in room air however, this population is significantly pruned (102, 103). This results in a significant decrease in the pool of alveolar type II cells later in life. Concomitant with the loss of type II cells, markers for type I alveolar epithelial cells increase during the same time frame. Currently, the source of these cells is unclear; however, evidence suggests that type II alveolar cells lost during recovery in room air are not the source of these cells (102). Further fate-mapping studies of type II and type I cells during and following exposure to hyperoxia should help to clarify the intricate balance and source of these cells. Regardless, the loss of type II cells may adversely impact alveolar repair as well as the production of innate immunity. Indeed, adult mice exposed to hyperoxia exhibit persistent and altered immune responses, fibrosis (**Figure 3**), and increased mortality compared to room air littermates when infected with a sublethal dose of IAV (32, 104, 105). The altered host response was not attributable to CD8 T cells and therefore the pathology is not likely due to a defect in viral clearance (106). While reduced numbers of type II cells did not negatively impact surfactant pools (107), it reduced expression of the antiviral protein eosinophil-associated RNase 1 (Ear1) detected in some type II cells (104). Reduced expression of Ear1, while conceptually attractive, does not solely account for the fibrotic phenotype observed in IAV-infected mice that have been previously exposed to hyperoxia as neonates. This is because neonatal hyperoxia has also been shown to enhance the severity of fibrosis in the neonatal hyperoxia model following bleomycin administration (108). Hypothetically, the loss of some type II cells may impact the orderly innate immune response releasing cytokines, chemokines, and SPs that are the first responders following IAV infection (109).

One example is monocyte chemoattractant protein-1 (MCP-1), which has been found to be selectively increased following IAV infection in a model of neonatal hyperoxia (105, 110). MCP-1 plays important roles in the recruitment of monocytes, T cells,

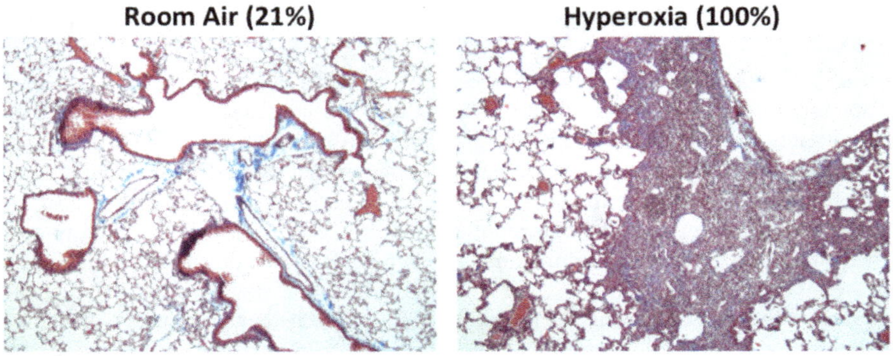

FIGURE 3 | Mice exposed to hyperoxia at birth develop fibrosis after influenza A infection. Adult (8-week old) C57Bl/6J mice exposed to room air (21% oxygen) or hyperoxia (100% oxygen) between postnatal days 0–4 were infected with 120 HAU of influenza A virus (H3N2).

Trichrome staining revealed extensive collagen deposition and inflammation in infected mice exposed to neonatal hyperoxia 14 days post infection. This pathology was not evidence in infected siblings exposed to room air at birth.

and NK cells to sites of infection and has been shown to protect against viral and bacterial challenges (111, 112). However, aberrant MCP-1 control has also been associated with lung disease in children and adults (113, 114). While MCP-1 is an attractive target, it has recently been shown that MCP-1 is not solely responsible for the enhanced respiratory sequelae observed following IAV infection in neonatal hyperoxia-treated mice (105). This suggests that increased MCP-1 production may be an effect rather than a driver of the mechanisms leading to enhanced respiratory disease due to neonatal oxygen exposure.

In addition to an imbalance in alveolar type II cells, there are many other pulmonary innate immune mechanisms that might be affected by oxygen at birth. Animal models have identified several innate immune factors common in BPD-like lung injury. These include alterations in IL-6, IL-8, TNF-α, TGF-β, macrophage inflammatory factor-1α, IL-1β, MCP-1 MCP-2, CXCL-1, and CXCL-2 (115). Recent work also has identified mast cells as being present in the lungs of pediatric subjects who were diagnosed with BPD prior to death (100). Members of the IL-6 cytokine family have been shown to have fibrotic potential, which could contribute to lung disease (116). The compliment subunit C5a plays a role in neutrophil recruitment to the mouse lung following IAV infection and may be a potent inducer of hyperoxia-mediated lung injury via recruitment of macrophages, neutrophils, and lymphocytes, and increased expression of IL-6, TNF-α, and MCP-1 occurs (117, 118). Furthermore, C5a has been shown to increase TGF-β1 in primary human small airway epithelial cells, which could then contribute to the development of fibrosis (119). Thus, multiple factors could lead to the accumulation of C5a, which could induce inflammation in the lungs of preterm infants. Some of these factors have been proposed targets to prevent the development or to treat patients with BPD (120).

Several recent studies illustrated effects that hyperoxic stress imparts on the innate immune system. For instance, macrophages exposed to hyperoxic conditions experience cell cycle arrest and showed impaired phagocytic and chemotactic activity (121, 122). GM-CSF is critical for the maintenance of alveolar macrophages and hyperoxic stress has been demonstrated to decrease levels of

GM-CSF via destabilization of mRNA in primary AEC cell cultures (123). Other studies indicate that the decrease in GM-CSF mRNA is due to upregulation of the microRNA molecule, miRNA 33 (124). This same publication illustrates the complex nature of hyperoxia by demonstrating that T cells actually up-regulate GM-CSF in response to hyperoxic stress (124). Taken together, this highlights the critical importance of macrophage balance on phenotype.

Macrophages have been shown to play a role in the development of alveoli (125). If these cells become more inflammatory in nature, such as experienced due to hyperoxic stress, they likely will contribute to lung pathology (126). A recent study illustrates that overexpression of TGF-β1 in the lung leads to the accumulation of inflammatory macrophages in a TGFβR2-dependent manner (127). Given the role for alveolar macrophages in activating T cells, it is possible that regulatory function of CD4 T cells could be compromised by pro-inflammatory macrophages found in the lung (128). In fact, active research is being conducted to try and target inflammatory macrophages to treat lung disease (129).

Neutrophils play a prominent role in the pathology of many lung diseases, including BPD (130). In a mouse model of hyperoxia, histological damage is preceded by neutrophil infiltration into the lung following a wave of macrophage recruitment (131). Several studies using animal models of hyperoxia show that reducing neutrophil infiltration correlates with decreased lung disease (132–134). Neutrophils play a complex role in the mechanism of inflammatory disease and it has recently been suggested that neutrophils can play an anti-inflammatory role in addition to their common pro-inflammatory role (135).

Human studies have reported an unexpected alteration in neutrophil counts in preterm infants, which could relate to the risk of preterm infants developing lung disease (136–138). Of note, one study reports that infants with respiratory distress syndrome born less than 32 weeks gestational age who develop BPD have elevated levels of IL-6 and IL-8 in tracheal aspirates prior to the influx of neutrophils versus those who do not develop BPD (139). A decrease in CD18 and CD62L on circulating neutrophils in the first 4 weeks of life in preterm infants was associated with the development of BPD (140). Additionally, increased serum levels of neutrophil-associated gelatinase-associated lipocalin in preterm infants born less than 31 weeks of gestation was predictive for the development of BPD (141). Of note, children who were born less than 32 weeks gestational age have higher IL-8 and neutrophil cell counts in sputum at the preschool age, which illustrates long-term consequences in lung inflammation due to preterm birth (142). Thus, more studies are needed to understand how hyperoxia could alter the function of neonatal neutrophil function, which could then affect the development of inflammatory lung disease later in life.

It is becoming more apparent that respiratory disease pathology varies greatly and that unique subtypes of disease exist. Many of these subtypes display unique alterations in the skewing of the immune system toward a Th1, Th2, or Th17 response (143). The endotype of disease tends to track with the type of T cell skewing with a Th17/neutrophilic response being more damaging than other types of disease, and this is intimately related to the stimulatory conditions of activated T cells (144). In a study of extremely preterm infants (born <32 weeks GA) RV infection was shown to induce a Th2 and Th17 response, and IL-4 production was related to severity respiratory morbidity (145). Furthermore, alterations in T regulatory cells have been described in humans with respiratory disease (146). An important consideration is that T regulatory cells are associated with inhibition of fibroblast proliferation and in vascular repair in the lung following injury (144). Given the surprising finding that cord blood contains T cells with an activated/memory phenotype, it is possible that these cells are poised to contribute to inflammatory lung disease (147). Recent work has also reported decreased CD4 T cells in cord blood from preterm infants who develop moderate BPD (148). Despite the finding that cytotoxic T cell function is not altered in mice exposed to hyperoxia followed by IAV infection (106), it is possible that CD4 T cells play a role in hyperoxia-mediated lung damage in humans and in the development of disease later in life. However, small animal models of oxygen effects on BPD do not support this hypothesis.

In adults, oxidative stress plays a role in COPD disease progression (149). It is possible that changes in the oxidative state of the lung due to chronic oxygen exposure in preterm infants could change how cells from the immune system respond to environmental exposures by altering cellular function or the types of cytokines that are produced (150–153). These cytokines could work in concert with cell types in the lung, including epithelial cells and innate lymphoid cells, known to produce pro-inflammatory and pro-fibrotic factors under certain conditions (154). One recent report demonstrates that reactive oxygen species in the lung can alter signaling of the inflammasome, leading to increased inflammation (155). One cell lineage receiving a great deal of attention is the innate lymphoid cell, which is a bone-marrow derived population found at mucosal surfaces, including the lung. They have the ability to generate high levels of cytokines that can influence the balance of the immune system (156). Much like cells in the adaptive immune system, they can be skewed to express transcription factors and produce cytokines consistent with Th1, Th2, and Th17 CD4 T cell lineages and play an essential role in responding to infection (157, 158). Of particular interest, ILC2

cells have been shown to play a role in the pathogenesis of lung disease by contributing to a Th2 T cell response (159, 160). IL-13 is a Th2 cytokine that, when overexpressed in the lung, results in oxidative damage to peripheral blood cells (161). Of note is that oxidized guanidine perpetuates the inflammatory response (162). A related inflammatory mechanism could be present with complexes of oxidized high-mobility group box protein 1, which has been shown to induce hyperoxia-mediated lung inflammation (136, 163). It is tempting to speculate that exposure to hyperoxia could contribute to this inflammatory loop of chronic lung disease through the induction of oxidized DNA.

Taken together, the balance of redox state within the lung is of critical importance in preventing chronic lung disease. It is very likely that early life exposure to hyperoxia changes this balance, which could result in permanent lung injury. Alterations in function of immune cells, including but not limited to CD4 T cells, neutrophils, and macrophages, likely play a major role in this development of lung disease. Importantly, pulmonary cells that produce innate immune molecules, like type II epithelial cells, might also be depleted or epigenetically modified in their ability to respond to injury (102). Taken together, it is likely that low levels of inflammation are present following exposure to hyperoxia, which could perpetually contribute to lung disease.

A Perspective on Oxygen as a Goldilock's Modifier of Respiratory Health

If we accept that high levels of oxygen at birth can alter children's health, does low levels of oxygen at birth also affect children's health? Indeed, there is growing evidence that gene–environment interactions influences health of people living at high altitude (low oxygen). Populations of Tibetans, Ethiopians, and Andeans living at >2.5 miles or between 11 and 13% oxygen exhibit resistance to hypoxemia, and develop larger lungs and hearts. These phenotypic changes appear to be genetically fixed in Tibetans and Ethiopians, but not in Andeans. Between 2010 and 2014, single-cell gene analysis and whole-exome sequencing identified haplotypes in the prolyl hydroxylase EGLN1, hypoxia-inducible factor (HIF)-2α, and peroxisome proliferator-activated receptor (PPAR)-α genes that correlated with lower hemoglobin levels in Tibetans (164–167). These haplotypes are not detected in Ethiopians. Instead, haplotype changes in the retinoic acid orphan receptor have been detected, which is interesting because this receptor dimerizes with HIF-2α (168). Taken together, this suggests that Tibetan and Ethiopian populations adapted separately to hypoxia through a common EGLN-HIF signaling pathway. Genetic changes conferring resistance to hypoxia have yet to be detected in Andeans and the hypoxic-resistant phenotype is only present in children born at high altitude (169). This implies Andeans acclimatize to an environmentally low level of oxygen at birth.

Regardless of how adaptation at high altitude is achieved, it maladaptively influences long-term health. When compared to people living at sea level, high-altitude natives have increased risk for cardiovascular disease particularly related to cardiac hypertrophy (169). A zip code study of children born at high altitude in Colorado suggests that birth at high altitude increases

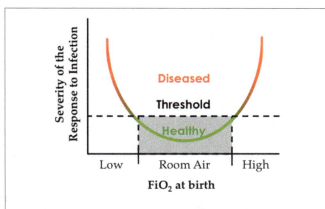

FIGURE 4 | **The oxygen environment at birth affects the severity of respiratory viral infection later in life.** Hypothetical graph depicting how exposure to low or high inspired oxygen at birth can increase respiratory morbidity following a respiratory viral infection.

re-hospitalization following infection with RSV (170). Living at high altitude may also reduce brain activity (171). High-altitude natives may have lower rates of obesity (172), but are often born small for gestational age and exhibit transient growth delay with compensatory catch-up growth (169, 173). Some of these health risks may mirror those seen in children who had sleep apnea, placental insufficiency, or cyanotic congenital heart disease as infants. Hence, adapting to low oxygen at birth causes similar maladaptive changes to children's health as high oxygen exposure.

This Goldilocks effect of oxygen reflects the convergence of an oxygen environment on genes present at birth, some of which have fixated changes that maintain the response to hypoxia even at sea level. Genetic changes that influence the response to high oxygen used to treat preterm infants have yet to be identified, perhaps because there is no evolutionary pressure or memory for adapting to hyperoxia. However, recognizing that the response to oxygen is non-linear, studying adaptation to low oxygen may help us understand adaptation to high oxygen (**Figure 4**).

In the preceding sections, we have highlighted the current understanding of normal pulmonary development and how it is perturbed due to premature birth. These changes become exasperated due to neonatal oxygen exposure that affects the pulmonary epithelium, angiogenesis, and the innate immune system in the developing infant. Great strides have recently been realized in both the treatment and understanding the mechanisms leading to sequelae later in life in this susceptible population. Our hope is that this review has left the reader with an appreciation for previous work as well as highlighting future areas of research that are warranted. These include but are not limited to gaining a more complete understanding of the molecular programing that drives development and regeneration of the respiratory epithelium that will allow for a better appreciation of the affects an immature lung experiences due to premature birth into an oxygen rich environment. Infants born prematurely, and likely provided oxygen, experience enhanced disease due to respiratory infections later in life. Understanding what pulmonary cell types are principally infected by various respiratory pathogens, like IAV, in healthy subjects precludes our understanding of the cell-specific alterations occurring in preterm infants later in life. Although cell-specific pulmonary tropism of IAV is unlikely to drastically change in this population, it may prove that a cell-specific imbalance in these aberrant lungs drives enhanced disease. It is also clear that genes involved in directing lung development overlap with those of the pulmonary innate immune system (97). It is therefore likely that overall respiratory health is accomplished by an interaction with oxygen at birth that influences the developmental trajectory of the lung and pulmonary innate immune system. A better understanding of how the oxygen environment at birth influences gene–innate immune interactions could help identify children at risk for disease and ideally treatments that improve their health.

Author Contributions

The design, writing, and editing of this manuscript was done with equal participation and intellectual contributions by WD, RM, and MO. Final editing and manuscript preparation was performed by WD.

Acknowledgments

Due to space limitations, we could not discuss all of the literature relevant to this topic and so apologize to those investigators whose research we did not present. We thank our colleagues, and the past and present members of the O'Reilly laboratory who have helped us understand how early life oxygen exposure alters lung development and function. We are grateful to support by the National Institutes of Health grants HL-067392 and HL-091968 (MO), training grant ES-07026 (WD), and a contract for the Respiratory Pathogens Research Center (HHSN27220100005C).

References

1. Barker DJ, Winter PD, Osmond C, Margetts B, Simmonds SJ. Weight in infancy and death from ischaemic heart disease. *Lancet* (1989) **2**:577–80. doi:10.1016/S0140-6736(89)90710-1
2. Plopper CG, Smiley-Jewell SM, Miller LA, Fanucchi MV, Evans MJ, Buckpitt AR, et al. Asthma/allergic airways disease: does postnatal exposure to environmental toxicants promote airway pathobiology? *Toxicol Pathol* (2007) **35**:97–110. doi:10.1080/01926230601132030
3. Pinkerton KE, Joad JP. The mammalian respiratory system and critical windows of exposure for children's health. *Environ Health Perspect* (2000) **108**(Suppl 3):457–62. doi:10.1289/ehp.00108s3457
4. Kajekar R. Environmental factors and developmental outcomes in the lung. *Pharmacol Ther* (2007) **114**:129–45. doi:10.1016/j.pharmthera.2007.01.011
5. Chandra RK. Nutrition and the immune system: an introduction. *Am J Clin Nutr* (1997) **66**:460S–3S.
6. Singh V. The burden of pneumonia in children: an Asian perspective. *Paediatr Respir Rev* (2005) **6**:88.93. doi:10.1016/j.prrv.2005.03.002
7. Le Souef PN. Adverse effects of maternal smoking during pregnancy on innate immunity in infants. *Eur Respir J* (2006) **28**:675–7. doi:10.1183/09031936.06.00101206
8. Lafeber HN, Westerbeek EA, Van Den Berg A, Fetter WP, Van Elburg RM. Nutritional factors influencing infections in preterm infants. *J Nutr* (2008) **138**:1813S–1817S.

9. Springer KW, Sheridan J, Kuo D, Carnes M. The long-term health outcomes of childhood abuse. An overview and a call to action. *J Gen Intern Med* (2003) **18**:864–70. doi:10.1046/j.1525-1497.2003.20918.x

10. Maeda Y, Dave V, Whitsett JA. Transcriptional control of lung morphogenesis. *Physiol Rev* (2007) **87**:219–44. doi:10.1152/physrev.00028.2006

11. Minoo P. Transcriptional regulation of lung development: emergence of specificity. *Respir Res* (2000) **1**:109–15. doi:10.1186/rr20

12. Morrisey EE, Hogan BL. Preparing for the first breath: genetic and cellular mechanisms in lung development. *Dev Cell* (2010) **18**:8–23. doi:10.1016/j.devcel.2009.12.010

13. Herriges M, Morrisey EE. Lung development: orchestrating the generation and regeneration of a complex organ. *Development* (2014) **141**:502–13. doi:10.1242/dev.098186

14. Kho AT, Bhattacharya S, Mecham BH, Hong J, Kohane IS, Mariani TJ. Expression profiles of the mouse lung identify a molecular signature of time-to-birth. *Am J Respir Cell Mol Biol* (2009) **40**:47–57. doi:10.1165/rcmb.2008-0048OC

15. Xu Y, Wang Y, Besnard V, Ikegami M, Wert SE, Heffner C, et al. Transcriptional programs controlling perinatal lung maturation. *PLoS One* (2012) **7**:e37046. doi:10.1371/journal.pone.0037046

16. Eber E, Zach MS. Long term sequelae of bronchopulmonary dysplasia (chronic lung disease of infancy). *Thorax* (2001) **56**:317–23. doi:10.1136/thorax.56.4.317

17. Chess PR, D'Angio CT, Pryhuber GS, Maniscalco WM. Pathogenesis of bronchopulmonary dysplasia. *Semin Perinatol* (2006) **30**:171–8. doi:10.1053/j.semperi.2006.05.003

18. Ehrenkranz RA, Walsh MC, Vohr BR, Jobe AH, Wright LL, Fanaroff AA, et al. Validation of the National Institutes of Health consensus definition of bronchopulmonary dysplasia. *Pediatrics* (2005) **116**:1353–60. doi:10.1542/peds.2005-0249

19. Merritt TA, Deming DD, Boynton BR. The 'new' bronchopulmonary dysplasia: challenges and commentary. *Semin Fetal Neonatal Med* (2009) **14**:345–57. doi:10.1016/j.siny.2009.08.009

20. Doyle LW, Faber B, Callanan C, Freezer N, Ford GW, Davis NM. Bronchopulmonary dysplasia in very low birth weight subjects and lung function in late adolescence. *Pediatrics* (2006) **118**:108–13. doi:10.1542/peds.2005-2522

21. Weisman LE. Populations at risk for developing respiratory syncytial virus and risk factors for respiratory syncytial virus severity: infants with predisposing conditions. *Pediatr Infect Dis J* (2003) **22**:S33–7. doi:10.1097/01.inf.0000053883.08663.e5

22. Doyle LW, Faber B, Callanan C, Morley R. Blood pressure in late adolescence and very low birth weight. *Pediatrics* (2003) **111**:252–7. doi:10.1542/peds.111.2.252

23. Roberts G, Anderson PJ, Doyle LW. Neurosensory disabilities at school age in geographic cohorts of extremely low birth weight children born between the 1970s and the 1990s. *J Pediatr* (2009) **154**(829–34):e1. doi:10.1016/j.jpeds.2008.12.036

24. Bream EN, Leppellere CR, Cooper ME, Dagle JM, Merrill DC, Christensen K, et al. Candidate gene linkage approach to identify DNA variants that predispose to preterm birth. *Pediatr Res* (2013) **73**:135–41. doi:10.1038/pr.2012.166

25. Ambalavanan N, Cotten CM, Page GP, Carlo WA, Murray JC, Bhattacharya S, et al. Integrated genomic analyses in bronchopulmonary dysplasia. *J Pediatr* (2015) **166**(531–537):e13. doi:10.1016/j.jpeds.2014.09.052

26. Wang H, St Julien KR, Stevenson DK, Hoffmann TJ, Witte JS, Lazzeroni LC, et al. A genome-wide association study (GWAS) for bronchopulmonary dysplasia. *Pediatrics* (2013) **132**:290–7. doi:10.1542/peds.2013-0533

27. Cruickshank MN, Oshlack A, Theda C, Davis PG, Martino D, Sheehan P, et al. Analysis of epigenetic changes in survivors of preterm birth reveals the effect of gestational age and evidence for a long term legacy. *Genome Med* (2013) **5**:96. doi:10.1186/gm500

28. Collard KJ, Godeck S, Holley JE, Quinn MW. Pulmonary antioxidant concentrations and oxidative damage in ventilated premature babies. *Arch Dis Child Fetal Neonatal Ed* (2004) **89**:F412–6. doi:10.1136/adc.2002.016717

29. Davis JM, Auten RL. Maturation of the antioxidant system and the effects on preterm birth. *Semin Fetal Neonatal Med* (2010) **15**:191–5. doi:10.1016/j.siny.2010.04.001

30. Jobe AJ. The new BPD: an arrest of lung development. *Pediatr Res* (1999) **46**:641–3. doi:10.1203/00006450-199912000-00007

31. Davis JM, Parad RB, Michele T, Allred E, Price A, Rosenfeld W, et al. Pulmonary outcome at 1 year corrected age in premature infants treated at birth with recombinant human CuZn superoxide dismutase. *Pediatrics* (2003) **111**:469–76. doi:10.1542/peds.111.3.469

32. Buczynski BW, Yee M, Martin KC, Lawrence BP, O'Reilly MA. Neonatal hyperoxia alters the host response to influenza A virus infection in adult mice through multiple pathways. *Am J Physiol Lung Cell Mol Physiol* (2013) **305**:L282–90. doi:10.1152/ajplung.00112.2013

33. Kinsella JP, Parker TA, Davis JM, Abman SH. Superoxide dismutase improves gas exchange and pulmonary hemodynamics in premature lambs. *Am J Respir Crit Care Med* (2005) **172**:745–9. doi:10.1164/rccm.200501-146OC

34. Auten RL, O'Reilly MA, Oury TD, Nozik-Grayck E, Whorton MH. Transgenic extracellular superoxide dismutase protects postnatal alveolar epithelial proliferation and development during hyperoxia. *Am J Physiol Lung Cell Mol Physiol* (2006) **290**:L32–40. doi:10.1152/ajplung.00133.2005

35. Buczynski BW, Maduekwe ET, O'Reilly MA. The role of hyperoxia in the pathogenesis of experimental BPD. *Semin Perinatol* (2013) **37**:69–78. doi:10.1053/j.semperi.2013.01.002

36. Berger J, Bhandari V. Animal models of bronchopulmonary dysplasia. The term mouse models. *Am J Physiol Lung Cell Mol Physiol* (2014) **307**:L936–47. doi:10.1152/ajplung.00159.2014

37. O'Reilly M, Thebaud B. Animal models of bronchopulmonary dysplasia. The term rat models. *Am J Physiol Lung Cell Mol Physiol* (2014) **307**:L948–58. doi:10.1152/ajplung.00160.2014

38. D'Angio CT, Ryan RM. Animal models of bronchopulmonary dysplasia. The preterm and term rabbit models. *Am J Physiol Lung Cell Mol Physiol* (2014) **307**:L959–69. doi:10.1152/ajplung.00228.2014

39. Yoder BA, Coalson JJ. Animal models of bronchopulmonary dysplasia. The preterm baboon models. *Am J Physiol Lung Cell Mol Physiol* (2014) **307**:L970–7. doi:10.1152/ajplung.00171.2014

40. Hilgendorff A, O'Reilly MA. Bronchopulmonary dysplasia early changes leading to long-term consequences. *Front Med* (2015) **2**:2. doi:10.3389/fmed.2015.00002

41. Warburton D, Schwarz M, Tefft D, Flores-Delgado G, Anderson KD, Cardoso WV. The molecular basis of lung morphogenesis. *Mech Dev* (2000) **92**:55–81. doi:10.1016/S0925-4773(99)00325-1

42. Hilfer SR. Morphogenesis of the lung: control of embryonic and fetal branching. *Annu Rev Physiol* (1996) **58**:93–113. doi:10.1146/annurev.ph.58.030196.000521

43. Mendelson CR. Role of transcription factors in fetal lung development and surfactant protein gene expression. *Annu Rev Physiol* (2000) **62**:875–915. doi:10.1146/annurev.physiol.62.1.875

44. Metzger RJ, Klein OD, Martin GR, Krasnow MA. The branching programme of mouse lung development. *Nature* (2008) **453**:745–50. doi:10.1038/nature07005

45. Bourbon JR, Boucherat O, Boczkowski J, Crestani B, Delacourt C. Bronchopulmonary dysplasia and emphysema: in search of common therapeutic targets. *Trends Mol Med* (2009) **15**:169–79. doi:10.1016/j.molmed.2009.02.003

46. Barletta KE, Cagnina RE, Wallace KL, Ramos SI, Mehrad B, Linden J. Leukocyte compartments in the mouse lung: distinguishing between marginated, interstitial, and alveolar cells in response to injury. *J Immunol Methods* (2012) **375**:100–10. doi:10.1016/j.jim.2011.09.013

47. Streets AM, Zhang X, Cao C, Pang Y, Wu X, Xiong L, et al. Microfluidic single-cell whole-transcriptome sequencing. *Proc Natl Acad Sci U S A* (2014) **111**:7048–53. doi:10.1073/pnas.1402030111

48. Treutlein B, Brownfield DG, Wu AR, Neff NF, Mantalas GL, Espinoza FH, et al. Reconstructing lineage hierarchies of the distal lung epithelium using single-cell RNA-seq. *Nature* (2014) **509**:371–5. doi:10.1038/nature13173

49. Rackley CR, Stripp BR. Building and maintaining the epithelium of the lung. *J Clin Invest* (2012) **122**:2724–30. doi:10.1172/JCI60519

50. Alanis DM, Chang DR, Akiyama H, Krasnow MA, Chen J. Two nested developmental waves demarcate a compartment boundary in the mouse lung. *Nat Commun* (2014) **5**:3923. doi:10.1038/ncomms4923

51. Giangreco A, Reynolds SD, Stripp BR. Terminal bronchioles harbor a unique airway stem cell population that localizes to the bronchoalveolar duct junction. *Am J Pathol* (2002) **161**:173–82. doi:10.1016/S0002-9440(10)64169-7

52. Hong KU, Reynolds SD, Giangreco A, Hurley CM, Stripp BR. Clara cell secretory protein-expressing cells of the airway neuroepithelial body microenvironment include a label-retaining subset and are critical for epithelial renewal after progenitor cell depletion. *Am J Respir Cell Mol Biol* (2001) 24:671–81. doi:10.1165/ajrcmb.24.6.4498

53. Kim CF, Jackson EL, Woolfenden AE, Lawrence S, Babar I, Vogel S, et al. Identification of bronchioalveolar stem cells in normal lung and lung cancer. *Cell* (2005) 121:823–35. doi:10.1016/j.cell.2005.03.032

54. Nolen-Walston RD, Kim CF, Mazan MR, Ingenito EP, Gruntman AM, Tsai L, et al. Cellular kinetics and modeling of bronchioalveolar stem cell response during lung regeneration. *Am J Physiol Lung Cell Mol Physiol* (2008) 294:L1158–65. doi:10.1152/ajplung.00298.2007

55. Ling TY, Kuo MD, Li CL, Yu AL, Huang YH, Wu TJ, et al. Identification of pulmonary Oct-4+ stem/progenitor cells and demonstration of their susceptibility to SARS coronavirus (SARS-CoV) infection in vitro. *Proc Natl Acad Sci U S A* (2006) 103:9530–5. doi:10.1073/pnas.0510232103

56. Perl AK, Tichelaar JW, Whitsett JA. Conditional gene expression in the respiratory epithelium of the mouse. *Transgenic Res* (2002) 11:21–9. doi:10.1023/A:1013986627504

57. Perl AK, Wert SE, Nagy A, Lobe CG, Whitsett JA. Early restriction of peripheral and proximal cell lineages during formation of the lung. *Proc Natl Acad Sci U S A* (2002) 99:10482–7. doi:10.1073/pnas.152238499

58. Rawlins EL, Okubo T, Xue Y, Brass DM, Auten RL, Hasegawa H, et al. The role of Scgb1a1+ Clara cells in the long-term maintenance and repair of lung airway, but not alveolar, epithelium. *Cell Stem Cell* (2009) 4:525–34. doi:10.1016/j.stem.2009.04.002

59. Zheng D, Limmon GV, Yin L, Leung NH, Yu H, Chow VT, et al. Regeneration of alveolar type I and II cells from Scgb1a1-expressing cells following severe pulmonary damage induced by bleomycin and influenza. *PLoS One* (2012) 7:e48451. doi:10.1371/journal.pone.0048451

60. Zheng D, Limmon GV, Yin L, Leung NH, Yu H, Chow VT, et al. A cellular pathway involved in Clara cell to alveolar type II cell differentiation after severe lung injury. *PLoS One* (2013) 8:e71028. doi:10.1371/journal.pone.0071028

61. Adamson IY, Bowden DH, Wyatt JP. Oxygen poisoning in mice. Ultrastructural and surfactant studies during exposure and recovery. *Arch Pathol* (1970) 90:463–72.

62. Bowden DH, Adamson IY, Wyatt JP. Reaction of the lung cells to a high concentration of oxygen. *Arch Pathol* (1968) 86:671–5.

63. Kapanci Y, Weibel ER, Kaplan HP, Robinson FR. Pathogenesis and reversibility of the pulmonary lesions of oxygen toxicity in monkeys. II. Ultrastructural and morphometric studies. *Lab Invest* (1969) 20:101–18.

64. Adamson IY, Bowden DH. The type 2 cell as progenitor of alveolar epithelial regeneration. A cytodynamic study in mice after exposure to oxygen. *Lab Invest* (1974) 30:35–42.

65. Evans MJ, Cabral LJ, Stephens RJ, Freeman G. Transformation of alveolar type 2 cells to type 1 cells following exposure to NO2. *Exp Mol Pathol* (1975) 22:142–50. doi:10.1016/0014-4800(75)90059-3

66. Tryka AF, Witschi H, Gosslee DG, McArthur AH, Clapp NK. Patterns of cell proliferation during recovery from oxygen injury. Species differences. *Am Rev Respir Dis* (1986) 133:1055–9.

67. Williams MC, Dobbs LG. Expression of cell-specific markers for alveolar epithelium in fetal rat lung. *Am J Respir Cell Mol Biol* (1990) 2:533–42. doi:10.1165/ajrcmb/2.6.533

68. Perl AK, Wert SE, Loudy DE, Shan Z, Blair PA, Whitsett JA. Conditional recombination reveals distinct subsets of epithelial cells in trachea, bronchi, and alveoli. *Am J Respir Cell Mol Biol* (2005) 33:455–62. doi:10.1165/rcmb.2005-0180OC

69. Gonzalez RF, Allen L, Dobbs LG. Rat alveolar type I cells proliferate, express OCT-4, and exhibit phenotypic plasticity in vitro. *Am J Physiol Lung Cell Mol Physiol* (2009) 297:L1045–55. doi:10.1152/ajplung.90389.2008

70. Garcia-Garcia ML, Gonzalez-Carrasco E, Quevedo S, Munoz C, Sanchez-Escudero V, Pozo F, et al. Clinical and virologic characteristics of early and moderate preterm infants readmitted with viral respiratory infections. *Pediatr Infect Dis J* (2015) 34(7):693–9. doi:10.1097/INF.0000000000000718

71. Olabarrieta I, Gonzalez-Carrasco E, Calvo C, Pozo F, Casas I, Garcia-Garcia ML. Hospital admission due to respiratory viral infections in moderate preterm, late preterm and term infants during their first year of life. *Allergol Immunopathol (Madr)* (2014). doi:10.1016/j.aller.2014.06.006

72. Carbonell-Estrany X, Perez-Yarza EG, Garcia LS, Guzman Cabanas JM, Boria EV, Atienza BB, et al. Long-term burden and respiratory effects of respiratory syncytial virus hospitalization in preterm infants-the SPRING study. *PLoS One* (2015) 10:e0125422. doi:10.1371/journal.pone.0125422

73. Miller EK, Bugna J, Libster R, Shepherd BE, Scalzo PM, Acosta PL, et al. Human rhinoviruses in severe respiratory disease in very low birth weight infants. *Pediatrics* (2012) 129:e60–7. doi:10.1542/peds.2011-0583

74. van Piggelen RO, Van Loon AM, Krediet TG, Verboon-Maciolek MA. Human rhinovirus causes severe infection in preterm infants. *Pediatr Infect Dis J* (2010) 29:364–5. doi:10.1097/INF.0b013e3181c6e60f

75. Drysdale SB, Alcazar-Paris M, Wilson T, Smith M, Zuckerman M, Broughton S, et al. Rhinovirus infection and healthcare utilisation in prematurely born infants. *Eur Respir J* (2013) 42:1029–36. doi:10.1183/09031936.00109012

76. Drysdale SB, Alcazar M, Wilson T, Smith M, Zuckerman M, Lauinger IL, et al. Respiratory outcome of prematurely born infants following human rhinovirus A and C infections. *Eur J Pediatr* (2014) 173:913–9. doi:10.1007/s00431-014-2262-1

77. Jackson DJ, Hartert TV, Martinez FD, Weiss ST, Fahy JV. Asthma: NHLBI workshop on the primary prevention of chronic lung diseases. *Ann Am Thorac Soc* (2014) 11(Suppl 3):S139–45. doi:10.1513/AnnalsATS.201312-448LD

78. American Academy of Pediatrics Committee on Infectious Diseases, American Academy of Pediatrics Bronchiolitis Guidelines Committee. Updated guidance for palivizumab prophylaxis among infants and young children at increased risk of hospitalization for respiratory syncytial virus infection. *Pediatrics* (2014) 134:415–20. doi:10.1542/peds.2014-1665

79. Iwane MK, Edwards KM, Szilagyi PG, Walker FJ, Griffin MR, Weinberg GA, et al. Population-based surveillance for hospitalizations associated with respiratory syncytial virus, influenza virus, and parainfluenza viruses among young children. *Pediatrics* (2004) 113:1758–64. doi:10.1542/peds.113.6.1758

80. Glezen WP, Taber LH, Frank AL, Gruber WC, Piedra PA. Influenza virus infections in infants. *Pediatr Infect Dis J* (1997) 16:1065–8. doi:10.1097/00006454-199711000-00012

81. Borchers AT, Chang C, Gershwin ME, Gershwin LJ. Respiratory syncytial virus – a comprehensive review. *Clin Rev Allergy Immunol* (2013) 45:331–79. doi:10.1007/s12016-013-8368-9

82. Bem RA, Domachowske JB, Rosenberg HF. Animal models of human respiratory syncytial virus disease. *Am J Physiol Lung Cell Mol Physiol* (2011) 301:L148–56. doi:10.1152/ajplung.00065.2011

83. Taubenberger JK, Kash JC. Influenza virus evolution, host adaptation, and pandemic formation. *Cell Host Microbe* (2010) 7:440–51. doi:10.1016/j.chom.2010.05.009

84. Manicassamy B, Manicassamy S, Belicha-Villanueva A, Pisanelli G, Pulendran B, Garcia-Sastre A. Analysis of in vivo dynamics of influenza virus infection in mice using a GFP reporter virus. *Proc Natl Acad Sci U S A* (2010) 107:11531–6. doi:10.1073/pnas.0914994107

85. Nogales A, Baker SF, Martinez-Sobrido L. Replication-competent influenza A viruses expressing a red fluorescent protein. *Virology* (2015) 476:206–16. doi:10.1016/j.virol.2014.12.006

86. Couceiro JN, Paulson JC, Baum LG. Influenza virus strains selectively recognize sialyloligosaccharides on human respiratory epithelium; the role of the host cell in selection of hemagglutinin receptor specificity. *Virus Res* (1993) 29:155–65. doi:10.1016/0168-1702(93)90056-S

87. Shinya K, Ebina M, Yamada S, Ono M, Kasai N, Kawaoka Y. Avian flu: influenza virus receptors in the human airway. *Nature* (2006) 440:435–6. doi:10.1038/440435a

88. van Riel D, Den Bakker MA, Leijten LM, Chutinimitkul S, Munster VJ, De Wit E, et al. Seasonal and pandemic human influenza viruses attach better to human upper respiratory tract epithelium than avian influenza viruses. *Am J Pathol* (2010) 176:1614–8. doi:10.2353/ajpath.2010.090949

89. van Riel D, Munster VJ, De Wit E, Rimmelzwaan GF, Fouchier RA, Osterhaus AD, et al. Human and avian influenza viruses target different cells in the lower respiratory tract of humans and other mammals. *Am J Pathol* (2007) 171:1215–23. doi:10.2353/ajpath.2007.070248

90. Nicholls JM, Chan MC, Chan WY, Wong HK, Cheung CY, Kwong DL, et al. Tropism of avian influenza A (H5N1) in the upper and lower respiratory tract. *Nat Med* (2007) 13:147–9. doi:10.1038/nm1529

91. Thompson CI, Barclay WS, Zambon MC, Pickles RJ. Infection of human airway epithelium by human and avian strains of influenza a virus. *J Virol* (2006) 80:8060–8. doi:10.1128/JVI.00384-06

92. Matrosovich MN, Matrosovich TY, Gray T, Roberts NA, Klenk HD. Human and avian influenza viruses target different cell types in cultures of human airway epithelium. *Proc Natl Acad Sci U S A* (2004) 101:4620–4. doi:10.1073/pnas.0308001101

93. Wang J, Nikrad MP, Phang T, Gao B, Alford T, Ito Y, et al. Innate immune response to influenza A virus in differentiated human alveolar type II cells. *Am J Respir Cell Mol Biol* (2011) 45:582–91. doi:10.1165/rcmb.2010-0108OC

94. Kumar PA, Hu Y, Yamamoto Y, Hoe NB, Wei TS, Mu D, et al. Distal airway stem cells yield alveoli in vitro and during lung regeneration following H1N1 influenza infection. *Cell* (2011) 147:525–38. doi:10.1016/j.cell.2011.10.001

95. Zuo W, Zhang T, Wu DZ, Guan SP, Liew AA, Yamamoto Y, et al. p63(+) Krt5(+) distal airway stem cells are essential for lung regeneration. *Nature* (2015) 517:616–20. doi:10.1038/nature13903

96. Smith LJ, McKay KO, Van Asperen PP, Selvadurai H, Fitzgerald DA. Normal development of the lung and premature birth. *Paediatr Respir Rev* (2010) 11:135–42. doi:10.1016/j.prrv.2009.12.006

97. Whitsett JA, Alenghat T. Respiratory epithelial cells orchestrate pulmonary innate immunity. *Nat Immunol* (2015) 16:27–35. doi:10.1038/ni.3045

98. Holtzman MJ. Asthma as a chronic disease of the innate and adaptive immune systems responding to viruses and allergens. *J Clin Invest* (2012) 122:2741–8. doi:10.1172/JCI60325

99. Felton JM, Lucas CD, Rossi AG, Dransfield I. Eosinophils in the lung – modulating apoptosis and efferocytosis in airway inflammation. *Front Immunol* (2014) 5:302. doi:10.3389/fimmu.2014.00302

100. Bhattacharya S, Go D, Krenitsky DL, Huyck HL, Solleti SK, Lunger VA, et al. Genome-wide transcriptional profiling reveals connective tissue mast cell accumulation in bronchopulmonary dysplasia. *Am J Respir Crit Care Med* (2012) 186:349–58. doi:10.1164/rccm.201203-0406OC

101. Thebaud B, Abman SH. Bronchopulmonary dysplasia: where have all the vessels gone? Roles of angiogenic growth factors in chronic lung disease. *Am J Respir Crit Care Med* (2007) 175:978–85. doi:10.1164/rccm.200611-1660PP

102. Yee M, Buczynski BW, O'Reilly MA. Neonatal hyperoxia stimulates the expansion of alveolar epithelial type II cells. *Am J Respir Cell Mol Biol* (2014) 50:757–66. doi:10.1165/rcmb.2013-0207OC

103. Yee M, Vitiello PF, Roper JM, Staversky RJ, Wright TW, McGrath-Morrow SA, et al. Type II epithelial cells are critical target for hyperoxia-mediated impairment of postnatal lung development. *Am J Physiol Lung Cell Mol Physiol* (2006) 291:L1101–11. doi:10.1152/ajplung.00126.2006

104. O'Reilly MA, Yee M, Buczynski BW, Vitiello PF, Keng PC, Welle SL, et al. Neonatal oxygen increases sensitivity to influenza A virus infection in adult mice by suppressing epithelial expression of Ear1. *Am J Pathol* (2012) 181:441–51. doi:10.1016/j.ajpath.2012.05.005

105. Buczynski BW, Yee M, Paige Lawrence B, O'Reilly MA. Lung development and the host response to influenza A virus are altered by different doses of neonatal oxygen in mice. *Am J Physiol Lung Cell Mol Physiol* (2012) 302:L1078–87. doi:10.1152/ajplung.00026.2012

106. Giannandrea M, Yee M, O'Reilly MA, Lawrence BP. Memory CD8+ T cells are sufficient to alleviate impaired host resistance to influenza A virus infection caused by neonatal oxygen supplementation. *Clin Vaccine Immunol* (2012) 19:1432–41. doi:10.1128/CVI.00265-12

107. Yee M, Chess PR, McGrath-Morrow SA, Wang Z, Gelein R, Zhou R, et al. Neonatal oxygen adversely affects lung function in adult mice without altering surfactant composition or activity. *Am J Physiol Lung Cell Mol Physiol* (2009) 297:L641–9. doi:10.1152/ajplung.00023.2009

108. Yee M, Buczynski BW, Lawrence BP, O'Reilly MA. Neonatal hyperoxia increases sensitivity of adult mice to bleomycin-induced lung fibrosis. *Am J Respir Cell Mol Biol* (2013) 48:258–66. doi:10.1165/rcmb.2012-0238OC

109. Kohlmeier JE, Woodland DL. Immunity to respiratory viruses. *Annu Rev Immunol* (2009) 27:61–82. doi:10.1146/annurev.immunol.021908.132625

110. O'Reilly MA, Marr SH, Yee M, McGrath-Morrow SA, Lawrence BP. Neonatal hyperoxia enhances the inflammatory response in adult mice infected with influenza A virus. *Am J Respir Crit Care Med* (2008) 177:1103–10. doi:10.1164/rccm.200712-1839OC

111. Deshmane SL, Kremlev S, Amini S, Sawaya BE. Monocyte chemoattractant protein-1 (MCP-1): an overview. *J Interferon Cytokine Res* (2009) 29:313–26. doi:10.1089/jir.2008.0027

112. Dessing MC, Van Der Sluijs KF, Florquin S, Van Der Poll T. Monocyte chemoattractant protein 1 contributes to an adequate immune response in influenza pneumonia. *Clin Immunol* (2007) 125:328–36. doi:10.1016/j.clim.2007.08.001

113. Hartl D, Griese M, Nicolai T, Zissel G, Prell C, Reinhardt D, et al. A role for MCP-1/CCR2 in interstitial lung disease in children. *Respir Res* (2005) 6:93. doi:10.1186/1465-9921-6-32

114. Suga M, Iyonaga K, Ichiyasu H, Saita N, Yamasaki H, Ando M. Clinical significance of MCP-1 levels in BALF and serum in patients with interstitial lung diseases. *Eur Respir J* (1999) 14:376–82. doi:10.1183/09031936.99.14237699

115. Bhandari V. Postnatal inflammation in the pathogenesis of bronchopulmonary dysplasia. *Birth Defects Res A Clin Mol Teratol* (2014) 100:189–201. doi:10.1002/bdra.23220

116. Knight DA, Ernst M, Anderson GP, Moodley YP, Mutsaers SE. The role of gp130/IL-6 cytokines in the development of pulmonary fibrosis: critical determinants of disease susceptibility and progression? *Pharmacol Ther* (2003) 99:327–38. doi:10.1016/S0163-7258(03)00095-0

117. Xu Y, Tian Z, Xie P. Targeting complement anaphylatoxin C5a receptor in hyperoxic lung injury in mice. *Mol Med Rep* (2014) 10:1786–92. doi:10.3892/mmr.2014.2394

118. Garcia CC, Weston-Davies W, Russo RC, Tavares LP, Rachid MA, Alves-Filho JC, et al. Complement C5 activation during influenza A infection in mice contributes to neutrophil recruitment and lung injury. *PLoS One* (2013) 8:e64443. doi:10.1371/journal.pone.0064443

119. Gu H, Mickler EA, Cummings OW, Sandusky GE, Weber DJ, Gracon A, et al. Crosstalk between TGF-beta1 and complement activation augments epithelial injury in pulmonary fibrosis. *FASEB J* (2014) 28:4223–34. doi:10.1096/fj.13-247650

120. Bhandari V. Drug therapy trials for the prevention of bronchopulmonary dysplasia: current and future targets. *Front Pediatr* (2014) 2:76. doi:10.3389/fped.2014.00076

121. Nyunoya T, Powers LS, Yarovinsky TO, Butler NS, Monick MM, Hunninghake GW. Hyperoxia induces macrophage cell cycle arrest by adhesion-dependent induction of p21Cip1 and activation of the retinoblastoma protein. *J Biol Chem* (2003) 278:36099–106. doi:10.1074/jbc.M304370200

122. Wang M, Gorasiya S, Antoine DJ, Sitapara RA, Wu W, Sharma L, et al. The compromise of macrophage functions by hyperoxia is attenuated by ethacrynic acid via inhibition of NF-kappaB-mediated release of high-mobility group box-1. *Am J Respir Cell Mol Biol* (2015) 52:171–82. doi:10.1165/rcmb.2013-0544OC

123. Sturrock A, Vollbrecht T, Mir-Kasimov M, McManus M, Wilcoxen SE, Paine R III. Mechanisms of suppression of alveolar epithelial cell GM-CSF expression in the setting of hyperoxic stress. *Am J Physiol Lung Cell Mol Physiol* (2010) 298:L446–53. doi:10.1152/ajplung.00161.2009

124. Sturrock A, Baker JA, Mir-Kasimov M, Paine R III. Contrasting effects of hyperoxia on GM-CSF gene transcription in alveolar epithelial cells and T cells. *Physiol Rep* (2015) 3(3):e12324. doi:10.14814/phy2.12324

125. Jones CV, Williams TM, Walker KA, Dickinson H, Sakkal S, Rumballe BA, et al. M2 macrophage polarisation is associated with alveolar formation during postnatal lung development. *Respir Res* (2013) 14:41. doi:10.1186/1465-9921-14-41

126. Syed MA, Bhandari V. Hyperoxia exacerbates postnatal inflammation-induced lung injury in neonatal BRP-39 null mutant mice promoting the M1 macrophage phenotype. *Mediators Inflamm* (2013) 2013:457189. doi:10.1155/2013/457189

127. Sureshbabu A, Syed MA, Boddupalli C, Dhodapkar MV, Homer RJ, Minoo P, et al. Conditional overexpression of TGFss1 promotes pulmonary inflammation, apoptosis and mortality via TGFssR2 in the developing mouse lung. *Respir Res* (2015) 16:4. doi:10.1186/s12931-014-0162-6

128. Duan W, Croft M. Control of regulatory T cells and airway tolerance by lung macrophages and dendritic cells. *Ann Am Thorac Soc* (2014) 11(Suppl 5):S306–13. doi:10.1513/AnnalsATS.201401-028AW

129. Costa A, Sarmento B, Seabra V. Targeted drug delivery systems for lung macrophages. *Curr Drug Targets* (2014). doi:10.2174/1389450115666141114152713

130. Grommes J, Soehnlein O. Contribution of neutrophils to acute lung injury. *Mol Med* (2011) **17**:293–307. doi:10.2119/molmed.2010.00138

131. Nagato AC, Bezerra FS, Lanzetti M, Lopes AA, Silva MA, Porto LC, et al. Time course of inflammation, oxidative stress and tissue damage induced by hyperoxia in mouse lungs. *Int J Exp Pathol* (2012) **93**:269–78. doi:10.1111/j.1365-2613.2012.00823.x

132. Min JH, Codipilly CN, Nasim S, Miller EJ, Ahmed MN. Synergistic protection against hyperoxia-induced lung injury by neutrophils blockade and EC-SOD overexpression. *Respir Res* (2012) **13**:58. doi:10.1186/1465-9921-13-58

133. Weichelt U, Cay R, Schmitz T, Strauss E, Sifringer M, Buhrer C, et al. Prevention of hyperoxia-mediated pulmonary inflammation in neonatal rats by caffeine. *Eur Respir J* (2013) **41**:966–73. doi:10.1183/09031936.00012412

134. Benipal B, Feinstein SI, Chatterjee S, Dodia C, Fisher AB. Inhibition of the phospholipase A2 activity of peroxiredoxin 6 prevents lung damage with exposure to hyperoxia. *Redox Biol* (2015) **4**:321–7. doi:10.1016/j.redox.2015.01.011

135. Kolaczkowska E, Kubes P. Neutrophil recruitment and function in health and inflammation. *Nat Rev Immunol* (2013) **13**:159–75. doi:10.1038/nri3399

136. Juul SE, Haynes JW, McPherson RJ. Evaluation of neutropenia and neutrophilia in hospitalized preterm infants. *J Perinatol* (2004) **24**:150–7. doi:10.1038/sj.jp.7211057

137. Nittala S, Subbarao GC, Maheshwari A. Evaluation of neutropenia and neutrophilia in preterm infants. *J Matern Fetal Neonatal Med* (2012) **25**:100–3. doi:10.3109/14767058.2012.715468

138. Del Vecchio A, Christensen RD. Neonatal neutropenia: what diagnostic evaluation is needed and when is treatment recommended? *Early Hum Dev* (2012) **88**(Suppl 2):S19–24. doi:10.1016/S0378-3782(12)70007-5

139. Munshi UK, Niu JO, Siddiq MM, Parton LA. Elevation of interleukin-8 and interleukin-6 precedes the influx of neutrophils in tracheal aspirates from preterm infants who develop bronchopulmonary dysplasia. *Pediatr Pulmonol* (1997) **24**:331–6. doi:10.1002/(SICI)1099-0496(199711)24:5<331::AID-PPUL5>3.0.CO;2-L

140. Ballabh P, Simm M, Kumari J, Krauss AN, Jain A, Califano C, et al. Neutrophil and monocyte adhesion molecules in bronchopulmonary dysplasia, and effects of corticosteroids. *Arch Dis Child Fetal Neonatal Ed* (2004) **89**:F76–83. doi:10.1136/fn.89.1.F76

141. Inoue H, Ohga S, Kusuda T, Kitajima J, Kinjo T, Ochiai M, et al. Serum neutrophil gelatinase-associated lipocalin as a predictor of the development of bronchopulmonary dysplasia in preterm infants. *Early Hum Dev* (2013) **89**:425–9. doi:10.1016/j.earlhumdev.2012.12.011

142. Teig N, Allali M, Rieger C, Hamelmann E. Inflammatory markers in induced sputum of school children born before 32 completed weeks of gestation. *J Pediatr* (2012) **161**:1085–90. doi:10.1016/j.jpeds.2012.06.007

143. Misra RS. A review of the CD4+ T cell contribution to lung infection, inflammation and repair with a focus on wheeze and asthma in the pediatric population. *EC Microbiol* (2014) **1**(1):4–14.

144. Vroman H, Van Den Blink B, Kool M. Mode of dendritic cell activation: the decisive hand in Th2/Th17 cell differentiation. Implications in asthma severity? *Immunobiology* (2015) **220**:254–61. doi:10.1016/j.imbio.2014.09.016

145. Perez GF, Pancham K, Huseni S, Jain A, Rodriguez-Martinez CE, Preciado D, et al. Rhinovirus-induced airway cytokines and respiratory morbidity in severely premature children. *Pediatr Allergy Immunol* (2015) **26**:145–52. doi:10.1111/pai.12346

146. Tan DB, Fernandez S, Price P, French MA, Thompson PJ, Moodley YP. Impaired function of regulatory T-cells in patients with chronic obstructive pulmonary disease (COPD). *Immunobiology* (2014) **219**:975–9. doi:10.1016/j.imbio.2014.07.005

147. Zhang X, Mozeleski B, Lemoine S, Deriaud E, Lim A, Zhivaki D, et al. CD4 T cells with effector memory phenotype and function develop in the sterile environment of the fetus. *Sci Transl Med* (2014) **6**:238ra72. doi:10.1126/scitranslmed.3008748

148. Misra RS, Shah S, Fowell DJ, Wang H, Scheible K, Misra SK, et al. Preterm cord blood CD4+ T cells exhibit increased IL-6 production in chorioamnionitis and decreased CD4+ T cells in bronchopulmonary dysplasia. *Hum Immunol* (2015) **76**(5):329–38. doi:10.1016/j.humimm.2015.03.007

149. Domej W, Oettl K, Renner W. Oxidative stress and free radicals in COPD – implications and relevance for treatment. *Int J Chron Obstruct Pulmon Dis* (2014) **9**:1207–24. doi:10.2147/COPD.S51226

150. Gostner JM, Becker K, Fuchs D, Sucher R. Redox regulation of the immune response. *Redox Rep* (2013) **18**:88–94. doi:10.1179/1351000213Y.0000000044

151. Circu ML, Aw TY. Reactive oxygen species, cellular redox systems, and apoptosis. *Free Radic Biol Med* (2010) **48**:749–62. doi:10.1016/j.freeradbiomed.2009.12.022

152. Schieber M, Chandel NS. ROS function in redox signaling and oxidative stress. *Curr Biol* (2014) **24**:R453–62. doi:10.1016/j.cub.2014.03.034

153. Secchi C, Carta M, Crescio C, Spano A, Arras M, Caocci G, et al. T cell tyrosine phosphorylation response to transient redox stress. *Cell Signal* (2015) **27**:777–88. doi:10.1016/j.cellsig.2014.12.014

154. Wynn TA. Integrating mechanisms of pulmonary fibrosis. *J Exp Med* (2011) **208**:1339–50. doi:10.1084/jem.20110551

155. Kim SR, Kim DI, Kim SH, Lee H, Lee KS, Cho SH, et al. NLRP3 inflammasome activation by mitochondrial ROS in bronchial epithelial cells is required for allergic inflammation. *Cell Death Dis* (2014) **5**:e1498. doi:10.1038/cddis.2014.460

156. Spits H, Artis D, Colonna M, Diefenbach A, Di Santo JP, Eberl G, et al. Innate lymphoid cells – a proposal for uniform nomenclature. *Nat Rev Immunol* (2013) **13**:145–9. doi:10.1038/nri3365

157. Sanos SL, Diefenbach A. Innate lymphoid cells: from border protection to the initiation of inflammatory diseases. *Immunol Cell Biol* (2013) **91**:215–24. doi:10.1038/icb.2013.3

158. Seillet C, Rankin LC, Groom JR, Mielke LA, Tellier J, Chopin M, et al. Nfil3 is required for the development of all innate lymphoid cell subsets. *J Exp Med* (2014) **211**:1733–40. doi:10.1084/jem.20140145

159. Roediger B, Weninger W. Group 2 innate lymphoid cells in the regulation of immune responses. *Adv Immunol* (2015) **125**:111–54. doi:10.1016/bs.ai.2014.09.004

160. DeKruyff RH, Yu S, Kim HY, Umetsu DT. Innate immunity in the lung regulates the development of asthma. *Immunol Rev* (2014) **260**:235–48. doi:10.1111/imr.12187

161. Chapman AM, Malkin DJ, Camacho J, Schiestl RH. IL-13 overexpression in mouse lungs triggers systemic genotoxicity in peripheral blood. *Mutat Res* (2014) **769**:100–7. doi:10.1016/j.mrfmmm.2014.06.007

162. Ba X, Aguilera-Aguirre L, Sur S, Boldogh I. 8-Oxoguanine DNA glycosylase-1-driven DNA base excision repair: role in asthma pathogenesis. *Curr Opin Allergy Clin Immunol* (2015) **15**:89–97. doi:10.1097/ACI.0000000000000135

163. Entezari M, Javdan M, Antoine DJ, Morrow DM, Sitapara RA, Patel V, et al. Inhibition of extracellular HMGB1 attenuates hyperoxia-induced inflammatory acute lung injury. *Redox Biol* (2014) **2**:314–22. doi:10.1016/j.redox.2014.01.013

164. Bigham A, Bauchet M, Pinto D, Mao X, Akey JM, Mei R, et al. Identifying signatures of natural selection in Tibetan and Andean populations using dense genome scan data. *PLoS Genet* (2010) **6**:e1001116. doi:10.1371/journal.pgen.1001116

165. Yi X, Liang Y, Huerta-Sanchez E, Jin X, Cuo ZX, Pool JE, et al. Sequencing of 50 human exomes reveals adaptation to high altitude. *Science* (2010) **329**:75–8. doi:10.1126/science.1190371

166. Simonson TS, Yang Y, Huff CD, Yun H, Qin G, Witherspoon DJ, et al. Genetic evidence for high-altitude adaptation in Tibet. *Science* (2010) **329**:72–5. doi:10.1126/science.1189406

167. Beall CM, Cavalleri GL, Deng L, Elston RC, Gao Y, Knight J, et al. Natural selection on EPAS1 (HIF2alpha) associated with low hemoglobin concentration in Tibetan highlanders. *Proc Natl Acad Sci U S A* (2010) **107**:11459–64. doi:10.1073/pnas.1002443107

168. Alkorta-Aranburu G, Beall CM, Witonsky DB, Gebremedhin A, Pritchard JK, Di Rienzo A. The genetic architecture of adaptations to high altitude in Ethiopia. *PLoS Genet* (2012) **8**:e1003110. doi:10.1371/journal.pgen.1003110

169. Frisancho AR. Developmental functional adaptation to high altitude: review. *Am J Hum Biol* (2013) **25**:151–68. doi:10.1002/ajhb.22367

170. Choudhuri JA, Ogden LG, Ruttenber AJ, Thomas DS, Todd JK, Simoes EA. Effect of altitude on hospitalizations for respiratory syncytial virus infection. *Pediatrics* (2006) **117**:349–56. doi:10.1542/peds.2004-2795

171. Yan X. Pro: all dwellers at high altitude are persons of impaired physical and mental powers. *High Alt Med Biol* (2013) **14**:208–11. doi:10.1089/ham.2013.1026

172. Voss JD, Allison DB, Webber BJ, Otto JL, Clark LL. Lower obesity rate during residence at high altitude among a military population with frequent migration: a quasi experimental model for investigating spatial causation. *PLoS One* (2014) **9**:e93493. doi:10.1371/journal.pone.0093493

173. Soria R, Julian CG, Vargas E, Moore LG, Giussani DA. Graduated effects of high-altitude hypoxia and highland ancestry on birth size. *Pediatr Res* (2013) **74**:633–8. doi:10.1038/pr.2013.150

17

Development and Functional Characterization of Fetal Lung Organoids

Mandy Laube[1]*, Soeren Pietsch[1], Thomas Pannicke[1], Ulrich H. Thome[1] and Claire Fabian[2]

[1] *Division of Neonatology, Department of Paediatrics, Center for Paediatric Research Leipzig, University of Leipzig, Leipzig, Germany,* [2] *Department of Vaccines and Infection Models, Fraunhofer Institute for Cell Therapy and Immunology, Leipzig, Germany*

*Correspondence:
Mandy Laube
mandy.laube@medizin.uni-leipzig.de

Preterm infants frequently suffer from pulmonary complications due to a physiological and structural lung immaturity resulting in significant morbidity and mortality. Novel *in vitro* and *in vivo* models are required to study the underlying mechanisms of late lung maturation and to facilitate the development of new therapeutic strategies. Organoids recapitulate essential aspects of structural organization and possibly organ function, and can be used to model developmental and disease processes. We aimed at generating fetal lung organoids (LOs) and to functionally characterize this *in vitro* model in comparison to primary lung epithelial cells and lung explants *ex vivo*. LOs were generated with alveolar and endothelial cells from fetal rat lung tissue, using a Matrigel-gradient and air-liquid-interface culture conditions. Immunocytochemical analysis showed that the LOs consisted of polarized epithelial cell adhesion molecule (EpCAM)-positive cells with the apical membrane compartment facing the organoid lumen. Expression of the alveolar type 2 cell marker, RT2-70, and the Club cell marker, CC-10, were observed. Na^+ transporter and surfactant protein mRNA expression were detected in the LOs. First time patch clamp analyses demonstrated the presence of several ion channels with specific electrophysiological properties, comparable to vital lung slices. Furthermore, the responsiveness of LOs to glucocorticoids was demonstrated. Finally, maturation of LOs induced by mesenchymal stem cells confirmed the convenience of the model to test and establish novel therapeutic strategies. The results showed that fetal LOs replicate key biological lung functions essential for lung maturation and therefore constitute a suitable *in vitro* model system to study lung development and related diseases.

Keywords: lung, 3D culture, organoids, patch clamp, fetal development, model system

INTRODUCTION

The study of fetal lung development is a challenging task. Any model system needs to reflect the biological properties such as morphology and function, while also being reproducible and, if possible, broadly accessible. Although many basic properties like cell morphology or protein localization can be modeled using classic 2-dimensional (2D) cell culture with cell lines or primary cells, their reflection of biological functions is often limited. The situation is further complicated by the highly complex nature of the pulmonary system with uniquely specialized cells. The lung is the central organ of the respiratory system, providing barrier function to facilitate oxygen delivery and carbon dioxide elimination. Severe clinical consequences can arise from a disruption of fetal lung development. Especially in preterm infants, pulmonary complications are common due to a physiological and structural lung immaturity leading to significant morbidity and mortality. Impaired perinatal transition from the liquid-filled to air-breathing lungs can result in respiratory distress syndrome (RDS), and possibly subsequent development of bronchopulmonary dysplasia (BPD). The pathology of BPD is based on an arrested lung development, including a reduced alveolar surface area and alveolar number, as well as impaired functions down to a cellular level. Functional disturbances of RDS mainly arise from a lack of differentiated alveolar type 2 (ATII) cells that are involved in surfactant synthesis and pulmonary fluid homeostasis. Alveolar fluid clearance (AFC) enables perinatal lung transition to air breathing that is accomplished by active Na^+ transport across the alveolar epithelium driven by epithelial Na^+ channels (ENaC). Importantly, ENaC expression is reduced in the preterm lungs (1), compromising AFC. These pathognomonic features must be reflected in model systems of fetal lung development. Animal models improved the understanding of lung development as well as the pathogenic mechanisms leading to RDS and BDP. Rats are a widely used animal model to reproduce the histopathology of human preterm infants with BPD. Exposing newborn rats to hyperoxia induces lung structural and functional impairment, accompanied by high levels of pulmonary inflammation (2). Thereby the critical relationship between oxygen toxicity and mechanical ventilation with lung injury and BPD development was demonstrated. However, rodent models are mainly used as endpoint models in which tissue damage and functional alterations are determined after sacrifice, preventing analysis of the disease course. Furthermore, newborn rodents are viable at birth and do not exhibit lung immaturity, which is of central importance in human BPD. Besides, respiratory distress in preterm infants is multifactorial, including congenital infection, growth restriction and placental dysfunction, and most preterm infants were exposed to clinical interventions like antenatal corticosteroids. This is not reflected in most animal models possibly leading to different responses to pathogenic challenges as well as therapeutic strategies. Therefore, novel model systems are required to study the underlying mechanisms of late lung maturation and to facilitate the development of novel therapeutic approaches. Moreover, any *in vitro* and *in vivo* model should replicate key features of lung development and maturation, and allow for a qualitative, quantitative, and most importantly, functional analysis. Immortalized lung cell lines were commonly used to determine gene expression and signaling pathways, but due to their immortalized nature, their differentiation capacity is limited. Instead, primary fetal distal lung epithelial (FDLE) cells represent a widely studied *in vitro* model due to their ability to differentiate into polarized and functional epithelia (3). FDLE cells are derived from fetal rat pups 24–48 h prior to birth. Studies showed that fetal rat pups born 24 h prior to term birth experience respiratory distress due to structural and functional lung immaturity (4). Na^+ transport as well as the expression and secretion of surfactant proteins were studied in FDLE cells before. Furthermore, FDLE cells enable analysis of sex-specific differences between male and female cells (5), and can be used for co-culture with other primary lung cell types. On the other hand, FDLE cells are limited in their lifetime and offer only a short time window for experiments of 2–3 days.

Lung organoids (LOs) offer the chance to bridge the gap between conventional *in vitro* and *in vivo* models. Organoids are self-organizing 3D structures that can be grown from stem cells or defined tissue-specific progenitor cells (6). They supposedly recapitulate the organs' structural organization, with multiple specialized cells, and function, although actual organ-like function has yet to be determined. The first 3D lung cell cultures, called organoids or "mass cultures," were generated using a crude cell mix derived from digested fetal lung tissue. This cell suspension consisted of epithelial, endothelial, mesenchymal and hematopoietic cells (7). By culturing the cell suspension at the air-liquid-interface (ALI) on a floating membrane filter, differentiation into mature ATII cells as well as connective tissue formation was achieved (7). This demonstrated the ability of fetal lung cells to self-organize in co-culture with other cells types and that ALI culture represents an important differentiation signal. However, lack of 3D growth limited the use of these early organoid cultures. The absence of a supporting structure, like hydrogels or a scaffold, resulted in a wide-stretched, multilayered and heterogeneous cell aggregation instead of the sophisticated 3D structures seen today. In addition, culture time was limited to a few days before mesenchymal cells overgrew and destroyed the epithelial cell structures. The culture of fetal and adult ATII cells on basement membrane extracts from Engelbreth-Holm-Swarm (EHS) tumor tissue (also known as matrix gel or Matrigel™) led to the establishment of organotypic cell cultures. ATII cell culture on polystyrol resulted in a loss of lamellar bodies, induced cell flattening and cell proliferation, while culture with EHS gels prevented the loss of lamellar bodies and the cells retained their cuboidal morphology (8, 9). These studies showed the importance of the biophysical environment, including the extracellular matrix (ECM) as well as the interface to air, to generate relevant *in vitro* lung models. The use of isolated and defined cell populations and the co-culture of lung epithelial cells with other lung-derived cell types like endothelial cells (10), mesenchymal stem cells (11), and fibroblasts (12), led to the development of self-organizing LOs reflecting morphological and cellular compositions of bronchial and alveolar tissue.

Our study focused on the generation of a biological relevant model system of fetal lung development that can be easily reproduced by other scientists. Furthermore, functional analyses demonstrated the opportunities this model offers for a variety of studies, including gene expression and patch clamp analyses. Fetal LOs were generated using FDLE and lung endothelial cells from fetal rat lungs. This allows a concise validation of the advantages and limitations of LOs as a model system for fetal lung development in comparison to the existing *in vitro* and *in vivo* studies done with rats.

MATERIALS AND METHODS
Cell Isolation
Sprague-Dawley rats (RGD Cat# 70508, RRID:RGD_70508) were obtained from the Medical Experimental Center (MEZ) of Leipzig University. Animals were kept in rooms with a 12 h

Development and Functional Characterization of Fetal Lung Organoids

light-dark cycle, constant temperature (22°C) and humidity (55%). Food and water were supplied *ad libitum*. At gestational day E20-21 (term E22) pregnant rats were anesthetized by CO_2 inhalation and euthanized by Pentobarbital injection. All experimental procedures were approved by the institutional review board (Landesdirektion Leipzig, permit number: T23/15). Fetal lungs were mechanically dissociated with razor blades. The resulting cell suspension was enzymatically digested with trypsin (0.125%, Fisher Scientific, Schwerte, Germany) and DNase (0.4 mg/mL, CellSystems, Troisdorf, Germany) in Hanks' Balanced Salt solution (HBSS, Fisher Scientific) for 10 min at 37°C, followed by MEM containing collagenase (0.1%, CellSystems) and DNase for 15 min at 37°C. FDLE cells, a model of fetal ATII cells, were isolated by plating the crude lung cell mix twice for 1.5 h to remove adjacent lung fibroblasts followed by differential centrifugation (3, 13). The supernatant contained FDLE cells with >95% purity (3). For the isolation of $CD31^+$ endothelial cells, fetal lungs were digested using the multi tissue dissociation kit II according to the manufacturer's recommendations, followed by Magnetic Activated Cell Sorting (MACS, GentleMACS Octo) using $CD31^+$ beads (all by Miltenyi Biotech, Bergisch Gladbach, Germany). The obtained cell mix was strained with a $70\,\mu m$ filter (Miltenyi). Resuspension and all subsequent labeling and washing steps were done using 0.5% BSA/OptiMEM (Fisher Scientific). The cells were incubated with an anti-CD31-PE antibody (1:50, #REA396, Miltenyi) for 10 min at 4°C, followed by incubation with anti-PE magnetic beads (20 $\mu l/10^7$ cells) for 15 min at 4°C. Up to 10^8 cells were loaded on a LS Column (Miltenyi), inserted in a QuadroMACS™ Separator (Miltenyi) and passed twice over the same column to enrich $CD31^+$ cells. To obtain a homogenous $CD31^+$ cell population, two rounds of subsequent antibody-mediated cell sorting were required. The first step enriched the $CD31^+$ cells to ~60–80% and the second step led to a purity of >90%. Enrichment was controlled by flow cytometry (BDAccuri, BD biosciences, San Jose, CA, USA). $CD31^+$ cells were cultured on gelatin-coated flasks with Endothelial Cell Growth Supplement (ECGS) medium containing DMEM (high glucose, GlutaMAX™, Fisher Scientific), 20% FCS (Biochrom, Berlin, Germany), 15 mM HEPES (Merck, Darmstadt, Germany), Heparin (100 $\mu g/mL$, Merck), ECGS (50 $\mu g/mL$, Corning, Corning, NY, USA), penicillin (100 units/mL, Fisher Scientific), streptomycin (100 $\mu g/mL$, Fisher Scientific), and amphotericin B (0.25 $\mu g/mL$, Fisher Scientific). After ~2 weeks in culture, confluent $CD31^+$ cells were used for LO generation up to passage 3 (**Supplementary Figure 1**). Subculture was done using TripLE™ Express (Fisher Scientific). A tube formation assay was done to determine the ability of $CD31^+$ cells to form tube-like structures to verify their endothelial cell character. The tube formation assay was done by plating $CD31^+$ cells at 5×10^4 cells on a Matrigel-coated well of a 24-well-plate in ECGS medium. Cell morphology was analyzed after 22 h (**Supplementary Figure 1**).

3D Culture

Transparent permeable transwell inserts (ThinCert, #662610, surface area 33.6 mm^2, Greiner Bio-One, Frickenhausen,

Germany) were first coated with growth-factor reduced (GFR) Matrigel (3 mg/mL, #356230, Corning) at 37°C. Matrigel GFR was dissolved in ice-cold LO medium (LO-Med) consisting of DMEM/F12 (#31330095, Fisher Scientific), 10% FCS, 1% insulin-transferrin-selenium-ethanolamine (ITS-X, #51500056, Fisher Scientific), 1 mM HEPES (#A1069,0250, AppliChem, Darmstadt, Germany), penicillin (100 units/mL), streptomycin (100 $\mu g/mL$) and amphotericin B (0.25 $\mu g/mL$). Freshly isolated FDLE cells (1.5 $\times$ 10^5 per well) were mixed with $CD31^+$ cells (0.375 $\times$ 10^5 per well), constituting an epithelial to endothelial cell ratio of 1:0.25. The defined cell mix was combined with Matrigel GFR (0.4 mg/mL in LO-Med) and transferred to the coated inserts. The lower compartment of the transwell insert was filled with LO-Med, while the upper compartment containing the cells in Matrigel was not submerged in medium enabling air-liquid interface (ALI) conditions. LOs were cultured at 37°C with medium exchange every 2 days. Live cell imaging was done using a microscope (CKX41, Olympus, Hamburg, Germany) with a temperature controller (ibidi, Graefelfing, Germany) and a CO_2 controller (The Brick Gas Mixer, Life Imaging Services, Basel, Switzerland) during the first day of FDLE and $CD31^+$ co-culture under submerged culture conditions to determine their initial self-organization. To analyze the effect of specific stimulating agents LO-Med was supplemented with dexamethasone (100 nM, Merck). Furthermore, the effect of mesenchymal stem cell-conditioned medium (MSC-CM) on LOs was determined after the organoids reached 15 days *in vitro* (div). The organoids were further cultured for 4 additional days in MSC-CM or the corresponding medium used for the culture of MSCs, which consisted of DMEM (low glucose, GlutaMAX™, Fisher Scientific) and 2% FCS. To subculture LOs or obtain them for further analyses, cell recovery solution (#354253, Corning) was used. To this end, all inserts were incubated on ice for ~2 h with ice cold cell recovery solution. Subsequently, the cell recovery solution was replaced by sterile 10% BSA (#8076.2, Carl Roth, Karlsruhe, Germany) in PBS. The digested Matrigel solution was centrifuged at 300 $\times$ g for 5 min, sedimented LOs were resuspended, washed twice in PBS and used for patch clamp analyses or fixed with 2% formaldehyde (#11586711, Fisher Scientific) in PBS for 20 min at room temperature followed by embedding in Tissue-Tek™ O.C.T. (#4583, Weckert, Kitzingen, Germany) for immunofluorescence staining. LO compactness was defined as the cellular area in proportion to the whole organoid area using Image J version 1.53c (ImageJ, RRID:SCR_003070) as published before (14). Compactness, also known as solidity, includes the packing density and the intercellular space cavities thereby indicating internal cellularity and external branching.

Immunofluorescence

Characterization of LOs was carried out with immunofluorescence staining of cryotome sections (5 μm). LO slices were washed with PBS and then treated with 5% BSA/PBS containing 0.5% Triton-X 100 (Merck) for 1 h at room temperature. Afterwards, the slices were incubated at 4°C overnight with the respective primary antibody, diluted in 5% BSA/PBS. LO slices were incubated with rabbit-anti-epithelial cell adhesion molecule (EpCAM) primary antibody (1:50; # ab71916, Abcam, Cambridge, UK, RRID:AB_1603782), mouse-anti-RT1-40 (1:150, #TB-11ART1-40, Terrace Biotech, San Francisco, CA, USA) for staining of ATI cells (15), rabbit-anti-aquaporin 5 (Aqp 5, 1:100, #178615, Merck, RRID:AB_211472), mouse-anti-RT2-70 (1:150, #TB-44ART2-70, Terrace Biotech) to detect ATII cells (16), rabbit-anti-Club cell secretary protein (CC-10, 1:100, #ab40873, Abcam, RRID:AB_778766), and rabbit-anti-Ki-67 (1:500, #9129, Cell Signaling Technology, Danvers, MA, USA, RRID:AB_2687446). Control slices were treated with 5% BSA/PBS without the primary antibody. The secondary antibody NL-493 (1:200; R&D Systems, Boston, USA, RRID:AB_663764) was used for primary rabbit IgG antibodies and NL-637 (1:200; R&D Systems, RRID:AB_663771) was used for primary mouse IgG antibodies. Nuclei were stained with DAPI (1 µg/ml, #D8417-1MG, Merck). For Live-Dead staining LOs were resuspended in fresh LO-Med containing 2 mg/mL Matrigel and plated on a glass bottom dish (#81218-200, ibidi). After 3 days, LO-Med was replaced by a solution containing Calcein-AM (5 µM, #sc-203865, Santa Cruz) and propidium iodide (PI, 1 µg/mL, #CN74.1, Carl Roth). Staining of actin filaments was performed with FITC-labeled phalloidin (2.5 µg/mL, #P1951, Merck, RRID:AB_2315148). All sections were covered with ProLong™ Glass Antifade Mountant (#P36980, Fischer Scientific). For image capturing a confocal laser-scanning microscope (LSM710, Laser: Diode 405, Argon 488, Helium-Neon 543; Objective: Plan- Apochromat 20 x, Zeiss, Goettingen, Germany) was used. Area and fluorescence calculation were done with Image J. Calculation of cell numbers was done by manual counting. Depending on the used antibodies, either whole positively stained cells (EpCAM) or in case of apical markers, cells with an adjacent positive staining (RT2-70), were counted as positive.

Gene Expression Analyses

RNA isolation was done at 15 div using the Purelink RNA Mini Kit (Fisher Scientific) according to the manufacturer's instructions. Reverse transcription was carried out using the Maxima H Minus First Strand cDNA Synthesis Kit with dsDNase (Fisher Scientific). Real-time quantitative PCR (RT-qPCR) was done in the CFX 96 Real-Time PCR Detection System (Bio-Rad, Munich, Germany) using the SYBR Select Master Mix (Fisher Scientific) and gene-specific primers listed in **Table 1**. A serial dilution of target-specific plasmid DNA was used for absolute quantification. Molecule concentrations were then normalized to a reference gene encoding for the mitochondrial ribosomal protein S18a (*Mrps18a*). Constant expression of *Mrps18a* was confirmed against other common reference genes. Using the relative standard curve method mRNA levels were calculated and expressed as relative fold change of the respective control. Melting curves and gel electrophoresis of PCR products were routinely performed to control the specificity of the PCR reaction.

Patch Clamp Analyses

Patch clamp studies were performed at 15 div. LOs were transferred to the recording chamber in a bath on the stage of a

microscope (BX61WI, Olympus), which was filled with a solution containing (mM): 135 KCl, 2 $MgCl_2$, 6 NaCl, 5.5 Glucose, 10 HEPES (pH 7.4). Cell attached currents were recorded with an EPC10 patch clamp amplifier (Heka Elektronik, Lambrecht, Germany). A standard personal computer running Patchmaster software (Heka, Patchmaster, RRID:SCR_000034) controlled the EPC10 and stored the current tracings. Patch pipettes were pulled from borosilicate capillaries with 1.5 mm outer diameter and 0.86 mm inner diameter (Science Products, #GB150-8P) using a P2000 laser puller (Sutter, Novato, CA). The pipettes were filled with a solution containing (mM): 140 NaCl, 5 KCl, 1 $MgCl_2$, 1.8 $CaCl_2$, 5.5 Glucose, 10 HEPES (pH 7.4), resulting in a tip resistance between 4 and 6 MΩ. ATII cells were identified using Lysotracker (1 µM, LysoTracker Green DND-26, Fisher Scientific), which selectively accumulates in their lamellar bodies (18). After forming a gigaohm seal, currents were recorded at membrane potentials between -100 and $+100$ mV in 10 mV increments, filtered at 2 kHz and sampled at 10 kHz. Cell attached recordings were analyzed with Fitmaster software (Heka, Fitmaster, RRID:SCR_016233). Voltages are given as the negative of the patch pipette potential, which represents the shift of the patch potential from the resting potential. Negative potentials represent hyperpolarization, and positive potentials represent depolarization of the cell membrane away from the resting potential. Highly selective cation (HSC) channels and non-selective cation (NSC) channels were identified by characteristic channel kinetics and the current-voltage relationship for the channel.

Ussing Chamber Measurements

Ussing chamber measurements of FDLE cells were performed 4 days after cell isolation, as previously reported (5). Only monolayers with a transepithelial resistance (R_{te}) exceeding 300 $\Omega \cdot cm^2$ were included in the analyses. Electrophysiological solutions consisted of: 145 mM Na^+, 5 mM K^+, 1.2 mM Ca^{2+}, 1.2 mM Mg^{2+}, 125 mM Cl^-, 25 mM HCO_3^-, 3.3 mM $H_2PO_4^-$, and 0.8 mM HPO_4^{2-} (pH 7.4). For the basolateral solution, 10 mM glucose was used, while 10 mM mannitol was used in the apical solution. During measurements, the solutions were continuously bubbled with carbogen (5% CO_2 and 95% O_2). Equivalent short-circuit currents (I_{SC}) were determined every 20 s by measuring transepithelial voltage (V_{te}) and R_{te} with a transepithelial current clamp (Physiologic instruments, San Diego, CA) and calculating the quotient $I_{SC} = V_{te}/R_{te}$. After the I_{SC} reached a stable plateau (I_{base}), amiloride (10 µM, # A7410, Sigma-Aldrich) was applied to the apical chamber to assess the amiloride-sensitive ΔI_{SC} (ΔI_{amil}). The current reduction induced by amiloride (ΔI_{amil}) was used as a measure of ENaC activity. Amiloride was dissolved in water.

Isolation of Human Mesenchymal Stem Cells

The study was approved by the ethical board of the medical faculty of Leipzig University. The umbilical cord tissue was collected after delivery from human newborns whose mothers granted informed consent. MSC isolation and characterization are described elsewhere (19). MSC-CM was produced by

Development and Functional Characterization of Fetal Lung Organoids

TABLE 1 | Primer sequences.

Gene	Primer (forward, 5′-3′)	Primer (reverse, 5′-3′)
α-ENaC NM_031548.2	TTCTGGGCGGTGCTGTGGCT	GCGTCTGCTCCGTGATGCGG
β-ENaC NM_012648.1	TGCAGGCCCAATGCCGAGGT	GGGCTCTGTGCCCTGGCTCT
γ-ENaC NM_017046.1	CACGCCAGCCGTGACCCTTC	CTCGGGACACCACGATGCGG
Na,K-ATPases-α₁ NM_012504.1	GGACGAGACAAGTATGAGCCCGC	CATGGAGAAGCCACCGAACAGC
Na,K-ATPases-β₁ NM_013113.2	GCGCAGCACTCGCTTTCCCT	GGGCCACACGGTCCTGGTACG
CFTR NM 031506.1	GCCTTCGCTGGTTGCACAGTAGTC	GCTTCTCCAGCACCCAGCACTAGA
Mrps18a NM_198756.2	GCGACCGGCTGGTTATGGCT	GGGCACTGGCCTGAGGGATTAG
Sftpa (17) NM_001270647.1	CCTCTTCTTGACTGTTGTCGCTGG	GCTGAGGACTCCCATTGTTTGCAG
Sftpb (17) NM_138842.1	GGAGCTAATGACCTGTGCCAAGAG	CTGGCCCTGGAAGTAGTCGATAAC
Sftpc (17) NM_017342.2	GATGGAGAGCCCACCGGATTACTC	GAACGATGCCAGTGGAGCCAATAG

incubating the culture medium with MSCs for 72 h, followed by sterile filtration.

Statistical Analyses

Differences between two groups were analyzed with the unpaired T-test or the Mann-Whitney test. A probability of $p < 0.05$ was considered significant for all statistical analyses. Statistical analysis was performed with GraphPad Prism software (GraphPad Software, La Jolla, CA, USA, RRID:SCR_002798).

RESULTS

Development of Fetal LOs

The generation of LOs is schematically illustrated in **Figure 1A**. The isolation of CD31$^+$ cells was done by antibody-mediated cell sorting using magnetic beads. This allowed analysis of cells during every step of the isolation process: the initial amount of CD31$^+$ cells in the total lung cell mix, the CD31$^+$ cells bound to the magnetic column as well as the non-bound cells in the flow-through. CD31$^+$ cells represented $5.2 \pm 2.6\%$ (Mean $\pm$ SD; $n = 16$) of total lung cells. CD31$^+$ cells were cultured for 7–14 days to increase their cell numbers. These CD31$^+$ cells were combined with freshly isolated FDLE cells and used for organoid generation. LO formation was compared between Matrigel-coated permeable inserts covered with cells in Matrigel exposed to air (ALI culture) and Matrigel-containing cell suspension plated at the bottom of a well and overlaid with LO-Med (submerged culture) (**Figure 1B**). The ALI condition resulted in more diverse and complex LO formation of branched and cystic morphology, while the submerged culture condition mainly led to the formation of cystic LOs. In some cystic

LOs, differentiated cells with beating cilia within the lumen were observed (data not shown). **Figure 1C** shows examples of the different morphologies observed. Cystic LOs exhibited one lumen and were mainly transparent. Branched morphology consisted of several cysts attached to each other, reminding of budding structures or even more condensed structures with opaque appearance. The discrimination between cystic and branched morphology was done according to published studies (20). Submerged cultures were not investigated further because of the morphology and presence of cilia. Testing different FDLE cell numbers demonstrated that at least 0.5×10^5 cells per well were required for 3D LO formation, otherwise only 2D cell layers were observed. Furthermore, without CD31$^+$ cells no 3D LOs were observed (**Figure 1D**). CD31$^+$ cells began to align themselves in the Matrigel and formed tube-like structures within the first 24 h of culture (**Supplementary Figures 1B,C**). Without CD31$^+$ cells, FDLE cells did not show active migration, but in co-culture cell-cell adhesive interactions between FDLE and CD31$^+$ cells led to initial cell aggregates (**Supplementary Figure 1C**). The 3D assembly was enhanced by direct interaction of FDLE cells with CD31$^+$ cells, while indirect co-culture delayed LO formation by ~1 week (**Figure 1D**). Different cell ratios were tested (FDLE to CD31$^+$ cells of 1:1, 1:0.5, and 1:0.25). Increasing the number of CD31$^+$ cells decreased LO area and number (**Figures 1E,F**). After 15 days in culture LOs reached mean sizes of $115.34 \pm 44.82\,\mu m$ (Mean $\pm$ SEM, $n = 22$). LO size increased during culture reaching a maximum at about 15 div, no further increase of LO size was observed at 43 div (**Figure 1G**). Prolonged LO culture led to overgrowth of a cell layer after ~1 month that consumed all medium and impaired organoid growth. Thus, splitting of LO cultures was necessary, which enabled further

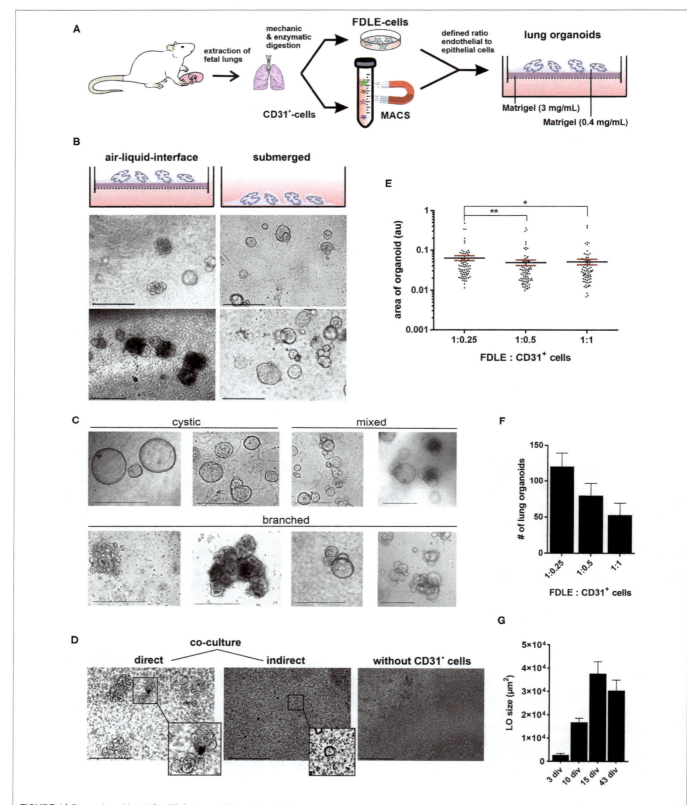

FIGURE 1 | Generation of fetal LOs. **(A)** Schematic illustration of LO generation. CD31+ cells were mixed with freshly isolated FDLE cells and used for LO generation. **(B)** LO formation was compared between ALI culture, in which LOs were cultured on permeable inserts exposed to air, and submerged culture without air exposure. ALI conditions resulted in more divers and complex LOs of branched and cystic morphology, while the submerged culture condition mainly led to the formation

(Continued)

Development and Functional Characterization of Fetal Lung Organoids

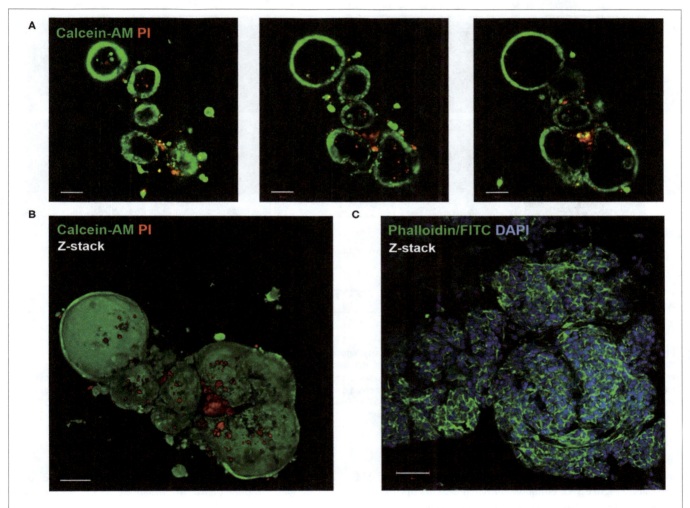

FIGURE 1 | of cystic LOs (pictures were taken at 15 div). **(C)** Exemplary demonstration of different morphologies (cystic, branched or a mixed appearance) observed during LO culture. **(D)** The 3D assembly was enhanced by direct interaction of FDLE cells with CD31$^+$ cells (3 div), while indirect co-culture delayed LO formation (3 div). Furthermore, without CD31$^+$ cells no LO formation was observed (4 div). **(E)** Different cell ratios were tested (FDLE to CD31$^+$ cells of 1:1, 1:0.5, and 1:0.25). Data of LO area are displayed in a scatter dot plot with mean (horizontal line) ± SEM. Increasing the number of CD31$^+$ cells decreased LO area ($n = 70-75$; **$p < 0.01$; *$p < 0.05$ by T-test). **(F)** Numbers of LOs are displayed as mean + SEM. Increasing the number of CD31$^+$ cells further decreased LO numbers. **(G)** LO size (μm^2) at 3, 10, 15, and 43 div ($n = 40$). div, days *in vitro*. Scale bar: 500 μm.

FIGURE 2 | Live-Dead and F-actin staining of fetal LOs. Fluorescence Z-stack serial images were taken by confocal microscopy. The bottom-to-top distance was 58 μm with 1 μm distance intervals between images. **(A)** Live-Dead staining with Calcein-AM (green) that accumulated in living cells and propidium iodide (PI, red) that accumulated in dead cells (23 div). Images of different optical sections through the LOs (11, 22, and 30 μm distance from bottom) demonstrated that the majority of cells were alive. **(B)** Z-stack image of **(A)** showed that dead cells were mainly attached to the LOs, while the LO structures consisted of living cells. **(C)** Z-stack image of F-actin staining that showed the structural organization of the LO (17 div) by phalloidin-FITC fluorescence (green). Nuclei were stained with DAPI (blue). div, days *in vitro*. Scale bar: 50 μm.

subculture, without the need to add additional CD31$^+$ cells. Using fetal adjacent lung fibroblasts or human umbilical vein-derived endothelial cells (HUVECs) instead of CD31$^+$ cells also resulted in the formation of 3D LOs.

Morphological Characterization of Fetal Lung Organoids

Live-Dead staining of passaged LOs showed that the majority of cells within the organoid were alive (**Figures 2A,B**). Staining with phalloidin-FITC was used to visualize the structural organization of filamentous actin (F-actin) with a cobblestone-like epithelial appearance of the LOs (**Figure 2C**). The cellular composition of the LOs consisted only of EpCAM$^+$ cells without direct integration of CD31$^+$ cells. We did not perform an additional staining of CD31$^+$ cells in the lung organoids at 15 div, since our initial experiments testing different medium conditions (data not shown) showed that the culture condition used for lung organoids was not supporting CD31$^+$ cells growth during

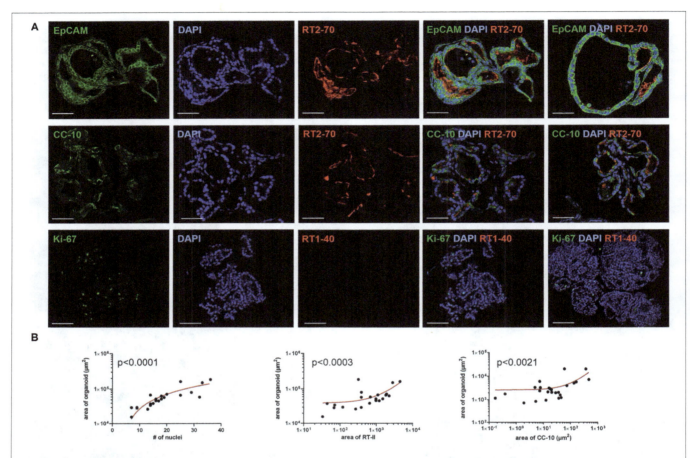

FIGURE 3 | Immunofluorescence characterization of fetal LOs. Fluorescence images of LO slices (15 div) were taken by confocal microscopy. **(A)** Organoids were strongly positive for EpCAM expression. Nuclei were stained with DAPI. Epithelial cells within the LOs polarized with the apical membrane compartment facing the lumen, as shown by the luminal expression of the RT2-70 antigen. Furthermore, expression of the Club cell marker CC-10 was detected. In contrast, the ATI cell marker RT1-40 was rarely observed in the LOs. Ki-67 staining showed that only a small subset of the total cells was actively proliferating. Scale bar: 50 μm. **(B)** The area of LOs positively correlated with the number of nuclei ($n = 21$; $p < 0.0001$). The area of RT2-70$^+$ cells positively correlated with LO area ($n = 21$; $p < 0.0003$). Furthermore, area of CC-10$^+$ expression positively correlated with LO area ($n = 25$; $p < 0.0021$). div, days *in vitro*.

long term culture. LOs were strongly positive for EpCAM expression (**Figure 3A**). Notably, epithelial cells within the LOs polarized with the apical membrane compartment facing the lumen of the organoid, as shown by the luminal expression of the RT2-70 antigen. Furthermore, expression of the Club cell marker CC-10 was detected. In contrast, the ATI cell markers, RT1-40 (T1α or podoplanin) and Aqp5 were not observed in the LOs. Notably, RT1-40 expression was also not detected in fetal rat lung slices (E21), while their pronounced and widespread expression was detected in adult rat lung tissue (**Supplementary Figure 2**). Ki-67 staining showed that only a small subset of the total cells was actively proliferating at 15 div.

The area of LOs positively correlated with the number of nuclei, determined by DAPI staining (Spearman $r = 0.89$; $p < 0.001$; **Figure 3B**). The positively stained area for ATII cells (RT2-70$^+$) positively correlated with LO area (in μm^2; Spearman $r = 0.703$; $p < 0.001$; **Figure 3B**), and $1.59 \pm 0.37\%$ of the LO area expressed the RT2-70 antigen, independent of organoid size. Furthermore, $1.38 \pm 0.30\%$ of total LO area was CC-10$^+$, whose expression also positively correlated with organoid size (Spearman $r = 0.619$; $p < 0.01$; **Figure 3B**). Notably, the positively stained area (in%) does not reflect the actual cell number.

Functional Characterization of Fetal Lung Organoids

Patch clamp analyses of LOs demonstrated the presence of ion channels of different conductance, open probability and open and closed time. First, ATII cells within the LOs were identified by fluorescence staining after incubation with Lysotracker (**Figure 4A**). Single as well as multiple channel activities were observed at different holding potentials, showing exemplary outward currents as demonstrated by the upward direction

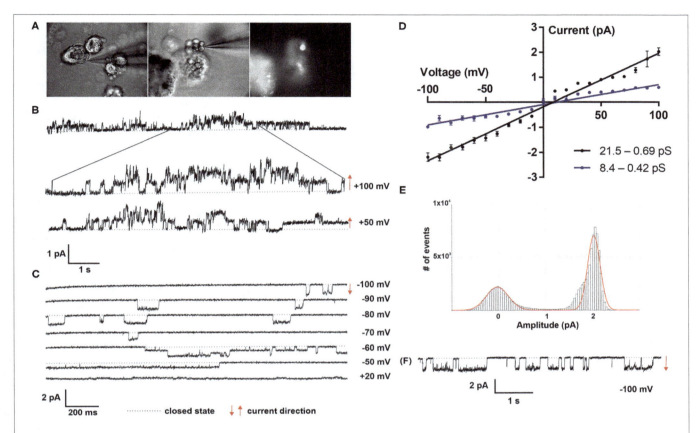

FIGURE 4 | Electrophysiological characterization of fetal LOs. Patch clamp analyses of LOs at 15 div demonstrated the presence of ion channels of different conductance, open probabilities and open and closed times. **(A)** ATII cells within the LOs were identified by fluorescence after incubation with Lysotracker. **(B)** Single as well as multiple channel activities were observed at different holding potentials (+100 and +50 mV), showing exemplary outward currents as demonstrated by the upward direction of openings from the closed state. **(C)** Furthermore, inward currents were observed at different negative holding potentials (−100 to +20 mV) as shown by the downward direction of the openings from the closed state. **(D)** Plotting the current-voltage relationship identified two types of channels: a channel with a conductance of 8.4 ± 0.42 pS (slope ± SE, $n = 18$ cells) and a reversal potential of 11.3 mV ($R^2 = 0.982$), and a second channel with a conductance of 21.5 ± 0.69 pS ($n = 15$ cells) that reversed at 9.2 mV ($R^2 = 0.955$). **(E,F)** Amplitude histogram and current tracing of single channel openings at −100 mV. Closed state is indicated by the dotted line. The arrows indicate the current direction with ↑ outward and ↓ inward currents.

of openings from the closed state (**Figure 4B**). Furthermore, inward currents were observed at different negative holding potentials as shown by the downward direction of the openings from the closed state (**Figure 4C**). Plotting the current-voltage relationship identified two types of channels: a channel with a slope conductance of 8.4 ± 0.42 pS (slope ± SE, $n = 18$ cells) and a reversal potential of 11.3 mV ($R^2 = 0.982$), and a second channel with a conductance of 21.5 ± 0.69 pS ($n = 15$ cells) that reversed at 9.2 mV ($R^2 = 0.955$) (**Figure 4D**). Thus, ATII cells within the LOs displayed functional epithelial Na$^+$ channels with HSC and NSC channel-like transport properties. **Figures 4E,F, 5A,B** further show the amplitude histograms of single and multiple channel openings on hyperpolarization. Different open times at different holding potentials are displayed in **Figure 5C**. Finally, high variability of channel kinetics (amplitude, open and closed times) are shown for a recording with voltage steps from −100 to +100 mV and a reversal potential close to 0 (**Figure 5D**). According to the strong rectifying properties of the illustrated recording, with smaller inward currents on hyperpolarization (28.41 pS) and larger outward currents when the patch membrane was depolarized (82.54 pS), an outwardly rectifying Cl$^-$ channel (ORCC) can be assumed.

Reviewing the Effect of Certain Lung-Stimulating Factors

Gene expression analysis of LOs demonstrated the mRNA expression of *ENaC* and the *Na,K-ATPase* as well as surfactant protein (*Sftp*)-A, B, and C, which exhibit essential functions in mature ATII cells. Dexamethasone is known to increase the mRNA expression of Na$^+$ transporters and surfactant genes *in vitro* and *in vivo*. Thus, LOs were incubated with dexamethasone (100 nM) for 48 h, prior to RNA isolation at 15 div. Dexamethasone significantly increased mRNA expression of the *ENaC* subunits (α, β, γ) and the *Na,K-ATPase subunit-β1* compared to control LOs cultured without dexamethasone (*p*

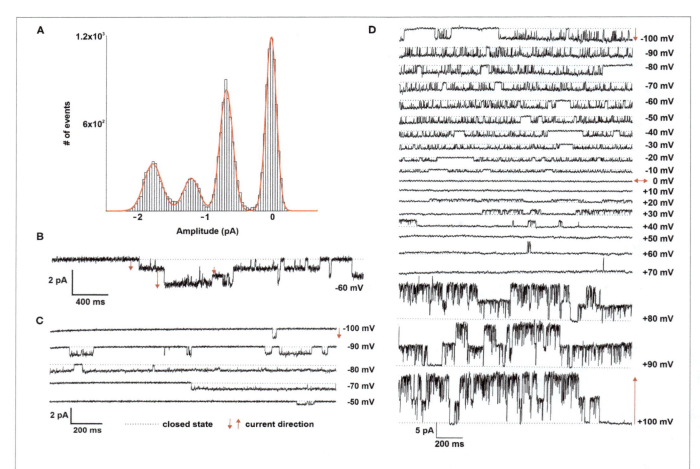

FIGURE 5 | Electrophysiological characterization of fetal LOs. (A,B) Amplitude histogram and current tracing of multiple channel openings at −60 mV. (C) Different open times at different holding potentials (−100 to −50 mV) are displayed. (D) High variability of channel kinetics (amplitude, open and closed times) are shown for a recording with voltage steps from −100 to +100 mV and a reversal potential close to 0. The strong rectifying properties of the illustrated recording, with smaller inward currents on hyperpolarization and larger outward currents when the patch membrane was depolarized, suggests an outwardly rectifying Cl⁻ channel (ORCC). Closed state is indicated by the dotted line. The arrows indicate the current direction with ↑ outward and ↓ inward currents.

< 0.01, $p < 0.05$; **Figure 6A**). In contrast, mRNA expression of the cystic fibrosis conductance regulator (*CFTR*) was significantly reduced by dexamethasone ($p < 0.05$). Furthermore, the mRNA expression of *Sftpb* (surfactant protein B) and *Sftpc* (surfactant protein C) were significantly increased by dexamethasone in LOs ($p < 0.01$, $p < 0.05$; **Figure 6A**). In agreement, dexamethasone significantly increased mRNA expression of ENaC and the Na,K-ATPase in primary FDLE cells grown on permeable inserts ($p < 0.001$; **Figure 6B**). Furthermore, Na⁺ transport was significantly enhanced by dexamethasone as determined in Ussing chambers (**Figure 6C**). Dexamethasone increased I_{base} from 3.67 ± 0.09 µA/cm² (Mean ± SEM) to 4.71 ± 0.13 µA/cm² and the ΔI_{amil} from 2.99 ± 0.08 µA/cm² to 4.06 ± 0.12 µA/cm² ($p < 0.001$; **Figure 6C**). These results show that the fetal LOs mimic the response to dexamethasone seen in primary fetal lung epithelia and that the observed increase of mRNA expression causes an elevated transepithelial Na⁺ transport activity. Furthermore, LOs were strongly positive for EpCAM expression (**Figure 7A**).

Notably, dexamethasone significantly increased expression of the EpCAM and RT2-70 antigen ($p < 0.01$; **Figure 7B**). Finally, morphology of LOs treated with dexamethasone was not altered compared to control LOs (**Supplementary Figure 3**).

Mesenchymal stem cells (MSCs) have demonstrated therapeutic potential in animal models of neonatal lung disease (21–23) and thus represent a promising future therapeutic approach to alleviate disease burden in preterm infants. In our previous study we determined the paracrine effect of MSCs on lung functional and structural development in FDLE cells and fetal lung explants (19). Herein we aimed at reproducing the reactivity of LOs in comparison to the prior study and to extend the knowledge about cellular effects of MSCs. The LOs (15 div) were cultured with mesenchymal stem cell-conditioned medium (MSC-CM) for 4 days. The respective LO control was incubated with medium used for MSC culture, without MSC conditioning. MSC-CM enhanced lumen formation and thinning of the epithelial layer, in contrast to the denser morphology of control

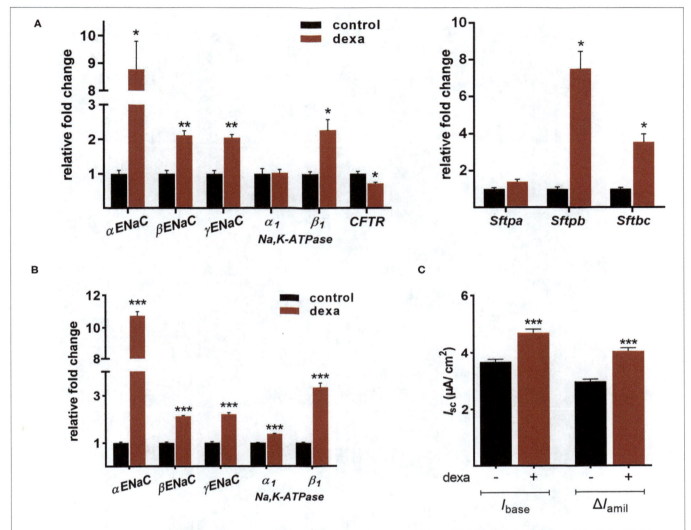

FIGURE 6 | Effects of dexamethasone on fetal LOs compared to FDLE cells. Data are displayed as Mean + SEM. (A) Gene expression analysis of LOs (15 div) stimulated with dexamethasone (100 nM) for 48 h. Dexamethasone significantly increased mRNA expression of the ENaC subunits (α, β, γ) and the Na,K-ATPase subunit-$\beta 1$ compared to control LOs cultured without dexamethasone ($n = 4/5$; **$p < 0.01$; *$p < 0.05$ by T-test). mRNA expression of CFTR was reduced by dexamethasone (*$p < 0.05$ by T-test). Furthermore, the mRNA expression of Sftpb and Sftpc were significantly increased by dexamethasone ($n = 4$; *$p < 0.05$ by T-test). (B) FDLE cells were also stimulated with dexamethasone (100 nM) for 48 h. In accordance to LOs, dexamethasone strongly increased the mRNA expression of the Na$^+$ transporters ($n = 12$; ***$p < 0.001$ by T-test). (C) The increased mRNA expression was accompanied by an enhanced Na$^+$ transport (I_{base}) and ENaC activity (ΔI_{amil}) in FDLE cells, as determined in Ussing chambers ($n = 78/92$; ***$p < 0.001$ by T-test). div, days in vitro.

LOs (**Figure 8A**). This was quantified by the compactness of the LOs, which is defined as the cellular area in proportion to the whole organoid area. Control LOs displayed a higher compactness compared to LOs treated with MSC-CM ($p < 0.01$; **Figure 8B**). These results show that MSC-CM-treated LOs exhibit a lower cellular packing density and higher intercellular space cavities in contrast to control LOs. Moreover, MSC-CM significantly increased the area of EpCAM and RT2-70 antigen expression, as shown by immunofluorescence and the percentage of RT2-70$^+$ cell area within the LOs ($p < 0.001$; **Figures 9A,B**). This was accompanied by an elevated RT2-70$^+$ cell number, which increased from 3.90 ± 3.67% (Mean ± SD) in control LOs to 11.78 ± 6.84% in MSC-CM-treated LOs ($p < 0.001$;

Figure 9B). While we could not detect T1α using the antibody RT1-40 in LOs at 15 div, staining of LOs treated with MSC-CM showed at least some RT1-40$^+$ ATI cells (**Figure 9C**). It is open whether this may be due to the four additional days in culture or the change of medium.

DISCUSSION

The study describes the establishment of fetal rat LOs as a relevant *in vitro* model of fetal lung development that allows scientists to replicate and functionally analyze key elements of lung maturation. For the first time, patch clamp

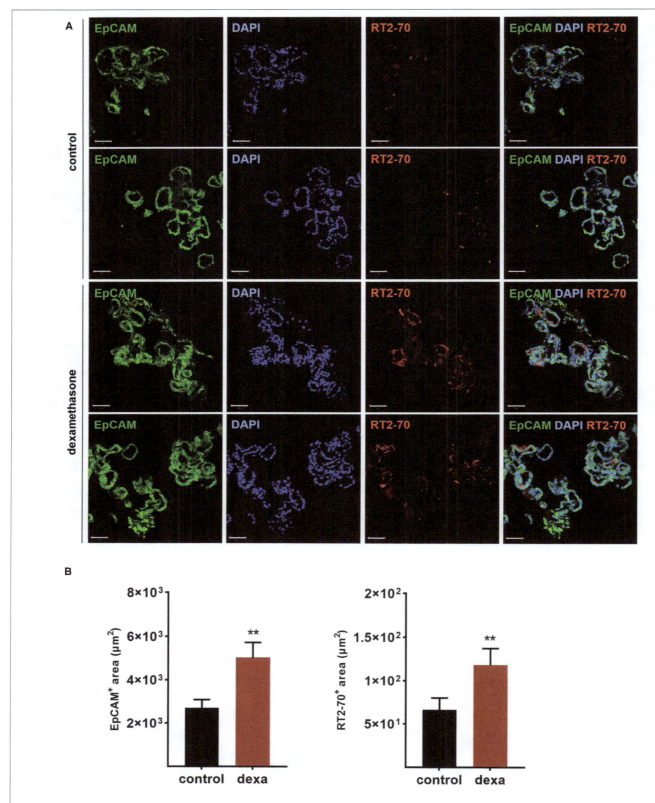

FIGURE 7 | Effects of dexamethasone on fetal LOs. LOs (15 div) were stimulated with dexamethasone (100 nM) for 48 h. Fluorescence images of LO slices were taken by confocal microscopy. (A) Organoids were strongly positive for EpCAM expression. Nuclei were stained with DAPI. Some epithelial cells showed luminal expression of the RT2-70 antigen. Scale bar: 50 μm. (B) Data are displayed as Mean + SEM. The area of EpCAM$^+$ area and RT2-70$^+$ area was higher in LOs stimulated with dexamethasone compared to control LOs ($n = 25$; **$p < 0.01$ by Mann-Whitney test). div, days in vitro.

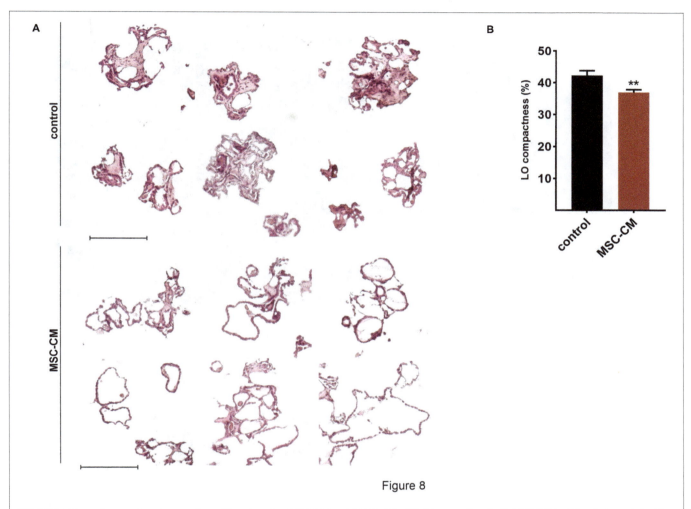

FIGURE 8 | Effects of mesenchymal stem cell-conditioned medium (MSC-CM) on fetal LOs. LOs (15 div) were cultured with MSC-CM for 96 h prior to analysis. **(A)** MSC-CM enhanced lumen formation and thinning of the epithelial layer, in contrast to the denser morphology of control LOs. Scale bar: 200 μm. **(B)** Data are displayed as Mean + SEM. Compactness was higher in control LOs compared to LOs treated with MSC-CM ($n = 56$; **$p < 0.01$ by T-test). div, days *in vitro*.

measurement demonstrated single ion channel activity in LOs. The responsiveness of fetal rat LOs to glucocorticoid mimicked the response *in vitro* and *in vivo*, thereby enhancing the relevance of the established model. Furthermore, the response of LOs to MSC-CM demonstrated the convenience of the model to test future therapeutic strategies to enhance maturation of immature lungs.

Even though the first described LOs were created using an undefined cell mix from fetal rat lungs (7), the further development of defined 3D organoid cultures in hydrogels was focusing on mouse and, later, human cells. Defined LOs were successfully generated from mouse and human cells, using primary fetal and adult lung cells as well as pluripotent cells, including embryonic stem cells (ESCs) and induced pluripotent stem cells (iPSCs) (10–12, 24–29). However, the rat is an important animal model and has been widely studied to gain a better understanding of physiological, developmental and pathophysiological mechanisms. Compared to rodent models, the use of human LOs harbors several limitations. Besides the limited availability of fetal lung tissue, its use is highly restricted due to ethical considerations. Similar ethical concerns can be raised for ESCs. ESCs or iPSCs possess great potential to model development and differentiation, but their use is accompanied by the need for a specialized laboratory and technical expertise, the high cost of cell culture, and the long time required for differentiation and production of respective LOs. In contrast, murine LO generation is feasible and can be easily reproduced. Another big obstacle of human fetal lung models and iPSCs is that they cannot be directly compared to the situation *in vivo*, while for rodents a comparison with animal models is possible. This may help to define the possibilities as well as limitations of the different *in vitro* fetal lung models, especially as basis for a future comparison with human fetal lung models. In addition, comparison of *in vivo* validated murine LOs with murine or human LOs from ESCs or iPSCs will show whether LOs from non-lung

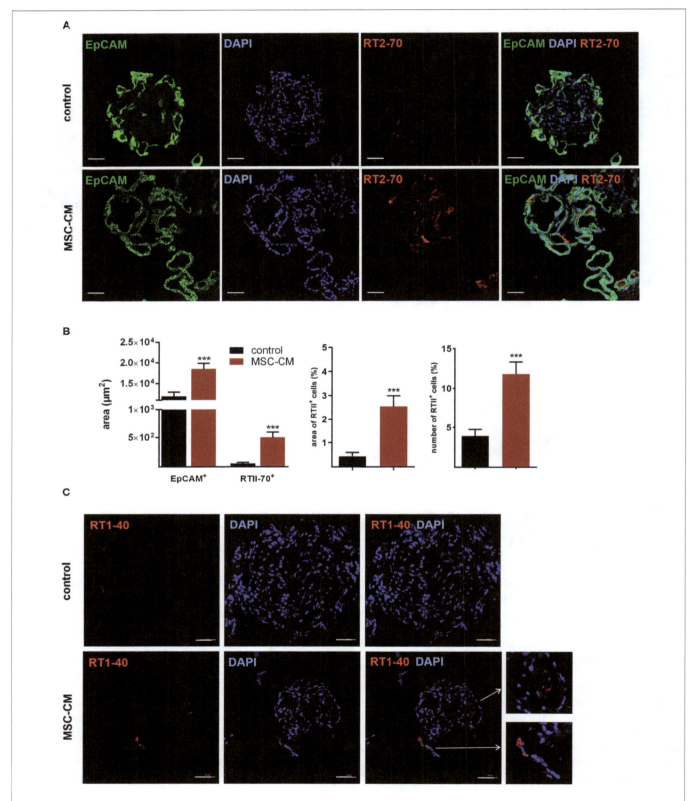

FIGURE 9 | Effects of mesenchymal stem cell-conditioned medium (MSC-CM) on fetal LOs. LOs (15 div) were cultured with MSC-CM for 96 h prior to analysis. Fluorescence images of LO slices were taken by confocal microscopy. (A) Organoids were strongly positive for EpCAM expression. Nuclei were stained with DAPI. Some epithelial cells showed luminal expression of the RT2-70 antigen. Scale bar: 50 μm. (B) Data are displayed as Mean + SEM. MSC-CM significantly increased

(Continued)

FIGURE 9 | the area of EpCAM and RT2-70 antigen expression, as shown by immunofluorescence and the percentage of RT2-70+ cell area within the LOs ($n = 20$; ***$p < 0.001$ by T-test with Welch's correction). Furthermore, RT2-70+ cell numbers were increased by MSC-CM ($n = 20$; ***$p < 0.001$ by Mann-Whitney test). **(C)** The ATI cell marker RT1-40 was observed in some individual cells of the MSC-CM-treated LOs. Scale bar: 50 μm. div, days in vitro.

sources can reflect essential lung functions and key elements of lung maturation.

Morphological Characterization of Fetal Lung Organoids

During their formation, fetal LOs demonstrated different morphologies of cystic, branched, and mixed appearance. Submerged culture mainly resulted in cystic LOs and cilia activity was observed in some of these cystic LOs. In contrast, ALI culture induced a heterogeneous cystic and branched morphology of LOs. Direct co-culture and interaction between CD31+ and FDLE cells was required for LO formation within 24 h, while indirect co-culture delayed the LO formation and reduced the efficacy. Furthermore, direct co-culture with lung mesenchymal cells like fetal lung fibroblasts as well as human CD31+ cells (HUVEC) could also support LO formation. Endothelial and mesenchymal cells were highly migratory in Matrigel, while FDLE cells did not show active migration. Direct cell-cell contact between endothelial/mesenchymal cells and FDLE cells facilitated initial cell aggregation required for organoid formation. Thus, the effect of helper cells may not be strictly cell-type specific, but rather based on their migratory capacity, and both endothelial and mesenchymal cells can support organoid growth. In addition, paracrine mechanisms might also be involved, since indirect co-culture with helper cells also resulted in, although delayed, LO formation, which is in contrast to FDLE cell-only culture that lacked LO formation. However, a big advantage of endothelial cells is that their proliferation is not supported under LO culture conditions, while mesenchymal cells proliferate and overgrow the whole cell culture. Notably, all cells in the LOs were positive for EpCAM staining, demonstrating that it consisted only of epithelial cells. Since culture conditions involved a rich serum-containing medium in combination with an ECM, CD31+ cells were probably not required as feeder cells, but rather for the 3D assembly of FDLE cells. CD31+ cells were highly migratory and provided early tube-like structures. The culture conditions allowed for formation and long-time persistence of vital LOs, showing only a few dead cells in the periphery. Although, these dead cells were not analyzed, the fact that LOs consisted of EpCAM+ cells only and CD31+ cells were not proliferating, these dead cells could well be leftover CD31+ cells. Concerning the maximal size reached at about 15 div, prior studies demonstrated that the ECM environment (Matrigel in our case) imposes solid stress on the growing organoid. Organoids in a mechanically resistant matrix grow until a growth-inhibitory threshold level of solid stress is attained. This is accompanied by an increase of cellular packing density, decreasing apoptosis with no significant changes in proliferation (30). It is therefore assumed that the maximum LO size depends on the mechanical properties of the ECM used.

Staining of LOs demonstrated the presence of EpCAM+ cells and cells being also positive for RT2-70 or CC-10, which are markers of ATII and Club cells, respectively. The EpCAM+ cells were polarized with the apical side facing the lumen, shown by the apical expression of RT2-70. In contrast to the ATII and Club cell markers, no ATI cells (RT1-40+ = T1α) were observed. T1α is expressed throughout lung morphogenesis although on a low and widespread level. T1α mRNA and protein expression increases during late fetal development and is then restricted to ATI cells in the distal epithelium (31, 32). We assume that the lack of RT1-40 staining in our fetal LOscould be based on an immature differentiation state with low T1α expression. Alveolarization start in rodents at postnatal day 4, while our FDLE cells are isolated at the saccular stage of lung development prior to actual development of alveoli. In our research context this immature LO mimics lung immaturity of fetal infants born prior to the start of alveolarization. We assume that the budding branched luminal structures we observe in the LOs possibly represent sacculi, a precursor which correspond to the later alveolar sacculi. In agreement, fetal rat lung slices of the same gestational age were negative for T1α protein staining, while adult rat lung slices were strongly positive for T1α.

Functional Characterization of Fetal Lung Organoids

Ion channel activity is important for lung growth in utero as well as for the perinatal adaptation to air breathing. The analysis of ion channels thus demonstrates a biological function of high physiological relevance with regard to fetal lung maturation. In general, the phenotype of isolated ATII cells under classical culture conditions differs from mature cells in vivo. They show differences with regard to cell-cell-communication, expression of tight junctions proteins, barrier function, and general morphology [reviewed by (33)]. Herein we show that fetal LOs represent a physiological model for AFC, as the contributing ion channels can be measured with patch clamp. We demonstrate the presence of ion channels with HSC and NSC channel-like properties in accordance with previous studies of vital lung slices, which showed an average conductance of 8.8 ± 3.2 pS (HSC) and 22.5 ± 6.3 pS (NSC) (34). We observed currents that reverse near 0 mV and exhibit little rectification, which is in contrast to the current-voltage relationship for HSC and NSC channels from ATII cells in primary culture (35). Therein, HSC channels strongly rectify and reverse at high depolarizing potentials, and NSC channels reverse at ~+40 mV (35). High K+ concentration in our bathing solution is supposed to depolarize the cell and to establish a resting membrane potential near 0 mV. Thereby the holding potential installed at the pipette should represent the actual patch potential. By their nature NSC channels must reverse at a patch potential of 0 mV, which means that the observed reversal potential is representative of the membrane potential. Thus, in primary ATII cells the membrane potential is $\sim$-40 mV, while in our depolarized LOs the membrane potential must be close to 0 mV, equal to the observed reverse potential. The same was reported for vital lung slices, which demonstrated HSC and NSC channels that reverse near 0 mV and HSC channels exhibiting little rectification (35, 36). Possible causes for the differences between cultured primary ATII cells and lung slices have been discussed in detail by the authors (35). It further underlines that LOs more closely represent vital lung tissue in contrast to primary ATII cells, which is important for studying ion transport in alveolar cells. Furthermore, anion channels with properties like ORCC were observed, which possibly contribute to balancing the electroneutrality of Na^+ transport in ATII cells. In our study, we did not aim at thoroughly depicting ion channel activities in fetal LOs, but to demonstrate the biological function and applicability of the model system. According to our observations, fetal LOs constitute a physiological model system to study the single channel activity of the (fetal) alveolar epithelia.

The Stimulating Effects of Dexamethasone and MSCs

After the characterization of LO function, we determined their responsiveness to established lung maturation-inducing hormones. Antenatal glucocorticoids accelerate late-gestation lung maturation in low doses by enhancing surfactant synthesis, increasing the volume density of ATII cells and upregulating AFC (37–39). Mice lacking intracellular glucocorticoid receptors died of respiratory failure shortly after birth (40). Their lung development was retarded, accompanied by a reduction of *ENaC* mRNA levels in total lung RNA (40). Several studies demonstrated the stimulation of *ENaC subunit* expression by glucocorticoids (13, 41). In accordance, dexamethasone strongly increased mRNA expression of all *ENaC subunits* and that of the rate-limiting *Na,K-ATPase* β_1-*subunit* in fetal LO. In contrast, *CFTR* mRNA expression was reduced by dexamethasone as previously shown in FDLE and human bronchial submucosal gland-derived Calu-3 cells (42, 43). Furthermore, dexamethasone stimulated mRNA expression of *Sftpb* and *Sftpc,* confirming the surfactant synthesis-stimulating effect. We complemented the analyses of mRNA expression in LOs with measurements done in our FDLE cell model. The comparison showed a similar increase of *ENaC* and *Na,K-ATPase* mRNA expression induced by dexamethasone. Furthermore, the elevated Na^+ transport and ENaC activity stimulated by dexamethasone was shown in Ussing chamber measurements, demonstrating the relevance of elevated mRNA expression for channel activity. These results confirm the validity of our fetal LO model reproducing the response to glucocorticoids seen *in vitro* and *in vivo*. Furthermore, dexamethasone increased the area of EpCAM and RT2-70 antigen expression, thereby underlining the stimulating effect of glucocorticoids on alveolar differentiation.

Regarding the immature state of lungs from preterm infants, developing and testing new therapeutic strategies is of high clinical relevance. Due to the immunomodulatory and regenerative potential of MSCs, MSC-based cell therapies represent an interesting therapeutic strategy to enhance lung maturation (23). The therapeutic potential of MSCs is mainly attributed to paracrine effects. In accordance, MSC-CM affected LO morphology with an enhanced lumen formation as well as an increased expression of EpCAM and RT2-70. The results showed that up to 15% of the cells expressed the RT2-70 antigen. This is close to the situation *in vivo*, where ATII cells comprise $\sim$15% of all lung cells, but cover only $\sim$2–5% of the internal surface area (44). These results suggest an enhanced maturation of LOs induced by MSC-CM, which is in line with a prior study of our group (19). Therein we showed that MSC-CM strongly stimulated functional and structural maturation of fetal lungs. Fetal lung explant growth and branching as well as surfactant protein mRNA expression were enhanced by MSC-CM (19). Furthermore, MSC-CM strongly increased the activity and mRNA expression of *ENaC* and the *Na,K-ATPase* in FDLE cells (19). These effects were at least partially mediated by the PI3-K/AKT (phosphoinositide 3-kinase/protein kinase B) and Rac1 (Ras-related C3 botulinum toxin substrate 1) signaling pathways (19). In agreement, we demonstrated changes in structural maturation in LOs stimulated with MSC-CM, as shown by reduced compactness, increased ATII cell number and area, and first detection of ATI cells. Therefore, results observed in fetal rat lung explants as well as primary FDLE culture were reproduced in fetal LOs, confirming its relevance as a functional *in vitro* model, which can be used to study novel therapeutic developments.

Limitations and Outlook

There are also several limitations of our fetal LOs as an *in vitro* model. An important aspect to consider is the undefined culture condition, which may affect research focused on differentiation and signaling pathways. The culture conditions applied in this study uses FCS and Matrigel, both complex, undefined, and batch-to-batch varying solutions isolated from primary tissue sources of different species, supplying growth factors or basement membrane proteins. Adapting the culture conditions of LOs in the future will possibly enable the generation of more complex co-culture systems to study direct and indirect cellular interactions.

In general, a detailed morphological analysis of fetal rat lung cells and tissues was challenging, since antibodies specific for rat lung tissue are rare. Furthermore, differences in antibody binding between fetal and adult lung tissue were observed and organ specific expression was also seen. Although several studies have shown that the monoclonal antibody RT2-70 is specific for the apical surfaces of rat ATII cells, the respective protein is largely unknown. It is therefore also unknown at which maturational state an ATII cell expresses this unknown protein and whether a lack of expression rules out an ATII cell identity. The target protein is expressed only at the apical membrane compartment, hence only a small area of the cell is stained, but most luminally located cells expressed the RT2-70 antigen. This is in contrast to the EpCAM staining, which can be found on the complete cell surface. Correlating the area positive for EpCAM to the whole LO area in comparison to the area positive for RT2-70 does not reflect the number of ATII cells and might underestimate the amount of ATII cells in our LOs. Despite these limitations FDLE cells are a physiologically well-characterized *in vitro* model that has been studied with Ussing chambers and patch clamp in addition to mRNA expression analyses. We have determined the effect of glucocorticoids, female and male sex hormones, insulin and many other factors on the maturity of FDLE cells in prior studies (45–49), which enabled us to compare the different *in vitro* fetal lung models and to evaluate if the generated 3D fetal LOs represent a novel *in vitro* model suitable for studies addressing developmental or therapeutic approaches. The FDLE cells are derived from fetal rat pups 24–48 h prior to birth. Studies showed that fetal rat pups born 24 h prior to term birth experience respiratory distress due to structural and functional lung immaturity, reflected in a survival rate of only 6% by 36 h after delivery if the pups were placed in air, which increased to 47% when they were placed in >95% oxygen (4). The authors concluded that the preterm rat is a suitable model for studies of acute and chronic neonatal lung disease, as structural and functional lung immaturity is a major risk factor for pulmonary complications. Due to this and other reports we believe that our model is suitable to study immaturity-associated complications arising from preterm birth.

While the CD31$^+$ cells used in this study were required for an efficient LO formation, their role and interactions seemed to be limited to the first days. It would be interesting to analyze how a combined co-culture of endothelial and mesenchymal cells may further enhance LO differentiation, especially with defined medium and ECM conditions. This could also provide an *in vitro* model to study the effects of inflammation on lung development by either applying proinflammatory stimuli or using a direct or indirect co-culture approach with cells of the innate immune system. Another aspect, which should be considered to enhance LOs as *in vitro* lung model, is the biophysical property of the environment, although this may be more technically challenging to adapt. This includes the defined elastic moduli of hydrogels, the oxygen concentration to present hyperoxia or hypoxia as well as biomechanical stimuli and stress induction by periodical stretching or acute pressure. Despite these limitations and currently unsolved challenges, LOs provide a fast and easy *in vitro* model that allows a faster screening procedure compared to animal models, while also providing a higher biological relevance compared to classical cell culture. LOs will allow for a broad range of manipulation and can be adjusted to the study needs like changing signal pathways using agonists or antagonists, adaption of the physical and chemical properties of the ECM, genetic manipulation of the cells used for LO formation, and/or co-culture with different cell types or pathogens. This could lead to more complex models with multiple and/or sequential impacts to recapitulate fetal and/or newborn lung injuries.

CONCLUSION

In conclusion, LOs generated from FDLE cells represent a fetal lung model that replicates key biological lung functions essential for lung maturation. In detail, the fetal LOs demonstrated the development of fetal lung alveoli, the expression of surfactant proteins, and most importantly the expression and electrophysiological activity of ion channels. For the first time electrophysiological analysis by patch clamp allowed the single cell measurement of ion channel activity in LOs. Furthermore, fetal LOs showed functional responsiveness to glucocorticoids and MSCs. The main goal was to develop an immature LO model to enable the study of maturation and how this can be enhanced to benefit preterm infants in the future. Thus, fetal LOs demonstrated the convenience of the model to test and establish new therapeutic strategies.

AUTHOR CONTRIBUTIONS

ML and CF: conceptualization, formal analysis, funding acquisition, resources, supervision, and writing-original draft. ML, SP, TP, and CF: data curation, investigation, and methodology. ML, SP, and CF: validation. All authors writing-review and editing.

ACKNOWLEDGMENTS

We wish to thank Jessica Loeffler and Annett Friedrich-Stoeckigt for excellent technical assistance. We acknowledge support from Leipzig University for Open Access Publishing.

REFERENCES

1. Barker PM, Gowen CW, Lawson EE, Knowles MR. Decreased sodium ion absorption across nasal epithelium of very premature infants with respiratory distress syndrome. *J Pediatr.* (1997) 130:373–7. doi: 10.1016/S0022-3476(97)70198-7
2. Hilgendorff A, Reiss I, Ehrhardt H, Eickelberg O, Alvira CM. Chronic lung disease in the preterm infant. Lessons learned from animal models. *Am J Respir Cell Mol Biol.* (2014) 50:233–45. doi: 10.1165/rcmb.2013-0014TR
3. Jassal D, Han RN, Caniggia I, Post M, Tanswell AK. Growth of distal fetal rat lung epithelial cells in a defined serum-free medium. *In Vitro Cell Dev Biol.* (1991) 27:625–32. doi: 10.1007/BF02631105

4. Tanswell AK, Wong L, Possmayer F, Freeman BA. The preterm rat: a model for studies of acute and chronic neonatal lung disease. *Pediatr Res.* (1989) 25:525–9. doi: 10.1203/00006450-198905000-00020
5. Kaltofen T, Haase M, Thome UH, Laube M. Male sex is associated with a reduced alveolar epithelial sodium transport. *PLoS ONE.* (2015) 10:e0136178. doi: 10.1371/journal.pone.0136178
6. Lancaster MA, Knoblich JA. Organogenesis in a dish: modeling development and disease using organoid technologies. *Science.* (2014) 345:1247125. doi: 10.1126/science.1247125
7. Zimmermann B, Barrach HJ, Merker HJ, Hinz N. Basement membrane formation and lung cell differentiation *in vitro. Eur J Cell Biol.* (1985) 36:66–73.

8. Rannels SR, Yarnell JA, Fisher CS, Fabisiak JP, Rannels DE. Role of laminin in maintenance of type II pneumocyte morphology and function. *Am J Physiol.* (1987) 253(6 Pt 1):C835–45. doi: 10.1152/ajpcell.1987.253.6.C835

9. Paine R, Ben-Ze'ev A, Farmer SR, Brody JS. The pattern of cytokeratin synthesis is a marker of type 2 cell differentiation in adult and maturing fetal lung alveolar cells. *Dev Biol.* (1988) 129:505–15. doi: 10.1016/0012-1606(88)90396-X

10. Lee J-H, Bhang DH, Beede A, Huang TL, Stripp BR, Bloch KD, et al. Lung stem cell differentiation in mice directed by endothelial cells via a BMP4-NFATc1-thrombospondin-1 axis. *Cell.* (2014) 156:440–55. doi: 10.1016/j.cell.2013.12.039

11. McQualter JL, Yuen K, Williams B, Bertoncello I. Evidence of an epithelial stem/progenitor cell hierarchy in the adult mouse lung. *Proc Natl Acad Sci U S A.* (2010) 107:1414–9. doi: 10.1073/pnas.0909207107

12. Barkauskas CE, Cronce MJ, Rackley CR, Bowie EJ, Keene DR, Stripp BR, et al. Type 2 alveolar cells are stem cells in adult lung. *J Clin Invest.* (2013) 123:3025–36. doi: 10.1172/JCI68782

13. Thome UH, Davis IC, Nguyen SV, Shelton BJ, Matalon S. Modulation of sodium transport in fetal alveolar epithelial cells by oxygen and corticosterone. *Am J Physiol Lung Cell Mol Physiol.* (2003) 284:L376–85. doi: 10.1152/ajplung.00218.2002

14. Drakhlis L, Biswanath S, Farr C-M, Lupanow V, Teske J, Ritzenhoff K, et al. Human heart-forming organoids recapitulate early heart and foregut development. *Nat Biotechnol.* (2021) 39:737–46. doi: 10.1038/s41587-021-00815-9

15. Gonzalez RF, Dobbs LG. Isolation and culture of alveolar epithelial Type I and Type II cells from rat lungs. *Methods Mol Biol.* (2013) 945:145–59. doi: 10.1007/978-1-62703-125-7_10

16. Dobbs LG, Pian MS, Maglio M, Dumars S, Allen L. Maintenance of the differentiated type II cell phenotype by culture with an apical air surface. *Am J Physiol.* (1997) 273(2 Pt 1):L347–54. doi: 10.1152/ajplung.1997.273.2.L347

17. Kirwin SM, Bhandari V, Dimatteo D, Barone C, Johnson L, Paul S, et al. Leptin enhances lung maturity in the fetal rat. *Pediatr Res.* (2006) 60:200–4. doi: 10.1203/01.pdr.0000227478.29271.52

18. van der Velden JL, Bertoncello I, McQualter JL. LysoTracker is a marker of differentiated alveolar type II cells. *Respir Res.* (2013) 14:123. doi: 10.1186/1465-9921-14-123

19. Obendorf J, Fabian C, Thome UH, Laube M. Paracrine stimulation of perinatal lung functional and structural maturation by mesenchymal stem cells. *Stem Cell Res Ther.* (2020) 11:525. doi: 10.1186/s13287-020-02028-4

20. Thalheim T, Quaas M, Herberg M, Braumann U, Kerner C, Loeffler M, et al. Linking stem cell function and growth pattern of intestinal organoids. *Dev Biol.* (2018) 433:254–61. doi: 10.1016/j.ydbio.2017.10.013

21. van Haaften T, Byrne R, Bonnet S, Rochefort GY, Akabutu J, Bouchentouf M, et al. Airway delivery of mesenchymal stem cells prevents arrested alveolar growth in neonatal lung injury in rats. *Am J Respir Crit Care Med.* (2009) 180:1131–42. doi: 10.1164/rccm.200902-0179OC

22. Di Bernardo J, Maiden MM, Jiang G, Hershenson MB, Kunisaki SM. Paracrine regulation of fetal lung morphogenesis using human placenta-derived mesenchymal stromal cells. *J Surg Res.* (2014) 190:255–63. doi: 10.1016/j.jss.2014.04.013

23. Laube M, Stolzing A, Thome UH, Fabian C. Therapeutic potential of mesenchymal stem cells for pulmonary complications associated with preterm birth. *Int J Biochem Cell Biol.* (2016) 74:18–32. doi: 10.1016/j.biocel.2016.02.023

24. Dye BR, Hill DR, Ferguson MA, Tsai Y-H, Nagy MS, Dyal R, et al. *In vitro* generation of human pluripotent stem cell derived lung organoids. *Elife.* (2015) 4:e05098. doi: 10.7554/eLife.05098

25. Hegab AE, Arai D, Gao J, Kuroda A, Yasuda H, Ishii M, et al. Mimicking the niche of lung epithelial stem cells and characterization of several effectors of their *in vitro* behavior. *Stem Cell Res.* (2015) 15:109–21. doi: 10.1016/j.scr.2015.05.005

26. Dye BR, Dedhia PH, Miller AJ, Nagy MS, White ES, Shea LD, et al. A bioengineered niche promotes *in vivo* engraftment and maturation of pluripotent stem cell derived human lung organoids. *Elife.* (2016) 5:e19732. doi: 10.7554/eLife.19732

27. Tan Q, Choi KM, Sicard D, Tschumperlin DJ. Human airway organoid engineering as a step toward lung regeneration and disease modeling. *Biomaterials.* (2016) 113:118–32. doi: 10.1016/j.biomaterials.2016.10.046

28. Ng-Blichfeldt J-P, Schrik A, Kortekaas RK, Noordhoek JA, Heijink IH, Hiemstra PS, et al. Retinoic acid signaling balances adult distal lung epithelial progenitor cell growth and differentiation. *EBioMedicine.* (2018) 36:461–74. doi: 10.1016/j.ebiom.2018.09.002

29. McQualter JL, Bertoncello I. Clonal culture of adult mouse lung epithelial stem/progenitor cells. *Methods Mol Biol.* (2015) 1235:231–41. doi: 10.1007/978-1-4939-1785-3_17

30. Helmlinger G, Netti P, Lichtenbeld H, Melder R, Jain R. Solid stress inhibits the growth of multicellular tumor spheroids. *Nat Biotechnol.* (1997) 15:778–83. doi: 10.1038/nbt0897-778

31. Ramirez MI, Millien G, Hinds A, Cao Y, Seldin DC, Williams MC. T1α, a lung type I cell differentiation gene, is required for normal lung cell proliferation and alveolus formation at birth. *Dev Biol.* (2003) 256:62–73. doi: 10.1016/S0012-1606(02)00098-2

32. Nikolić MZ, Caritg O, Jeng Q, Johnson J-A, Sun D, Howell KJ, et al. Human embryonic lung epithelial tips are multipotent progenitors that can be expanded *in vitro* as long-term self-renewing organoids. *Elife.* (2017) 6:e26575. doi: 10.7554/eLife.26575

33. Dobbs LG, Johnson MD. Alveolar epithelial transport in the adult lung. *Respir Physiol Neurobiol.* (2007) 159:283–300. doi: 10.1016/j.resp.2007.06.011

34. Helms MN, Jain L, Self JL, Eaton DC. Redox regulation of epithelial sodium channels examined in alveolar type 1 and 2 cells patch-clamped in lung slice tissue. *J Biol Chem.* (2008) 283:22875–83. doi: 10.1074/jbc.M801363200

35. Trac PT, Thai TL, Linck V, Zou L, Greenlee M, Yue Q, et al. Alveolar nonselective channels are ASIC1a/α-ENaC channels and contribute to AFC. *Am J Physiol Lung Cell Mol Physiol.* (2017) 312:L797–811. doi: 10.1152/ajplung.00379.2016

36. Shlyonsky V, Goolaerts A, Mies F, Naeije R. Electrophysiological characterization of rat type II pneumocytes *in situ*. *Am J Respir Cell Mol Biol.* (2008) 39:36–44. doi: 10.1165/rcmb.2007-0227OC

37. Ballard PL, Ning Y, Polk D, Ikegami M, Jobe AH. Glucocorticoid regulation of surfactant components in immature lambs. *Am J Physiol.* (1997) 273(5 Pt 1):L1048–57. doi: 10.1152/ajplung.1997.273.5.L1048

38. Folkesson HG, Norlin A, Wang Y, Abedinpour P, Matthay MA. Dexamethasone and thyroid hormone pretreatment upregulate alveolar epithelial fluid clearance in adult rats. *J Appl Physiol.* (2000) 88:416–24. doi: 10.1152/jappl.2000.88.2.416

39. Snyder JM, Rodgers HF, O'Brien JA, Mahli N, Magliato SA, Durham PL. Glucocorticoid effects on rabbit fetal lung maturation *in vivo*: an ultrastructural morphometric study. *Anat Rec.* (1992) 232:133–40. doi: 10.1002/ar.1092320115

40. Cole TJ, Blendy JA, Monaghan AP, Krieglstein K, Schmid W, Aguzzi A, et al. Targeted disruption of the glucocorticoid receptor gene blocks adrenergic chromaffin cell development and severely retards lung maturation. *Genes Dev.* (1995) 9:1608–21. doi: 10.1101/gad.9.13.1608

41. Tchepichev S, Ueda J, Canessa C, Rossier BC, O'Brodovich H. Lung epithelial⁺ Na channel subunits are differentially regulated during development and by steroids. *Am J Physiol.* (1995) 269(3 Pt 1):C805–12. doi: 10.1152/ajpcell.1995.269.3.C805

42. Prota LFM, Cebotaru L, Cheng J, Wright J, Vij N, Morales MM, et al. Dexamethasone regulates CFTR expression in Calu-3 cells with the involvement of chaperones HSP70 and HSP90. *PLoS ONE.* (2012) 7:e47405. doi: 10.1371/journal.pone.0047405

43. Laube M, Bossmann M, Thome UH. Glucocorticoids distinctively modulate the CFTR channel with possible implications in lung development and transition into extrauterine life. *PLoS ONE.* (2015) 10:e0124833. doi: 10.1371/journal.pone.0124833

44. Dobbs LG. Isolation and culture of alveolar type II cells. *Am J Physiol Lung Cell Mol Physiol.* (1990) 258:L134–7. doi: 10.1152/ajplung.1990.258.4.L134

45. Schmidt C, Klammt J, Thome UH, Laube M. The interaction of glucocorticoids and progesterone distinctively affects epithelial sodium transport. *Lung.* (2014) 192:935–46. doi: 10.1007/s00408-014-9640-3

46. Haase M, Laube M, Thome UH. Sex-specific effects of sex steroids on alveolar epithelial Na+ transport. *Am J Physiol Lung Cell Mol Physiol.* (2017) 312:L405–14. doi: 10.1152/ajplung.00275.2016

47. Laube M, Küppers E, Thome UH. Modulation of sodium transport in alveolar epithelial cells by estradiol and progesterone. *Pediatr Res.* (2011) 69:200–5. doi: 10.1203/PDR.0b013e3182070ec8

48. Laube M, Riedel D, Ackermann B, Haase M, H Thome U. Glucocorticoids equally stimulate epithelial Na+ transport in male and female fetal alveolar cells. *Int J Mol Sci.* (2019) 21:57. doi: 10.3390/ijms21010057

49. Mattes C, Laube M, Thome UH. Rapid elevation of sodium transport through insulin is mediated by AKT in alveolar cells. *Physiol Rep.* (2014) 2:e00269. doi: 10.1002/phy2.269

18

Imaging Bronchopulmonary Dysplasia—A Multimodality Update

Thomas Semple[1,2], Mohammed R. Akhtar[3] and Catherine M. Owens[2]*

[1] The Royal Brompton Hospital, London, United Kingdon, [2] Great Ormond Street Hospital, London, United Kingdom,
[3] St Bartholomews and The Royal London Hospital, London, United Kingdom

*Correspondence:
Catherine M. Owens
owenscatherine.5@gmail.com

Bronchopulmonary dysplasia is the most common form of infantile chronic lung disease and results in significant health-care expenditure. The roles of chest radiography and computed tomography (CT) are well documented but numerous recent advances in imaging technology have paved the way for newer imaging techniques including structural pulmonary assessment *via* lung magnetic resonance imaging (MRI), functional assessment *via* ventilation, and perfusion MRI and quantitative imaging techniques using both CT and MRI. New applications for ultrasound have also been suggested. With the increasing array of complex technologies available, it is becoming increasingly important to have a deeper knowledge of the technological advances of the past 5–10 years and particularly the limitations of some newer techniques currently undergoing intense research. This review article aims to cover the most salient advances relevant to BPD imaging, particularly advances within CT technology, postprocessing and quantitative CT; structural MRI assessment, ventilation and perfusion imaging using gas contrast agents and Fourier decomposition techniques and lung ultrasound.

Keywords: bronchopulmonary dysplasia, structural characterization, imaging techniques, quantitative pulmonary magnetic resonance imaging, lung parenchymal magnetic resonance imaging, hyperpolarized gas imaging, lung ultrasound

BRONCHOPULMONARY DYSPLASIA (BPD)

Bronchopulmonary dysplasia is the most common form of infantile chronic lung disease and is reported to occur in between 10.2 and 24.8% of European infants born between 24 + 0 and 31 + 6 weeks of gestation (1). While only representing 8% of births in population-based data from the US, preterm or low-birth weight infants accounted for 47% of the total annual expenditure for all births (2, 3).

The clinical definition of BPD is the requirement of supplemental oxygen for at least 28 days in an infant born at less than 32 weeks of gestation (4).

The classic form of BPD was described in premature infants exposed to prolonged high-pressure mechanical ventilation and high concentrations of inspired oxygen (5). Pathological findings include alternating regions of overinflation and atelectasis, airway smooth muscle hypertrophy, squamous metaplasia of the airway epithelium, peribronchial fibrosis, constrictive obliterative bronchiolitis, and hypertensive pulmonary vascular changes (6).

While the current widespread administration of antenatal steroids, adoption of lower pressure ventilatory support, and reduction in the use of high concentration inspired oxygen have led to a decreased incidence of classical BPD, the increased survival of extremely premature (24–26 weeks of gestation) low-birth weight (<1,000 g) neonates has produced a new variant of BPD (7). Extremely premature neonates tend to respond well to the administration of exogenous surfactant and require relatively low-pressure mechanical ventilation with low to moderate oxygen concentrations. However, they are more prone to infection and pulmonary edema from physiological shunts (e.g., patent ductus arteriosus) leading to increased respiratory support needs (8). The lungs of neonates born at 24–28 weeks of gestation are still undergoing significant development and maturation, transitioning from the canalicular stage (formation of acina and invasion of capillaries into the pulmonary mesenchyme), through the saccular stage (formation of alveolar saccules from the terminal bronchioles) toward the alveolar phase at around 32 weeks of gestation, where the first true alveoli are formed (9). Birth and premature initiation of gas exchange will interrupt this development, with studies demonstrating the presence of fewer, larger (simplified) alveoli with reduced vascularity in the lungs of neonates born prematurely (10, 11). Pathologic specimens demonstrate a lower incidence of airway and vascular diseases and less interstitial fibrosis than in the more severe classic form of BPD (12).

In the longer term, alongside other disorders related to prematurity, BPD can lead to recurrent hospitalizations with lower respiratory tract infections, reduced lung function, severe obstructive airways disease, and pulmonary hypertension with right heart dysfunction (13, 14) with neurological and cognitive impairment causing further morbidity (15). Interestingly, a recent study has suggested an association with pulmonary vein stenosis (PVS) with 4.6% of a 213-patient cohort of infants with BPD affected, more frequently those with lower birth weights. Those with associated PVS experienced higher rates of mortality (16).

ROLE OF IMAGING IN BPD

During their initial neonatal intensive care unit (NICU) admission the imaging modality most commonly utilized in premature infants is chest radiography, allowing simultaneous assessment of support apparatus (endotracheal tubes, umbilical arterial, venous catheters, etc.), pulmonary parenchymal status [degree of respiratory distress syndrome (RDS) related change, edema from persistent shunting *via* a patent ductus arteriosus, etc.], and complications of mechanical ventilation (pneumothorax, pulmonary interstitial emphysema, etc.).

Chest radiographic features of established BPD include interstitial thickening, focal or generalized hyperexpansion, and atelectasis (**Figure 1**) (17). Computed tomography (CT) is more sensitive to the abnormalities of BPD demonstrating abnormalities in over 85% of patients with BPD including regions of decreased attenuation, emphysema-like change, linear and subpleural opacities, and bronchial wall thickening (**Figure 2**). Furthermore, the extent of structural abnormality on CT has been shown to correlate with the clinical severity of BPD (18).

There have been many developments within pediatric thoracic imaging (and indeed medical imaging in general) over the past 5–10 years with great potential to shed further light on the pathogenesis and temporal evolution of respiratory conditions such as BPD, further guide the treatment of RDS with the goal of reducing the subsequent development of BPD, and in the long-term follow-up of chronic respiratory disease. Some of the more significant developments are discussed below.

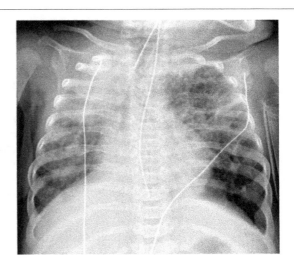

FIGURE 1 | Chest radiograph demonstrating widespread coarse interstitial markings, atelectasis, and regions of hyperexpansion (particularly at the left lung base), typical of bronchopulmonary dysplasia. Note also the right upper lobe consolidation and malposition of the NG tube.

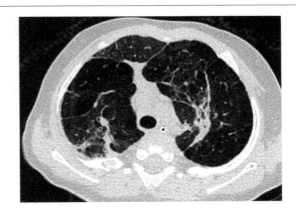

FIGURE 2 | Axial computed tomography section through the upper lobes on lung window settings demonstrates linear and subpleural opacities, bronchial wall thickening, and areas of low attenuation (indicative of small airways disease) in a patient with bronchopulmonary dysplasia.

EVOLUTION OF IMAGING TECHNIQUES RELEVANT TO BPD

Computed Tomography

Traditional "step and shoot" high-resolution computed tomography produced non-contiguous (interrupted) high spatial resolution images that could only be viewed in a single (axial) anatomical plane. This method has now largely been replaced with spiral/volumetric acquisitions that produce continuous volumetric data sets with isotropic voxels (each voxel—three-dimensional pixel—is the same length in x, y, and z axis). This allows reconstruction of the data in any plane (multiplanar reconstruction) and is essential for the more advanced postprocessing techniques discussed below.

Recent advances in CT technology have resulted in faster (subsecond) CT X-ray tube rotation speeds and smaller, more sensitive radiation detectors resulting in significant improvements in both temporal and spatial resolution (19). Current state of the art CT scanners are available with a single 320-row detector array, allowing the coverage of 16 cm in the z-axis (craniocaudal length) in a single tube rotation. An alternative arrangement (dual source CT) consists of two X-ray tubes (rather than the traditional single tube) with two arrays of detector banks mounted at 95° to each other such that two interlocking spiral data sets are formed around the patient, thus scanning the same volume of tissue in half the time as a single source scanner. Both these methods allow an infant's entire chest to be imaged in a fraction of a second (19, 20). This combination of faster tube rotation speeds, greater numbers of detectors and dual source systems, alongside the use of immobilization devices, such as vacuum splints (**Figure 3**) to keep the child still reducing the effects of patient body movement, has resulted in a paradigm shift within pediatric chest imaging, from scans requiring general anesthetic and breath-holding maneuvers, to ultrafast scans that produce diagnostic quality images, with minimal respiratory and cardiac motion artifact without the need for light sedation (21). Even at the high heart rates typical within the neonatal population, high-pitch CT, following the administration of intravenous (IV) contrast material has been proven capable of demonstrating small, fast-moving structures, such as the pulmonary veins, in diagnostically acceptable detail (22).

It is well known that the radiation burden of conventional thoracic CT is greater than that of chest radiography; however, technological advances (including rotational tube current modulation, adaptive array detectors and the introduction of iterative reconstruction techniques), alongside departmental dose optimization programs, have resulted in a significant reduction in CT radiation dose, while maintaining and even improving diagnostic image quality. There is also work in progress regarding the feasibility of ultralow dose thoracic CT with equivalent doses of the same order as chest radiography. Shi et al demonstrated a drop in equivalent dose from 0.89 to 0.61 mSv with no statistically significant difference in perceived image quality, and only a 14.8% decrease in measured signal to noise ratio when reducing tube voltage from 80 to 70 kV (23).

Postprocessing techniques are playing an increasingly important role within cardiothoracic imaging. Basic reconstruction into multiple orthogonal planes allows for easy differentiation of pulmonary vessels from parenchymal nodules. Increasing the slice thickness (average intensity projection) can reduce image noise in low dose examinations of small infants. Maximum and minimum intensity projection images (MIP and MinIP, respectively) can be utilized to better demonstrate vasculature and low attenuation regions such as regions of air trapping, respectively (24, 25). MinIP images are particularly well suited to demonstrating the areas of low attenuation alternating with higher attenuation lung (variegate mosaic attenuation) seen in patients with a small airways component of BPD (**Figure 4**).

More advanced postprocessing techniques such as volume rendering techniques allow the formation of 3D images of lungs and airways that can aid discussion with the wider multidisciplinary respiratory team and with families in clinic. There is further on-going research into the possible role of quantitative CT measures of lung volume, assessment of bronchial wall thickness, and quantification of abnormally low attenuation lung allowing potentially more robust and reproducible measures of airway and lung parenchymal disease (26).

As quantitative CT measures of respiratory tract disease become more mainstream, the necessity for protocol standardization will become more important, particularly in young infants who cannot follow breathing instructions, resulting in scan acquisitions during variable phases of the respiratory cycle. Attempts

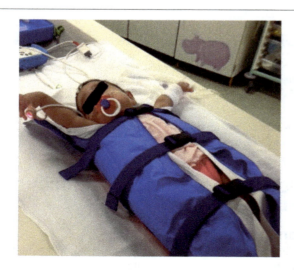

FIGURE 3 | Vacuum immobilization device used to limit gross patient movement. Use of these devices, alongside ultrafast, high-pitch computed tomography, has dramatically reduced the need for general anesthetic or sedation for cardiothoracic CT at our institution.

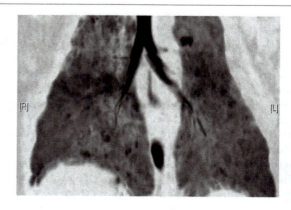

FIGURE 4 | Minimum intensity projection CT reconstruction demonstrating airway morphology and regions of heterogeneous (mosaic) attenuation in a child with bronchopulmonary dysplasia.

to overcome this problem, including spirometer-triggered CT, are currently in use in several specialist centers (27, 28).

Magnetic Resonance Imaging (MRI)

As a cross-sectional imaging technique that does not rely on ionizing radiation exposure, MRI seems the ideal modality for cross-sectional imaging in the pediatric population. However, the significant inherent limitations of conventional MRI severely limit its use in pediatric thoracic imaging. The lung parenchyma is inherently low in proton density and contains many air–tissue interfaces. As such, it returns extremely low levels of rapidly decaying signal, resulting in the formation of extremely low-resolution images of the lung parenchyma and all tissues save for the most central airways. Long examination times necessitate general anesthesia or heavy sedation and produce significant respiratory and cardiac motion artifacts (29). Further limitations result from the overall large size and reasonably small inner bore of the scanner, the need to transfer an unwell infant from the NICU to the MRI scanner, and the magnetic field strength which limits the level of medical support an infant can be provided without the use of specific MRI safe monitoring and anesthetic equipment.

More robust respiratory and ECG/pulse gating techniques, along with new RF pulse sequences, and sampling and reconstruction techniques have significantly improved the visualization of the pulmonary parenchyma and airways resulting in renewed interest in structural lung assessment *via* MRI. Faster MRI sequences such as T2-HASTE (single shot half-Fourier turbo spin echo) and T1 3D gradient recalled echo with parallel imaging algorithms (e.g., generalized autocalibrating partially parallel acquisition) have been employed with more recent interest in radial acquisitions [e.g., Periodically Rotated Overlapping ParallEL Lines with Enhanced Reconstruction (PROPELLER)], which are less sensitive to respiratory motion artifact, and ultrashort echotime sequences such as pointwise encoding time reduction with radial acquisition (PETRA)—a noiseless, free breathing sequence capable of isometric data acquisition at a submillimeter voxel size (30–32).

While significant headway has been made in improving structural lung assessment *via* MRI, the spatial resolution remains poor relative to CT (**Figures 5A,B**) [PETRA achieved a voxel size of 0.86 mm³ compared to 0.2 mm³ from a state of the art CT scanner (19)] and image acquisition time remains high [8–12 min for PETRA (33), 7–10 min for respiratory triggered PROPELLER (31) compared to a fraction of a second *via* CT]. Lung MRI may, however, have far more to offer in terms of quantitative and functional data output. Multiple acquisitions following the administration of IV contrast material (gadolinium chelate) allow the study of regional pulmonary perfusion over time (**Figure 6**). Newer techniques allow the formation of similar perfusion "maps" without the administration of contrast media and the associated risk in the presence of renal dysfunction (particularly relevant in premature infants). A variant of arterial spin labeling (ASL-FAIRER arterial spin labeling-flow sensitive alternating inversion recovery with an extra radiofrequency pulse) techniques involving the use of magnetic "tagging" of inflowing blood as a contrast medium has been used to study regional pulmonary perfusion without the

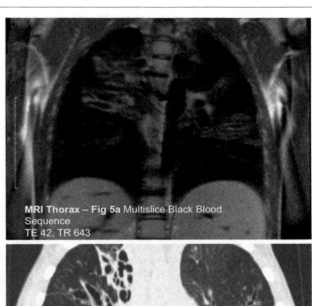

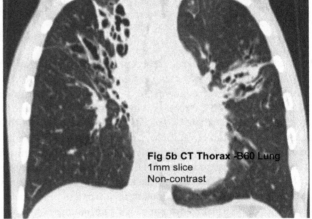

FIGURE 5 | **(A)** Coronal black blood SSFP magnetic resonance (MR) image and **(B)** coronal computed tomography (CT) reconstruction in a child with cystic fibrosis. Although the spatial resolution of MRI is relatively poor compared to CT, MRI is capable of demonstrating gross airway pathology.

need for IV administration of contrast medium (32). A second mathematically derived technique, Fourier decomposition, enables the formation of both perfusion and ventilation maps, again without the need for IV contrast administration, by extracting (decomposing) signal acquired throughout the respiratory cycle at respiratory and pulse frequencies, and has been shown to be feasible in children with cystic fibrosis (34).

Ventilation imaging *via* MRI has been extensively investigated with the highest resolution images obtained *via* the administration of hyperpolarized noble gases (typically He^3 or Xe^{129}) (35). Similar direct imaging of ventilation is also possible through the inhalation of fluorinated gases (e.g., sulfur hexafluoride and hexafluoroethane) (36). It is also possible to measure the degree of diffusion of these gases using multiple rapidly acquired diffusion-weighted images at differing B-values to provide a "short range" apparent diffusion coefficient (37). The free diffusivity of ^{3}He makes it ideal for ventilation imaging, but the solubility of ^{129}Xe and oxygen allows imaging of not only the inhalational phase but

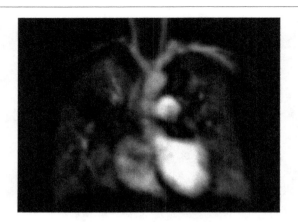

FIGURE 6 | Magnetic resonance imaging angiogram in a child with bronchopulmonary dysplasia demonstrating poor perfusion of the right upper lobe related to severe small airways disease and reflex vasoconstriction.

also the tissue and blood phases, giving further potentially useful information regarding the whole gas-exchange process (38).

Oxygen imparts a concentration-dependent paramagnetic effect on the rate of T1 recovery in adjacent tissue. Rapid T1 mapping *via* low flip angle GRE or "FLASH" (fast low angle shot) sequences before and at multiple concentrations of inhaled oxygen can thence produce an imaging measure of oxygen transfer (the oxygen transfer function—OTF) (39). The ready availability of oxygen as a medical gas and lack of the need for expensive hyperpolarization equipment make this a particularly attractive option for MR ventilation imaging. A combination of inversion pulses and single shot fast spin echo sequences, with prospective respiratory gating and retrospective deformable image registration, interleaved 2D slices with parallel imaging and half-Fourier reconstruction, allows whole lung oxygen-enhanced imaging of adult patients within 8–13 min (40).

While many of the abovementioned methods of ventilation/perfusion MRI have yet to be reported in the context of BPD, the development of a small footprint 1.5 T MRI unit installed on the neonatal unit of Cincinnati Children's Hospital has allowed several studies of MRI utilization in the investigation of neonatal lung disease. One such study identified a significantly higher volume of "high signal lung" in infants with BPD than was demonstrated in premature infants without BPD and healthy term infants. However, it should be noted that small numbers of infants were included (six term, six premature without BPD, and six infants with BPD) and that the infants with BPD were significantly lower weight and gestational age than the premature non-BPD and term groups. Also that "high signal" was defined as signal over 45% of the patient's mean chest wall signal without any mention of differing muscle mass/fat composition between groups. The study also assumes that the T1, T2, and T2* relaxation times of lung parenchyma and chest wall soft tissues are identical. While quantitative measurements of MRI signal in small neonates are in their infancy and should be interpreted with caution, this group did produce diagnostic-quality cross-sectional images of the lung parenchyma with no general anesthetic or sedation, with infants scanned during a 1.5-h period of free breathing. Two infants with BPD also underwent CT. In comparison with 3 mm CT sections (as opposed to more conventional 1 mm sections), CT demonstrated a greater number of regions of hyperlucent "emphysema-like" change and more severe bronchovascular distortion than MRI (Ochiai structural BPD score *via* CT of 12 vs 9 *via* MRI) (41).

Clearly significant headway has been made in pulmonary MRI, both in terms of structural and quantitative/functional imaging capability; however, further work, particularly regarding reproducibility and the clinical significance of quantitative/functional measures, remains to be done, before MRI can become a part of routine clinical care.

Ultrasound

Studies have suggested a role for ultrasound in the assessment of premature neonates with RDS (also known as hyaline membrane disease—HMD) in predicting the development of BPD. Avni et al. reported homogeneous hyperechogenicity of the lung bases, obscuring the diaphragm on transhepatic/transsplenic ultrasound in the setting of HMD with hyperechoic reverberation artifacts, beyond that expected at the diaphragmatic position. This "HMD-pattern" was found to transform to a "BPD pattern" of streaky, irregular areas of lower echogenicity, seen at day 18 of life in all patients subsequently diagnosed with BPD, with a negative predictive value of 95% (42). A further study by Pieper et al. demonstrated similar changes with the greatest predictive value of subsequent BPD diagnosis achieved *via* ultrasound at day 9 of life. They did, however, also observe a false positive case with the "BPD pattern" caused by bilateral lower lobe pneumonia (as demonstrated *via* chest radiography) (43). Clearly, there may be a specific role of lung ultrasound in the prediction of the development of BPD, however, these appearances (essentially artifacts) cannot be interpreted in isolation, and overall ultrasound is not a safe alternative to chest radiography. Complications of mechanical ventilation such as the misplacement of tubes and lines, air leaks (pneumothorax, pneumomediastinum, and pulmonary interstitial emphysema), and central pathology that do not abut the pleural surface can be completely invisible *via* ultrasound. There are, however potential roles in the setting of longitudinal research studies (as utilized in the Drakenstein Child Health Study), particularly in resource-poor areas (44).

CONCLUSION

Despite numerous significant advances within imaging technology, especially in CT and MRI, the simple chest radiograph remains the cornerstone of pediatric parenchymal lung imaging, particularly in the setting of premature neonates receiving complex support on a NICU. CT is reserved for specific clinical questions, including the presence of complex pathology and the more recently recognized association of prematurity with PVS.

New low and ultra-low dose CT techniques have brought the radiation exposure associated with CT closer to that of plain radiography and faster CT scanners have significantly reduced the need for general anesthetic and sedation use when imaging small children.

Improvements in respiratory and pulse gating in MRI alongside newer faster sequences and acceleration techniques have significantly improved the spatial resolution of pulmonary parenchymal MRI; however, the resolution remains inferior to that of CT. Coupled with long examination times, the role of MRI in pediatric pulmonary parenchymal imaging therefore remains predominantly as a research tool.

Ventilation MRI with hyperpolarized noble gases, fluorinated gases, oxygen, or *via* Fourier decomposition is making significant potential but again remains a research tool at this time.

Quantitative imaging by CT (lung volume calculation, bronchial wall thickness measurement, and low attenuation mapping) and MRI (OTF, quantification of regional signal) is showing significant promise, but still needs to be interpreted with care. It is clear that if imaging moves away from a traditional structural assessment toward a quantitative assessment, significant care will have to be taken to standardize examination techniques both within and between institutions. There is a very real risk that without a high level of standardization these techniques amount to a poor attempt at functional imaging, at a spatial resolution far below that of conventional nuclear medicine without its established robust clinical correlation.

Ultrasound has potentially established a niche use within risk assessment of premature neonates and may guide the future treatment of infants deemed to be at higher risk following the first few weeks of life. It should, however be noted that it does not constitute a potential replacement for plain radiography as suggested by some authors (45), as central pathology and important complications arising from misplaced support apparatus or air leaks can be completely missed *via* ultrasound alone.

Clearly, we are at an exciting crossroads between conventional structural and novel quantitative and functional imaging assessment, with ample room for new technology to significantly influence the future of neonatal pulmonary imaging. As progressively more sophisticated and complex technology is introduced it becomes increasingly important to stay up to date with advances and to maintain a detailed understanding of each technique. Novel techniques need validation within large cohorts of patients paying careful attention to protocol standardization. In the meantime, the humble chest radiograph is here to stay.

AUTHOR CONTRIBUTIONS

Imaging bronchopulmonary dysplasia—a multimodality update. All persons who meet authorship criteria are listed as authors, and all the authors certify that they have participated sufficiently in the work to take public responsibility for the content, including participation in the concept, design, analysis, writing, or revision of the manuscript. Authorship contributions: Category 1, conception and design of study: TS, CO, MA; acquisition of data: TS, CO, MA; analysis and/or interpretation of data: TS, CO, MA; Category 2, drafting the manuscript: TS, CO, MA; revising the manuscript critically for important intellectual content: TS, CO, MA; category 3, approval of the version of the manuscript to be published (the names of all authors must be listed): TS, CO, MA.

ACKNOWLEDGMENTS

All persons who have made substantial contributions to the work reported in the manuscript (e.g., technical help, writing and editing assistance, general support), but who do not meet the criteria for authorship, are named in the Acknowledgements and have given us their written permission to be named.

REFERENCES

1. Gortner L, Misselwitz B, Milligan D, Zeitlin J, Kollée L, Boerch K, et al. Rates of bronchopulmonary dysplasia in very preterm neonates in Europe: results from the MOSAIC cohort. *Neonatology* (2011) 99(2):112–7. doi:10.1159/000313024
2. Russell RB, Green NS, Steiner CA, Meikle S, Howse JL, Poschman K, et al. Cost of hospitalization for pre-term and low birth weight infants in the United States. *Pediatrics* (2007) 120:e1–9. doi:10.1542/peds.2006-2386
3. Barradas DT, Wasserman MP, Daniel-Robinson L, Bruce MA, DiSantis KI, Navarro FH, et al. Hospital utilization and costs among preterm infants by payer: nationwide inpatient sample, 2009. *Matern Child Health J* (2016) 20:808–18. doi:10.1007/s10995-015-1911-y
4. Jobe AH. Bronchopulmonary dysplasia. *Am J Respir Crit Care Med* (2001) 163:1723–9. doi:10.1164/ajrccm.163.7.2011060
5. Cherukupalli K, Larson JE, Rotschild A, Thurlbeck WM. Biochemical, clinical and morphologic studies on lungs of infants with bronchopulmonary dysplasia. *Pediatr Pulmonol* (1996) 22:215–29. doi:10.1002/(SICI)1099-0496(199610)22:4<215::AID-PPUL1>3.0.CO;2-L
6. Coalson JJ. Pathology of bronchopulmonary dysplasia. *Semin perinatol* (2006) 30:179–84. doi:10.1053/j.semperi.2006.05.004
7. Northway WH Jr. Bronchopulmonary dysplasia: twenty-five years later. *Pediatrics* (1992) 89:969–73.
8. Rojas MA, Gonzalez A, Bancalari E, Claure N, Poole C, Silva-Neto G. Changing trends in the epidemiology and pathogenesis of neonatal chronic lung disease. *J Pediatr* (1995) 126:605–10. doi:10.1016/S0022-3476(95)70362-4
9. Langston C, Kida K, Reed M, Thurlbeck WM. Human lung growth in late gestation and in the neonate. *Am Rev Respir Dis* (1984) 129: 607–13.
10. Husain AN, Siddiqui NH, Stocker JT. Pathology of arrested acinar development in postsurfactant bronchopulmonary dysplasia. *Hum Pathol* (1998) 29:710–7. doi:10.1016/S0046-8177(98)90280-5
11. Hislop AA, Haworth SG. Pulmonary vascular damage and the development of cor pulmonale following hyaline membrane disease. *Pediatr Pulmonol* (1990) 9:152–61. doi:10.1002/ppul.1950090306
12. Jobe AJ. The new BPD: an arrest of lung development. *Pediatr Res* (1999) 46:641–3. doi:10.1203/00006450-199912000-00007
13. Mourani PM, Ivy DD, Gao D, Abman SH. Pulmonary vascular effects of inhaled nitric oxide and oxygen tension in bronchopulmonary dysplasia. *Am J Respir Crit Care Med* (2004) 170(9):1006–13. doi:10.1164/rccm.200310-1483OC
14. Eber E, Zach MS. Long term sequelae of bronchopulmonary dysplasia (chronic lung disease of infancy). *Thorax* (2001) 56:317–23. doi:10.1136/thorax.56.4.317
15. Baraldi E, Carraro S, Filippone M. Bronchopulmonary dysplasia: definitions and long-term respiratory outcome. *Early Hum Dev* (2009) 85:S1–3. doi:10.1016/j.earlhumdev.2009.08.002
16. Swier NL, Richards B, Cua CL, Lynch SK, Yin H, Nelin LD, et al. Pulmonary vein stenosis in neonates with severe bronchopulmonary dysplasia. *Am J Perinatol* (2016) 33:671–7. doi:10.1055/s-0035-1571201
17. Griscom NT, Wheeler WB, Sweezey NB, Kim YC, Lindsey JC, Wohl ME. Bronchopulmonary dysplasia: radiographic appearance in middle childhood. *Radiology* (1989) 171:811–4. doi:10.1148/radiology.171.3.2717757

18. van Mastrigt E, Logie K, Ciet P, Reiss IK, Duijts L, Pijnenburg MW, et al. Lung CT imaging in patients with bronchopulmonary dysplasia: a systematic review. *Pediatr Pulmonol* (2016) 51:975–86. doi:10.1002/ppul.23446

19. SiemensUK.Availablefrom:https://www.healthcare.siemens.co.uk/computed-tomography/dual-source-ct/somatom-force/technical-specifications (accessed June 7, 2017).

20. Toshiba EU. Available from: http://www.toshiba-medical.eu/eu/product-solutions/computed-tomography/aquilion-one/# (accessed June 7, 2017).

21. Golan A, Marco R, Raz H, Shany E. Imaging in the newborn: infant immobilizer obviates the need for anaesthesia. *Isr Med Assoc J* (2011) 13(11):663–5.

22. Sriharan M, Lazoura O, Pavitt CW, Castellano I, Owens CM, Rubens MB, et al. Evaluation of high-pitch ungated pediatric cardiovascular computed tomography for the assessment of cardiac structures in neonates. *J Thorac Imaging* (2016) 31(3):177–82. doi:10.1097/RTI.0000000000000201

23. Shi JW, Xu DF, Dai HZ, Shen L, Ji YD. Evaluation of chest CT scan in low-weight children with ultralow tube voltage (70kVp) combined with Flash scan technique. *Br J Radiol* (2016) 89(1059):20150184. doi:10.1259/bjr.20150184

24. Siegel MJ. Multiplanar and three-dimensional multidetector row CT of the thoracic vessels and airways in the paediatric population. *Radiology* (2003) 229:641–50. doi:10.1148/radiol.2293020999

25. Remy J, Remy-Jardin M, Artaud D, Fribourg M. Multiplanar and threedimensional reconstruction techniques in CT: impact on chest diseases. *Eur Radiol* (2003) 8:335–51. doi:10.1007/s003300050391

26. Washko GR, Parraga G, Coxson HO. Quantitative pulmonary imaging using computed tomography and magnetic resonance imaging. *Respirology* (2012) 17:432–44. doi:10.1111/j.1440-1843.2011.02117.x

27. Robinson TE, Goris ML, Zhu HJ, Chen X, Bhise P, Sheikh F, et al. Dornase alfa reduces air trapping in children with mild cystic fibrosis lung disease: a quantitative analysis. *Chest* (2005) 128(4):2327–35. doi:10.1378/chest.128.4.2327

28. Bonnel AS, Song SM, Kesavarju K, Newaskar M, Paxton CJ, Bloch DA, et al. Quantitative air-trapping analysis in children with mild cystic fibrosis lung disease. *Pediatr Pulmonol* (2004) 38(5):396–405. doi:10.1002/ppul.20091

29. Mulkern R, Haker S, Mamata H, Lee E, Mitsouras D, Oshio K, et al. Lung parenchymal signal intensity in MRI: a technical review with educational aspirations regarding reversible versus irreversible transverse relaxation effects in common pulse sequences. *Concepts Magn Reson Part A Bridg Educ Res* (2014) 43A(2):29–53. doi:10.1002/cmr.a.21297

30. Puderbach M, Hintze C, Ley S, Eichinger M, Kauczor HU, Biederer J. MR imaging of the chest: a practical approach at 1.5T. *Eur J Radiol* (2007) 64:345–55. doi:10.1016/j.ejrad.2007.08.009

31. Ciet P, Serra G, Bertolo S, Spronk S, Ros M, Fraioli F, et al. Assessment of CF lung disease using motion corrected PROPELLER MRI: a comparison with CT. *Eur Radiol* (2016) 26(3):780–7. doi:10.1007/s00330-015-3850-9

32. Miller GW, Mugler JP III, Sá RC, Altes TA, Prisk GK, Hopkins SR. Advances in functional and structural imaging of the human lung using proton MRI. *NMR Biomed* (2014) 27(12):1542–56. doi:10.1002/nbm.3156

33. Dournes G, Grodzki D, Macey J, Girodet PO, Fayon M, Chateil JF, et al. Quiet submillimeter MR imaging of the lung is feasible with a PETRA sequence at 1.5T. *Radiology* (2015) 276(1):258–65. doi:10.1148/radiol.15141655

34. Bauman G, Puderbach M, Heimann T, Kopp-Schneider A, Fritzsching E, Mall MA, et al. Validation of Fourier decomposition MRI with dynamic contrast-enhanced MRI using visual and automated scoring of pulmonary perfusion in young cystic fibrosis patients. *Eur Radiol* (2013) 82(12):2371–7. doi:10.1016/j.ejrad.2013.08.018

35. Fain S, Schiebler ML, McCormack DG, Parraga G. Imaging of lung function using hyperpolarized helium-3 magnetic resonance imaging: review of current and emerging translational methods and applications. *J Magn Reson Imaging* (2010) 32:1398–408. doi:10.1002/jmri.22375

36. Ruiz-Cabello J, Barnett BP, Bottomley PA, Bulte JW. Fluorine (19F) MRS and MRI in biomedicine. *NMR Biomed* (2011) 24:114–29. doi:10.1002/nbm.1570

37. Saam BT, Yablonskiy DA, Kodibagkar VD, Leawoods JC, Gierada DS, Cooper JD, et al. MR imaging of diffusion of (3)He gas in healthy and diseased lungs. *Magn Reson Med* (2000) 44:174–9. doi:10.1002/1522-2594(200008)44:2<174::AID-MRM2>3.0.CO;2-4

38. Kaushik SS, Freeman MS, Cleveland ZI, Davies J, Stiles J, Virgincar RS, et al. Probing the regional distribution of pulmonary gas exchange through single-breath gas- and dissolved-phase 129Xe MR imaging. *J Appl Physiol* (2013) 115:850–60. doi:10.1152/japplphysiol.00092.2013

39. Arnold JF, Fidler F, Wang T, Pracht ED, Schmidt M, Jakob PM. Imaging lung function using rapid dynamic acquisition of T1-maps during oxygen enhancement. *MAGMA* (2004) 16:246–53. doi:10.1007/s10334-004-0034-z

40. Dietrich O, Losert C, Attenberger U, Fasol U, Peller M, Nikolaou K, et al. Fast oxygen-enhanced multislice imaging of the lung using parallel acquisition techniques. *Magn Reson Med* (2005) 53:1317–25. doi:10.1002/mrm.20495

41. Walkup LL, Tkach JA, Higano NS, Thomen RP, Fain SB, Merhar SL, et al. Quantitative magnetic resonance imaging of bronchopulmonary dysplasia in the neonatal intensive care unit environment. *Am J Respir Crit Care Med* (2015) 192(10):1215–22. doi:10.1164/rccm.201503-0552OC

42. Avni EF, Cassart M, de Maertelaer V, Rypens F, Vermeylen D, Gevenois PA. Sonographic prediction of chronic lung disease in the premature undergoing mechanical ventilation. *Pediatr Radiol* (1996) 26:463–9. doi:10.1007/BF01377203

43. Pieper CH, Smith J, Brand EJ. The value of ultrasound examination of the lungs in predicting bronchopulmonary dysplasia. *Pediatr Radiol* (2004) 34:227–31. doi:10.1007/s00247-003-1102-7

44. Zar HJ, Barnett W, Myer L, Stein DJ, Nicol MP. Investigating the early-life determinants of illness in Africa: the Drakenstein Child Health Study. *Thorax* (2015) 70:592–4. doi:10.1136/thoraxjnl-2014-206242

45. Caiulo VA, Gargani L, Caiulo S, Fisicaro A, Moramarco F, Latini G, et al. Lung ultrasound in bronchiolitis: comparison with chest X-ray. *Eur J Pediatr* (2011) 170:1427–33. doi:10.1007/s00431-011-1461-2

Mitochondrial Fission-Mediated Lung Development in Newborn Rats with Hyperoxia-Induced Bronchopulmonary Dysplasia with Pulmonary Hypertension

Yuanyuan Dai[1†], Binyuan Yu[1†], Danyang Ai[2], Lin Yuan[2], Xinye Wang[1], Ran Huo[1], Xiaoqin Fu[1], Shangqin Chen[1*] and Chao Chen[1,2*]

[1] Department of Neonatology, The Second Affiliated Hospital, Yuying Children's Hospital of Wenzhou Medical University, Zhejiang, China, [2] Department of Neonatology, The Children's Hospital of Fudan University, Shanghai, China

*Correspondence:
Chao Chen
chen6010@163.com
Shangqin Chen
chensq5725@163.com

†These authors have contributed equally to this work and share first authorship

Background: Bronchopulmonary dysplasia (BPD) is the most common chronic respiratory disease in premature infants. Oxygen inhalation and mechanical ventilation are common treatments, which can cause hyperoxia-induced lung injury, but the underlying mechanism is not yet understood. Mitochondrial fission is essential for mitochondrial homeostasis. The objective of this study was to determine whether mitochondrial fission (dynamin-related protein 1, Drp1) is an important mediator of hyperoxia lung injury in rats.

Methods: The animal model of BPD was induced with high oxygen (80–85% O_2). Pulmonary histological changes were observed by hematoxylin-eosin (HE) staining. Pulmonary microvessels were observed by immunofluorescence staining of von Willebrand Factor (vWF). Protein expression levels of Drp1 and p-Drp1 (Ser616) were observed using Western Blot. We used echocardiography to measure pulmonary artery acceleration time (PAT), pulmonary vascular resistance index (PVRi), peak flow velocity of the pulmonary artery (PFVP), pulmonary arteriovenous diameter, and pulmonary vein peak velocity. Mitochondrial division inhibitor-1 (Mdivi-1) was used as an inhibitor of Drp1, and administered through intraperitoneal injection (25 mg/kg).

Results: Pulmonary artery resistance of the hyperoxide-induced neonatal rat model of BPD increased after it entered normoxic convalescence. During the critical stage of alveolar development in neonatal rats exposed to high oxygen levels for an extended period, the expression and phosphorylation of Drp1 increased in lung tissues. When Drp1 expression was inhibited, small pulmonary vessel development improved and PH was relieved.

Conclusion: Our study shows that excessive mitochondrial fission is an important mediator of hyperoxia-induced pulmonary vascular injury, and inhibition of mitochondrial fission may be a useful treatment for hyperoxia-induced related pulmonary diseases.

Keywords: bronchopulmonary dysplasia, pulmonary hypertension, mitochondrial fission, Mdivi-1, Drp1, echocardiography, pulmonary vascular resistance

INTRODUCTION

Bronchopulmonary dysplasia (BPD) is a chronic lung disease that occurs in preterm infants who require respiratory support and oxygen therapy at birth (1). It is caused by a variety of molecular factors such as genetic predisposition, oxygen toxicity, and inflammatory injury, whose complex interactions are still not fully understood; and the prevention and treatment strategies for BPD are still limited (2–4). Impaired intrauterine lung development and post-partum injury can impair angiogenesis and alveolar formation, resulting in simplification of the distal alveoli. These characteristic histological changes of BPD clinically manifest as persistent respiratory diseases, requiring long-term oxygen supplementation (5), and pulmonary hypertension (PH). Approximately 15–25% of BPD cases will develop PH (6). Among severe cases of BPD, the incidence of PH is higher (7). Furthermore, the existence of PH is closely related to adverse outcomes of BPD, and the mortality rate of BPD combined with PH is as high as 48% (8).

It is generally believed that mitochondrial dynamics play a vital role in mitochondrial homeostasis (9). Mitochondrial fission is mediated mainly by dynamin-related protein 1 (Drp1), a GTPase associated with cytoplasmic dynamin-related proteins, which belongs to the dynamin-related family and was the first fission protein discovered (10). When activated, cytoplasmic Drp1 is transported to the mitochondrial outer membrane, where GTPase is hydrolyzed and polymerized (9). Accumulating data also suggest that Drp1 is a key molecule in mitochondrial dynamics that controls mitochondrial fusion and fission (11), and abnormal expression of it may lead to abnormal changes in chronic lung diseases such as PH and lung cancer (12, 13). Besides, post-translational modification of Drp1, such as phosphorylation at Ser616, is an important mechanism for modulating mitochondrial fission (14). Recent studies have found that hypoxia can lead to mitochondrial fission of pulmonary artery smooth muscle (15), but the changes in pulmonary vascular mitochondrial dynamics induced by excessive oxygen have not been studied.

Echocardiography is a common method of PH examination in adults and children (16). Echocardiography can show direct signs of PH due to increased tricuspid regurgitation. However, the tricuspid regurgitation velocity used in adult pulmonary artery pressure estimations cannot be used in children, particularly infants, because it is difficult to obtain a good and clear image, and this measurement may not have good agreement with the data measured using a cardiac catheter (17). Therefore, indirect signs, such as changes in right ventricular function and changes in pulmonary artery acceleration time, are indispensable.

In this study, we hypothesized that hyperoxia would induce mitochondrial fission and thus impact lung development, resulting in the occurrence of BPD combined with PH. We found that after excessive oxygen stimulation, alveolar simplification, PH, and p-Drp1 mitochondrial translocation increased mitochondrial fission. Mdivi-1 is a Drp1 inhibitor that decreases mitochondrial fragmentation (18). Our results also suggest that inhibition of mitochondrial fission may be a useful treatment strategy for hyperoxia-associated pulmonary endothelial injury and related diseases.

MATERIALS AND METHODS
Hyperoxia-Induced Lung Injury

All animal experiments were performed in accordance with the policies and guidelines of the Laboratory Animal Ethics Committee of Wenzhou Medical University. A total of 10 pregnant Sprague Dawley rats were purchased from the Experimental Animal Center of Wenzhou Medical University. The dams were maintained in humidity- and temperature-controlled rooms on a 12:12-h light-dark cycle and were allowed food and water *ad libitum*. On the final day of pregnancy, the dams delivered naturally (120 pups). Seventy-two pups from six pregnant rats were pooled, randomized, and returned to the nursing dams and then divided into two groups: the control ($n = 36$) and hyperoxia ($n = 36$) groups. The hyperoxia group of pups was exposed to 80–85% oxygen in a sealed Plexiglass box for 14 days, while the control group was maintained in room air (21% oxygen). Over the 14 days, the nursing dams were exchanged between the two groups every 24 h to avoid oxygen toxicity. The oxygen level of the Plexiglass box was monitored continuously using an oxygen analyzer.

The pups from the other four pregnant rats (48 pups) were experimentally divided into four groups: control + vehicle ($n = 12$), control + Mdivi-1 ($n = 12$), hyperoxia + vehicle ($n = 12$), and hyperoxia + Mdivi-1 ($n = 12$). Mdivi-1 (25 mg/kg) was given to the pups on days 7–14 by intraperitoneal injection. The pups in the control + vehicle and hyperoxia + vehicle groups were injected with the same volume of vehicle (corn oil, Sohrab Biotechnology, Beijing, China).

Lung Histology and Morphometric Analyses

After 14 days, all hyperoxia groups (hyperoxia alone, hyperoxia + vehicle, and hyperoxia + Mdivi-1) were maintained in room air. Sixty pups in total from the control and hyperoxia groups were sacrificed on days 3, 7, 14, 21, and 28 by injection of 1% pentobarbital. The left lungs were removed and fixed in 4% paraformaldehyde for 48 h. The sections were then embedded into paraffin and sliced into 4-μm sections for hematoxylin-eosin (HE) staining (Sohrab Biotechnology, Beijing, China). At the same time, the right lungs were stored at $-80°C$ for western blot.

The radial alveolar count (RAC, the number of alveoli contained in the terminal respiratory unit), which reflects the degree of alveolation, and Mean alveolar diameter (MAD) was the average alveolar diameter (19). And they were important indicators for the evaluation of non-development. Briefly, six lung sections were taken for HE staining on days 3, 7, 14, 21, and 28 from the control and hyperoxia groups, five fields were randomly selected for imaging under a 100x magnification lens, and the number of alveoli passing from the center of the respiratory bronchioles to the nearest interpleural line were counted as the RAC. The MAD was measured by Image-Pro Plus 6.0 software (Media Cybernetics, Rockville, MD, USA).

Immunofluorescence

On day 14, the lung tissue sections from 24 rats [control + vehicle ($n = 6$), control + Mdivi-1($n = 6$), hyperoxia + vehicle ($n = 6$), and hyperoxia + Mdivi-1 ($n = 6$)] were dried overnight at $37°C$ and then hydrated in xylene and an ethanol gradient series. The sections were then heated in a microwave in $10\,mM$ citric acid buffer (pH 6.0) for 20 min for antigen retrieval. The sections were then incubated in 5% bovine serum albumin at $37°C$ for 1 h. The sections were incubated at $4°C$ overnight with a rabbit polyclonal anti-vWF (AF3000; 1:200 dilution; Affinity Biosciences. OH. USA), while the negative control group was incubated with phosphate-buffered saline. The sections were then incubated with Alexa Fluor-594 sheep anti-rabbit IgG (AB150076; diluted 1:500; Abcam) at room temperature for 4 h and subsequently with $4'$,6-diamidino-2-phenylindole (DAPI). Dual immunophotography images were acquired using a scanning microscope (C1; Nikon, Tokyo, Japan).

Western Blotting

Protein was extracted from frozen lung tissue samples from 36 rats in the control and hyperoxia groups on days 3, 7, and 14, and mixed with the loading buffer. Equal amounts of protein were separated by 10% sodium dodecyl sulfate-polyacrylamide gel electrophoresis at $100\,V$ for $3\,h$ and transferred to polyacrylamide difluoride membranes at $100\,V$ for $50\,min$. Membranes were then blocked in 5% skimmed milk for $3\,h$ at room temperature ($20–25°C$). Membranes were then incubated with rabbit monoclonal anti-Drp1 (ab184247; 1:500 dilution; Abcam, Cambridge, UK) or rabbit Phospho-Drp1 (Ser616) Antibody (#3455; 1:1,000 dilution; Cell Signaling Technology, Boston, USA) and gently shaken at $4°C$ overnight. The next day, the membranes were incubated with horseradish peroxidase-conjugated goat anti-rabbit or anti-mouse secondary antibody (1:5,000 dilution; Cell Signaling Technology, Boston, USA) for $2\,h$ after being washed three times in Tris-buffered saline and tween-20, and developed using enhanced chemiluminescence reagents (Thermo Scientific Pierce; Thermo Fisher Scientific, Waltham, MA, USA). Densitometry values of each sample were calculated by Image Lab 5.0 software (Bio-Rad, Hercules, CA, USA) for all bands and standardized relative to β-actin.

Echocardiographic Imaging

On days 14, 21, 28, and 42, six pups from the control and hyperoxia groups and 24 rats from other four groups on days 21 and 28 were prepared for ultrasonic imaging. The rats were anesthetized with isoflurane using a small animal respiratory anesthesia machine (R620-S1, RWD life science, Shenzhen, China). After full chest hair removal, the rats received continuous isoflurane anesthesia, were fixed in the supine position on the examination table, and connected with electrocardiogram electrodes. Their chests were coated with coupling agent.

The probe was slightly adjusted upwards to obtain a minor axial view of the aorta, and the probe was slightly tilted cephalically to obtain a major axial view of the pulmonary artery. The left atrial pulmonary vein junction was located, and the Doppler sampling point was placed at the junction to measure the pulmonary vein flow velocity.

To measure the hemodynamics of the pulmonary arteries and veins, the short-axis view of the aortic valve was obtained first, and the pulmonary artery was identified using a color Doppler instrument. The diameter of the pulmonary artery was measured at the attachment point of the pulmonary valve. The pulsed Doppler gate was placed at the proximal end of the pulmonary valve at an incident angle $<20°$ to maximize laminar flow. Pulmonary acceleration time (PAT), pulmonary ejection time (PET), and peak flow velocity of the pulmonary artery (PFVP) were measured. PAT was measured as the time from the beginning of systolic blood flow to the peak flow rate, while PET was measured as the time from the beginning of systolic blood flow to the completion of pulmonary blood flow. The pulmonary vascular resistance index (PVRi) was calculated as the ratio of PET to PAT. Similarly, the size of the left atrial pulmonary vein junction was measured as the value of the pulmonary vein diameter, and the peak velocity of the pulmonary vein was measured according to the pulmonary vein flow velocity curve. To measure right ventricular load, short-axis views of the right and left ventricles were obtained at the level of the distal mitral valve.

Right and left ventricular diastolic area (RVEDA and LVEDA, respectively) were measured by manual endocardial boundary tracing. The ratio between RVEDA and LVEDA (RVEDA/LVEDA) was calculated as the measurement index of the right ventricular load (20).

Statistical Analysis

The experiments were performed in triplicate and repeated at least three times. The data are presented as the mean $\pm$ SD or SEM and were analyzed using one-way analysis of variance (ANOVA) followed by Tukey's *post-hoc* test (equal variance) or Dunnett T3's *post-hoc* test (unequal variance) for multiple comparisons. Correlation analyses were performed using Spearman's rank correlation. Statistical analysis was carried out using SPSS Statistics 19.0 (SPSS Inc., Chicago, USA) or GraphPad 6.0 (GraphPad Software, San Diego, USA). Values of $P < 0.05$ were considered statistically significant.

RESULTS

Hyperoxia Stunts Alveolar Development, Which Is Restored After Recovery in Room Air

Hyperoxia causes substantial morphological simplification in the lung tissue, including a visible decrease in alveolar numbers and increase in alveolar size. These negative changes in the hyperoxia group can be quantified by the decrease in RAC and MAD, an important indicator of lung development. Significant histological differences between the hyperoxia and control groups were found in day 3, 7, 14, 21, and 28 (**Figure 1A**). This result indicated that chronic exposure to hyperoxia interrupts alveolar

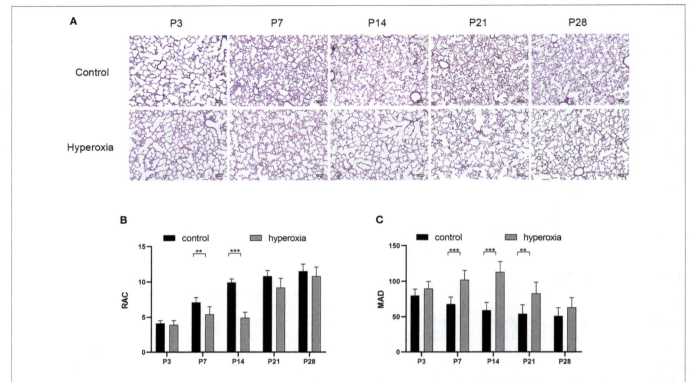

FIGURE 1 | Morphological changes in rat lungs after hyperoxia. Newborn pups (P0) were exposed to 21% O₂ (control) or 80–85% O₂ (hyperoxia) for 14 days. **(A)** Hematoxylin and eosin staining of rat lungs exposed to hyperoxia or control group on day 3, 7, 14, 21, and 28. Scale bar: 100 μm. **(B)** Compared with the controls, the radial alveolar counts (RACs) of hyperoxia group were significantly reduced on five periods. **(C)** The Mean alveolar diameter (MAD) of hyperoxia group were significantly increased on five periods. $n = 6$ per group. Data are shown as mean ± SD; **$P < 0.01$, ***$P < 0.001$.

formation, as evidenced by a decrease in alveolar numbers and increase in alveolar diameter. On day 7 (**Figure 1B**), the RAC number of control group was higher than hyperoxia group ($P < 0.01$), and on day 14 this number in control group was much higher than in hyperoxia group ($P < 0.001$). However, these developmental abnormalities in the hyperoxia group were reversed after recovery in room air for 14 days. As for the MAD (**Figure 1C**), the MAD value of control group was significantly lower than hyperoxia group on day 7 ($P < 0.001$), on day 14 ($P < 0.001$), and on day 21 ($P < 0.01$).

Hyperoxia Causes Drp1 Overexpression in Newborn Rat Lungs

To investigate whether hyperoxia altered the expression of Drp1 in rat lung tissues, we examined the levels of Drp1 and p-Drp1 over time by western blotting (**Figure 2A**). On the third day of hyperoxia (**Figure 2B**), the expression of Drp1 in the hyperoxia group was higher than that in the control group ($P < 0.05$). On the seventh day of hyperoxia, the levels of Drp1 ($P < 0.05$) and p-Drp1 (Ser616) ($P < 0.001$) in the hyperoxia group were both significantly elevated (**Figures 2B,C**), although the ratios of p-Drp1 (Ser616)/Drp1 were not different between the two groups, suggesting that the elevated p-Drp1 (Ser616) levels increased concomitantly with Drp1 levels (**Figure 2D**). After 14 days of hyperoxia, Drp1 levels in the hyperoxia group were still high ($P < 0.01$). Furthermore, the ratio of p-Drp1 (Ser616) to Drp1 ($P < 0.001$) was significantly increased compared to the controls, indicating that the phosphorylation of Drp1 at Ser616 (**Figure 2C**) was actively upregulated ($P < 0.001$).

Pharmacological Inhibition of Drp1 With Mdivi-1 During Hyperoxia Mitigates Pulmonary Vascular Complications

Mdivi-1 is a specific inhibitor of Drp1. Based on the results that DRP1 started to increase in the hyperoxia group on P7 and the high level persisted until P14, the Drp1 inhibitor, mdivi-1, was injected intraperitoneally daily from days 7 to 14 to investigate whether mdivi-1 had protective effects on chronic hyperoxia-induced lung injury. To evaluate vascular development, vWF-positive small blood vessels were visualized using immunofluorescence staining and counted (**Figure 3**). We found that long-term hyperoxia significantly decreased the number of pulmonary small blood vessels at day 14 ($P < 0.001$), whereas mdivi-1 treatment in the hyperoxia group (**Figure 3B**) partially rescued this decrease at day 14 ($P < 0.001$), indicating that mdivi-1 can alleviate hyperoxia-induced obstruction of pulmonary vascular development. To evaluate the long-term effects on

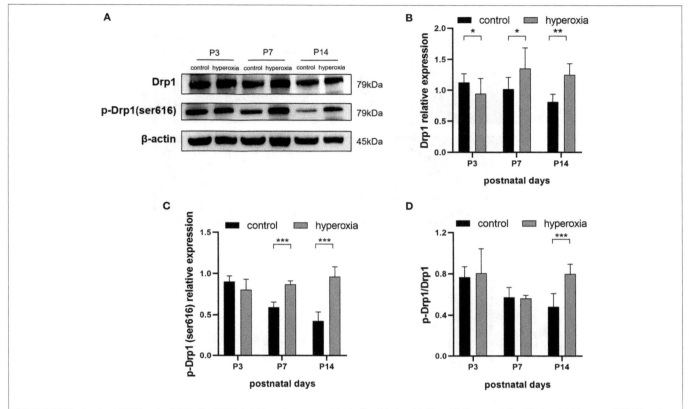

FIGURE 2 | The levels of DRP1 and p-DRP1 (Ser616) in total lung tissues are detected by Western blotting. **(A)** Representative Western blot images of DRP1 and p-DRP1 (Ser616) in lung tissues from controls or from hyperoxia group on day 3, 7, or 14. **(B,C)** Protein levels of DRP1 **(B)** or p-DRP1 (Ser616) **(C)** in arbitrary units (AU) normalized to β-actin levels. **(D)** The ratios of p-DRP1 (Ser616)/DRP1 was calculated based on Western blot results. β-actin was the loading control. $n = 6$ animals/group; Values are expressed as means ± SD; *$P < 0.05$, **$P < 0.01$, ***$P < 0.001$.

blood vessels, ultrasonic echocardiogram monitoring revealed that the pulmonary vascular resistance index (**Figure 3C**) of the hyperoxia + mdivi-1 group was significantly lower than that of the hyperoxia + vehicle group on P21 ($P < 0.05$). The peak pulmonary flow velocity was measured on P28 (**Figure 3D**). The results showed that the pulmonary artery peak flow velocity decreased after administration of mdivi-1, indicating an improvement in pulmonary artery pressure. In addition, the heart tissue was weighed and Fulton index was calculated on P28. The Fulton index of the hyperoxia + vehicle group was significantly higher than that of the control + vehicle group (**Figure 3E**), indicating that the right ventricle was hypertrophic. Compared to the hyperoxia + vehicle group, the Fulton index of the hyperoxia + mdivi-1 group was lower, suggesting that right ventricular hypertrophy had improved (**Figure 3E**).

Recovery in Room Air Leaves Hyperoxia-Exposed Rats With Abnormal Pulmonary Hemodynamics Until Adolescence

Although the alveolar developmental obstruction caused by hyperoxia had no significant difference in lung morphology between the control and hyperoxia groups after 7 days of normal oxygen recovery, the pulmonary vessels showed significant abnormalities in the hyperoxia group during the recovery period. We performed continuous pulmonary vascular-related cardiac ultrasonography on rats released from the hypertoxic environment on post-natal day 14, P21, P28, and P42 (**Figure 4**). After measuring indexes from the Doppler ultrasound trace of the pulmonary artery (**Figures 4A,B**), the results showed that the PAT (**Figure 4C**) reflecting the pulmonary circulation resistance was markedly shortened on day 14 ($P < 0.05$), day 21 ($P < 0.01$), and day 28 ($P < 0.001$). The other two indicators: PVRi and peak pulmonary flow velocity were significantly increased (**Figures 4D,E**). PVRi were significantly increased on day 21 ($P < 0.001$) and day 28 ($P < 0.001$) in the hyperoxia group compared to the control group. and the peak pulmonary flow velocity were increased on day 21 ($P < 0.001$), day 28 ($P < 0.001$), and day 42 ($P < 0.05$). In addition, cardiac ultrasound-related features of the pulmonary veins were also detected. After hyperoxia, the diameter of the pulmonary vein (**Figure 4F**) decreased on day 21 ($P < 0.05$), whereas the diameter of the pulmonary artery (**Figure 4G**) was not significantly changed at day 21. In order to observe the effect of this pulmonary hemodynamic abnormality on the heart, particularly on the right ventricular load, we acquired a short-axis image of the

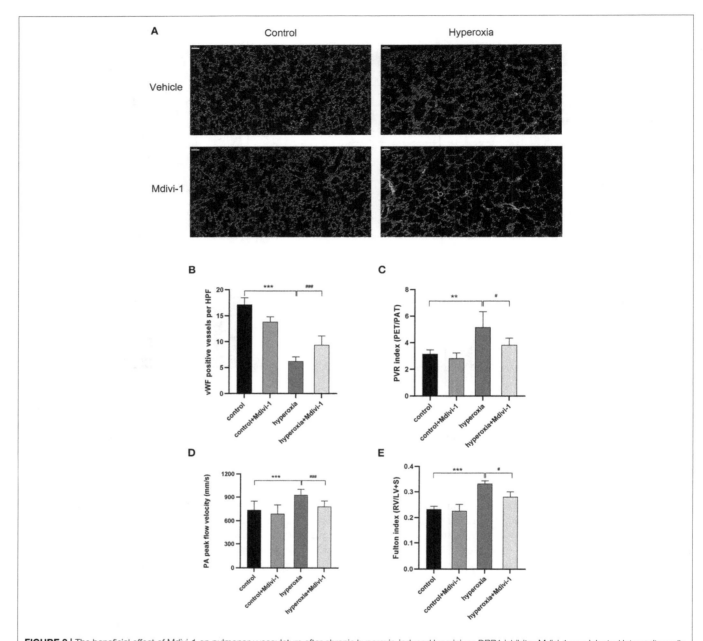

FIGURE 3 | The beneficial effect of Mdivi-1 on pulmonary vasculature after chronic hyperoxia-induced lung injury. DRP1 inhibitor Mdivi-1 was injected intraperitoneally daily to the rats from day 7 to 14. (A) Representative images of immunofluorescence staining. Green fluorescence represented vWF expression. Scale bar = 50 μm. (B) vWF-positive vessels whose diameters were < 50 μm were calculated accordingly. (C) The pulmonary vascular resistance index (PVRi) measured on day 21. (D) The peak pulmonary flow velocity was measured on P28 (E) the Fulton's index was measured on day 28. $n = 6$ animals/group; Values are presented as mean ± SD. **$P < 0.01$, ***$P < 0.001$, hyperoxia vs. control; #$P < 0.05$, ###$P < 0.001$, hyperoxia+Mdivi-1 vs. hyperoxia.

end-diastolic ventricle at the mitral valve level, and outlined the cross-sections of the right and left ventricular cavities. The area ratio (RVEDA/LVEDA) is a measurement of the right ventricular load. We found that the area ratio was higher in the hyperoxia group on day 14 ($P < 0.05$) and on day 21 ($P < 0.01$), suggesting that the right ventricle was dilated, and this trend continued for 7 days (up to day 21) in the hyperoxia group (**Figure 4H**). A representative two-dimensional echocardiography image of the left and right ventricular dimensions on day 21 demonstrated right ventricular dilation in the hyperoxia group compared to the control group, indicative of diastolic right ventricle dysfunction (**Figures 4I,J**).

DISCUSSION

In this study, we attempted to explore the relationship between BPD and mitochondrial fission induced by hyperoxia. To simulate severe BPD in rodent models, we

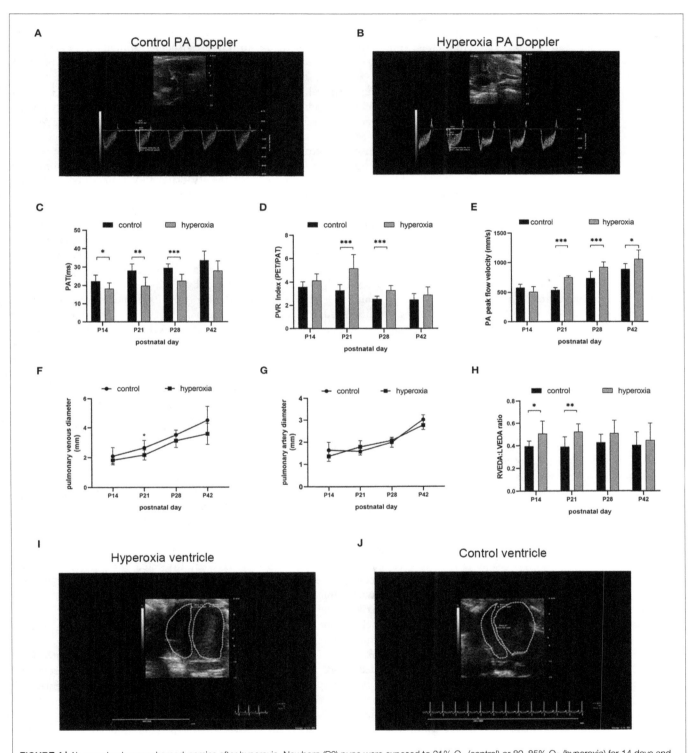

FIGURE 4 | Abnormal pulmonary hemodynamics after hyperoxia. Newborn (P0) pups were exposed to 21% O_2 (control) or 80–85% O_2 (hyperoxia) for 14 days and returned to air to receive echocardiography detection on post-natal day 14, 21, 28, and 42. (A) Representative Doppler ultrasound images of the pulmonary artery (PA) on day 21 after exposure to either normoxia or hyperoxia for 14 days from birth. (B) Representative 2-dimensional echocardiography images of left and right ventricular dimensions on day 21 was shown by comparing the difference between exposure to normoxia and hyperoxia for 14 days after birth. (C–H) Echocardiography and pulse-wave Doppler-derived indexes of pulmonary acceleration time (PAT) (C), pulmonary vascular resistance (PVR) index (D), peak flow velocity of pulmonary artery (E), pulmonary venous diameter (F), pulmonary artery diameter (G), and right ventricular end-diastolic area (RVEDA)-to-left ventricular end-diastolic area ratio (LVEDA) (H) were analyzed and compared between hyperoxia group and control group on P14, P21, P28, and P42. (I,J) Representative two-dimensional echocardiography images of the left and right ventricular dimensions on control and hyperoxia group on day 21. $n = 6$ animals/group; Values are expressed as means ± SD; *$P < 0.05$, **$P < 0.01$, ***$P < 0.001$, compared with hyperoxia and control group.

first exposed rats to 80–85% oxygen for a long period (14 days). The results showed that the lung morphology was seriously damaged and alveolar structure was simplified, which was consistent with the pathology of BPD. Protein expression of Drp1/p-Drp1 in the hyperoxia group was significantly higher compared to in the control group. We then applied the Drp1 inhibitor, Mdivi-1, and found an improvement in the reduction of pulmonary microvasculature under hyperoxia. Finally, we discussed whether hyperoxia-induced BPD would have adverse effects on pulmonary circulation function and followed up with echocardiography.

In recent years, many studies have shown that mitochondrial dysfunction plays an important role in BPD and PH (21). Mitochondrial dynamics are essential for maintaining mitochondrial integrity and regulating apoptosis (22). Drp1 is a mitochondrial outer membrane protein that mediates fission of mitochondria and controls mitochondrial morphology (23). The latest research shows that by inducing overexpression of hypoxia inducible factor-1, hypoxia stimuli can promote the expression of Drp1 to regulate mitochondrial dynamics in pulmonary vascular remodeling (24). In this study Drp1 changes were investigated after hyperoxia exposure in newborn rats to further our understanding of the relationship between hyperoxia and Drp1. We found that Drp1 reached its peak on day 7 in the hyperoxia group and maintained this level until day 14. These results showed that Drp1 protein expression could be enhanced by hyperoxia. Many studies have suggested that abnormally high expression of Drp1 in the lungs is an indicator of poor prognosis, particularly in chronic malignant diseases (25, 26). Drp1 has been regarded as an attractive therapeutic target.

Mitochondrial oxidative stress is a component of general oxidative stress, and excessive reactive oxygen species would lead to increased mitochondrial fission (27). Studies have found that particulate matter ($PM_{2.5}$) can lead to oxidative stress in lung epithelial cells, increasing mitochondrial fission, resulting in cell apoptosis (28), and Drp1 and oxidative stress are essential mediators in cigarette smoke-induced pulmonary endothelial Injury (29). Combined with our findings, we speculated that lung injury caused by hyperoxia in newborn rats would increase mitochondrial fission, namely the expression of Drp1, due to oxidative stress. In addition, experiments have confirmed the relationship between hypoxia and Drp1, studies were not only involved in animal models about Lung Ischemia-reperfusion Injury (30) and lung vascular ischemic/hypoxic injury (31), but also in others like hepatocellular carcinoma cells in hypoxia (32), and Hypoxia-Reoxygenation Injury of Cardiomyocytes (33). Although hypoxia or hyperoxia can trigger similar pathological responses, such as oxidative stress and inflammation, these underlying mechanisms need to be further studied at the cellular level.

Mdivi-1, a specific inhibitor of DRP1 (34) is reported to be effective in suppressing the pulmonary artery smooth muscle cells in lungs with PH (35). Because of the changes in Drp1 after hyper oxygen in this study, the rats were injected intraperitoneally with Mdivi-1 (25 mg/kg) from days 7 to 14 to explore whether inhibition of Drp1 has protective effects on hyperoxia-induced lung injury. It was found that long-term hyperoxia severely hindered the development of small pulmonary vessels, and after mdivi-1 administration, the number of small pulmonary vessels significantly increased. These results indicate that Mdivi-1 can relieve hyperoxia-induced obstruction of pulmonary microvascular development. From the perspective of the long-term effects on blood vessels, ultrasonic monitoring results showed that the PVR and PFVP measured during the recovery period were lower after the administration of Mdivi-1, suggesting improvements in pulmonary artery pressure. In addition, the heart tissue was weighed on 28 days after birth to calculate the Fulton index the results showed that the right ventricular hypertrophy index in the hyperoxia group was significantly higher than that in the control group, suggesting right ventricular hypertrophy.

To investigate whether this BPD model would have an adverse effect on pulmonary circulation function, follow-up detection was carried out by echocardiography in rats at 14, 21, 28, and 42 days after birth. It was demonstrated that PAT in the hyperoxia group was shortened, while the PVRi and PFVP increased significantly compared to the control group. These parameters all reflected higher pulmonary pressure after exposure to hyperoxia for 2 weeks. In addition, by measuring the area ratio and Fulton index, we found that over-circulation influenced right ventricular structure and function.

It is worth mentioning that in this study, in addition to focusing on the pulmonary artery, cardiac echocardiography indicators related to the pulmonary vein were also detected, and it was found that the pulmonary vein diameter showed signs of narrowing after exposure to hyperoxia, while there was no significant difference in pulmonary artery diameter between the two groups. Pulmonary vein stenosis is a rare problem that is often neglected (36); however, it is a severe and increasingly common complication of preterm infants with BPD (37). Although this study identified the manifestations of pulmonary vein stenosis, it did not elucidate the underlying mechanisms, which require further investigation.

Lastly, there are some limitations present in this study. First, we did not further explore the mechanism between hyperoxia and Drp1. Secondly, we did not carry out in *vitro* experiments, such as on pulmonary epithelial cells and microvascular endothelial cells. Thirdly, this experiment only discussed the development of pulmonary vessels after hyperoxia stimulation, but future studies will focus on the effects of Drp1 and Mdivi-1 on alveolar development.

In conclusion, the present study identified the echocardiographic features of hyperoxia-induced BPD-PH models and confirmed that the expression of Drp1 is increased in hyperoxia-induced lung injury. Treatment with Mdivi-1 during hyperoxia was protective against pulmonary vasculature development and function. However, further studies are required to determine the precise mechanism of Drp1 in BPD and BPD-PH.

AUTHOR CONTRIBUTIONS

YD conceived and designed the experiments. YD and BY performed the experiments and wrote the paper. YD, DA, and LY analyzed the data. XW, RH, and XF contributed materials and analysis tools. CC and SC edited and approved final draft. All authors contributed to the article and approved the submitted version.

REFERENCES

1. Jobe AH, Bancalari E. Bronchopulmonary dysplasia. *Am J Respir Crit Care Med.* (2001) 163:1723–9. doi: 10.1164/ajrccm.163.7.2011060
2. Baraldi E, Filippone M. Chronic lung disease after premature birth. *N Engl J Med.* (2007) 357:1946–55. doi: 10.1056/NEJMra067279
3. Hilgendorff A, Reiss I, Ehrhardt H, Eickelberg O, Alvira CM. Chronic lung disease in the preterm infant. Lessons learned from animal models. *Am J Respir Cell Mol Biol.* (2014) 50:233–45. doi: 10.1165/rcmb.2013-0014TR
4. McEvoy CT, Jain L, Schmidt B, Abman S, Bancalari E, Aschner JL. Bronchopulmonary dysplasia: NHLBI workshop on the primary prevention of chronic lung diseases. *Ann Am Thorac Soc.* (2014) 11(Suppl. 3):S146–53. doi: 10.1513/AnnalsATS.201312-424LD
5. Smith VC, Zupancic JA, McCormick MC, Croen LA, Greene J, Escobar GJ, et al. Rehospitalization in the first year of life among infants with bronchopulmonary dysplasia. *J Pediatr.* (2004) 144:799–803. doi: 10.1016/j.jpeds.2004.03.026
6. Arjaans S, Zwart EAH, Ploegstra MJ, Bos AF, Kooi EMW, Hillege HL, et al. Identification of gaps in the current knowledge on pulmonary hypertension in extremely preterm infants: a systematic review and meta-analysis. *Paediatr Perinat Epidemiol.* (2018) 32:258–67. doi: 10.1111/ppe.12444
7. Mirza H, Ziegler J, Ford S, Padbury J, Tucker R, Laptook A. Pulmonary hypertension in preterm infants: prevalence and association with bronchopulmonary dysplasia. *J Pediatr.* (2014) 165:909–14.e1. doi: 10.1016/j.jpeds.2014.07.040
8. Khemani E, McElhinney DB, Rhein L, Andrade O, Lacro RV, Thomas KC, et al. Pulmonary artery hypertension in formerly premature infants with bronchopulmonary dysplasia: clinical features and outcomes in the surfactant era. *Pediatrics.* (2007) 120:1260–9. doi: 10.1542/peds.2007-0971
9. Archer SL. Mitochondrial dynamics–mitochondrial fission and fusion in human diseases. *N Engl J Med.* (2013) 369:2236–51. doi: 10.1056/NEJMra1215233
10. Jahani-Asl A, Slack RS. The phosphorylation state of Drp1 determines cell fate. *EMBO Rep.* (2007) 8:912–3. doi: 10.1038/sj.embor.7401077
11. Losón OC, Song Z, Chen H, Chan DC. Fis1, Mff, MiD49, and MiD51 mediate Drp1 recruitment in mitochondrial fission. *Mol Biol Cell.* (2013) 24:659–67. doi: 10.1091/mbc.e12-10-0721
12. Kim YY, Yun SH, Yun J. Downregulation of Drp1, a fission regulator, is associated with human lung and colon cancers. *Acta Biochim Biophys Sin.* (2018) 50:209–15. doi: 10.1093/abbs/gmx137
13. Chiang YY, Chen SL, Hsiao YT, Huang CH, Lin TY, Chiang IP, et al. Nuclear expression of dynamin-related protein 1 in lung adenocarcinomas. *Mod Pathol.* (2009) 22:1139–50. doi: 10.1038/modpathol.2009.83
14. Kim YM, Youn SW, Sudhahar V, Das A, Chandhri R, Cuervo Grajal H, et al. Redox regulation of mitochondrial fission protein Drp1 by protein disulfide isomerase limits endothelial senescence. *Cell Rep.* (2018) 23:3565–78. doi: 10.1016/j.celrep.2018.05.054
15. Liu X, Tan H, Liu X, Wu Q. Correlation between the expression of Drp1 in vascular endothelial cells and inflammatory factors in hypertension rats. *Exp Ther Med.* (2018) 15:3892–98. doi: 10.3892/etm.2018.5899
16. Krishnan U, Feinstein JA, Adatia I, Austin ED, Mullen MP, Hopper RK, et al. Evaluation and management of pulmonary hypertension in children with bronchopulmonary dysplasia. *J Pediatr.* (2017) 188:24–34.e1. doi: 10.1016/j.jpeds.2017.05.029
17. Keller RL. Pulmonary hypertension and pulmonary vasodilators. *Clin Perinatol.* (2016) 43:187–202. doi: 10.1016/j.clp.2015.11.013
18. Cassidy-Stone A, Chipuk JE, Ingerman E, Song C, Yoo C, Kuwana T, et al. Chemical inhibition of the mitochondrial division dynamin reveals its role in Bax/Bak-dependent mitochondrial outer membrane permeabilization. *Dev Cell.* (2008) 14:193–204. doi: 10.1016/j.devcel.2007.11.019
19. Bhaskaran M, Xi D, Wang Y, Huang C, Narasaraju T, Shu W, et al. Identification of microRNAs changed in the neonatal lungs in response to hyperoxia exposure. *Physiol Genomics.* (2012) 44:970–80. doi: 10.1152/physiolgenomics.00145.2011
20. Kantores C, McNamara PJ, Teixeira L, Engelberts D, Murthy P, Kavanagh BP, et al. Therapeutic hypercapnia prevents chronic hypoxia-induced pulmonary hypertension in the newborn rat. *Am J Physiol Lung Cell Mol Physiol.* (2006) 291:L912–22. doi: 10.1152/ajplung.00480.2005
21. Shah D, Das P, Bhandari V. Mitochondrial dysfunction in bronchopulmonary dysplasia. *Am J Respir Crit Care Med.* (2018) 197:1363. doi: 10.1164/rccm.201711-2197LE
22. Suen DF, Norris KL, Youle RJ. Mitochondrial dynamics and apoptosis. *Genes Dev.* (2008) 22:1577–90. doi: 10.1101/gad.1658508
23. Westermann B. Mitochondrial fusion and fission in cell life and death. *Nat Rev Mol Cell Biol.* (2010) 11:872–84. doi: 10.1038/nrm3013
24. Chen X, Yao JM, Fang X, Zhang C, Yang YS, Hu CP, et al. Hypoxia promotes pulmonary vascular remodeling via HIF-1α to regulate mitochondrial dynamics. *J Geriatr Cardiol.* (2019) 16:855–71. doi: 10.11909/j.issn.1671-5411.2019.12.003
25. Zhao J, Zhang J, Yu M, Xie Y, Huang Y, Wolff DW, et al. Mitochondrial dynamics regulates migration and invasion of breast cancer cells. *Oncogene.* (2013) 32:4814–24. doi: 10.1038/onc.2012.494
26. Shen F, Gai J, Xing J, Guan J, Fu L, Li Q. Dynasore suppresses proliferation and induces apoptosis of the non-small-cell lung cancer cell line A549. *Biochem Biophys Res Commun.* (2018) 495:1158–66. doi: 10.1016/j.bbrc.2017.11.109
27. Pradeepkiran JA, Reddy PH. Defective mitophagy in Alzheimer's disease. *Ageing Res Rev.* (2020) 64:101191. doi: 10.1016/j.arr.2020.101191
28. Liu X, Zhao X, Li X, Lv S, Ma R, Qi Y, et al. PM$_{2.5}$ triggered apoptosis in lung epithelial cells through the mitochondrial apoptotic way mediated by a ROS-DRP1-mitochondrial fission axis. *J Hazard Mater.* (2020) 397:122608. doi: 10.1016/j.jhazmat.2020.122608
29. Wang Z, White A, Wang X, Ko J, Choudhary G, Lange T, et al. Mitochondrial fission mediated cigarette smoke-induced pulmonary endothelial injury. *Am J Respir Cell Mol Biol.* (2020) 63:637–51. doi: 10.1165/rcmb.2020-0008OC
30. Lin KC, Yeh JN, Chen YL, Chiang JY, Sung PH, Lee FY, et al. Xenogeneic and allogeneic mesenchymal stem cells effectively protect the lung against ischemia-reperfusion injury through downregulating the inflammatory, oxidative stress, and autophagic signaling pathways in rat. *Cell Transplant.* (2020) 29:963689720954140. doi: 10.1177/0963689720954140
31. Duan C, Wang L, Zhang J, Xiang X, Wu Y, Zhang Z, et al. Mdivi-1 attenuates oxidative stress and exerts vascular protection in ischemic/hypoxic injury by a mechanism independent of Drp1 GTPase activity. *Redox Biol.* (2020) 37:101706. doi: 10.1016/j.redox.2020.101706
32. Lin XH, Qiu BQ, Ma M, Zhang R, Hsu SJ, Liu HH, et al. Suppressing DRP1-mediated mitochondrial fission and mitophagy increases mitochondrial apoptosis of hepatocellular carcinoma cells in the setting of hypoxia. *Oncogenesis.* (2020) 9:67. doi: 10.1038/s41389-020-00251-5
33. Luo H, Song S, Chen Y, Xu M, Sun L, Meng G, et al. Inhibitor 1 of protein phosphatase 1 regulates Ca^{2+}/calmodulin-dependent protein kinase II to alleviate oxidative stress in hypoxia-reoxygenation injury of cardiomyocytes. *Oxid Med Cell Longev.* (2019) 2019:2193019. doi: 10.1155/2019/2193019

34. Bordt EA, Clerc P, Roelofs BA, Saladino AJ, Tretter L, Adam-Vizi V, et al. The putative Drp1 inhibitor mdivi-1 is a reversible mitochondrial complex I inhibitor that modulates reactive oxygen species. *Dev Cell.* (2017) 40:583–94.e6. doi: 10.1016/j.devcel.2017.02.020

35. Marsboom G, Toth PT, Ryan JJ, Hong Z, Wu X, Fang YH, et al. Dynamin-related protein 1-mediated mitochondrial mitotic fission permits hyperproliferation of vascular smooth muscle cells and offers a novel therapeutic target in pulmonary hypertension. *Circ Res.* (2012) 110:1484–97. doi: 10.1161/CIRCRESAHA.111.263848

36. Mahgoub L, Kaddoura T, Kameny AR, Lopez Ortego P, Vanderlaan RD, Kakadekar A, et al. Pulmonary vein stenosis of ex-premature infants with pulmonary hypertension and bronchopulmonary dysplasia, epidemiology, and survival from a multicenter cohort. *Pediatr Pulmonol.* (2017) 52:1063–70. doi: 10.1002/ppul.23679

37. Nasr VG, Callahan R, Wichner Z, Odegard KC, DiNardo JA. Intraluminal pulmonary vein stenosis in children: a "New" lesion. *Anesth Analg.* (2019) 129:27–40. doi: 10.1213/ANE.0000000000003924

20

Aberrant Pulmonary Vascular Growth and Remodeling in Bronchopulmonary Dysplasia

Cristina M. Alvira*

Department of Pediatrics, Division of Critical Care Medicine, Stanford University School of Medicine, Stanford, CA, USA

*Correspondence:
Cristina M. Alvira
calvira@stanford.edu

In contrast to many other organs, a significant portion of lung development occurs after birth during alveolarization, thus rendering the lung highly susceptible to injuries that may disrupt this developmental process. Premature birth heightens this susceptibility, with many premature infants developing the chronic lung disease, bronchopulmonary dysplasia (BPD), a disease characterized by arrested alveolarization. Over the past decade, tremendous progress has been made in the elucidation of mechanisms that promote postnatal lung development, including extensive data suggesting that impaired pulmonary angiogenesis contributes to the pathogenesis of BPD. Moreover, in addition to impaired vascular growth, patients with BPD also frequently demonstrate alterations in pulmonary vascular remodeling and tone, increasing the risk for persistent hypoxemia and the development of pulmonary hypertension. In this review, an overview of normal lung development will be presented, and the pathologic features of arrested development observed in BPD will be described, with a specific emphasis on the pulmonary vascular abnormalities. Key pathways that promote normal pulmonary vascular development will be reviewed, and the experimental and clinical evidence demonstrating alterations of these essential pathways in BPD summarized.

Keywords: pulmonary angiogenesis, pulmonary hypertension, alveolarization, chronic lung disease, VEGF, HIF, nitric oxide

INTRODUCTION

A significant portion of lung development occurs after birth during the alveolar stage of development. During this final stage, the alveolar ducts divide into alveolar sacs by secondary septation, and the pulmonary capillary bed expands *via* angiogenesis to markedly increase the gas exchange surface area of the lung (1). However, postnatal completion of growth renders the lung highly susceptible to insults that disrupt this developmental program. This is particularly evident in the setting of preterm birth, where disruption of alveolarization causes bronchopulmonary dysplasia (BPD), the most common complication of prematurity (2). While advances in the supportive care of extremely premature infants have reduced mortality, the morbidities associated with severe BPD persist (3). Accompanying this increase in survival, the clinical and pathologic features of BPD have changed significantly. In contrast to the severe lung injury characterizing "old BPD" as originally described by Northway (4), premature birth earlier in gestation appears to disrupt the normal program of alveolar and vascular development, resulting in the "new BPD," characterized by an arrest in alveolar and vascular development (5).

The impaired pulmonary angiogenesis observed in patients with BPD appears to be the key to the pathogenesis. Proangiogenic factors are decreased in the lungs of infants dying from BPD (6) and in animal models of BPD induced by hyperoxia (7). Administration of anti-angiogenic agents to neonatal rats impairs both pulmonary angiogenesis and alveolarization (8, 9), and overexpression of proangiogenic factors, such as vascular endothelial growth factor (VEGF), rescues the adverse effects of hyperoxia on alveolarization (7). Moreover, in addition to simple decreases in pulmonary microvascular growth, the pulmonary vascular abnormalities in BPD may also include pathologic remodeling and heightened tone, leading to the development of pulmonary hypertension (PH), as well as an increase in the development of abnormal aorto–pulmonary communications, potentially promoting intrapulmonary shunting.

This review presents an overview of lung development and details the pathology of the "new" BPD, characterized by an arrest in normal lung development. Specific focus will be centered upon the pulmonary vascular abnormalities in BPD including impaired pulmonary angiogenesis, abnormal pulmonary vascular remodeling, heightened pulmonary vascular tone, and development of abnormal collateral circulations. Key pathways that promote normal pulmonary vascular development will be reviewed, and the experimental and clinical evidence demonstrating how these pathways are altered in BPD summarized.

OVERVIEW OF NORMAL AIRWAY AND PULMONARY VASCULAR DEVELOPMENT

Lung development begins when the primitive lung bud emerges from the ventral foregut and divides during the embryonic stage of development (4–7 weeks gestation), forming two lung buds lying on either side of the future esophagus and surrounded by splanchnic mesenchyme (10). The remaining four stages follow sequentially, beginning with the development of the pre-acinar airways *via* branching morphogenesis during the pseudoglandular stage (7–17 weeks gestation). During the canalicular stage (17–25 weeks gestation), the airways divide further to form the alveolar ducts, and the distal lung mesenchyme thins to allow close approximation of the developing respiratory epithelium and vascular endothelium. Widening and branching of these distal air sacs occurs in the saccular stage (26–36 weeks gestation), and finally, during the alveolar stage (36 weeks gestation onward), the terminal alveoli form by the process of secondary septation and rapidly increase in number throughout early childhood (11).

The mature lung contains approximately 500 million alveoli (12), each surrounded by a network of pulmonary capillaries allowing close proximity of the air filled alveolus with the blood-filled capillary. This intimate association of the pulmonary microcirculation with the terminal airspaces is imperative for efficient gas exchange. Therefore, the pulmonary blood supply must develop in close relationship to the airways throughout lung development (10). Early recognition that the branching of the pre-acinar arteries (formed by the end of the pseudoglandular stage) occurs at the same time and along a similar pattern, as the branching of the airways, suggested that the airways may provide

a template for the development of the pulmonary arteries and veins (13).

The pulmonary circulation likely forms through a combination of vasculogenesis, the *de novo* formation of vessels from the differentiation of primitive angioblasts and hemangioblasts, and angiogenesis, the sprouting and branching of new vessels from existing vessels (14, 15). However, the degree to which each process contributes to the formation of the pulmonary vasculature at each stage of development remains a source for debate. Early evidence supported the notion that the proximal arteries form by angiogenic sprouting from the main pulmonary trunk and that distal branches form *de novo* in the distal mesenchyme *via* vasculogenesis. Using a method to make a cast of the developing pulmonary vasculature in fetal rats (from E9 to E20), deMelo et al. showed that isolated "blood lakes" form in the periphery of the lung (presumably by vasculogenesis) as early as E9. This was followed by the central sprouting of the proximal arteries, with the formation of five to seven generations of branching by E14, and connections between the proximal and distal vessels by E13–14 (16). In contrast, using transgenic reporter mice that express LacZ under the control of an endothelial specific promoter, Schachtner et al. found evidence of connections between the proximal, branching pulmonary arteries, and endothelial cells located in the distal mesenchyme as early as E10.5, several days before patency of the central pulmonary arteries has occurred. These findings suggested the authors that vasculogenesis may contribute to the development of the proximal pulmonary vasculature as well (17).

Prior to term birth, the density of the peripheral pulmonary vessels markedly increases in density, suggesting expansion of the capillary network by angiogenesis (16). After birth, the pulmonary capillary network continues to expand, resulting in a 35-fold increase by adulthood (13). Airway and vascular development are closely linked, with the disruption of one process impairing the other, and each culminating in a global disruption of lung development (18). Moreover, pulmonary vascular development continues throughout all stages of lung development in a manner proportional to the overall growth of the lung, rendering it vulnerable to perturbations occurring in both embryonic and postnatal life (17).

EXTREME LUNG IMMATURITY AND ARRESTED LUNG DEVELOPMENT: THE "NEW" BPD

In 1967, Northway et al. used the term BPD to describe a novel form of chronic lung disease that developed in preterm infants (mean gestational age of 32 weeks) who had a history of neonatal respiratory distress (4). This original form of BPD was associated with positive-pressure ventilation and prolonged oxygen therapy, and characterized by histologic evidence of severe lung injury (e.g., inflammation, protein-rich edema, airway epithelial metaplasia, and peribronchial fibrosis) and marked airway and pulmonary vascular smooth muscle hypertrophy (19, 20). Abnormalities in the pulmonary vasculature were also a feature of the disease. Pathologic examination of post-mortem lung tissue from a small group of infants with BPD who survived for at least 1 month demonstrated decreased density of peripheral pulmonary arteries as compared to control patients, both by barium angiogram and histologic measures (21).

However, advances in medical therapy, including antenatal steroids, surfactant replacement therapy, and the institution of lung protective strategies of ventilation, have permitted the survival of extremely immature, very low birth weight (VLBW) infants. Accompanying this increase in survival, the clinical, radiographic, and pathological features of BPD have changed significantly. In contradistinction to the original form of BPD, birth of VLBW infants during the late canalicular or early saccular stages of lung development appears to disrupt the normal alveolar and vascular development, resulting in the "new BPD." Margraf et al. described the lung pathology of this new, post-surfactant form of BPD in a small case series of infants who died with severe BPD. One of the most striking findings observed by the authors was the severely reduced alveolar number in the infants with BPD compared to controls, with little evidence of the normal, physiologic increases in alveolar number typically observed with advancing age (22). Similarly, Husain et al. also showed evidence of arrested acinar development in a series of infants with post-surfactant BPD, including both reductions in acinar number and increases in acinar size (23).

Pathologic data obtained from autopsy specimens can be difficult to interpret and generalize to the entire disease population, as these samples often represent the most severe lung disease in patients with BPD (24). This is particularly true now that key advances in the medical care of preterm infants have markedly decreased mortality, such that infants who die from BPD in this era truly represent an extremely ill subset of patients. However, Coalson et al. obtained important information surrounding the evolving histopathology in infants with this "new" form of BPD in a small series that examined open lung biopsies from low-birth weight babies on ventilator support who received surfactant but not steroids. Those infants also demonstrated alveolar simplification but minimal metaplasia, and variable degrees of inflammation and abnormal extracellular matrix deposition (25).

ABNORMALITIES IN PULMONARY VASCULAR DEVELOPMENT AND REMODELING

Dysmorphic Pulmonary Microvascular Development

In addition to alveolar simplification (i.e., decreased complexity of distal lung septation), the pathology of this "new" form of BPD also appears to include abnormalities in the development of the pulmonary microvasculature. A comparison of autopsy specimens taken from infants dying from BPD compared to infants dying without lung disease at similar post-conceptional ages demonstrated that the lungs of infants with BPD had an overall reduction in immunostaining for the endothelial specific marker CD31, suggesting a decrease in pulmonary microvascular density. Moreover, the pulmonary capillaries, when present, appeared to be abnormally dilated and frequently located within thickened

alveolar septa, rather than immediately adjacent to the alveolar epithelium (6). These reductions in the growth of the distal pulmonary vasculature were in keeping with the pathologic findings observed in specimens obtained from patients dying of BPD in the pre-surfactant era, where decreases in arterial number and cross-sectional area were thought to contribute to the increased dead space ventilation observed in those infants (26).

However, additional studies have suggested that rather than a simple decrease in pulmonary vascular growth, the vascular abnormalities observed in patients with BPD might be more accurately described as "dysmorphic." In the open lung biopsy samples obtained by Coalson et al., evidence of abnormal capillary development was apparent, with CD31 immunostaining demonstrating an "adaptive dysmorphic pattern of vascular organization." This pattern included a paucity of capillaries within the walls of the thinned abnormally enlarged alveoli, and dilated, more abundant capillaries in other sites (25). In contrast, a stereology-based assessment of endothelial cell volume in short- and long-term ventilated preterm infants demonstrated that total endothelial cell volume increased in ventilated infants as compared to age-matched controls, in association with an increase in total parenchymal volume, suggesting an expansion of the pulmonary microvasculature. However, in the long-term ventilated patients, the capillary network was simplified, had decreased branching, and retained the dual capillary pattern characteristic of the saccular lung, features predicted to decrease gas exchange efficiency (27). Taken together, these studies suggest that variable abnormalities in the pulmonary capillaries may be observed in BPD, with suppressed vascular growth at some stages of the disease, and excessive, dysmorphic growth at other stages, perhaps representing a maladaptive compensatory response.

Abnormal Muscularization, Heightened Vascular Tone, and the Development of Pulmonary Hypertension

In his original description of BPD, Northway noted that some patients had evidence of medial hypertrophy of the pulmonary arteries, suggesting the development of PH (4). This histologic finding was confirmed by clinical studies demonstrating elevations in pulmonary arterial pressures (PAPs) and pulmonary vascular resistance (PVR) by either cardiac catheterization or enchocardiography in survivors of BPD. In one such study, Fouron et al. found that the majority of patients with BPD in the "acute phase" had echocardiographic evidence of PH, and that pulmonary pressures remained high in those infants who eventually died, but normalized in infants who recovered (28). However, long-term follow-up of patients with pre-surfactant BPD and PH showed that in many patients, elevations in PAPs persisted through early childhood (29).

With the evolution of BPD in the post-surfactant era, the development of PH remains a significant feature of the disease for a subgroup of patients and significantly impacts long-term prognosis. In a prospective study of preterm infants using a broad echocardiogram-based definition of PH, early evidence of PH was found in more than 40% of patients at 7 days of age, and late PH found in almost 15% of patients at 36 weeks PMA. In patients who develop severe BPD, the incidence of late PH appears to be significantly higher ranging from 30 to 50% of patients (30–32). Moreover, the presence of PH in patients with BPD is independently associated with a greater increase in the odds of death (30, 32), with mortality rates as high as 40% in some studies (33). Of note, the risk of death appears to be highest in the first 6 months after the diagnosis of PH, and the majority of infants with BPD and PH who survive beyond a mean of 10 months of age demonstrate an improvement in the severity of PH (33). Numerous risk factors have been associated with an increased incidence of PH in patients with BPD including: oligohydramnios (32, 34), low apgar scores (32, 34), postnatal sepsis (34), small for gestational age (33), and prolonged use of positive-pressure ventilation (31). Of note, while the risk of developing PH is significantly higher in patients with severe versus moderate BPD (32), a smaller percentage of infants with no, mild, or moderate BPD also develop late PH. This suggests that the risk for developing late PH may not be primarily dictated by the severity of lung disease (31). In addition, early PH appears to predict the development of BPD (35), again highlighting the link between abnormalities in the pulmonary circulation and impairments in distal lung development (**Figure 1**). While a complete understanding of the mechanisms leading to PH in a subset of patients is lacking, the data suggest that patients with BPD and PH demonstrate abnormalities in both distal pulmonary artery muscularization and tone.

Abnormalities in Pulmonary Arterial Muscularization

In his original report, Northway et al. identified "early vascular lesions of the pulmonary hypertensive type" in the cohort of infants in the later stages of the disease, which comprised medial hypertrophy and characteristic breakdown of the elastic lamina (4). Later studies demonstrated similar pathologic remodeling of small pulmonary arteries in patients with the pre-surfactant form of BPD. In a small study of preterm infants with severe BPD and cor pulmonale, affected patients demonstrated an increase in the percent medial thickness of distal arteries and an extension of arterial smooth muscle into peripheral arteries such that the majority of alveolar wall arteries were completely muscularized (26). Further, abnormal muscularization of the pulmonary arteries was often a feature of pre-surfactant BPD even in patients that did not develop cor pulmonale. In premature infants with respiratory distress syndrome (RDS) who died early in life while still requiring mechanical support, many demonstrated increased medial thickness of distal arteries, appearing similar to the muscularized small arteries characteristic of a term infant on the first day of life (20). Moreover, in keeping with the findings of Bush et al., those infants with BPD who developed cor pulmonale had evidence of marked muscularization of small arteries, with complete muscularization of arteriolar wall arteries, and some patients with intimal proliferation of larger arteries (20). In a separate study, the combination of abnormal muscularization

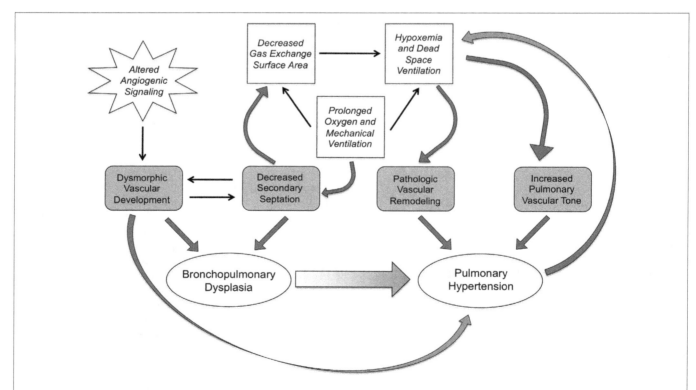

FIGURE 1 | The interplay of pathologic and clinical factors that lead to pulmonary hypertension in bronchopulmonary dysplasia. Dysmorphic vascular development as a result of altered angiogenic signaling combines with impairments in secondary septation, leading to the development of BPD. These events set the stage, pre- and postnatally, for the development of pulmonary hypertension. The decrease in gas exchange surface area resulting from the impaired secondary septation also sets up a vicious cycle of hypoxemia and dead space ventilation that prolongs the need for mechanical ventilation and oxygen therapy, and induces pathologic changes in pulmonary vascular remodeling and tone, further increasing the risk of pulmonary hypertension.

of distal arteries with variable degrees of either increased or decreased pulmonary capillary density suggested a "dual process of adaptation and response to injury in a hypoplastic lung" (36).

In the post-surfactant era, mortality of premature infants has decreased, thus limiting the availability of autopsy specimens that would allow careful characterization of the pulmonary arterial histopathologic changes in the "new" form of BPD. However, in at least one study, it appears that the abnormal muscularization of peripheral arteries remains a consistent pathologic feature. In a study of post-mortem tissue obtained from surfactant-treated preterm infants with BPD, there was evidence of increased arterial wall thickness and muscularization of distal vessels in preterm infants with severe BPD, although these histologic changes were less marked than those observed in specimens obtained from infants who developed PH in the setting of persistent pulmonary hypertension of the newborn (PPHN) and premature rupture of membranes (PROM) (37). While the mechanisms that specifically induce pathologic pulmonary vascular remodeling in BPD are unknown, they are hypothesized to include some of the well recognized injurious stimuli that disrupt distal lung growth including hyperoxia, mechanical ventilation, and inflammation (38).

Abnormalities in Pulmonary Vascular Tone

In addition to abnormal pulmonary arterial remodeling, heightened pulmonary arterial tone also appeared to be an important component of the PH observed in patients with pre-surfactant BPD. Survivors of BPD with persistent oxygen requirements and evidence of right ventricular hypertrophy (RVH) on ECG had evidence of PH on cardiac catheterization, with pulmonary vascular beds that were responsive to even low levels of oxygen (39). In a prospective study of 15 patients with moderate to severe BPD and PH undergoing cardiac catheterization, all patients demonstrated a reduction in PA pressure with supplemental oxygen, and variable responses to vasodilator therapy depending on the presence or absence of systemic–pulmonary collaterals (40).

Elevated pulmonary vascular tone remains a key feature of the PH in BPD survivors in the post-surfactant era. A study examining BPD survivors with PH who underwent cardiac catheterization found that most patients have significant pulmonary vascular reactivity, demonstrating elevations in mean PAP with hypoxia, and conversely, decreased mean PAP with the combination of hyperoxia and inhaled nitric oxide (iNO) (41). Similarly, in a study reporting data from the cardiac catheterization of 13 patients with BPD and PH, PAP and PVR decreased significantly with vasodilator therapy (100% O_2 or iNO) in the majority of patients, but still remained elevated above normal levels (33).

Abnormal Collateral Circulations

In an early report, cardiac catheterization of two premature infants who required prolonged mechanical ventilation found that although these infants had normal pulmonary pressures, they both had evidence of large systemic collaterals with left to right shunts, a finding the authors hypothesized likely contributed to their persistent ventilator dependence (42). This report was followed by the description of similar collateral vessels in a subgroup of patients with severe BPD and PH, in whom the administration of vasodilators had deleterious results, inducing respiratory acidosis, pulmonary edema, and more severe hypoxemia (40). However, it was not clear from either report whether these abnormal vessels were congenital in nature or acquired, resulting from persistent hypoxemia, pathologic alterations in pulmonary blood flow, or disrupted lung development (43).

More recently, histologic examination of lung tissue from a number of patients dying with severe BPD demonstrated the presence of numerous smaller intrapulmonary arteriovenous anastomotic vessels (IAAV) that appear similar to the "misalignment of veins" seen in alveolar capillary dysplasia. These vascular channels are located in the lobar periphery and extend toward the pulmonary arteries, appearing to connect with the microvascular plexus surrounding the pulmonary arteries and airways (44). Of note, these intrapulmonary anastomotic vessels are not unique to BPD, but observed in other diseases of impaired alveolarization. For example, in a similar study examining the lung tissue of infants dying from severe congenital diaphragmatic hernia (CDH) and associated PH, the lungs of all patients demonstrated prominent, engorged intrapulmonary vessels connecting the pulmonary veins to the microvessels surrounding the pulmonary arteries (45). Similar, intrapulmonary, bronchopulmonary anastomoses have also been noted in infants dying from meconium aspiration syndrome (46). These prominent IAAV may represent the failure of the normal fetal IAAV circulation to close after birth and have the potential to permit right to left intrapulmonary shunting, thus contributing to the hypoxemia observed in patients with severe BPD.

KEY PATHWAYS DIRECTING NORMAL PULMONARY VASCULAR DEVELOPMENT AND FUNCTION

Extensive clinical evidence obtained from patients with BPD in both the pre- and post-surfactant era has identified impaired and dysmorphic pulmonary vascular development as a key feature of the disease. These data suggest that the normal pathways that promote postnatal pulmonary vascular growth are disrupted in BPD. In this section, a number of key pathways that direct normal pulmonary vascular growth and function will be reviewed, and evidence demonstrating alterations in these pathways in experimental models of BPD (**Table 1**) and clinical studies will be summarized.

Vascular Endothelial Growth Factor

The endothelial cell mitogen and survival factor, VEGF, is essential for normal blood vessel development. Alternate splicing from a single gene produces three distinct isoforms: $VEGF_{120}$, $VEGF_{164}$, and $VEGF_{188}$. These three isoforms demonstrate differential binding to heparin sulfate and affinities for the two predominant receptors: tyrosine kinases fms-like-tyrosine kinase-1 (FLT-1) and fetal liver kinase-1 (FLK-1) (47). The lung expression of the two heparin-binding isoforms, $VEGF_{164}$ and $VEGF_{188}$, increases during the late saccular stage of development in the mouse and remains high through adulthood (47), with $VEGF_{188}$ becoming

TABLE 1 | Molecular mechanisms contributing to impaired alveolar and pulmonary vascular growth in animal models.

Molecule	Physiologic functions and disruption in animal models of BPD	Reference
VEGF	Global deletion delays endothelial cell differentiation, impairs vascular development, and induces lethality at E8.5	(55, 56)
	Isoform-specific deletion (VEGF$_{164}$ and VEGF$_{188}$) impairs lung microvascular development and delays airspace maturation	(57)
	Postnatal inhibition decreases somatic growth and impairs alveolarization	(58)
	Decreased expression in response to hyperoxia and mechanical ventilation in numerous animal models	(60–64)
	Overexpression promotes lung angiogenesis, and inhibits hyperoxia-induced alveolar simplification and mortality in rats	(66)
FLK-1	Homozygous deletion prevents endothelial cell differentiation and blood vessel formation, and induces embryonic lethality	(53)
	Decreased expression in response to mechanical ventilation in neonatal mice	(63, 64)
	Postnatal inhibition impairs lung angiogenesis and alveolarization and induces pulmonary hypertension in neonatal rats	(8, 9)
FLT-1	Homozygous deletion causes disorganization of vascular development and induces embryonic lethality	(54)
	Decreased expression in response to mechanical ventilation in preterm baboons	(63)
NFκB	Pharmacologic inhibition in neonatal mice impairs lung angiogenesis and alveolarization and decreases *Flk-1* expression, and exaggerates the impairment in angiogenesis and alveolarization induced by systemic endotoxin	(65, 66)
HIF-1α	Global deletion results in numerous cardiac and vascular abnormalities and embryonic lethality at E10.5	(71, 72)
	Decreased expression in response to mechanical ventilation in preterm baboons and lambs	(69, 75)
	Stabilization of HIF improves alveolar growth in preterm baboons and neonatal rats exposed to combined endotoxin/hyperoxia	(78–80)
HIF-2α	Global deletion results in perinatal mortality due to respiratory failure, decreased VEGF expression, and decreased surfactant	(73)
	Decreased expression in mechanical ventilation of preterm baboons and lambs, and in neonatal rats exposed to chronic hypoxia	(69, 75)
NO/eNOS	Deletion of eNOS impairs VEGF-mediated angiogenesis and neovascularization, worsens pulmonary hypertension in adult mice exposed to chronic hypoxia, and increases susceptibility of neonatal mice to the impaired alveolarization induced by hyperoxia	(88, 90, 91, 99, 100)
	Decreased eNOS expression in mechanically ventilated preterm baboons and lambs, in fetal lambs exposed to intrauterine endotoxin	(94–96)
	Decreased NO production in pulmonary arteries from fetal lambs with intrauterine growth restriction	(97)
H$_2$S	Deletion of enzymes that produce H$_2$S impairs alveolarization, decrease lung vascular growth, and induce pathologic vascular remodeling	(104)
	Exogenous administration improves alveolarization, limits pulmonary hypertension, and decreases lung inflammation in neonatal rats and mice exposed to hyperoxia	(105, 106)
Retinoic acid	Deletion of the RA receptor-gamma impairs alveolarization and decreases lung elastin	(110)
	Promotes alveolar regeneration in adult mice with elastase-induced emphysema and limits the impaired alveolarization induced by glucocorticoids in neonatal mice	(108, 109)
LPA	Deletion of the LPA-receptor 1 limits lung inflammation and fibrosis, and improves survival in neonatal rats exposed to hyperoxia	(116)
	Pharmacologic blockade of LPA receptors -1 and -3 limits pulmonary hypertension in newborn rats exposed to hyperoxia	(116)
EC-SOD	Deletion impairs alveolarization and lung angiogenesis, and decreases FLK-1 protein expression in neonatal mice	(118)
	Alveolar epithelial overexpression preserves alveolar and vascular growth of neonatal mice exposed to hyperoxia	(119)

the predominant isoform by late alveolarization (48). Paralleling the expression pattern observed with VEGF, FLT-1 and FLK-1 are highly expressed by endothelial cells during lung development (49), and in the murine lung, the expression of both receptors increase during alveolarization and remain high in the adult lung (47, 48). In addition to the full-length, membrane-bound form of FLT-1, a soluble form, comprised of the extracellular ligand binding domain, can be produced by alternative splicing from a single gene transcript (50, 51). It is thought that this soluble form (sFLT-1) may function as a physiologic inhibitor of angiogenesis given its ability to sequester VEGF ligands and prevent them from binding to the active transmembrane receptors (52).

The absolute requirement of intact VEGF signaling for vascular development is underscored by the severe phenotypes observed in mice containing targeted disruptions of discrete components of the pathway. Homozygous deletion of *Flk-1* in mice results in early embryonic lethality, complete absence of blood vessel formation, and a failure of endothelial differentiation (53). In contrast, while homozygous deletion of *Flt-1* also results in embryonic lethality, endothelial cell differentiation is

preserved, and the vasculature develops but is very disorganized (54). Targeted deletion of *Vegf* in mice delays endothelial cell differentiation and severely impairs vascular development, resulting in embryonic lethality between E8.5 and 9.5 (55). Of note, even the absence of a single allele of *Vegf* impairs vascular development and induces embryonic lethality (56). Absence of the two heparin-bound isomers, VEGF$_{164}$ and VEGF$_{188}$, impairs lung microvascular development and delays airspace maturation in mice, suggesting that these isoforms which are bound tightly in the extracellular matrix may provide a source of local VEGF specifically essential for pulmonary vascular development (57).

In addition to these indispensable roles for VEGF during embryonic development, VEGF is also an important mediator of postnatal organ growth and development. Partial inhibition of VEGF in mice during the first week of life using an inducible gene targeting strategy decreases somatic growth and impairs organ development, while complete inhibition by the administration of a soluble VEGF receptor chimeric protein exaggerates these effects on organ development and growth and specifically impairs alveolarization (58). Moreover, the spatial expression of VEGF during late development is critical. Expression of $VEGF_{164}$ in the alveolar type II (ATII) cells using the SP-C promoter induces earlier and higher levels of VEGF in the developing lung and increases pulmonary blood vessel growth, but disrupts branching morphogenesis and inhibits alveolar type I cell differentiation (59). Taken together, these studies demonstrate the importance of tightly regulated temporal and spatial expression of VEGF for normal vascular development.

Abnormalities in VEGF signaling appear to be a key mechanism in the impaired alveolarization and angiogenesis observed in experimental models of BPD. Chronic exposure to hyperoxia in neonatal rabbits decreases VEGF gene and protein expression by alveolar epithelial cells (60). In neonatal rats, high levels of hyperoxia decrease *Vegf* gene expression (61), and sustained hyperoxia from postnatal day (P)4–14 impairs alveolarization, and suppresses *Vegf* and *Hif-2α* gene expression and VEGF receptor protein expression (61, 62). In the preterm baboon model of BPD, mechanical ventilation and oxygen reduce pulmonary capillary volume, impair alveolarization, and repress the physiologic increase in VEGF and FLT-1 observed in control animals (63). Similarly, mechanical ventilation of neonatal mice during the late saccular stage of development induces alveolar simplification and reduces lung expression of VEGF and FLK-1 (64). Inhibiting constitutive activation of nuclear factor-κB, a direct regulator of *Flk-1* during alveolarization, impairs pulmonary angiogenesis and disrupts alveolarization in neonatal mice (65), and exaggerates the impairment in angiogenesis and alveolarization induced by systemic endotoxin (66). Moreover, blocking angiogenesis in neonatal rats directly using either non-specific anti-angiogenic compounds, or a selective FLK-1 inhibitor, decreases pulmonary arterial density and impairs alveolarization, thus providing some of the first direct, experimental evidence to support the notion that angiogenesis actively promotes distal lung growth (8). In fact, even the administration of a single dose of the FLK-1 inhibitor significantly decreases pulmonary arterial density, impairs alveolarization, and induces pulmonary artery muscularization and RVH that persist into adulthood (9). Consistent with these studies, overexpression of VEGF in newborn rats is effective in increasing survival, promoting lung angiogenesis, and preventing hyperoxia-induced alveolar simplification (67).

Hypoxia-Inducible Factor

Fetal development occurs at low oxygen tension. The hypoxia-inducible factor (HIF) family of transcription factors is a key regulator of O_2 homeostasis, activating genes critical for energy metabolism, oxygen transport, and angiogenesis. The HIFs are heterodimeric transcription factors comprised of oxygen sensitive subunits (HIF-1α, HIF-2α, and HIF-3) paired with the constitutively expressed HIF-1β (previously known as ARNT) subunit. Under normal oxygen tension, the O_2 sensitive subunits are continuously degraded. However, under conditions of low oxygen tension, HIF degradation is inhibited, resulting in HIF protein stabilization and accumulation, thereby promoting the binding of HIF to hypoxia-response elements (HREs) located within the promoters of downstream target genes, including *VEGF*. During lung development, HIF-1α is expressed in the branching epithelium, and HIF-2 expressed in both the epithelium and the mesenchyme (68). In the primate lung, expression of both HIF-1α and HIF-2 is high in the third trimester of pregnancy; however, at term birth, HIF-2 expression remains high while HIF-1α is absent (69). In mouse lung, HIF-2α expression also increases immediately after birth and remains high throughout alveolarization, with production predominantly by ATII cells and colocalizing with VEGF expression (70).

The importance of this pathway in vascular development was highlighted by studies that performed targeted deletions of HIF family members in mice. Loss of *Hif-1α* results in embryonic lethality at E10.5, with null embryos demonstrating numerous cardiac and vascular malformations including vascular regression and abnormal vascular remodeling (71, 72). Interestingly, although this phenotype was similar to that seen in the VEGF null mice, *Hif-1α⁻/⁻* mice were found to have normal levels of *Vegf* mRNA, suggesting that the vascular malformations observed were independent of impairments in VEGF expression. In contrast, *Hif-2α⁻/⁻* mice die from RDS during the perinatal period in association with decreases in ATII-mediated expression of VEGF and insufficient surfactant production (73). Moreover, a similar phenotype is induced in mice by specifically deleting the HRE located within the *Vegf* promoter. Targeted deletion of ARNT, the dimerization partner for both HIF-1α and HIF-2α, as well as for other transcription factors, also results in embryonic lethality at E10.5, with affected embryos displaying defective angiogenesis of the yolk sac and branchial arteries (74).

Experimental studies in animal models of BPD suggest that HIF family members are important for late lung development in general and, in specific, that HIF plays an important role in both normal pulmonary vascular development and abnormal pulmonary vascular remodeling. HIF-1α and HIF-2α protein are decreased in the lungs of preterm baboon and lambs undergoing mechanical ventilation (69, 75). Expression of HIF-2α is also decreased in the lungs of neonatal rats exposed to chronic hypoxia, another stimulus that impairs alveolar development and decreases pulmonary vascular growth in mice (76). Enhancement of HIF signaling by either selective or non-selective inhibition of PHD-mediated HIF degradation increases angiogenesis of lung microvascular endothelial cells *in vitro*, in association with increases in PECAM-1, VEGF, and FLT-1 (77). A similar strategy to stabilize HIFs *in vivo* increases VEGF and PECAM expression in the lungs of preterm baboons (78), and improves alveolarization, oxygenation, and lung compliance (79). In a newborn rat model of BPD induced by intra-amniotic LPS followed by hyperoxia, non-selective inhibition of PHDs stabilizes HIF-1α in the whole lung, and attenuates the disrupted alveolar and vascular growth observed in this model (80). Interestingly, sildenafil, a phosphodiesterase inhibitor that has been used clinically to treat PH by increasing cGMP levels, improves alveolarization in neonatal mice exposed to hyperoxia and directly activates HIF-1α-mediated signaling in airway epithelial cells (81).

Nitric Oxide

Nitric oxide (NO) is a free radical gas that functions as a second messenger, regulating diverse physiologic processes such as angiogenesis, vasodilation, and anticoagulation (82). NO is produced by the nitric oxide synthase (NOS) family of proteins, which contains three isoforms: neuronal NOS (*NOS1*), inducible NOS (*NOS2*), and endothelial NOS (*NOS3*). After release from the endothelium, NO can diffuse to the luminal side of the vessel to inhibit platelet aggregation and adhesion or to the abluminal side of the vessel where it regulates vascular smooth muscle contraction and proliferation (83). Many of the downstream effects of NO on vascular tone result from the ability of NO to activate soluble guanylyl cyclase, thereby increasing cGMP and decreasing intracellular calcium.

Endothelial nitric oxide synthase (eNOS), initially believed to be expressed solely by endothelial cells in a constitutive fashion, is now known to be expressed by additional cell types (84) and dynamically regulated in response to hypoxia, inflammation, and other factors (84, 85). Importantly, VEGF induces eNOS expression *via* a FLK-1-dependent mechanism (86, 87), and loss of eNOS impairs VEGF-mediated angiogenesis (88). NO is a downstream effector of VEGF-mediated angiogenesis but not fibroblast growth factor (FGF)-mediated angiogenesis (89), and *eNOS*$^{-/-}$ mice demonstrate impaired VEGF-mediated angiogenesis (88) and neovascularization during wound healing and after ischemia (90, 91). Expression of eNOS is modulated by changes in oxygen tension both *in vitro* and *in vivo*. NOS activity in pulmonary artery endothelial cells increases at higher oxygen concentrations and decreases at lower oxygen concentrations (92), an effect mediated by both transcriptional and posttranscriptional mechanisms (93).

Decreased expression of eNOS is observed in a number of animal models of BPD. Chronic ventilation of preterm lambs increases pulmonary vascular and airway resistance, and decreases eNOS protein expression in the endothelium of the small intrapulmonary arteries and the airway epithelium (94). Similarly, chronic ventilation of extremely preterm fetal baboons also decreases lung eNOS expression (95). Intra-amniotic endotoxin also decreases eNOS expression in the lungs of fetal lambs, particularly in small pulmonary arteries (96). In an ovine model, intrauterine growth restriction decreases pulmonary vascular density and alveolarization, in association with decreases in VEGF-induced NO production in large proximal pulmonary arteries (97).

In adult mice, compensatory lung growth after pneumonectomy is severely impaired by targeted deletion of eNOS or inhibition of NO production with a NOS inhibitor (98). Exposing adult *eNOS*$^{-/-}$ mice to mild hypoxia induces more severe PH than that seen in control mice (99), and exposing neonatal *eNOS*$^{-/-}$ mice to mild hypoxia impairs alveolarization and decreases pulmonary vascular density (100). In both models, these detrimental effects on pulmonary pressures and lung structure are rescued by iNO (99, 101). Further, iNO appears to have beneficial effect in other experimental models of BPD. Treatment of neonatal rats with a single dose of the FLK-1 inhibitor, SU-5416, impairs alveolarization and induces RVH, and iNO administration prevents RVH development and significantly increases radial alveolar counts (102). Prolonged iNO therapy also prevents RVH and partially rescues the severe defect in alveolarization induced by bleomycin in neonatal rats (103).

ADDITIONAL MOLECULAR MECHANISMS THAT MAY INFLUENCE ALVEOLAR AND VASCULAR GROWTH

In addition to the well-established molecular pathways described above that are central regulators of normal pulmonary vascular development and function, a number of additional molecules and pathways have been recently identified that also appear play a role in the aberrant vascular growth observed in BPD.

Hydrogen Sulfide

In addition to NO, hydrogen sulfide (H_2S) is an additional gasotransmitter that appears to have an important role in late lung development. H_2S is produced by two main enzymes: cystathionine β-synthase (Cbs) and cystathionine γ-lyase (Cth). Deletion of either *Cbs* or *Cth* decreases alveolar number by 50%, reduces the pulmonary vascular supply, and increases the number of muscularized small and medium-sized pulmonary arteries (104). In addition, H_2S appears to have important, direct effects on the angiogenic function of pulmonary endothelial cells. Silencing or pharmacologic inhibition of Cbs and Cth, respectively, impairs *in vitro* tube formation in human lung endothelial cells, and conversely, exogenous administration of H_2S enhances tube formation *in vitro* (104). Further, exogenous administration of H_2S improves alveolarization *in vivo* and limits PH in hyperoxia-exposed neonatal rats (105); and improves epithelial repair and decreases inflammation in hyperoxia-exposed neonatal mice (106).

Retinoic Acid

Retinoic acid (RA) is a biologically active derivative of vitamin A. Early studies identified a role for vitamin A and RA in enhancing limb regeneration in amphibians after amputation (107). Subsequently, RA was shown to promote alveolar regeneration in adult rats in elastase-induced emphysema (108) and to blunt the impaired alveolarization induced by dexamethasone in neonatal rats (109). Mice with genetic deletion in the RA-receptor-gamma have decreased lung elastin and impaired alveolarization (110). Pulmonary endothelial cells are a source of RA in the developing lung, where it appears to promote pulmonary angiogenesis by increasing the expression of VEGF-A and to regulate elastin synthesis by increasing FGF-18 expression (111).

Lysophosphatidic Acid

Lysophosphatidic acid is a small glycerophospholipid that exerts multiple biologic effects on cell proliferation, migration, survival, and cell–cell interactions by binding to G-protein coupled receptors on the cell membrane (112). LPA appears to have an important role in many lung diseases, functioning to regulate airway inflammation, remodeling, and fibrosis (113–115). In the vasculature, LPA can function as either a vasodilator or a vasopressor depending on context. For example, in the thoracic aorta, LPA causes NOS-dependent vasodilation by acting through the LPA receptor-1 (LPAR1). Mice containing mutations in the LPAR1 demonstrate decreased lung inflammation and fibrosis and improved survival in an experimental model of BPD, and pharmacologic blockade of the LPAR-1 and -3 protects against pathologic vascular remodeling, limiting muscularization and RVH in newborn rats exposed to chronic hyperoxia (116). Although there were some phenotypic differences between the mice with genetic deletions of LPAR-1 and pharmacologic blockade that require future study, these studies suggest that the LPA pathway may prove to be a promising new target for BPD.

Extracellular Superoxide Dismutase

Extracellular superoxide dismutase (EC-SOD) is a potent antioxidant that catalyzes the dismutation of superoxide to hydrogen peroxide and oxygen (117). EC-SOD is highly expressed in the lung and vasculature, and EC-SOD expression and activity is suppressed in experimental models of BPD (118). Alveolar epithelial overexpression of EC-SOD preserves alveolar surface and volume density, decreases inflammation in newborn mice exposed to hyperoxia (119), and attenuates pathologic vascular remodeling and PH in adult mice exposed to chronic hypoxia (120). Conversely, deletion of EC-SOD impairs alveolarization in neonatal mice and decreases pulmonary vascular density and Flk-1 protein expression (118). Taken together, these studies highlight the importance of tight control of the oxidative balance in the lung in promoting physiologic alveolar and vascular growth, and preventing pathologic airway and vascular remodeling.

Stem and Progenitor Cells

A number of resident stem and progenitor cell populations have been identified in the lung, deriving from epithelial, mesenchymal, and endothelial origins. Each population is unique in its defining characteristics and putative functions, which are comprehensively discussed in a number of excellent, recent reviews (121–123). Accumulating evidence from clinical and experimental studies have suggested that alterations in circulating and/or resident lung stem and progenitor cells may contribute to the pathogenesis of BPD, sparking great interest in the investigation of cell-based therapeutic strategies as a potential treatment for BPD. Hyperoxia decreases lung and circulating endothelial progenitor cells in neonatal mice (124), and diminishes the number of lung side population (SP) progenitor cells, a population believed to have both epithelial and mesenchymal potential (125). Further, studies in experimental models suggest that mesenchymal stem cell therapy may have beneficial effects on preserving alveolar and vascular growth during injury. Intratracheal administration of mesenchymal stem cells attenuates induced lung cell apoptosis and inflammation, and improves alveolarization in neonatal rats exposed to hyperoxia (126). Intravenous administration of bone marrow-derived mesenchymal stem cells (BMSCs) in neonatal mice prevents PH and blunts the impaired alveolarization induced by hyperoxia despite a low level of engraftment. Importantly, in that study, the administration of conditioned media of these stem cells had an even greater beneficial effect, preserving normal alveolarization and preventing pathologic vascular remodeling (127). A similar improvement in alveolar and vascular growth is observed in hyperoxia-exposed neonatal rats after intratracheal

administration of BMSCs (128), and this beneficial effect is evident even if the MSCs are administered after the initiation of lung injury (129). Moreover, MSC treatment results in durable improvements in lung structure, with sustained improvement in lung structure and exercise tolerance in adult mice at 6 months of age, and an absence of any evidence of long-term detrimental side effects. These exciting data prompted clinical studies to assess whether alterations in lung progenitor cells play a role in BPD, discussed in the following section.

ALTERATIONS IN ANGIOGENIC PATHWAYS IN PATIENTS WITH BRONCHOPULMONARY DYSPLASIA

These data, obtained from experimental models demonstrating disruption of key pathways known to promote physiologic pulmonary angiogenesis, appear to have some fidelity with the human disease. The impaired pulmonary vascular development observed in infants dying of severe BPD is associated with decreased expression of VEGF and FLT-1 (6). In response to short-term ventilation, the expression of classic angiogenic growth factors, such as VEGF and angiopoietin-1, decreases in the lungs of preterm infants, while expression of endoglin increases, suggesting that endoglin may be one important regulator of the vascular remodeling which occurs in BPD (130). In a similar, but separate, study by the same group, short-term ventilation decreases the gene expression of proangiogenic factors such as *FLK-1*, TEK tryrosine kinase, endothelial (*TIE-2*), and angiogenin, yet increases the expression of anti-angiogenic mediators such as thrombospondin-1 (131). Taken together, these two studies suggest that even short-term mechanical ventilation causes widespread alterations in a variety of angiogenic signaling pathways in the developing lung.

In contrast to these studies demonstrating changes in the gene and protein expression of angiogenic mediators from whole lung tissue of patients dying with BPD, studies evaluating levels of VEGF in the tracheal fluid have not shown clear differences between preterm infants who develop and those who do not develop BPD. Lassus et al. found that the levels of VEGF in tracheal fluid obtained during the first 10 days of life are not significantly different in preterm infants who developed BPD versus those who do not develop BPD (132). In keeping with these results, two additional studies demonstrated that tracheal fluid VEGF levels obtained during the first month of life also did not correlate with the development of BPD (133). However, it is not clear whether the absence of positive findings in these studies represent differences between the pathogenesis of experimental BPD and the human disease, a lack of statistical power, or the inability of tracheal aspirates to reflect the true microenvironment present in the developing lung.

Similarly, despite strong experimental evidence demonstrating the importance of both the HIF and NO signaling pathways in physiologic pulmonary angiogenesis, data assessing the integrity of the HIF of NO signaling in patients with BPD remain scarce. In the developing human lung, both *HIF-2α* and *VEGFA* gene expression demonstrate a positive correlation as lung development progresses; however, little is known regarding how HIF activity or expression is altered in preterm infants with BPD. Similarly, there is an absence of data directly demonstrating decreased NOS expression or NO production in infants with BPD. However, the levels of the endogenous NOS inhibitor, asymmetric dimethylarginine (ADMA), are increased in patients with BPD and PH, suggesting that heightened levels of ADMA may contribute to the increased PVR observed in patients with BPD and PH by limiting NO production (134). Yet, despite extensive experimental evidence demonstrating disruptions in NO signaling and the therapeutic benefit of iNO therapy in animal models, a number of recent, prospective, and randomized trials have failed to demonstrate beneficial effects of iNO therapy in the prevention of BPD in preterm infants (135–137).

Given the accumulating evidence from experimental models that demonstrated the beneficial role of stem and progenitor cells in promoting alveolar and vascular growth during injury, clinical studies aimed to determine whether disruption of angiogenic progenitors might contribute to the pathophysiology of BPD. Late outgrowth endothelial colony-forming cells (ECFCs), a sub-type of EPCs that are highly proliferative, self-renewing, and capable of forming blood vessels de novo in vivo (138). ECFCs obtained from preterm infants are more proliferative than those obtained from term infants, yet more highly susceptible to the growth inhibiting effects of hyperoxia (139). In a small, early prospective study, ECFCs were found to be low in extremely premature infants and to increase with increasing gestation. Further, extremely preterm infants with lower numbers of ECFC were found to be at increased risk of developing BPD (140). In keeping with these results, a subsequent study confirmed that cord blood ECFCs are significantly lower in preterm infants who go onto develop moderate or severe BPD (141). Taken together, these studies lend further support to the notion that antenatal events may influence later respiratory outcomes, and suggest that ECFC may represent a biomarker for the identification of patients at greatest risk for the development of BPD. In addition to these endothelial progenitors, another small clinical study demonstrated the presence of fibroblast-like cells with colony-forming potential and cell surface marked similar to MSCs in the tracheal aspirates of premature infants with RDS. After adjusting for numerous potential confounders, including gestational age, duration of mechanical ventilation, and others, the presence of these tracheal MSC predicted the development of BPD (142). Although clinical evidence regarding the role of MSC in patients with BPD is limited, the strong experimental evidence demonstrating the benefit of MSC therapy on alveolar and vascular growth in animal models has already lead the way for phase 1 clinical trails for testing this therapy in preterm infants at high risk for BPD (143).

CONCLUSION

Over the past three decades, significant advances in the supportive care of extremely premature infants, including surfactant replacement therapy, have significantly decreased mortality from BPD, yet, the morbidity associated with BPD remains high. Numerous abnormalities of the pulmonary circulation are observed in patients with BPD, influencing long-term prognosis, including dysmorphic pulmonary capillary development, maladaptive pulmonary vascular remodeling, heighted pulmonary vascular tone, and the development of abnormal collateral circulation. Extensive experimental and clinical data derived form studies over the last decade have advanced our understanding of the pathobiology contributing to BPD, including the recognition that pulmonary angiogenesis is essential for alveolarization, and that disrupted pulmonary angiogenesis likely contributes to BPD. Given the limited availability of human lung tissue from patients with BPD, much of our understanding of the molecular mechanisms involved have been derived from experimental animal models (144), and definitive clinical evidence demonstrating that these same mechanisms are causative in the human disease are lacking. Nonetheless, these studies suggest that replacement of angiogenic factors and/or stem cell-based therapies could prove to be beneficial for the treatment of BPD. Moving forward, the development of innovative non-invasive diagnostic technologies that may permit an accurate assessment of the molecular pathways that are dysregulated in patients at risk for BPD will be required in order to foster the development of targeted biologic therapies that can effectively stimulate lung growth and regeneration.

AUTHOR CONTRIBUTIONS

Dr. CA composed the manuscript and designed the figure and table.

REFERENCES

1. Galambos C, Demello DE. Regulation of alveologenesis: clinical implications of impaired growth. *Pathology* (2008) **40**(2):124–40. doi:10.1080/00313020701818981
2. Jobe AH, Bancalari E. Bronchopulmonary dysplasia. *Am J Respir Crit Care Med* (2001) **163**(7):1723–9. doi:10.1164/ajrccm.163.7.2011060
3. Kinsella JP, Greenough A, Abman SH. Bronchopulmonary dysplasia. *Lancet* (2006) **367**(9520):1421–31. doi:10.1016/S0140-6736(06)68615-7
4. Northway WH Jr, Rosan RC, Porter DY. Pulmonary disease following respirator therapy of hyaline-membrane disease. Bronchopulmonary dysplasia. *N Engl J Med* (1967) **276**(7):357–68. doi:10.1056/NEJM196702162760701

5. Jobe AJ. The new BPD: an arrest of lung development. *Pediatr Res* (1999) **46**(6):641–3. doi:10.1203/00006450-199912000-00007
6. Bhatt AJ, Pryhuber GS, Huyck H, Watkins RH, Metlay LA, Maniscalco WM. Disrupted pulmonary vasculature and decreased vascular endothelial growth factor, Flt-1, and TIE-2 in human infants dying with bronchopulmonary dysplasia. *Am J Respir Crit Care Med* (2001) **164**(10 Pt 1):1971–80. doi:10.1164/ajrccm.164.10.2101140
7. Thébaud B, Ladha F, Michelakis ED, Sawicka M, Thurston G, Eaton F, et al. Vascular endothelial growth factor gene therapy increases survival, promotes lung angiogenesis, and prevents alveolar damage in hyperoxia-induced lung injury: evidence that angiogenesis participates in alveolarization. *Circulation* (2005) **112**(16):2477–86. doi:10.1161/CIRCULATIONAHA.105.541524

8. Jakkula M, Le Cras TD, Gebb S, Hirth KP, Tuder RM, Voelkel NF, et al. Inhibition of angiogenesis decreases alveolarization in the developing rat lung. *Am J Physiol Lung Cell Mol Physiol* (2000) 279(3):L600–7.

9. Le Cras TD, Markham NE, Tuder RM, Voelkel NF, Abman SH. Treatment of newborn rats with a VEGF receptor inhibitor causes pulmonary hypertension and abnormal lung structure. *Am J Physiol Lung Cell Mol Physiol* (2002) 283(3):L555–62. doi:10.1152/ajplung.00408.2001

10. Hislop AA. Airway and blood vessel interaction during lung development. *J Anat* (2002) 201(4):325–34. doi:10.1046/j.1469-7580.2002.00097.x

11. Hislop A. Developmental biology of the pulmonary circulation. *Paediatr Respir Rev* (2005) 6(1):35–43. doi:10.1016/j.prrv.2004.11.009

12. Ochs M, Nyengaard JR, Jung A, Knudsen L, Voigt M, Wahlers T, et al. The number of alveoli in the human lung. *Am J Respir Crit Care Med* (2004) 169(1):120–4. doi:10.1164/rccm.200308-1107OC

13. Hislop AA, Pierce CM. Growth of the vascular tree. *Paediatr Respir Rev* (2000) 1(4):321–7. doi:10.1053/prrv.2000.0071

14. Flamme I, Risau W. Induction of vasculogenesis and hematopoiesis in vitro. *Development* (1992) 116(2):435–9.

15. Risau W. Mechanisms of angiogenesis. *Nature* (1997) 386(6626):671–4. doi:10.1038/386671a0

16. deMello DE, Sawyer D, Galvin N, Reid LM. Early fetal development of lung vasculature. *Am J Respir Cell Mol Biol* (1997) 16(5):568–81. doi:10.1165/ajrcmb.16.5.9160839

17. Schachtner SK, Wang Y, Scott Baldwin H. Qualitative and quantitative analysis of embryonic pulmonary vessel formation. *Am J Respir Cell Mol Biol* (2000) 22(2):157–65. doi:10.1165/ajrcmb.22.2.3766

18. Stenmark KR, Abman SH. Lung vascular development: implications for the pathogenesis of bronchopulmonary dysplasia. *Annu Rev Physiol* (2005) 67:623–61. doi:10.1146/annurev.physiol.67.040403.102229

19. Chambers HM, van Velzen D. Ventilator-related pathology in the extremely immature lung. *Pathology* (1989) 21(2):79–83. doi:10.3109/00313028909059539

20. Hislop AA, Haworth SG. Pulmonary vascular damage and the development of cor pulmonale following hyaline membrane disease. *Pediatr Pulmonol* (1990) 9(3):152–61. doi:10.1002/ppul.1950090306

21. Gorenflo M, Vogel M, Obladen M. Pulmonary vascular changes in bronchopulmonary dysplasia: a clinicopathologic correlation in short- and long-term survivors. *Pediatr Pathol* (1991) 11(6):851–66. doi:10.3109/15513819109065482

22. Margraf LR, Tomashefski JF Jr, Bruce MC, Dahms BB. Morphometric analysis of the lung in bronchopulmonary dysplasia. *Am Rev Respir Dis* (1991) 143(2):391–400. doi:10.1164/ajrccm/143.2.391

23. Husain AN, Siddiqui NH, Stocker JT. Pathology of arrested acinar development in postsurfactant bronchopulmonary dysplasia. *Hum Pathol* (1998) 29(7):710–7. doi:10.1016/S0046-8177(98)90280-5

24. O'Brodovich HM, Mellins RB. Bronchopulmonary dysplasia. Unresolved neonatal acute lung injury. *Am Rev Respir Dis* (1985) 132(3):694–709.

25. Coalson JJ. *Chronic Lung Disease in Early Infancy*. New York: Marcel Dekker (2000).

26. Bush A, Busst CM, Knight WB, Hislop AA, Haworth SG, Shinebourne EA. Changes in pulmonary circulation in severe bronchopulmonary dysplasia. *Arch Dis Child* (1990) 65(7):739–45. doi:10.1136/adc.65.7.739

27. De Paepe ME, Mao Q, Powell J, Rubin SE, DeKoninck P, Appel N, et al. Growth of pulmonary microvasculature in ventilated preterm infants. *Am J Respir Crit Care Med* (2006) 173(2):204–11. doi:10.1164/rccm.200506-927OC

28. Fouron JC, Le Guennec JC, Villemant D, Perreault G, Davignon A. Value of echocardiography in assessing the outcome of bronchopulmonary dysplasia of the newborn. *Pediatrics* (1980) 65(3):529–35.

29. Berman W Jr, Katz R, Yabek SM, Dillon T, Fripp RR, Papile LA. Long-term follow-up of bronchopulmonary dysplasia. *J Pediatr* (1986) 109(1):45–50. doi:10.1016/S0022-3476(86)80570-4

30. Slaughter JL, Pakrashi T, Jones DE, South AP, Shah TA. Echocardiographic detection of pulmonary hypertension in extremely low birth weight infants with bronchopulmonary dysplasia requiring prolonged positive pressure ventilation. *J Perinatol* (2011) 31(10):635–40. doi:10.1038/jp.2010.213

31. Mourani PM, Sontag MK, Younoszai A, Miller JI, Kinsella JP, Baker CD, et al. Early pulmonary vascular disease in preterm infants at risk for bronchopulmonary dysplasia. *Am J Respir Crit Care Med* (2015) 191(1):87–95. doi:10.1164/rccm.201409-1594OC

32. Kim DH, Kim HS, Choi CW, Kim EK, Kim BI, Choi JH. Risk factors for pulmonary artery hypertension in preterm infants with moderate or severe bronchopulmonary dysplasia. *Neonatology* (2012) 101(1):40–6. doi:10.1159/000327891

33. Khemani E, McElhinney DB, Rhein L, Andrade O, Lacro RV, Thomas KC, et al. Pulmonary artery hypertension in formerly premature infants with bronchopulmonary dysplasia: clinical features and outcomes in the surfactant era. *Pediatrics* (2007) 120(6):1260–9. doi:10.1542/peds.2007-0971

34. Kumar VH, Hutchison AA, Lakshminrusimha S, Morin FC III, Wynn RJ, Ryan RM. Characteristics of pulmonary hypertension in preterm neonates. *J Perinatol* (2007) 27(4):214–9. doi:10.1038/sj.jp.7211673

35. Mirza H, Ziegler J, Ford S, Padbury J, Tucker R, Laptook A. Pulmonary hypertension in preterm infants: prevalence and association with bronchopulmonary dysplasia. *J Pediatr* (2014) 165(5):909.e–14.e. doi:10.1016/j.jpeds.2014.07.040

36. Tomashefski JF Jr, Oppermann HC, Vawter GF, Reid LM. Bronchopulmonary dysplasia: a morphometric study with emphasis on the pulmonary vasculature. *Pediatr Pathol* (1984) 2(4):469–87. doi:10.3109/15513818409025895

37. Thibeault DW, Truog WE, Ekekezie II. Acinar arterial changes with chronic lung disease of prematurity in the surfactant era. *Pediatr Pulmonol* (2003) 36(6):482–9. doi:10.1002/ppul.10349

38. Parker TA, Abman SH. The pulmonary circulation in bronchopulmonary dysplasia. *Semin Neonatol* (2003) 8(1):51–61. doi:10.1016/S1084-2756(02)00191-4

39. Abman SH, Wolfe RR, Accurso FJ, Koops BL, Bowman CM, Wiggins JW Jr. Pulmonary vascular response to oxygen in infants with severe bronchopulmonary dysplasia. *Pediatrics* (1985) 75(1):80–4.

40. Goodman G, Perkin RM, Anas NG, Sperling DR, Hicks DA, Rowen M. Pulmonary hypertension in infants with bronchopulmonary dysplasia. *J Pediatr* (1988) 112(1):67–72. doi:10.1016/S0022-3476(88)80125-2

41. Mourani PM, Ivy DD, Gao D, Abman SH. Pulmonary vascular effects of inhaled nitric oxide and oxygen tension in bronchopulmonary dysplasia. *Am J Respir Crit Care Med* (2004) 170(9):1006–13. doi:10.1164/rccm.200310-1483OC

42. Ascher DP, Rosen P, Null DM, de Lemos RA, Wheller JJ. Systemic to pulmonary collaterals mimicking patent ductus arteriosus in neonates with prolonged ventilatory courses. *J Pediatr* (1985) 107(2):282–4. doi:10.1016/S0022-3476(85)80150-5

43. Covert RF, Drummond WH, Gessner IH. Collateral vessels complicating bronchopulmonary dysplasia. *J Pediatr* (1988) 113(3):617–8. doi:10.1016/S0022-3476(88)80672-3

44. Galambos C, Sims-Lucas S, Abman SH. Histologic evidence of intrapulmonary anastomoses by three-dimensional reconstruction in severe bronchopulmonary dysplasia. *Ann Am Thorac Soc* (2013) 10(5):474–81. doi:10.1513/AnnalsATS.201305-124OC

45. Acker SN, Mandell EW, Sims-Lucas S, Gien J, Abman SH, Galambos C. Histologic identification of prominent intrapulmonary anastomotic vessels in severe congenital diaphragmatic hernia. *J Pediatr* (2015) 166(1):178–83. doi:10.1016/j.jpeds.2014.09.010

46. Ali N, Abman SH, Galambos C. Histologic evidence of intrapulmonary bronchopulmonary anastomotic pathways in neonates with meconium aspiration syndrome. *J Pediatr* (2015) 167:1445–7. doi:10.1016/j.jpeds.2015.08.049

47. Ng YS, Rohan R, Sunday ME, Demello DE, D'Amore PA. Differential expression of VEGF isoforms in mouse during development and in the adult. *Dev Dyn* (2001) 220(2):112–21. doi:10.1002/1097-0177(2000)9999:9999<::AID-DVDY1093>3.0.CO;2-D

48. Hara A, Chapin CJ, Ertsey R, Kitterman JA. Changes in fetal lung distension alter expression of vascular endothelial growth factor and its isoforms in developing rat lung. *Pediatr Res* (2005) 58(1):30–7. doi:10.1203/01.PDR.0000163614.20031.C5

49. Kaipainen A, Korhonen J, Pajusola K, Aprelikova O, Persico MG, Terman BI, et al. The related FLT4, FLT1, and KDR receptor tyrosine kinases show distinct expression patterns in human fetal endothelial cells. *J Exp Med* (1993) 178(6):2077–88. doi:10.1084/jem.178.6.2077

50. Kendall RL, Thomas KA. Inhibition of vascular endothelial cell growth factor activity by an endogenously encoded soluble receptor. *Proc Natl Acad Sci U S A* (1993) 90(22):10705–9. doi:10.1073/pnas.90.22.10705

51. Roda JM, Sumner LA, Evans R, Phillips GS, Marsh CB, Eubank TD. Hypoxia-inducible factor-2alpha regulates GM-CSF-derived soluble vascular

endothelial growth factor receptor 1 production from macrophages and inhibits tumor growth and angiogenesis. *J Immunol* (2011) **187**(4):1970–6. doi:10.4049/jimmunol.1100841

52. Kendall RL, Wang G, Thomas KA. Identification of a natural soluble form of the vascular endothelial growth factor receptor, FLT-1, and its heterodimerization with KDR. *Biochem Biophys Res Commun* (1996) **226**(2):324–8. doi:10.1006/bbrc.1996.1355

53. Shalaby F, Rossant J, Yamaguchi TP, Gertsenstein M, Wu XF, Breitman ML, et al. Failure of blood-island formation and vasculogenesis in Flk-1-deficient mice. *Nature* (1995) **376**(6535):62–6. doi:10.1038/376062a0

54. Fong GH, Rossant J, Gertsenstein M, Breitman ML. Role of the Flt-1 receptor tyrosine kinase in regulating the assembly of vascular endothelium. *Nature* (1995) **376**(6535):66–70. doi:10.1038/376066a0

55. Carmeliet P, Ferreira V, Breier G, Pollefeyt S, Kieckens L, Gertsenstein M, et al. Abnormal blood vessel development and lethality in embryos lacking a single VEGF allele. *Nature* (1996) **380**(6573):435–9. doi:10.1038/380435a0

56. Ferrara N, Carver-Moore K, Chen H, Dowd M, Lu L, O'Shea KS, et al. Heterozygous embryonic lethality induced by targeted inactivation of the VEGF gene. *Nature* (1996) **380**(6573):439–42. doi:10.1038/380439a0

57. Galambos C, Ng YS, Ali A, Noguchi A, Lovejoy S, D'Amore PA, et al. Defective pulmonary development in the absence of heparin-binding vascular endothelial growth factor isoforms. *Am J Respir Cell Mol Biol* (2002) **27**(2):194–203. doi:10.1165/ajrcmb.27.2.4703

58. Gerber HP, Hillan KJ, Ryan AM, Kowalski J, Keller GA, Rangell L, et al. VEGF is required for growth and survival in neonatal mice. *Development* (1999) **126**(6):1149–59.

59. Zeng X, Wert SE, Federici R, Peters KG, Whitsett JA. VEGF enhances pulmonary vasculogenesis and disrupts lung morphogenesis in vivo. *Dev Dyn* (1998) **211**(3):215–27. doi:10.1002/(SICI)1097-0177(199803)211:3<215::AID-AJA3>3.0.CO;2-K

60. Maniscalco WM, Watkins RH, D'Angio CT, Ryan RM. Hyperoxic injury decreases alveolar epithelial cell expression of vascular endothelial growth factor (VEGF) in neonatal rabbit lung. *Am J Respir Cell Mol Biol* (1997) **16**(5):557–67. doi:10.1165/ajrcmb.16.5.9160838

61. Perkett EA, Klekamp JG. Vascular endothelial growth factor expression is decreased in rat lung following exposure to 24 or 48 hours of hyperoxia: implications for endothelial cell survival. *Chest* (1998) **114**(1 Suppl):52S–3S. doi:10.1378/chest.114.1_Supplement.52S

62. Hosford GE, Olson DM. Effects of hyperoxia on VEGF, its receptors, and HIF-2alpha in the newborn rat lung. *Am J Physiol Lung Cell Mol Physiol* (2003) **285**(1):L161–8. doi:10.1152/ajplung.00285.2002

63. Maniscalco WM, Watkins RH, Pryhuber GS, Bhatt A, Shea C, Huyck H. Angiogenic factors and alveolar vasculature: development and alterations by injury in very premature baboons. *Am J Physiol Lung Cell Mol Physiol* (2002) **282**(4):L811–23. doi:10.1152/ajplung.00325.2001

64. Bland RD, Mokres LM, Ertsey R, Jacobson BE, Jiang S, Rabinovitch M, et al. Mechanical ventilation with 40% oxygen reduces pulmonary expression of genes that regulate lung development and impairs alveolar septation in newborn mice. *Am J Physiol Lung Cell Mol Physiol* (2007) **293**(5):L1099–110. doi:10.1152/ajplung.00217.2007

65. Iosef C, Alastalo TP, Hou Y, Chen C, Adams ES, Lyu SC, et al. Inhibiting NF-kappaB in the developing lung disrupts angiogenesis and alveolarization. *Am J Physiol Lung Cell Mol Physiol* (2012) **302**(10):L1023–36. doi:10.1152/ajplung.00230.2011

66. Hou Y, Liu M, Husted C, Chen C, Thiagarajan K, Johns JL, et al. Activation of the nuclear factor-kappaB pathway during postnatal lung inflammation preserves alveolarization by suppressing macrophage inflammatory protein-2. *Am J Physiol Lung Cell Mol Physiol* (2015) **309**(6):L593–604. doi:10.1152/ajplung.00029.2015

67. Thebaud B, Ladha F, Michelakis ED, Sawicka M, Thurston G, Eaton F, et al. Vascular endothelial growth factor gene therapy increases survival, promotes lung angiogenesis, and prevents alveolar damage in hyperoxia-induced lung injury: evidence that angiogenesis participates in alveolarization. *Circulation* (2005) **112**(16):2477–86. doi:10.1161/CIRCULATIONAHA.105.541524

68. Groenman F, Rutter M, Caniggia I, Tibboel D, Post M. Hypoxia-inducible factors in the first trimester human lung. *J Histochem Cytochem* (2007) **55**(4):355–63. doi:10.1369/jhc.6A7129.2006

69. Asikainen TM, Ahmad A, Schneider BK, White CW. Effect of preterm birth on hypoxia-inducible factors and vascular endothelial growth factor in primate lungs. *Pediatr Pulmonol* (2005) **40**(6):538–46. doi:10.1002/ppul.20321

70. Ema M, Taya S, Yokotani N, Sogawa K, Matsuda Y, Fujii-Kuriyama Y. A novel bHLH-PAS factor with close sequence similarity to hypoxia-inducible factor 1alpha regulates the VEGF expression and is potentially involved in lung and vascular development. *Proc Natl Acad Sci U S A* (1997) **94**(9):4273–8. doi:10.1073/pnas.94.9.4273

71. Iyer NV, Kotch LE, Agani F, Leung SW, Laughner E, Wenger RH, et al. Cellular and developmental control of O_2 homeostasis by hypoxia-inducible factor 1 alpha. *Genes Dev* (1998) **12**(2):149–62. doi:10.1101/gad.12.2.149

72. Kotch LE, Iyer NV, Laughner E, Semenza GL. Defective vascularization of HIF-1alpha-null embryos is not associated with VEGF deficiency but with mesenchymal cell death. *Dev Biol* (1999) **209**(2):254–67. doi:10.1006/dbio.1999.9253

73. Compernolle V, Brusselmans K, Acker T, Hoet P, Tjwa M, Beck H, et al. Loss of HIF-2alpha and inhibition of VEGF impair fetal lung maturation, whereas treatment with VEGF prevents fatal respiratory distress in premature mice. *Nat Med* (2002) **8**(7):702–10. doi:10.1038/nm1102-1329b

74. Maltepe E, Schmidt JV, Baunoch D, Bradfield CA, Simon MC. Abnormal angiogenesis and responses to glucose and oxygen deprivation in mice lacking the protein ARNT. *Nature* (1997) **386**(6623):403–7. doi:10.1038/386403a0

75. Grover TR, Asikainen TM, Kinsella JP, Abman SH, White CW. Hypoxia-inducible factors HIF-1alpha and HIF-2alpha are decreased in an experimental model of severe respiratory distress syndrome in preterm lambs. *Am J Physiol Lung Cell Mol Physiol* (2007) **292**(6):L1345–51. doi:10.1152/ajplung.00372.2006

76. Truog WE, Xu D, Ekekezie II, Mabry S, Rezaiekhaligh M, Svojanovsky S, et al. Chronic hypoxia and rat lung development: analysis by morphometry and directed microarray. *Pediatr Res* (2008) **64**(1):56–62. doi:10.1203/PDR.0b013e31817289f2

77. Asikainen TM, Schneider BK, Waleh NS, Clyman RI, Ho WB, Flippin LA, et al. Activation of hypoxia-inducible factors in hyperoxia through prolyl 4-hydroxylase blockade in cells and explants of primate lung. *Proc Natl Acad Sci U S A* (2005) **102**(29):10212–7. doi:10.1073/pnas.0504520102

78. Asikainen TM, Waleh NS, Schneider BK, Clyman RI, White CW. Enhancement of angiogenic effectors through hypoxia-inducible factor in preterm primate lung in vivo. *Am J Physiol Lung Cell Mol Physiol* (2006) **291**(4):L588–95. doi:10.1152/ajplung.00098.2006

79. Asikainen TM, Chang LY, Coalson JJ, Schneider BK, Waleh NS, Ikegami M, et al. Improved lung growth and function through hypoxia-inducible factor in primate chronic lung disease of prematurity. *FASEB J* (2006) **20**(10):1698–700. doi:10.1096/fj.06-5887fje

80. Choi CW, Lee J, Lee HJ, Park HS, Chun YS, Kim BI. Deferoxamine improves alveolar and pulmonary vascular development by upregulating hypoxia-inducible factor-1alpha in a rat model of bronchopulmonary dysplasia. *J Korean Med Sci* (2015) **30**(9):1295–301. doi:10.3346/jkms.2015.30.9.1295

81. Park HS, Park JW, Kim HJ, Choi CW, Lee HJ, Kim BI, et al. Sildenafil alleviates bronchopulmonary dysplasia in neonatal rats by activating the hypoxia-inducible factor signaling pathway. *Am J Respir Cell Mol Biol* (2013) **48**(1):105–13. doi:10.1165/rcmb.2012-0043OC

82. Sessa WC. Molecular control of blood flow and angiogenesis: role of nitric oxide. *J Thromb Haemost* (2009) **7**(Suppl 1):35–7. doi:10.1111/j.1538-7836.2009.03424.x

83. Mitchell JA, Ali F, Bailey L, Moreno L, Harrington LS. Role of nitric oxide and prostacyclin as vasoactive hormones released by the endothelium. *Exp Physiol* (2008) **93**(1):141–7. doi:10.1113/expphysiol.2007.038588

84. Sase K, Michel T. Expression and regulation of endothelial nitric oxide synthase. *Trends Cardiovasc Med* (1997) **7**(1):28–37. doi:10.1016/S1050-1738(96)00121-1

85. Arnal JF, Dinh-Xuan AT, Pueyo M, Darblade B, Rami J. Endothelium-derived nitric oxide and vascular physiology and pathology. *Cell Mol Life Sci* (1999) **55**(8–9):1078–87. doi:10.1007/s000180050358

86. Kroll J, Waltenberger J. VEGF-A induces expression of eNOS and iNOS in endothelial cells via VEGF receptor-2 (KDR). *Biochem Biophys Res Commun* (1998) **252**(3):743–6. doi:10.1006/bbrc.1998.9719

87. Shen BQ, Lee DY, Zioncheck TF. Vascular endothelial growth factor governs endothelial nitric-oxide synthase expression via a KDR/Flk-1 receptor and a

88. protein kinase C signaling pathway. *J Biol Chem* (1999) **274**(46):33057–63. doi:10.1074/jbc.274.46.33057

88. Fukumura D, Gohongi T, Kadambi A, Izumi Y, Ang J, Yun CO, et al. Predominant role of endothelial nitric oxide synthase in vascular endothelial growth factor-induced angiogenesis and vascular permeability. *Proc Natl Acad Sci U S A* (2001) **98**(5):2604–9. doi:10.1073/pnas.041359198

89. Ziche M, Morbidelli L, Choudhuri R, Zhang HT, Donnini S, Granger HJ, et al. Nitric oxide synthase lies downstream from vascular endothelial growth factor-induced but not basic fibroblast growth factor-induced angiogenesis. *J Clin Invest* (1997) **99**(11):2625–34. doi:10.1172/JCI119451

90. Murohara T, Asahara T, Silver M, Bauters C, Masuda H, Kalka C, et al. Nitric oxide synthase modulates angiogenesis in response to tissue ischemia. *J Clin Invest* (1998) **101**(11):2567–78. doi:10.1172/JCI1560

91. Lee PC, Salyapongse AN, Bragdon GA, Shears LL II, Watkins SC, Edington HD, et al. Impaired wound healing and angiogenesis in eNOS-deficient mice. *Am J Physiol* (1999) **277**(4 Pt 2):H1600–8.

92. Liao JK, Zulueta JJ, Yu FS, Peng HB, Cote CG, Hassoun PM. Regulation of bovine endothelial constitutive nitric oxide synthase by oxygen. *J Clin Invest* (1995) **96**(6):2661–6. doi:10.1172/JCI118332

93. McQuillan LP, Leung GK, Marsden PA, Kostyk SK, Kourembanas S. Hypoxia inhibits expression of eNOS via transcriptional and posttranscriptional mechanisms. *Am J Physiol* (1994) **267**(5 Pt 2):H1921–7.

94. MacRitchie AN, Albertine KH, Sun J, Lei PS, Jensen SC, Freestone AA, et al. Reduced endothelial nitric oxide synthase in lungs of chronically ventilated preterm lambs. *Am J Physiol Lung Cell Mol Physiol* (2001) **281**(4):L1011–20.

95. Afshar S, Gibson LL, Yuhanna IS, Sherman TS, Kerecman JD, Grubb PH, et al. Pulmonary NO synthase expression is attenuated in a fetal baboon model of chronic lung disease. *Am J Physiol Lung Cell Mol Physiol* (2003) **284**(5):L749–58. doi:10.1152/ajplung.00334.2002

96. Kallapur SG, Bachurski CJ, Le Cras TD, Joshi SN, Ikegami M, Jobe AH. Vascular changes after intra-amniotic endotoxin in preterm lamb lungs. *Am J Physiol Lung Cell Mol Physiol* (2004) **287**(6):L1178–85. doi:10.1152/ajplung.00049.2004

97. Rozance PJ, Seedorf GJ, Brown A, Roe GB, O'Meara MC, Gien J, et al. Intrauterine growth restriction decreases pulmonary alveolar and vessel growth and causes pulmonary artery endothelial cell dysfunction in vitro in fetal sheep. *Am J Physiol Lung Cell Mol Physiol* (2011) **301**:L860–71. doi:10.1152/ajplung.00197.2011

98. Leuwerke SM, Kaza AK, Tribble CG, Kron IL, Laubach VE. Inhibition of compensatory lung growth in endothelial nitric oxide synthase-deficient mice. *Am J Physiol Lung Cell Mol Physiol* (2002) **282**(6):L1272–8. doi:10.1152/ajplung.00490.2001

99. Fagan KA, Fouty BW, Tyler RC, Morris KG Jr, Hepler LK, Sato K, et al. The pulmonary circulation of homozygous or heterozygous eNOS-null mice is hyperresponsive to mild hypoxia. *J Clin Invest* (1999) **103**(2):291–9. doi:10.1172/JCI3862

100. Balasubramaniam V, Tang JR, Maxey A, Plopper CG, Abman SH. Mild hypoxia impairs alveolarization in the endothelial nitric oxide synthase-deficient mouse. *Am J Physiol Lung Cell Mol Physiol* (2003) **284**(6):L964–71. doi:10.1152/ajplung.00421.2002

101. Balasubramaniam V, Maxey AM, Morgan DB, Markham NE, Abman SH. Inhaled NO restores lung structure in eNOS-deficient mice recovering from neonatal hypoxia. *Am J Physiol Lung Cell Mol Physiol* (2006) **291**(1):L119–27. doi:10.1152/ajplung.00395.2005

102. Tang JR, Markham NE, Lin YJ, McMurtry IF, Maxey A, Kinsella JP, et al. Inhaled nitric oxide attenuates pulmonary hypertension and improves lung growth in infant rats after neonatal treatment with a VEGF receptor inhibitor. *Am J Physiol Lung Cell Mol Physiol* (2004) **287**(2):L344–51. doi:10.1152/ajplung.00291.2003

103. Tourneux P, Markham N, Seedorf G, Balasubramaniam V, Abman SH. Inhaled nitric oxide improves lung structure and pulmonary hypertension in a model of bleomycin-induced bronchopulmonary dysplasia in neonatal rats. *Am J Physiol Lung Cell Mol Physiol* (2009) **297**(6):L1103–11. doi:10.1152/ajplung.00293.2009

104. Madurga A, Golec A, Pozarska A, Ishii I, Mizikova I, Nardiello C, et al. The H2S-generating enzymes cystathionine beta-synthase and cystathionine gamma-lyase play a role in vascular development during normal lung alveolarization. *Am J Physiol Lung Cell Mol Physiol* (2015) **309**(7):L710–24. doi:10.1152/ajplung.00134.2015

105. Vadivel A, Alphonse RS, Ionescu L, Machado DS, O'Reilly M, Eaton F, et al. Exogenous hydrogen sulfide (H_2S) protects alveolar growth in experimental O_2-induced neonatal lung injury. *PLoS One* (2014) **9**(3):e90965. doi:10.1371/journal.pone.0090965

106. Madurga A, Mizikova I, Ruiz-Camp J, Vadasz I, Herold S, Mayer K, et al. Systemic hydrogen sulfide administration partially restores normal alveolarization in an experimental animal model of bronchopulmonary dysplasia. *Am J Physiol Lung Cell Mol Physiol* (2014) **306**(7):L684–97. doi:10.1152/ajplung.00361.2013

107. Maden M. Vitamin A and pattern formation in the regenerating limb. *Nature* (1982) **295**(5851):672–5. doi:10.1038/295672a0

108. Massaro GD, Massaro D. Retinoic acid treatment abrogates elastase-induced pulmonary emphysema in rats. *Nat Med* (1997) **3**(6):675–7. doi:10.1038/nm0697-675

109. Massaro GD, Massaro D. Retinoic acid treatment partially rescues failed septation in rats and in mice. *Am J Physiol Lung Cell Mol Physiol* (2000) **278**(5):L955–60.

110. McGowan S, Jackson SK, Jenkins-Moore M, Dai HH, Chambon P, Snyder JM. Mice bearing deletions of retinoic acid receptors demonstrate reduced lung elastin and alveolar numbers. *Am J Respir Cell Mol Biol* (2000) **23**(2):162–7. doi:10.1165/ajrcmb.23.2.3904

111. Yun EJ, Lorizio W, Seedorf G, Abman SH, Vu TH. VEGF and endothelium-derived retinoic acid regulate lung vascular and alveolar development. *Am J Physiol Lung Cell Mol Physiol* (2016) **310**(4):L287–98. doi:10.1152/ajplung.00229.2015

112. Choi JW, Herr DR, Noguchi K, Yung YC, Lee CW, Mutoh T, et al. LPA receptors: subtypes and biological actions. *Annu Rev Pharmacol Toxicol* (2010) **50**:157–86. doi:10.1146/annurev.pharmtox.010909.105753

113. Toews ML, Ediger TL, Romberger DJ, Rennard SI. Lysophosphatidic acid in airway function and disease. *Biochim Biophys Acta* (2002) **1582**(1–3):240–50. doi:10.1016/S1388-1981(02)00177-4

114. Tager AM, LaCamera P, Shea BS, Campanella GS, Selman M, Zhao Z, et al. The lysophosphatidic acid receptor LPA1 links pulmonary fibrosis to lung injury by mediating fibroblast recruitment and vascular leak. *Nat Med* (2008) **14**(1):45–54. doi:10.1038/nm1685

115. Zhao J, He D, Su Y, Berdyshev E, Chun J, Natarajan V, et al. Lysophosphatidic acid receptor 1 modulates lipopolysaccharide-induced inflammation in alveolar epithelial cells and murine lungs. *Am J Physiol Lung Cell Mol Physiol* (2011) **301**(4):L547–56. doi:10.1152/ajplung.00058.2011

116. Chen X, Walther FJ, van Boxtel R, Laghmani EH, Sengers RM, Folkerts G, et al. Deficiency or inhibition of lysophosphatidic acid receptor 1 protects against hyperoxia-induced lung injury in neonatal rats. *Acta Physiol (Oxf)* (2016) **216**(3):358–75. doi:10.1111/apha.12622

117. Nozik-Grayck E, Suliman HB, Piantadosi CA. Extracellular superoxide dismutase. *Int J Biochem Cell Biol* (2005) **37**(12):2466–71. doi:10.1016/j.biocel.2005.06.012

118. Delaney C, Wright RH, Tang JR, Woods C, Villegas L, Sherlock L, et al. Lack of EC-SOD worsens alveolar and vascular development in a neonatal mouse model of bleomycin-induced bronchopulmonary dysplasia and pulmonary hypertension. *Pediatr Res* (2015) **78**(6):634–40. doi:10.1038/pr.2015.166

119. Ahmed MN, Suliman HB, Folz RJ, Nozik-Grayck E, Golson ML, Mason SN, et al. Extracellular superoxide dismutase protects lung development in hyperoxia-exposed newborn mice. *Am J Respir Crit Care Med* (2003) **167**(3):400–5. doi:10.1164/rccm.200202-108OC

120. Nozik-Grayck E, Suliman HB, Majka S, Albietz J, Van Rheen Z, Roush K, et al. Lung EC-SOD overexpression attenuates hypoxic induction of Egr-1 and chronic hypoxic pulmonary vascular remodeling. *Am J Physiol Lung Cell Mol Physiol* (2008) **295**(3):L422–30. doi:10.1152/ajplung.90293.2008

121. Collins JJ, Thebaud B. Progenitor cells of the distal lung and their potential role in neonatal lung disease. *Birth Defects Res A Clin Mol Teratol* (2014) **100**(3):217–26. doi:10.1002/bdra.23227

122. Pierro M, Thebaud B. Mesenchymal stem cells in chronic lung disease: culprit or savior? *Am J Physiol Lung Cell Mol Physiol* (2010) **298**(6):L732–4. doi:10.1152/ajplung.00099.2010

123. Hogan BL, Barkauskas CE, Chapman HA, Epstein JA, Jain R, Hsia CC, et al. Repair and regeneration of the respiratory system: complexity, plasticity, and mechanisms of lung stem cell function. *Cell Stem Cell* (2014) **15**(2):123–38. doi:10.1016/j.stem.2014.07.012

124. Balasubramaniam V, Mervis CF, Maxey AM, Markham NE, Abman SH. Hyperoxia reduces bone marrow, circulating, and lung endothelial progenitor cells in the developing lung: implications for the pathogenesis of bronchopulmonary dysplasia. *Am J Physiol Lung Cell Mol Physiol* (2007) **292**(5):L1073–84. doi:10.1152/ajplung.00347.2006

125. Irwin D, Helm K, Campbell N, Imamura M, Fagan K, Harral J, et al. Neonatal lung side population cells demonstrate endothelial potential and are altered in response to hyperoxia-induced lung simplification. *Am J Physiol Lung Cell Mol Physiol* (2007) **293**(4):L941–51. doi:10.1152/ajplung.00054.2007

126. Chang YS, Oh W, Choi SJ, Sung DK, Kim SY, Choi EY, et al. Human umbilical cord blood-derived mesenchymal stem cells attenuate hyperoxia-induced lung injury in neonatal rats. *Cell Transplant* (2009) **18**(8):869–86. doi:10.3727/096368909X471189

127. Aslam M, Baveja R, Liang OD, Fernandez-Gonzalez A, Lee C, Mitsialis SA, et al. Bone marrow stromal cells attenuate lung injury in a murine model of neonatal chronic lung disease. *Am J Respir Crit Care Med* (2009) **180**(11):1122–30. doi:10.1164/rccm.200902-0242OC

128. van Haaften T, Byrne R, Bonnet S, Rochefort GY, Akabutu J, Bouchentouf M, et al. Airway delivery of mesenchymal stem cells prevents arrested alveolar growth in neonatal lung injury in rats. *Am J Respir Crit Care Med* (2009) **180**(11):1131–42. doi:10.1164/rccm.200902-0179OC

129. Pierro M, Ionescu L, Montemurro T, Vadivel A, Weissmann G, Oudit G, et al. Short-term, long-term and paracrine effect of human umbilical cord-derived stem cells in lung injury prevention and repair in experimental bronchopulmonary dysplasia. *Thorax* (2013) **68**(5):475–84. doi:10.1136/thoraxjnl-2012-202323

130. De Paepe ME, Patel C, Tsai A, Gundavarapu S, Mao Q. Endoglin (CD105) up-regulation in pulmonary microvasculature of ventilated preterm infants. *Am J Respir Crit Care Med* (2008) **178**(2):180–7. doi:10.1164/rccm.200608-1240OC

131. De Paepe ME, Greco D, Mao Q. Angiogenesis-related gene expression profiling in ventilated preterm human lungs. *Exp Lung Res* (2010) **36**(7):399–410. doi:10.3109/01902141003714031

132. Lassus P, Turanlahti M, Heikkila P, Andersson LC, Nupponen I, Sarnesto A, et al. Pulmonary vascular endothelial growth factor and Flt-1 in fetuses, in acute and chronic lung disease, and in persistent pulmonary hypertension of the newborn. *Am J Respir Crit Care Med* (2001) **164**(10 Pt 1):1981–7. doi:10.1164/ajrccm.164.10.2012036

133. Ambalavanan N, Novak ZE. Peptide growth factors in tracheal aspirates of mechanically ventilated preterm neonates. *Pediatr Res* (2003) **53**(2):240–4. doi:10.1203/00006450-200302000-00007

134. Trittmann JK, Peterson E, Rogers LK, Chen B, Backes CH, Klebanoff MA, et al. Plasma asymmetric dimethylarginine levels are increased in neonates with bronchopulmonary dysplasia-associated pulmonary hypertension. *J Pediatr* (2015) **166**(2):230–3. doi:10.1016/j.jpeds.2014.09.004

135. Mercier JC, Hummler H, Durrmeyer X, Sanchez-Luna M, Carnielli V, Field D, et al. Inhaled nitric oxide for prevention of bronchopulmonary dysplasia in premature babies (EUNO): a randomised controlled trial. *Lancet* (2010) **376**(9738):346–54. doi:10.1016/S0140-6736(10)60664-2

136. Cole FS, Alleyne C, Barks JD, Boyle RJ, Carroll JL, Dokken D, et al. NIH Consensus Development Conference statement: inhaled nitric-oxide therapy for premature infants. *Pediatrics* (2011) **127**(2):363–9. doi:10.1542/peds.2010-3507

137. Kinsella JP, Cutter GR, Steinhorn RH, Nelin LD, Walsh WF, Finer NN, et al. Noninvasive inhaled nitric oxide does not prevent bronchopulmonary dysplasia in premature newborns. *J Pediatr* (2014) **165**(6):1104.e–8.e. doi:10.1016/j.jpeds.2014.06.018

138. Yoder MC, Mead LE, Prater D, Krier TR, Mroueh KN, Li F, et al. Redefining endothelial progenitor cells via clonal analysis and hematopoietic stem/progenitor cell principals. *Blood* (2007) **109**(5):1801–9. doi:10.1182/blood-2006-08-043471

139. Baker CD, Ryan SL, Ingram DA, Seedorf GJ, Abman SH, Balasubramaniam V. Endothelial colony-forming cells from preterm infants are increased and more susceptible to hyperoxia. *Am J Respir Crit Care Med* (2009) **180**(5):454–61. doi:10.1164/rccm.200901-0115OC

140. Borghesi A, Massa M, Campanelli R, Bollani L, Tzialla C, Figar TA, et al. Circulating endothelial progenitor cells in preterm infants with bronchopulmonary dysplasia. *Am J Respir Crit Care Med* (2009) **180**(6):540–6. doi:10.1164/rccm.200812-1949OC

141. Baker CD, Balasubramaniam V, Mourani PM, Sontag MK, Black CP, Ryan SL, et al. Cord blood angiogenic progenitor cells are decreased in bronchopulmonary dysplasia. *Eur Respir J* (2012) **40**(6):1516–22. doi:10.1183/09031936.00017312

142. Popova AP, Bozyk PD, Bentley JK, Linn MJ, Goldsmith AM, Schumacher RE, et al. Isolation of tracheal aspirate mesenchymal stromal cells predicts bronchopulmonary dysplasia. *Pediatrics* (2010) **126**(5):e1127–33. doi:10.1542/peds.2009-3445

143. Chang YS, Ahn SY, Yoo HS, Sung SI, Choi SJ, Oh WI, et al. Mesenchymal stem cells for bronchopulmonary dysplasia: phase 1 dose-escalation clinical trial. *J Pediatr* (2014) **164**(5):966.e–72.e. doi:10.1016/j.jpeds.2013.12.011

144. Hilgendorff A, Reiss I, Ehrhardt H, Eickelberg O, Alvira CM. Chronic lung disease in the preterm infant. Lessons learned from animal models. *Am J Respir Cell Mol Biol* (2014) **50**(2):233–45. doi:10.1165/rcmb.2013-0014TR

Permissions

All chapters in this book were first published by Frontiers; hereby published with permission under the Creative Commons Attribution License or equivalent. Every chapter published in this book has been scrutinized by our experts. Their significance has been extensively debated. The topics covered herein carry significant findings which will fuel the growth of the discipline. They may even be implemented as practical applications or may be referred to as a beginning point for another development.

The contributors of this book come from diverse backgrounds, making this book a truly international effort. This book will bring forth new frontiers with its revolutionizing research information and detailed analysis of the nascent developments around the world.

We would like to thank all the contributing authors for lending their expertise to make the book truly unique. They have played a crucial role in the development of this book. Without their invaluable contributions this book wouldn't have been possible. They have made vital efforts to compile up to date information on the varied aspects of this subject to make this book a valuable addition to the collection of many professionals and students.

This book was conceptualized with the vision of imparting up-to-date information and advanced data in this field. To ensure the same, a matchless editorial board was set up. Every individual on the board went through rigorous rounds of assessment to prove their worth. After which they invested a large part of their time researching and compiling the most relevant data for our readers.

The editorial board has been involved in producing this book since its inception. They have spent rigorous hours researching and exploring the diverse topics which have resulted in the successful publishing of this book. They have passed on their knowledge of decades through this book. To expedite this challenging task, the publisher supported the team at every step. A small team of assistant editors was also appointed to further simplify the editing procedure and attain best results for the readers.

Apart from the editorial board, the designing team has also invested a significant amount of their time in understanding the subject and creating the most relevant covers. They scrutinized every image to scout for the most suitable representation of the subject and create an appropriate cover for the book.

The publishing team has been an ardent support to the editorial, designing and production team. Their endless efforts to recruit the best for this project, has resulted in the accomplishment of this book. They are a veteran in the field of academics and their pool of knowledge is as vast as their experience in printing. Their expertise and guidance has proved useful at every step. Their uncompromising quality standards have made this book an exceptional effort. Their encouragement from time to time has been an inspiration for everyone.

The publisher and the editorial board hope that this book will prove to be a valuable piece of knowledge for researchers, students, practitioners and scholars across the globe.

List of Contributors

Celien Kuiper-Makris and Jaco Selle
Department of Pediatric and Adolescent Medicine, Translational Experimental Pediatrics — Experimental Pulmonology, Faculty of Medicine and University Hospital Cologne, University of Cologne, Cologne, Germany

Eva Nüsken and Jörg Dötsch
Department of Pediatric and Adolescent Medicine, Faculty of Medicine and University Hospital Cologne, University of Cologne, Cologne, Germany

Miguel A. Alejandre Alcazar
Department of Pediatric and Adolescent Medicine, Translational Experimental Pediatrics — Experimental Pulmonology, Faculty of Medicine and University Hospital Cologne, University of Cologne, Cologne, Germany
Center for Molecular Medicine Cologne (CMMC), Faculty of Medicine and University Hospital Cologne, University of Cologne, Cologne, Germany
Excellence Cluster on Stress Responses in Aging-associated Diseases (CECAD), Faculty of Medicine and University Hospital Cologne, University of Cologne, Cologne, Germany
Member of the German Centre for Lung Research (DZL), Institute for Lung Health, University of Giessen and Marburg Lung Centre (UGMLC), Gießen, Germany

Daphne S. Mous, Rene M. H. Wijnen and Dick Tibboel
Department of Pediatric Surgery, Erasmus Medical Center – Sophia Children's Hospital, Rotterdam, Netherlands

Marjon J. Buscop-van Kempen and Robbert J. Rottier
Department of Pediatric Surgery, Erasmus Medical Center – Sophia Children's Hospital, Rotterdam, Netherlands
Department of Cell Biology, Erasmus Medical Center, Rotterdam, Netherlands

Rory E. Morty
Department of Lung Development and Remodelling, Max Planck Institute for Heart and Lung Research, Bad Nauheim, Germany
Department of Internal Medicine (Pulmonology), University of Giessen and Marburg Lung Center (UGMLC), Giessen, Germany

Lakshanie C. Wickramasinghe, Evelyn Tsantikos and Margaret L. Hibbs
Leukocyte Signalling Laboratory, Department of Immunology and Pathology, Central Clinical School, Monash University, Melbourne, VIC, Australia

Peter van Wijngaarden
Department of Surgery - Ophthalmology, University of Melbourne, Melbourne, VIC, Australia
Centre for Eye Research Australia, Royal Victorian Eye and Ear Hospital, East Melbourne, VIC, Australia

Chad Johnson
Monash Micro Imaging, Alfred Research Alliance, Monash University, Melbourne, VIC, Australia

Anne Greenough
Division of Asthma, Allergy and Lung Biology, MRC and Asthma UK Centre in Allergic Mechanisms of Asthma, King's College London, London, UK
NIHR Biomedical Research Centre, Guy's and St. Thomas NHS Foundation Trust, London, UK

Anoop Pahuja
Neonatal Intensive Care Centre, King's College Hospital NHS Foundation Trust, London, UK

Jack O. Kalotas, Carolyn J. Wang and Peter B. Noble
School of Human Sciences, The University of Western Australia, Crawley, WA, Australia

Kimberley C. W. Wang
School of Human Sciences, The University of Western Australia, Crawley, WA, Australia
Telethon Kids Institute, The University of Western Australia, Nedlands, WA, Australia

Marius A. Möbius
Department of Neonatology and Pediatric Critical Care Medicine, Medical Faculty, University Hospital Carl Gustav Carus, Technische Universität Dresden, Dresden, Germany
DFG Research Center and Cluster of Excellence for Regenerative Therapies (CRTD), Technische Universität Dresden, Dresden, Germany
Regenerative Medicine Program, Sprott Centre for Stem Cell Research, Ottawa Hospital Research Institute, University of Ottawa, Ottawa, ON, Canada

Bernard Thébaud
Regenerative Medicine Program, Sprott Centre for Stem Cell Research, Ottawa Hospital Research Institute, University of Ottawa, Ottawa, ON, Canada
Division of Neonatology, Department of Pediatrics, Children's Hospital of Eastern Ontario, University of Ottawa, Ottawa, ON, Canada

List of Contributors

Helene Widowski
Department of Pediatrics, Maastricht University Medical Center, Maastricht, Netherlands
Department of BioMedical Engineering, Maastricht University Medical Center, Maastricht, Netherlands
GROW School for Oncology and Developmental Biology, Maastricht University Medical Center, Maastricht, Netherlands

Niki L. Reynaert
Department of Respiratory Medicine, Maastricht University, Maastricht, Netherlands
NUTRIM School of Nutrition and Translational Research in Metabolism, Maastricht University Medical Center, Maastricht, Netherlands

Daan R. M. G. Ophelders
Department of Pediatrics, Maastricht University Medical Center, Maastricht, Netherlands
GROW School for Oncology and Developmental Biology, Maastricht University Medical Center, Maastricht, Netherlands

Matthias C. Hütten
Neonatology, Pediatrics Department, Faculty of Health, Medicine and Life Sciences, Maastricht University Medical Center, Maastricht, Netherlands
University Children's Hospital Würzburg, University of Würzburg, Würzburg, Germany

Peter G. J. Nikkels
Department of Pathology, University Medical Center Utrecht, Utrecht, Netherlands

Carmen A. H. Severens-Rijvers
Department of Pathology, Maastricht University Medical Center, Maastricht, Netherlands

Jack P. M. Cleutjens
Department of Pathology, Maastricht University Medical Center, Maastricht, Netherlands
CARIM School for Cardiovascular Diseases, Maastricht University Medical Center, Maastricht, Netherlands

Matthew W. Kemp, John P. Newnham and Matthew S. Payne
Division of Obstetrics and Gynecology, The University of Western Australia, Crawley, WA, Australia

Masatoshi Saito and Haruo Usuda
Division of Obstetrics and Gynecology, The University of Western Australia, Crawley, WA, Australia
Tohoku University Centre for Perinatal and Neonatal Medicine, Tohoku University Hospital, Sendai, Japan

Alan H. Jobe
Division of Obstetrics and Gynecology, The University of Western Australia, Crawley, WA, Australia
Perinatal Institute Cincinnati Children's Hospital Medical Center, Cincinnati, OH, United States

Boris W. Kramer
Department of Pediatrics, Maastricht University Medical Center, Maastricht, Netherlands
Perinatal Institute Cincinnati Children's Hospital Medical Center, Cincinnati, OH, United States
School for Mental Health and Neuroscience, Maastricht University, Maastricht, Netherlands

Tammo Delhaas
Department of BioMedical Engineering, Maastricht University Medical Center, Maastricht, Netherlands
CARIM School for Cardiovascular Diseases, Maastricht University Medical Center, Maastricht, Netherlands

Tim G. A. M. Wolfs
Department of Pediatrics, Maastricht University Medical Center, Maastricht, Netherlands
GROW School for Oncology and Developmental Biology, Maastricht University Medical Center, Maastricht, Netherlands

Jennifer J. P. Collins
Department of Pediatric Surgery, Sophia Children's Hospital, Erasmus University Medical Centre, Rotterdam, Netherlands

Ismé M. de Kleer
Division of Pediatric Pulmonology, Department of Pediatrics, Sophia Children's Hospital, Erasmus University Medical Centre, Rotterdam, Netherlands

Irwin K. M. Reiss
Division of Neonatology, Department of Pediatrics, Sophia Children's Hospital, Erasmus University Medical Centre, Rotterdam, Netherlands

Xueyu Chen, Junyan Zhong and Dongshan Han
Laboratory of Neonatology, Department of Neonatology, Affiliated Shenzhen Maternity and Child Healthcare Hospital, Southern Medical University, Shenzhen, China

Fang Yao, Jie Zhao and Chuanzhong Yang
Department of Neonatology, Shenzhen Maternity and Child Healthcare Hospital, The First School of Clinical Medicine, Southern Medical University, Shenzhen, China

Gerry. T. M. Wagenaar
Faculty of Science, VU University Amsterdam, Amsterdam, Netherlands

Frans J. Walther
Department of Pediatrics, David Geffen School of Medicine, University of California, Los Angeles, Los Angeles, CA, United States
The Lundquist Institute for Biomedical Innovation at Harbor-UCLA Medical Center, Torrance, CA, United States

Ivana Mižíková and Rory E. Morty
Department of Lung Development and Remodelling, Max Planck Institute for Heart and Lung Research, Bad Nauheim, Germany
Pulmonology, Department of Internal Medicine, University of Giessen and Marburg Lung Center, Giessen, Germany

Longli Yan, Zhuxiao Ren, Jianlan Wang, Xin Xia, Liling Yang, Jiayu Miao, Fang Xu, Weiwei Gao and Jie Yang
Department of Neonatology, Guangdong Women and Children Hospital, Guangzhou Medical University, Guangzhou, China

Cho-Ming Chao
Department of General Pediatrics and Neonatology, University Children's Hospital Giessen, Giessen, Germany
Department of Internal Medicine II, Universities of Giessen and Marburg Lung Center, Giessen, Germany
Member of the German Center for Lung Research (DZL), Giessen, Germany

Elie El Agha
Department of Internal Medicine II, Universities of Giessen and Marburg Lung Center, Giessen, Germany
Member of the German Center for Lung Research (DZL), Giessen, Germany

Caterina Tiozzo
Division of Neonatology, Department of Pediatrics, Columbia University, New York, NY, USA

Parviz Minoo
Division of Newborn Medicine, Department of Pediatrics, Children's Hospital Los Angeles, University of Southern California, Los Angeles, CA, USA

Saverio Bellusci
Department of Internal Medicine II, Universities of Giessen and Marburg Lung Center, Giessen, Germany
Member of the German Center for Lung Research (DZL), Giessen, Germany

Saban Research Institute, Childrens Hospital Los Angeles, University of Southern California, Los Angeles, CA, USA
Kazan Federal University, Kazan, Russia

Andressa Daronco Cereta and Letícia Lopes Guimarães
School of Veterinary Medicine and Animal Sciences, University of São Paulo, São Paulo, Brazil

Vinícius Rosa Oliveira
Department of Physical Therapy, EUSES University School, University of Barcelona-University of Girona (UB-UdG), Barcelona, Spain
Research Group on Methodology, Methods, Models and Outcomes of Health and Social Sciences (M3O), University of VIC-Central University of Catalonia, Vic, Spain

Ivan Peres Costa
Master's and Doctoral Programs in Rehabilitation Sciences, Nove de Julho University, São Paulo, Brazil

João Pedro Ribeiro Afonso, Adriano Luís Fonseca, Alan Robson Trigueiro de Sousa, Guilherme Augusto Moreira Silva, Diego A. C. P. G. Mello and Luis Vicente Franco de Oliveira
Human Movement and Rehabilitation, Post Graduation Program Medical School, University Center of Anápolis-UniEVANGELICA, Anápolis, Brazil

Renata Kelly da Palma
School of Veterinary Medicine and Animal Sciences, University of São Paulo, São Paulo, Brazil
Department of Physical Therapy, EUSES University School, University of Barcelona-University of Girona (UB-UdG), Barcelona, Spain
Institute for Bioengineering of Catalonia, Barcelona, Spain

Jherna Balany and Vineet Bhandari
Section of Neonatology, Department of Pediatrics, St. Christopher's Hospital for Children, Drexel University College of Medicine, Philadelphia, PA, USA

Sainan Chen, Yuqing Wang, Anrong Li, Wujun Jiang, Min Wu, Zhengrong Chen, Chuangli Hao, Xunjun Shao and Jun Xu
Department of Respiratory Medicine, Children's Hospital of Soochow University, Suzhou, China

Qiuyan Xu
Department of Pediatrics, Affiliated Suzhou Science and Technology Town Hospital of Nanjing Medical University, Suzhou, China

List of Contributors

William Domm and Michael A. O'Reilly
Department of Pediatrics, School of Medicine and Dentistry, The University of Rochester, Rochester, NY, USA
Department of Environmental Medicine, School of Medicine and Dentistry, The University of Rochester, Rochester, NY, USA

Ravi S. Misra
Department of Pediatrics, School of Medicine and Dentistry, The University of Rochester, Rochester, NY, USA

Mandy Laube, Soeren Pietsch, Thomas Pannicke and Ulrich H. Thome
Division of Neonatology, Department of Paediatrics, Center for Paediatric Research Leipzig, University of Leipzig, Leipzig, Germany

Claire Fabian
Department of Vaccines and Infection Models, Fraunhofer Institute for Cell Therapy and Immunology, Leipzig, Germany

Thomas Semple
The Royal Brompton Hospital, London, United Kingdon
Great Ormond Street Hospital, London, United Kingdom

Mohammed R. Akhtar
St Bartholomews and The Royal London Hospital, London, United Kingdom

Catherine M. Owens
Great Ormond Street Hospital, London, United Kingdom

Yuanyuan Dai, Binyuan Yu, Xinye Wang, Ran Huo, Xiaoqin Fu and Shangqin Chen
Department of Neonatology, The Second Affiliated Hospital, Yuying Children's Hospital of Wenzhou Medical University, Zhejiang, China

Danyang Ai and Lin Yuan
Department of Neonatology, The Children's Hospital of Fudan University, Shanghai, China

Chao Chen
Department of Neonatology, The Second Affiliated Hospital, Yuying Children's Hospital of Wenzhou Medical University, Zhejiang, China
Department of Neonatology, The Children's Hospital of Fudan University, Shanghai, China

Cristina M. Alvira
Department of Pediatrics, Division of Critical Care Medicine, Stanford University School of Medicine, Stanford, CA, USA

Index

A
Aeroallergen, 51, 56, 58

Alveolar Regeneration, 91, 97, 110, 144, 148, 228, 230

Alveolarization, 1-2, 6, 11, 13, 18, 23, 29, 34, 37, 41-42, 69-70, 73, 83-84, 87, 89, 97-99, 101, 103-104, 106, 108-110, 113-114, 116-127, 140-146, 148-149, 157-160, 162-165, 201, 223-224, 227-235

Antenatal Steroids, 45, 47, 88, 97, 139-140, 157-158, 206

Aortic Valve, 215

Asthma, 1-2, 4-6, 9-10, 12-16, 18-20, 32, 39, 41, 43, 51-52, 56-59, 64, 69, 86, 92, 94, 107, 132, 150-155, 175, 177, 181, 183-185

B
Bleomycin, 63, 66, 69, 71, 93, 101, 126, 149, 176, 178, 183-184, 230, 235

Blood Flow, 215, 227, 234

Bronchiolitis, 60-61, 166-168, 170-173, 183, 206, 212

Bronchodilators, 43, 47-48, 50

Bronchopulmonary Dysplasia, 1, 18-20, 31-32, 41-43, 47-50, 60-61, 67-70, 72-73, 83-87, 90, 92, 96-104, 110-111, 115, 124-128, 131-132, 134, 136-139, 146, 148-149, 156-157, 162-165, 167, 175, 182, 184-185, 188, 206-208, 211-214, 221-223, 226, 231-236

C
Cell Culture, 88, 177, 187-188, 199, 201, 203

Choroidal Thinning, 31, 35, 39

Chronic Inflammation, 4-6, 8, 11, 31, 39

Chronic Lung Disease, 1, 6, 11, 15, 18, 20, 41-43, 48-50, 64, 68, 84, 86, 93, 97, 99, 101, 103, 124, 127, 139, 146, 148-149, 156, 162, 164-165, 178, 180, 182, 184, 206, 211-212, 214, 221, 223-224, 233-236

Coinfection, 166, 168-173

Computed Tomography, 45, 49, 206-207, 209, 212

Corticosteroids, 37, 43-44, 83, 86, 88, 93, 96-97, 101, 146, 185, 188

Cystic Fibrosis, 10, 20, 94, 123, 130, 196, 209, 212

Cytokines, 4-6, 13, 15, 20, 39, 42, 52, 59, 63, 65-66, 88, 92, 119, 136, 156-162, 178, 180, 184-185

D
Dexamethasone, 48, 50, 88, 93, 117, 125, 148, 163, 189, 195-198, 202, 204, 230

Disease Progression, 36, 129, 166

Diuretics, 43, 47-49

Dysbiosis, 10, 13, 20, 92, 96, 150-151, 153-155

E
Echocardiography, 213-214, 218-220, 233

Elastin, 62, 87, 97, 111-128, 140-144, 148-149, 159, 163-164, 228, 230, 235

Embryonic Development, 3, 145, 228

Endothelial Cell
Endothelial Cell, 17, 60, 96, 135, 145, 149, 189, 225, 227-228, 233-235

Endotoxin, 63, 73, 82-85, 159, 163, 165, 228-230, 235

F
Fatty Acids, 2, 5-6, 10, 16, 92, 154-155

Fetal Development, 145, 149, 187, 201, 229, 233

Fibrosis, 4, 10, 15, 20, 31-32, 34, 36-37, 44-45, 60, 62, 64, 66, 71, 94, 107, 114, 123, 125-127, 129-130, 139-140, 143-144, 148-149, 178-179, 184-185, 196, 206-207, 209, 212, 224, 228, 230, 235

G
Gestation, 9, 17, 19, 21, 23, 29, 32, 44, 72, 74, 82, 97, 102, 132, 134, 139-140, 146, 159, 163, 175, 180, 185, 202, 206-207, 211, 223-224, 232

H
Hyperoxia, 19-20, 31, 34, 36-37, 39, 41-42, 61-63, 65-70, 82, 84, 86, 88-89, 91-94, 96-105, 107-111, 114-124, 126-127, 129, 136, 142, 144-145, 148-149, 156-157, 160-165, 174, 176, 178-182, 184-185, 188, 203, 213-221, 224, 227-232, 234-236

I
Imaging Technique, 209

Inflammasome, 93, 101, 180, 185

Innate Immunity, 157, 174, 178, 181, 184-185

Intrauterine Growth Restriction, 1-3, 6, 10-11, 17-21, 51-54, 56-59, 89, 94, 228, 230, 235

Intubation, 88, 105, 160, 164

L
Leptin, 2, 4-5, 8-9, 11-16, 18-20, 144, 148, 204

Leukocyte Count, 166-168, 171-172

Ligands, 24, 42, 109, 116, 119-120, 141, 143-144, 147, 228

Lung Development, 1-2, 4-8, 12-13, 16-17, 22-23, 30-32, 38, 41-42, 62, 68, 72-73, 78-80, 82-84, 86-92, 94, 96-97, 99-104, 107, 109, 111-114, 116-130, 135, 138-143, 145-149, 156, 159-165, 174-176, 178, 181-182, 184, 187-188, 197, 203, 211, 213-215, 223-230, 232-235

Lung Diseases, 1-4, 10, 12, 20, 34, 61, 73, 88, 93-94, 97, 102, 121, 129, 175, 179, 183-184, 214, 221, 230

Lung Injury, 4-5, 9, 39, 42, 62-71, 80, 84, 86-92, 94, 96-103, 107, 109, 124-127, 129, 137, 139, 142, 144, 148-149, 156, 158-165, 178-180, 183-185, 188, 204, 213-214, 216, 218, 220, 223-224, 231, 233-236

Lung Microbiome, 9-10, 20, 91-92, 150

Lung Pathology, 2, 32, 39, 78, 127, 179, 225

Lung Ultrasound, 206, 210

M
Maternal Obesity, 1-3, 5, 7, 9-14, 17, 19

Index 243

Mechanical Ventilation, 1, 43-46, 60-61, 69, 79, 82, 84, 86, 88-89, 93, 98, 101, 111, 115-119, 122, 124, 126, 132, 136, 139, 141, 156-157, 159, 163, 206-207, 212, 226-229, 231-232, 234

Mesenchymal Cells, 67, 91, 94, 99, 120, 140-142, 144-145, 147, 188, 201, 203

Metabolic Programming, 1-2, 5-6, 12-14, 16

Mitochondrial Fission, 213-214, 218, 220-221

Muscularization, 22, 225-227, 229, 231

Myofibroblasts, 17, 87, 90-91, 104, 117, 144, 146

N
Non-invasive Ventilation, 88, 159-160, 164

Nutrient Availability, 8, 10

O
Organoids, 187-189, 193-194, 198, 200-201, 204

Oxidative Stress, 32, 42, 66, 93, 101, 124, 153, 155, 165, 175, 178, 180, 185, 220-221

Oxygen Toxicity, 1, 32-33, 89, 112, 142, 183, 188, 214

Oxygenation, 47-48, 50, 60, 94, 110, 229

P
Patch Clamp, 187-190, 194-195, 197, 201, 203

Perinatal Inflammation, 21, 82, 89, 92, 100, 163

Perinatal Nutrition, 1, 8, 12

Postnatal Period, 2, 32, 39, 42, 128, 150, 153

Prematurity, 1-2, 4, 9, 15, 18-19, 31-32, 41-44, 61, 67, 86, 88-89, 97-98, 103, 125, 127, 134, 136, 146, 149, 157, 165, 174, 207, 210, 223, 233-234

Prevention Strategies, 12, 150, 152-153

Pulmonary Angiogenesis, 1, 8, 223-224, 230-232

Pulmonary Disease, 2, 13, 19-20, 31-32, 42, 58, 60, 96, 107, 124, 136, 141, 146-147, 185, 207, 232

Pulmonary Hypertension, 15-16, 18, 20, 22-23, 29-30, 62-63, 66-67, 69-70, 86-87, 93, 107, 121, 123, 130, 137, 139, 149, 162, 207, 213-214, 221-228, 233, 235-236

Pulmonary Valve, 215

Pulmonary Vasculature, 22, 24, 26, 29, 65, 70, 80, 84, 97, 112, 146, 162, 218, 220, 224, 232

Pulmonary Vessels, 22, 24, 26-29, 80, 208, 217, 220, 224

R
Retinopathy, 31-32, 40, 42, 44, 96, 175

Risk Factors, 59, 87, 90, 96, 127, 136, 139, 146, 150-153, 163, 172-173, 182, 233

S
Sepsis, 73, 79, 88, 92, 94, 105, 156-159, 162-163, 226

W
Wheezing, 1, 3, 14, 49, 155, 167

Printed in the USA
CPSIA information can be obtained
at www.ICGtesting.com
LVHW081337061023
760215LV00004B/164